T0344758

EMERGING INFECTIONS 10

EMERGING INFECTIONS 10

Edited by
W. Michael Scheld
Department of Infectious Diseases
University of Virginia Health System
Charlottesville, VA

James M. Hughes
Division of Infectious Diseases
Department of Medicine
Emory University School of Medicine
Atlanta, GA

Richard J. Whitley
Department of Pediatrics
University of Alabama at Birmingham
Birmingham, AL

ASM PRESS *Washington, DC*

Library of Congress Cataloging-in-Publication Data

Names: Scheld, W. Michael, editor. | Hughes, James M., 1945- editor. | Whitley, Richard J., editor.
Title: Emerging infections 10 / edited by W. Michael Scheld, Department of Infectious Diseases, University of Virginia Health System; James M. Hughes, Division of Infectious Diseases, Department of Medicine, Emory University School of Medicine; Richard J. Whitley, Department of Pediatrics, University of Alabama at Birmingham.
Other titles: Emerging infections ten
Description: Washington, DC : ASM Press, [2016] | Includes index.
Identifiers: LCCN 2016018788 (print) | LCCN 2016020453 (ebook) | ISBN 9781555819446 (hardcover) | ISBN 9781555819453 (ebook)
Subjects: LCSH: Emerging infectious diseases. | Communicable diseases--Epidemiology.
Classification: LCC RA643 .E44 2016 (print) | LCC RA643 (ebook) | DDC 616.9--dc23
LC record available at https://lccn.loc.gov/2016018788

SKY10025034_021821

Address editorial correspondence to
ASM Press, 1752 N St., N.W.,
Washington, DC 20036-2904, USA

Send orders to ASM Press, P.O. Box 605, Herndon, VA 20172, USA
Phone: 800-546-2416; 703-661-1593
Fax: 703-661-1501
E-mail: books@asmusa.org
Online: http://www.asmscience.org

Cover: Zika virus, TEM. Credit: AMI Images/Science Photo Library.

In memory of William A. Craig (1939-2015) and Robert C. Moellering, Jr. (1936-2014), two highly esteemed colleagues, clinicians, educators, investigators, and mentors. We thank them for their friendship, inspiration, and collective contributions to the development of nearly every new antibacterial agent in the last four decades.

Contents

Contributors   ix
Foreword   xv
Preface   xvii
Acknowledgments   xix

1   **West Africa 2013: Re-examining Ebola   1**
    Daniel G. Bausch and Amanda Rojek

2   **Preparing for Serious Communicable Diseases in the United States: What the Ebola Virus Epidemic Has Taught Us   39**
    Jay B. Varkey and Bruce S. Ribner

3   **Ebola Virus Disease: Therapeutic and Potential Preventative Opportunities   53**
    Robert Fisher and Luciana Borio

4   **Middle East Respiratory Syndrome (MERS)   73**
    Sonja A. Rasmussen, Amelia K. Watson, and David L. Swerdlow

5   **The Emergence of Enterovirus D-68   105**
    Kevin Messacar, Mark J. Abzug, and Samuel R. Dominguez

6   **The Role of Punctuated Evolution in the Pathogenicity of Influenza Viruses   121**
    Jonathan A. McCullers

7   **Measles in the United States since the Millennium: Perils and Progress in the Postelimination Era   131**
    Anne Schuchat, Amy Parker Fiebelkorn, and William Bellini

8   **Chikungunya Virus: Current Perspectives on a Reemerging Virus   143**
    Clayton R. Morrison, Kenneth S. Plante, and Mark T. Heise

9   **Zika Virus Disease   163**
    Werner Slenczka

10   **West Nile Virus Infection   175**
     James J. Sejvar

11   **Mobilization of Carbapenemase-Mediated Resistance in *Enterobacteriaceae*   201**
     Amy Mathers

12   **Antimicrobial Resistance Expressed by *Neisseria gonorrhoeae*: A Major Global Public Health Problem in the 21st Century   213**
     Magnus Unemo, Carlos del Rio, and William M. Shafer

13 *Bordetella holmesii*: Still Emerging and Elusive 20 Years On 239
Laure F. Pittet and Klara M. Posfay-Barbe

14 *Cronobacter* spp. 255
Brian P. Blackwood and Catherine J. Hunter

15 *Clostridium difficile* Infection 265
Jae Hyun Shin, Esteban Chaves-Olarte, and Cirle A. Warren

16 Emerging Tick-Borne Bacterial Pathogens 295
Tahar Kernif, Hamza Leulmi, Didier Raoult, and Philippe Parola

17 *Bordetella pertussis* 311
Delma J. Nieves and Ulrich Heininger

18 Invasive Infections with Nontyphoidal *Salmonella* in Sub-Saharan
Africa 341
Barbara E. Mahon and Patricia I. Fields

19 Fungal Infections Associated with Contaminated Steroid
Injections 359
Carol A. Kauffman and Anurag N. Malani

20 Emerging Fungal Infections in the Pacific Northwest:
The Unrecognized Burden and Geographic Range of
Cryptococcus gattii and *Coccidioides immitis* 375
Shawn R. Lockhart, Orion Z. McCotter, and Tom M. Chiller

21 The Emerging Amphibian Fungal Disease, Chytridiomycosis:
A Key Example of the Global Phenomenon of Wildlife Emerging
Infectious Diseases 385
Jonathan E. Kolby and Peter Daszak

22 Artemisinin-Resistant *Plasmodium falciparum* Malaria 409
Rick M. Fairhurst and Arjen M. Dondorp

Index 431

Contributors

Mark J. Abzug
University of Colorado School of Medicine
Department of Pediatrics
Section of Infectious Disease
Aurora, CO 80045

Daniel G. Bausch
Tulane School of Public Health and Tropical Medicine
Department of Tropical Medicine
New Orleans, LA 70112

William Bellini
Division of Viral Diseases
The National Center for Immunization and
Respiratory Diseases
Centers for Disease Control and Prevention
Atlanta, GA 30329

Brian P. Blackwood
Ann and Robert H. Lurie Children's Hospital of Chicago
Chicago, IL 60611

Luciana Borio
Food and Drug Administration
Office of the Chief Scientist
Silver Spring, MD 20993

Esteban Chaves-Olarte
Universidad de Costa Rica
San Pedro, Costa Rica

Tom M. Chiller
Mycotic Diseases Branch
Centers for Disease Control and Prevention
Atlanta, GA 30333

Peter Daszak
EcoHealth Alliance
New York, NY 10001

Carlos del Rio
Hubert Department of Global Health
Rollins School of Public Health of Emory University
and Department of Medicine
Division of Infectious Diseases
Emory University School of Medicine
Atlanta, GA 30322

Samuel R. Dominguez
University of Colorado School of Medicine
Department of Pediatrics
Section of Infectious Disease
Aurora, CO 80045

Arjen M. Dondorp
Mahidol-Oxford Tropical Medicine Research Unit
Faculty of Tropical Medicine
Mahidol University
Bangkok 10400, Thailand;
Centre for Tropical Medicine
Nuffield Department of Medicine
University of Oxford
Oxford OX3 7BN, United Kingdom

Rick M. Fairhurst
Laboratory of Malaria and Vector Research
National Institute of Allergy and Infectious Diseases
National Institutes of Health
Rockville, MD 20852

Patricia I. Fields
Division of Foodborne, Waterborne, and Environmental Diseases
National Center for Emerging and Zoonotic Infectious Diseases
Centers for Disease Control and Prevention
Atlanta, GA 30329

Robert Fisher
Food and Drug Administration
Office of Counterterrorism and Emerging Threats
Silver Spring, MD 20993

Ulrich Heininger
Universitäts-Kinderspital beider Basel (UKBB)
CH-4031 Basel, Switzerland

Mark T. Heise
Department of Genetics
The University of North Carolina
Chapel Hill, NC 27599

Catherine J. Hunter
Ann and Robert H. Lurie Children's Hospital of Chicago
Chicago, IL 60611

Carol A. Kauffman
Division of Infectious Diseases
Department of Internal Medicine
Veterans Affairs Ann Arbor Healthcare System;
University of Michigan Medical School
Ann Arbor, MI 48105

Tahar Kernif
Aix Marseille Université
Unité de Recherche sur les Maladies Infectieuses Transmissibles
et Emergentes (URMITE)
UM63, CNRS 7278, IRD 198,
Inserm 1095, Faculté de Médecine,
13385 Marseille cedex 5, France;
Institut Pasteur d'Algérie
Algiers, Algeria

Jonathan E. Kolby
One Health Research Group, College of Public Health, Medical,
and Veterinary Sciences
James Cook University, Townsville
Queensland, Australia

Hamza Leulmi
Aix Marseille Université
Unité de Recherche sur les Maladies Infectieuses Transmissibles
et Emergentes (URMITE)
UM63, CNRS 7278, IRD 198,
Inserm 1095, Faculté de Médecine,
13385 Marseille cedex 5, France;
Ecole Nationale Supérieure Vétérinaire d'Alger
El Aliya Alger, Algérie

Shawn R. Lockhart
Mycotic Diseases Branch
Centers for Disease Control and Prevention
Atlanta, GA 30333

Barbara E. Mahon
Division of Foodborne, Waterborne, and Environmental Diseases
National Center for Emerging and Zoonotic Infectious Diseases
Centers for Disease Control and Prevention
Atlanta, GA 30329

Anurag N. Malani
St. Joseph Mercy Hospital;
University of Michigan Medical School
Ann Arbor, MI 48105

Amy Mathers
Division of Infectious Diseases and International Health
Department of Medicine
University of Virginia Health System;
Clinical Microbiology
Department of Pathology
University of Virginia Health System
Charlottesville, VA 22911

Orion Z. McCotter
Mycotic Diseases Branch
Centers for Disease Control and Prevention
Atlanta, GA 30333

Jonathan A. McCullers
Department of Pediatrics
The University of Tennessee Health Sciences Center
Memphis, TN 38103

Kevin Messacar
University of Colorado School of Medicine
Department of Pediatrics
Sections of Infectious Disease and Section of Hospital Medicine
Aurora, CO 80045

Clayton R. Morrison
Department of Genetics
The University of North Carolina
Chapel Hill, NC 27599

Delma J. Nieves
Pediatric Infectious Diseases
CHOC Children's
Orange, CA 92868

Amy Parker Fiebelkorn
Division of Viral Diseases
The National Center for Immunization
and Respiratory Diseases
Centers for Disease Control and Prevention
Atlanta, GA 30329

Philippe Parola
Aix Marseille Université
Unité de Recherche sur les Maladies Infectieuses Transmissibles
et Emergentes (URMITE)
UM63, CNRS 7278, IRD 198,
Inserm 1095, Faculté de Médecine,
13385 Marseille cedex 5, France

Laure F. Pittet
Pediatric Infectious Diseases Unit
Children's Hospital of Geneva
University Hospitals of Geneva
1211 Geneva 14, Switzerland

Kenneth S. Plante
Department of Genetics
The University of North Carolina
Chapel Hill, NC 27599

Klara M. Posfay-Barbe
Pediatric Infectious Diseases Unit
Children's Hospital of Geneva
University Hospitals of Geneva
1211 Geneva 14, Switzerland

Didier Raoult
Aix Marseille Université
Unité de Recherche sur les Maladies Infectieuses Transmissibles
et Emergentes (URMITE)
UM63, CNRS 7278, IRD 198,
Inserm 1095, Faculté de Médecine,
13385 Marseille cedex 5, France

Sonja A. Rasmussen
Centers for Disease Control and Prevention
Atlanta, GA

Bruce S. Ribner
Emory University School of Medicine
Atlanta, GA 30307

Amanda Rojek
University of Oxford
Epidemic Diseases Research Group, Centre for Tropical Medicine
and Global Health
Oxford, United Kingdom

Anne Schuchat
The National Center for Immunization and Respiratory Diseases
Centers for Disease Control and Prevention
Atlanta, GA 30329

James J. Sejvar
Division of High-Consequence Pathogens and Pathology
National Center for Emerging and Zoonotic Infectious Diseases (NCEZID)
Centers for Disease Control and Prevention (CDC)
Atlanta, GA 30333

William M. Shafer
Department of Microbiology and Immunology
Emory University School of Medicine
Atlanta, GA 30322;
Veterans Affairs Medical Center (Atlanta)
Decatur, GA 30033

Jae Hyun Shin
Department of Medicine
University of Virginia
Charlottesville, VA 22908

Werner Slenczka
Philipps-University Marburg
Institute of Virology
35037 Marburg, Germany

David L. Swerdlow
Centers for Disease Control and Prevention
Atlanta, GA 30602

Magnus Unemo
WHO Collaborating Centre for Gonorrhoea and Other STIs
Department of Laboratory Medicine, Microbiology
Örebro University Hospital
SE-701 85 Örebro, Sweden

Jay B. Varkey
Emory University School of Medicine
Atlanta, GA 30307

Cirle A. Warren
Department of Medicine
University of Virginia
Charlottesville, VA 22908

Amelia K. Watson
The University of Georgia
Athens, GA 30602

Foreword

The field of emerging and re-emerging infectious diseases has traveled from A (anthrax) to Z (Zika) in less than 15 years. Fortuitously, over that same interval, the insights, tools, and investments needed to address these challenges to medicine and public health have kept pace. The One Health Initiative has its roots in antiquity but only began to gather momentum with the appearance of West Nile virus in the Americas in 1999. Investigators now prospect wildlife and domesticated animals worldwide looking for novel agents and hints for origins of the next pandemic.

Molecular strategies for microbial surveillance, diagnosis and discovery have largely supplanted more laborious and expensive classical methods, resulting in an explosive expansion of genetic data that require increasingly complex and powerful resources for bioinformatic and biostatistical analysis. Discovery, an activity once focused in the West, is becoming decentralized as costs and expertise required for sequencing decrease. Governments and foundations invest in support of the United Nations International Health Regulations of 2005—a document signed by all member states "designed to prevent, protect against, control and provide a public health response to the international spread of disease in ways that are commensurate with and restricted to public health risks, and which avoid unnecessary interference with international traffic and trade." The importance of this document and of the commitment of the scientific and communities to transparency has been underscored by the emergence of pandemic strains of influenza, antibiotic-resistant bacteria, Nipah, SARS, chikungunya, MERS, Ebola, and most recently Zika, which threaten regional and global public health as well as economic security.

The U.S. Supreme Court decision in the *Association for Molecular Pathology v. Myriad Genetics* that challenged the patentability of sequences existing in nature had ramifications far beyond the field of diagnostic oncology that prompted the initial litigation. It effectively ended the race to simply recover, claim and license microbial sequences of emerging pathogens. The result has been to encourage more mechanistic science. The number of laboratories focused on work in high-level biocontainment has dramatically increased. This has enabled more investigators to contribute to research into the biology, pathogenesis, diagnosis, prevention and treatment of emerging infectious diseases. It has also driven concerns about gain-of-function and dual use research as well as inadvertent release of high threat agents. An appropriate balance will be essential if the needs of all stakeholders are to be met.

Emerging Infections 10 is the latest in an American Society for Microbiology series initiated in 1998. My dear friend and mentor, the late Josh Lederberg, who wrote the foreword to *Emerging Infections* 1, would be pleased to see that the series is alive and well and that the authors include an international cast of veterinarians, physicians, basic scientists, and public health practitioners. He would have anticipated the emergence of novel agents and the re-emergence of old foes like measles. In channeling Josh and his propensity for driving the field with predictions, I expect that volume 11 will feature chapters on modeling and the role of social media in biosecurity.

W. Ian Lipkin
New York, NY
2016

Preface

Despite progress in the prevention and control of infectious diseases during the past several decades, the first 15 years of the 21st century continue to provide evidence of the persistence and tenacity of emerging microbial threats. The interplay of rapid globalization, demographic shifts, ecological changes, environmental degradation, climate change, and unprecedented movement of people, animals, and commodities yield unexpected risks to health, often with attendant social, economic, and political repercussions. The emergence and rapid global spread of diseases such as MERS, Ebola virus disease, chikungunya, and Zika virus disease provide dramatic evidence of the continued ability of microbes to emerge, spread, adapt, and challenge the global infectious diseases, microbiology, and public health communities. In addition, the resurgence of long recognized diseases such as measles and pertussis and the spread of diseases such as coccidioidomycosis beyond endemic areas pose additional challenges.

Since 1995, annual infectious diseases meetings including those organized by the Infectious Diseases Society of America and the American Society for Microbiology have included updates on emerging infectious diseases. The 22 chapters in *Emerging Infections 10* provide important updates on a broad range of emerging and re-emerging bacterial, viral, parasitic, and fungal infectious diseases in the United States and globally. Highlights include timely chapters on MERS, Ebola virus disease, chikungunya, and Zika virus disease which have recently been the focus of clinicians, researchers, and public health officials around the world and have received extensive media attention. The global threat of antimicrobial resistance is addressed in chapters on carbapenem-resistant *Enterobacteriaceae*, multiply-resistant gonococcal infections, non-typhoidal *Salmonella* infections in sub-Saharan Africa, and artemisinin-resistant *Plasmodium falciparum* malaria. Topics range from recently recognized diseases to long-recognized diseases posing current challenges to the clinical, laboratory, research, public health, and animal health communities.

Our experiences in responding to recent outbreaks, many of which are of vectorborne or zoonotic origin, provide important lessons for the future and highlight the relevance and importance of the One Health concept which emphasizes the importance of closer collaboration among the human, animal (both domestic and wildlife), and environmental and ecosystem health sectors. Recent experience emphasizes the importance of preparedness to respond to domestic and global threats with a co-ordinated, evidence-based, interdisciplinary response guided by strong, effective leadership at the national and global levels and accelerated implementation of a research agenda to provide tools to support diagnostic, therapeutic, and prevention strategies.

Because weak health systems in many areas of the world pose threats to all, investments in health system strengthening, national public health institutions, response capacity, and workforce development can yield substantial returns for the health and security of the global community. Recent experiences with and lessons learned from MERS, Ebola virus disease, chikungunya, and Zika virus disease have highlighted the importance of strengthening national capacities in support of the International Health Regulations and the Global Health Security Agenda. Fortunately, important scientific and prevention opportunities in the future are likely to result from advances in molecular diagnostics, next generation sequencing, utilization of big data, microbiome research, pathogen discovery, and epidemic modeling.

Future infectious disease challenges are difficult to predict but certainly include antimicrobial-resistant infections in healthcare and community settings, foodborne and waterborne diseases, influenza and other respiratory diseases, and vectorborne and zoonotic diseases, as well as new threats for immunocompromised and disadvantaged populations. Additional links between chronic diseases and infectious agents and between the microbiome and human health and disease will certainly be identified, providing new prevention and treatment opportunities. We hope the tenth volume in the *Emerging Infections* series will serve as a valuable resource for those currently working to address emerging infectious disease threats to national and global health and security as well as for the next generation of talented, committed professionals needed to confront these threats in the future.

W. Michael Scheld
James M. Hughes
Richard J. Whitley

Acknowledgments

We thank all of our colleagues who have helped us in preparing this volume. Most importantly, we thank all of the authors for their outstanding contributions. As editors, we are particularly grateful to the members of the Interscience Conference on Antimicrobial Agents and Chemotherapy (ICAAC) and the Infectious Diseases Society of America (IDSA) Program Committees who assisted us in coordinating topic and speaker selection for and/or moderating the joint symposia on emerging infections during previous ICAAC and IDSA meetings. As past presidents of IDSA, we would especially like to thank Mark Leasure, the soon to retire CEO of IDSA, for nearly 20 years of outstanding service to the Society and the infectious diseases profession. Numerous other colleagues provided helpful discussion, advice, and criticisms. We are also grateful to our assistants, Lisa Cook, Dianne Miller, and Dunia Ritchey. We also want to thank Lauren Luethy, Megan Angelini, and their colleagues at ASM Press for their superb work in coordinating production of the book. And finally, we thank our families for their understanding and support during this undertaking.

West Africa 2013: Re-examining Ebola

DANIEL G. BAUSCH[1] and AMANDA ROJEK[2]

INTRODUCTION

The outbreak of Ebola virus disease (EVD) that began in Guinea in 2013 and then rapidly spread through Liberia and Sierra Leone lasted over 2 years and resulted in over 28,500 cases and at least 11,000 deaths in West Africa, with 27 imported or medically evacuated cases and 5 deaths in the United States and Europe (Fig. 1) (1, 2). By comparison, fewer than 3,000 cases of EVD have been registered for *all* previous outbreaks combined (Table 1). The previous largest outbreak on record, which occurred in Gulu, Uganda, in 2000–2001, lasted only three and a half months and consisted of 425 cases with 224 deaths. But the impact of an outbreak of EVD or other emerging viruses cannot be measured simply by tallying cases and deaths. In 2015 the West Africa EVD outbreak resulted in $2.2 billion in lost economic growth in the region, stalling fledgling economies that were struggling to recover from civil war. On a personal level, such sterile-sounding statistics translate to extreme personal suffering—upward of 3,000 orphaned children, children's education and development jeopardized as school is cancelled for a year, job loss, smaller harvests and hungry families, and deep but less easily measurable mental health and socio-cultural impacts. Furthermore, as the region's

[1]Tulane School of Public Health and Tropical Medicine, New Orleans, LA 70112; [2]University of Oxford, Oxford, UK.

Emerging Infections 10
Edited by W. Michael Scheld, James M. Hughes and Richard J. Whitley
© 2016 American Society for Microbiology, Washington, DC
doi:10.1128/microbiolspec.EI10-0022-2016

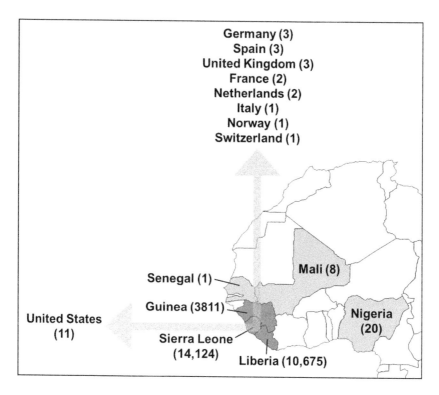

Germany (3)
Spain (3)
United Kingdom (3)
France (2)
Netherlands (2)
Italy (1)
Norway (1)
Switzerland (1)

Senegal (1)
Mali (8)
Guinea (3811)
United States (11)
Nigeria (20)
Sierra Leone (14,124)
Liberia (10,675)

FIGURE 1 Map of West Africa showing the epicenter of the 2013–2016 outbreak of Ebola virus disease (red) and imported cases (orange and arrows). The total number of cases seen in each country is shown in parentheses.

resources were funneled to EVD, there were an estimated 10,000 excess deaths due to untreated malaria, HIV/AIDS, and tuberculosis. Reductions in vaccination coverage and a rise in teenage pregnancy were also noted (3).

The unprecedented scale of West Africa 2013 took the world by surprise and sadly added another tragic event to a region already struggling to escape decades of poverty and war. The outbreak also shook the international response community, laying bare deficiencies in our response capacity to complex humanitarian disasters of highly infectious and lethal pathogens. It also has taught the world many new things about EVD, previously considered so mysterious and usually seen only in small numbers and in remote and resource-poor locations that hindered systematic study. Here we re-examine EVD, reviewing the unique features of West Africa

2013, contrasting them with the prior assumptions and classical teachings, and identifying what they have taught us and what we still have to learn.

WHY WAS THE WEST AFRICA 2013 OUTBREAK SO BIG?

The reasons for the unprecedented size of West Africa 2013 are undoubtedly multifactorial. Many of the challenges had been encountered in previous EVD outbreaks but certainly not on the scale and with the intensity noted in West Africa. Whether the end result was just bad luck, or the perfect storm, is in the eye of the beholder. Although much will forever remain speculation, any attempt to understand the events requires a detailed look at a complex web of interrelated biological, economic, ecological, and social determinants viewed in the context of the overall geopolitical history of the region.

Resource-Poor Countries with Fragile Health Care and Disease Surveillance and Response Systems

Much remains to be understood regarding the factors that dictate Ebola virus introduction into humans at a given time (4). However, once introduced, an almost invariable underlying determinant of large outbreaks is a backdrop of previous civil conflict or failed development resulting in fragile health care and disease surveillance and response systems (4, 5–9). Guinea, Liberia, and Sierra Leone sadly fit the bill, with all three countries working to recover from decades of civil war and unrest. All three rank near the bottom of the 187 nations on the United Nations Development Program Human Development Index, with a majority of their populations living below the national poverty lines. Thus, when Ebola virus was introduced, it unfortunately found not only an immunologically susceptible population, but also surveillance and health care systems that were unable to readily detect it or contain it.

The introduction of Ebola virus that initiated West Africa 2013 likely occurred in the town of Meliandou in a remote, largely deforested, and resource-poor region of Guinea in December 2013 (10, 11). However, with no organized surveillance or reporting system for hemorrhagic fever syndromes and no laboratory in all of West Africa with the standing capacity to diagnose EVD (Fig. 1), diagnostic confirmation and the first notification by Guinean health authorities to the World Health Organization (WHO) of a "rapidly evolving outbreak" did not occur until over three months later (11). By this time at least 49 cases with multiple but often poorly defined chains of transmission had occurred in Guinea, with the disease already slipping quietly across the border into Liberia (12, 13).

The West African countries also lacked the trained personnel (see below), disease surveillance and response systems, and physical infrastructure and materials to contain the outbreak. Infection prevention and control (IPC) practices were undeveloped at best, with simple medical necessities such as soap, clean water, and sterile needles being far from given, much less the costly personal protective equipment (PPE) needed to safely care for EVD patients (14–18). Disease reporting and response systems for case identification, isolation, and treatment; contact tracing; and safe burials were close to nonexistent, as were ambulances to transport patients to health facilities.

Delayed Response by the International Community

Given the evident incapacity of the local response from West African countries, international assistance was clearly needed. The first order of business required recognition of the gravity of the situation by WHO and the international community. Much has been made of WHO's slow response (19). Although they contributed personnel and resources from the onset, WHO did not formally declare the outbreak in West Africa to be a Public Health Emergency of International Concern (PHEIC), as outlined under the International Health Regulations, until 8 August 2015, 6 months after the first notice of EVD in the region. The reasons for the long delay are much debated but may include a true underestimate of the gravity of the situation (despite many organizations making vocal calls for an international response by this time), political pressures from the affected countries, and being "gun shy" in the wake of significant criticism that WHO overreacted in declaring the 2009 "swine flu" (H1N1 influenza virus) to be a public health emergency of international concern.

With case numbers rapidly mounting, including imported cases into the United States and Europe, and projections of millions of cases of EVD in West Africa if no aggressive response was taken (20), the international

TABLE 1 Laboratory-confirmed outbreaks of Ebola virus disease since discovery of the virus in 1976 through April 2016. Cases related to laboratory infections are not shown[a]

Year of onset	Virus species	Country	Epicenter(s)	No. of cases (CFR [%])	Source of primary infection	Factors contributing to secondary spread	No. of cases in health care workers[b]	Reference
1976	Zaire	Zaire (present day DRC)	Yambuku	318 (88)	Unknown	Nosocomial transmission	≥13	141
1976	Sudan	Sudan	Maridi and Nzara	284 (53)	Unknown	Nosocomial transmission	70	23
1977	Zaire	Zaire	Tandala	1 (100)	Unknown	None	0	142
1979	Sudan	Sudan	Maridi and Nzara	34 (65)	Unknown	Nosocomial transmission	≥2	143
1994	Zaire	Gabon	Mékouka, Ogooué-Ivindo Province	52 (60)	Infection in gold mining camps	Traditional healing practices, nosocomial and community-based transmission	None reported	144
1994	Taï Forest	Côte d'Ivoire	Taï Forest	1 (0)	Scientist conducting autopsy on wild chimpanzee	None	0	145
1995	Zaire	DRC	Kikwit	315 (81)	Unknown	Nosocomial and community-based transmission	None reported	26
1996	Zaire	Gabon	Mayibout, Ogooué-Ivindo Province	21 (57)	Consumption of dead chimp	Community-based transmission	None reported	144
1996	Zaire	Gabon	Booué, Ogooué-Ivindo Province	45 (74)	Consumption of chimp?	Nosocomial and community-based transmission	None reported	144
1996	Zaire	South Africa	Johannesburg	2 (50)	Imported from Gabon by infected doctor	Nosocomial transmission	2	146
2000	Sudan	Uganda	Gulu	425 (53)	Unknown	Nosocomial and community-based transmission, traditional burial practices	≥3	146
2001	Zaire	Gabon and ROC	Ogooué-Ivindo Province (Gabon)	65 (82)	Hunting and consumption of NHPs	Nosocomial transmission and community-based transmission, traditional healing practices	2	148

Year							Community-based transmission	
2001	Zaire	Gabon and ROC	Cuvette Ouest Region (ROC)	57 (75)	Unknown		0	148
2002	Zaire	ROC	Mbomo and Kéllé, Cuvette Ouest Region	143 (89)	Hunting and consumption of NHPs	Nosocomial and community-based transmission, traditional healing practices	None reported	28
2003	Zaire	ROC	Mbomo and Mbandza, Cuvette Ouest Region	35 (83)	Hunting and consumption of NHPs	Traditional healing practices	None reported	149
2004	Sudan	South Sudan	Yambio	17 (41)	Exposure to baboon meat?	Nosocomial transmission and community-based transmission	None reported	150
2007	Zaire	DRC	Kasai Occidental Province	264 (71)	Exposure to local wildlife, including bats	Nosocomial and community-based transmission	None reported	28
2007	Bundibugyo	Uganda	Bundibugyo	149 (25)	Unknown	Nosocomial transmission and community-based transmission	None reported	29
2008	Zaire	DRC	Mweka and Luebo	32 (47)	Exposure to fruit bats through hunting?	Unknown	None reported	151
2011	Sudan	Uganda	Luwero	1 (100)	Unknown	None	0	152
2012	Sudan	Uganda	Kibaale	11 (36)	Unknown	Community-based transmission	None reported	153
2012	Bundibugyo	DRC	Province Orientale	36 (36)	Hunted bushmeat?	Community-based transmission	≥13	141
2012	Sudan	Uganda	Luwero	6 (50)	Unknown	Unknown	None reported	154
2013	Zaire	Multiple, mostly Republic of Guinea, Liberia, and Sierra Leone	Southeast forest region of Guinea	Ongoing, ≥28,646 cases at this writing (31–76)	Unknown, suspected exposure to bats	Nosocomial and community-based transmission, unsafe burial practices	≥874	155
2014	Zaire	DRC	Province Equateur	66 (74)	Hunted bushmeat?	Community-based transmission	≥8	141

ᵃAbbreviations: CFR, case fatality rate; DRC, Democratic Republic of the Congo; ROC, Republic of the Congo; NHP, nonhuman primate.
ᵇMay include cleaners and other ancillary staff working in Ebola treatment units.

community finally stirred to action. Responses generally aligned with historical connections between the United States and European countries and their colonial-era African counterparts. In September 2014 U.S. President Obama committed to the construction of 17 100-bed Ebola treatment units (ETUs) in Liberia, deployment of up to 3,000 medical military and support personnel, and support to train 500 health care workers (HCWs) a week. The United Kingdom and France soon followed with commitments to combat EVD in their ex-colonies of Sierra Leone and Guinea, respectively. Ultimately, a vast array of government and nongovernmental organizations contributed. However, the response remained agonizingly slow, hampered by the logistical challenges of operationalizing work in the poorest countries in the world with fledgling governments and poor infrastructure. Even after laboratories began being rapidly established, the steep increase in the number of samples exceeded local diagnostic capacities in many areas until well into the outbreak. In addition, the response operations were initially poorly coordinated, with each organization acting independently or in bilateral concert with the government. In August 2014 the United Nations appointed a special envoy on Ebola, followed by the creation in September 2014 of a coordination body, the United Nations Mission for Ebola Emergency, headquartered in Ghana (Fig. 2). Opinions vary on the efficacy of these measures. Without doubt, the enormous scale and complexity of the outbreak and the sheer number of organizations involved (far more than had ever been involved in an EVD outbreak before and at times compounded by historical frictions between them) made seamless coordination a substantial challenge.

The Labor Problem

Certainly the greatest single impediment to controlling the West Africa EVD outbreak was the lack of skilled labor in the health sciences. Caring for patients with EVD and controlling transmission require experience and resources that most health care systems and HCWs do not possess. Furthermore, as discussed above, EVD outbreaks almost invariably occur in areas with inadequate human resources in general. Before the outbreak, Guinea, Liberia, and Sierra Leone had less than 1 doctor per 1,000 population, among the lowest HCW coverages in the world (21). The ranks were then further thinned by the estimated 500 HCW deaths due to EVD (14) (see below).

International support for EVD outbreaks is almost invariably needed and has traditionally come from a relatively small group of organizations with the necessary expertise, including WHO, the U.S. Centers for Disease Control and Prevention (CDC), Médecins Sans Frontières (MSF), the International Federation of the Red Cross, and Public Health Agency of Canada. However, the number of people in each of these organizations with experience responding to EVD outbreaks was small and was further complicated in some cases by significant turnover of personnel between outbreaks, with consequent loss of institutional memory. With the exception of MSF, none of the traditionally responding organizations had ever focused on providing clinical care (in fact, most made a specific decision against it). Nevertheless, these organizations had a collective successful history of supporting national governments to contain EVD outbreaks to usually at most a few hundred cases and a few months duration (Table 1). And they responded in a typical manner in West Africa, no doubt expecting the same outcome. But as the case counts skyrocketed, it became clear that a much greater investment of personnel, time, and funds would be needed.

Recognizing the shortage of personnel, many governments and international organizations implemented training programs (22). But who was there to be trained? The West African HCWs were already maximally deployed, and then their numbers were

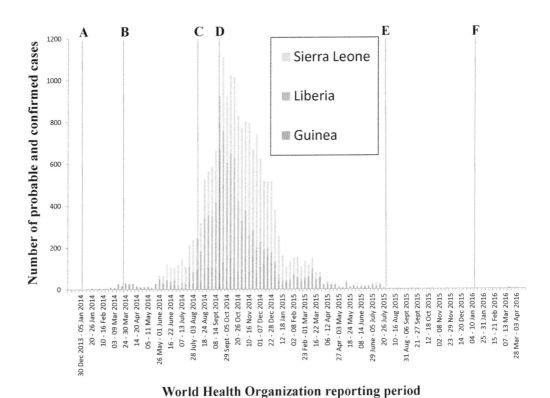

World Health Organization reporting period

FIGURE 2 Epidemiologic curve of the West Africa 2013 Ebola virus disease (EVD) outbreak. The dashed vertical lines indicate key events during the outbreak: (A) First suspected case in Meliandou, Guinea. (B) Laboratory confirmation of EVD and disease reported by Guinean Health Authorities. (C) WHO declares public health emergency of international concern. (D) U.S. President Obama announces major initiative to help control EVD in Liberia; creation of the United Nations Mission for Ebola Emergency. (E) Publication of preliminary results from first EVD phase III vaccine efficacy study (rVSV-EBOV). (F) Publication of preliminary results of first EVD phase III therapeutic efficacy trial (convalescent plasma). Adapted from WHO Ebola Response Roadmap Situation Reports with publicly available data. World Health Organization: http://apps.who.int/gho/data/node.ebola-sitrep.main-countries?lang=en.

further thinned by EVD. In addition, pulling the few remaining local HCWs into EVD care threatened to further degrade the already very significant loss of general health services for so many other important conditions. The handful of international experts on EVD had already been deployed for months and were exhausted, with few qualified and trained replacements waiting in the wings. Military personnel were deployed, but very few had clinical experience with EVD. Certainly, a theoretical international pool of new HCWs was there, but who would be interested and able to leave their families,

jobs, and patients for months to manage patients with EVD in West Africa? The situation was further complicated by questions of legal and financial liability if an international HCW became infected.

The potential labor pool from the United States was thinned even more by draconian, largely politically motivated quarantine policies in some states that mandated 3 weeks of strict isolation (the maximum incubation period of EVD), and thus another 3 weeks away from work, of all people returning from West Africa, regardless of possible exposures or symptoms. This was despite the lack of evidence of risk of virus transmission from asymptomatic people or even during the first few days of disease. The phrase "out of an abundance of caution" became a well-worn preface to the subsequent expression of a strict policy or decision without scientific evidence to support it. The contradictory messages (e.g., "Ebola virus cannot be transmitted from an asymptomatic person but, out of an abundance of caution, we will require strict quarantine of all asymptomatic persons.") ultimately gave the impression that we were operating in a complete scientific vacuum, despite 40 years' experience with the disease—fomenting, rather than quelling panic.

Although the international community committed to and ultimately did provide the necessary infrastructure and labor to help combat EVD in West Africa, the process was too slow. At the height of the epidemic, the beds for patients with EVD, the HCWs to care for them, and the field workers to trace their contacts simply were not there (Table 2). Thus, highly infectious patients remained untreated in the community, and patients who were admitted to the drastically understaffed ETUs could expect little more than palliative care. Furthermore, with cases of EVD in HCWs mounting, some ETUs opted to enhance safety by proscribing close contact with patients, including the controversial measure of not placing IVs for fluid repletion. This move likely further under-

TABLE 2 **Bed capacity and bed requirements for patients with Ebola virus disease in West Africa in October, 2014**[a]

Country	Current number of beds	Estimated number of beds required	Current capacity/estimated demand (%)
Guinea	160	210	76%
Liberia	620	2,930	21%
Sierra Leone	304	1,148	26%

[a]Bed capacity in each district was planned on the basis of a needs assessment carried out by the relevant Ministry of Health. Source: WHO: Ebola Response Roadmap Situation Report, October 8, 2014, World Health Organization: http://apps.who.int/iris/bitstream/10665/136020/1/roadmapsitrep_8Oct2014_eng.pdf?ua=1.

mined the local population's already shaky faith in the response operation.

High Population Density and Frequent Travel, Including Across Borders and to Large Urban Areas

EVD outbreaks have usually occurred in remote and sparsely populated areas of Central Africa (23–29). While the remoteness may add logistical complexity to mounting the outbreak response, the large distance between the epicenter and other populations also presents a barrier to virus transmission. In contrast, Guinea, Liberia, and Sierra Leone are generally very densely populated countries, with a surface area much smaller and more navigable than the vast expanses of Central Africa (Fig. 3). Furthermore, the Guinean Prefecture of Guéckédou where the outbreak began is a point where borders of the three countries converge (Fig. 1).

The geopolitical historical context is again important here; in reality, borders in this area of the world exist more on maps, originally drawn by former colonial powers, than as a barrier on the ground. The region is highly polyglot, dotted with small towns, dispersed on all sides of the "border," comprised of populations who often self-identify just as readily by ethnic group as by nationality. While there may be a degree of passport control at the few major roads (or, just as often, rivers) that traverse borders, in most places the borders are crossed at will. And crossed they are, quite readily—for weekly market days, to see friends and family, even for the daily walk to school. However, while individuals readily cross back and forth, the governmental jurisdictions and corresponding operational capacity for outbreak response are fixed along the national boundaries. Surprisingly, especially considering the very frequent influx of refugees into Guinea from both Liberia and Sierra Leone in recent decades, prior to the outbreak there was very little communication or coordination between local government authorities on different

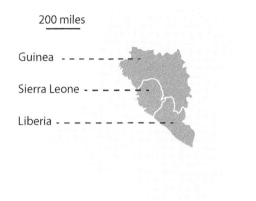

200 miles

Guinea - - - - - - - - - -

Sierra Leone - - - - - -

Liberia - - - - - - - - - - -

	Republic of the Congo	Guinea-Liberia-Sierra Leone
Population	68 million	22 million
Surface Area (Km²)	2.3 million	430,000
Population Density (persons/ Km²)	30	51

FIGURE 3 Sizes and population densities of Guinea, Liberia, and Sierra Leone combined compared with the Democratic Republic of the Congo. To illustrate the difference in size, the three West African countries are shown superimposed on the Democratic Republic of the Congo.

sides of the borders. The challenge to communication was exacerbated by the fact that government functionaries were often assigned to regions distant from their places of upbringing, making communication difficult since they spoke the national language (French in Guinea and English in Liberia and Sierra Leone) but little of the local dialects or the national language of the country on the other side of the border. Consequently, in the early stages of the outbreak, cases or contacts of EVD patients who crossed the border were effectively lost to follow-up. Cross-border meetings and communication were eventually established, but not until the virus was already widely disseminated on all sides of the borders.

In addition to the porous borders and frequent local crossings, the relatively short distances and low cost of travel between even

the farthest reaches of Guinea, Liberia, and Sierra Leone and their major urban centers was a major factor. Go to any bus or taxi station in any village early any morning in Guinea, Liberia, and Sierra Leone and you will see vehicles being overloaded with people and goods destined to arrive late that night at densely populated capital cities of millions of people (Fig. 4). The constant back-and-forth travel, be it for commerce or social visits, ultimately resulted in the introduction of Ebola virus into the capital cities and posed a major impediment to case finding and contact tracing. From there, it was just a matter of time until international air travelers carried the virus to neighboring, and occasionally more distant, countries (30–38) (Fig. 1).

Cultural Clashes and Community Resistance to Control Measures

In the absence of effective therapeutics and vaccines (a work in progress; see below), control of EVD is almost completely based on the classic control measures of thorough case identification, isolation, and contact tracing. Since the early symptoms of EVD (fever, headache, myalgia) are undetectable from casual observation, this approach is completely dependent on individual cooperation both to agree to follow-up and to report symptoms should they occur. Crucial to this cooperation is a common understanding of the nature of the disease threat and the appropriateness of the measures advocated to mitigate it—an understanding unfortunately lacking throughout much of West Africa 2013.

Community resistance to biomedical explanations for EVD outbreaks and proposed control measures is not unique to West Africa 2013, but the scale and tenacity of the distrust and resistance were more than had ever been met before. Again, an understanding of the geopolitical history of the region is essential; after four centuries of colonialism, much of it involving the slave trade, Guinea and Sierra

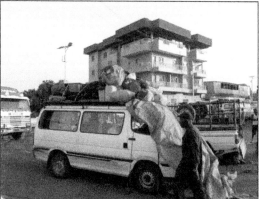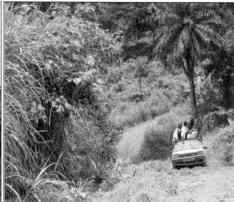

FIGURE 4 "Bush taxis" in Guinea traveling back and forth between remote areas and major cities. Photos by Frederique Jacquerioz.

Leone were granted independence from France (1958) and the United Kingdom (1961), respectively. Liberia was founded as an independent nation in 1847 after originating as a haven for resettled slaves from the United States. Unfortunately, colonial rule was generally replaced by weak and often corrupt governments. The situation ultimately deteriorated to civil war in Liberia (1989–1996) and Sierra Leone (1991–2002), fueled largely not by a desire for good governance by rebels or government soldiers (who were often thought to change sides at night), but rather by the desire to control the region's rich mineral wealth, especially diamonds. The civilian population was caught in the middle. While never formally embroiled in civil war, Guinea's governance was also suspect, a situation that culminated in widespread violence after the death of strong-man leader Lansana Conteh in 2008. In the past few decades, all three countries were struggling to overcome the decades of war and government neglect, with some significant progress until they were hit by EVD in 2013. Given this history, it is hardly surprising or illogical (in fact, the opposite) that a deep distrust of authority was pervasive, creating from the beginning an exceptionally challenging sociocultural backdrop in which outbreak control must take place.

In more concrete terms on the ground, this distrust fueled misconceptions, denial, and fear surrounding EVD, occasionally culminating in violence. The practice of isolating patients with EVD who, due to the high case fatality rates (CFRs), often die, frequently translates to the perception of causality to the local population; that is, "If you go into the ETU, they will kill you and you will die." Other often invoked and arguably effective control measures such as roadblocks for health and temperature checks and quarantine of individuals, households, or whole villages reinforced the impression of a desire for control and the nefarious intentions of the health authorities, especially when the measures exacerbated the developing problem of food insecurity as a result of the outbreak. With the outbreak control teams viewed as a threat and the ETU as a mortuary, not surprisingly, sick people and their contacts frequently opted to hide or abscond.

Another challenging and delicate issue was that of burials of EVD victims, which proved to be a major source of transmission during the outbreak (39–41). The importance of respecting traditional burial ceremonies, which in many African cultures often involve touching the corpse, can hardly be overstated. On the surface, slight changes to ceremony to avoid such contact and virus transmission would seem to be a simple matter. But while Western cultures tend to draw a very distinct line between life and death, this is not always so in West Africa, where varying from proper burial practices may be believed to have very real consequences on the living, including bringing future bad luck, disease, and crop failures. Faced with such consequences, is it any wonder that advice from distrusted authorities to change centuries-old customs (including Liberia's well-intended but ultimately disastrous policy of cremation of the corpses of EVD victims) to avoid transmission of an invisible and previously unheard of viral threat often went unheeded?

The perhaps inevitable cultural clashes inherent in response to an EVD outbreak have been increasingly recognized by the international community over the past few decades, prompting routine inclusion of anthropologists and social scientists to lead community engagement, education, and social mobilization efforts. These efforts typically include working with village chiefs, religious leaders, traditional healers, and other prominent leaders in the community to come to common ground on the approach to the outbreak. But changing beliefs and mindsets rapidly, especially those cultivated across centuries, is never easy, and it becomes harder as distress and fear grow in a community. The task is often oversimplified by outbreak response teams that sometimes have a mindset more oriented toward dictating steps that communities must follow rather than working with communities to develop solutions. Clearly, there is still much more to be learned and work to be done to put local populations and outbreak response teams in reasonable concert in the control of EVD.

Funding for Global Health Preparedness and Response

While not absolving the international community and WHO from responsibility, it must be noted that funding for general global health preparedness and response has not kept pace over the past decade of global economic downturn. Global health funding increased significantly from 2000 to 2009, but growth has been minimal since that time (42). The majority of funding since 2000 has been focused on specific Millennium Development Goal areas (HIV/AIDS, malaria, and tuberculosis) and has not passed through WHO. Funding for WHO specifically has plateaued or decreased since 2010 (43), challenging the organization to maintain capacity for response to disease outbreaks while simultaneously addressing the ever increasing burden of noncommunicable disease in low- and middle-income countries (LMICs). This prompted Dr. Oyewale Tomori, an international expert on emerging viruses and long-time WHO collaborator, to declare, "They killed WHO and then blamed it for being dead" (44). In addition, over 70% of WHO's annual budget typically comes from voluntary contributions from donor counties. This money is generally earmarked for specific projects. Whether the new Global Health Security Agenda led by the United States can rejuvenate investment in broader global health preparedness and response remains to be seen.

Too Many Fronts

In the fight to control EVD, it is difficult to resist war analogies; it is a war against a dangerous and stealthy enemy. Victory requires manpower and material resources strategically organized for efficiency and speed. In the Ebola war, each battle front requires an ETU and appropriately trained and equipped HCWs to isolate and treat patients; field teams for case identification, contact tracing, social mobilization, and safe burials; laboratory diagnostics; and logistical and financial support for communications and travel to coordinate the operation. The international community has successfully fought this battle and won Ebola wars before, but only on a few fronts at a time. West Africa 2013 ultimately presented too many fronts, quickly outstripping both local and international capacity. We eventually caught up, but only after heavy losses, too late to prevent an international humanitarian disaster.

CLINICAL PRESENTATION

The enormous size of West Africa 2013 has provided the opportunity for much more detailed clinical observation (45–48). Perhaps the most definitive conclusion in this regard is confirming observations from recent outbreaks that hemorrhage occurs in a minority (less than 20%) of patients, prompting the renaming of the disease from "Ebola hemorrhagic fever" to "Ebola virus disease." The contribution of volume loss from diarrhea to the pathogenesis of EVD, with the potential for almost cholera-type fluid losses of up to 10 liters per day, has also become clear. Debate persists over whether this is something specific to the Makona variant of Ebola virus that is the etiology of West Africa 2013 or is common to EVD from all virus species and variants but was previously poorly documented and underappreciated. Enteropathy may extend beyond severe diarrhea, based on the frequency of abdominal pain and peritoneal signs as well as ultrasound evidence of paralytic ileus (49–51). Hiccups, previously considered an end-stage manifestation, have also often been recognized in early disease, the pathogenesis of which remains unclear.

Relatively newly described, or at least described in significantly greater detail, severe complications of acute EVD include meningoencephalitis (with evidence of microvascular occlusion and ischemia on magnetic resonance imaging), renal and respiratory failure, and rhabdomyolysis (48, 52–54; M. Lado, personal communication). Cardiac arrhythmias have been reported in high-income settings (50) and inferred as the cause of sudden death in some patients in West Africa (48), but it is not clear whether this reflects direct myocardial pathology or is secondary to electrolyte disturbances or systemic inflammatory response syndrome. Another possible cause of sudden death may be thrombotic cardiac or cerebrovascular accidents related to thrombocytosis and a hypercoaguable state that have been documented in early EVD recovery (55). Some of the more severe complications have been described primarily in medically evacuated cases, raising questions as to whether they are truly common manifestations in all infected people, but perhaps go undetected or unreported in West Africa, or are rather a consequence of the intensive care and/or investigational drugs received by patients treated in resource-rich areas of the world.

While the expanded clinical observations from West Africa 2013 help refine our understanding of EVD, the noted variation in clinical presentation also poses challenges to surveillance and case identification. Given the public health implications of missed cases, case definitions for suspected EVD have always been designed to maximize sensitivity at the expense of specificity. Fever has always been a central feature, augmented through the addition of various equally nonspecific symptoms and a history of contact with another person with EVD (56). However, during West Africa 2013, patients with confirmed EVD were frequently noted who did not meet this broad case definition; in one study, 9% of confirmed cases reported neither a history of fever nor a risk factor for Ebola virus exposure (57, 58). The sensitivity and specificity of the standard WHO case definition for EVD were only 79.7% and 31.5%, respectively. Given the frequent reluctance of local populations in West Africa to be identified as possibly having EVD, inaccurate histories could perhaps underlie these findings. Nevertheless, since such reluctance, and perhaps inaccurate reporting, are unfortunately likely to be encountered in future outbreaks, these results are very concerning and create operational challenges to field surveillance and clinical triage alike. Whether the enormous amount of clinical data gathered during West Africa 2013 can be harmonized and analyzed to further refine and improve sensitivity and specificity of the EVD case definition remains to be seen. The task can be facilitated by standardized minimum data collection protocols and forms for EVD generated by the International Severe Acute Respiratory and Emerging Infection Consortium with support from WHO (59). Such data standardization and coordination should be an early consideration in all outbreaks of EVD and other emerging infections to facilitate real-time improvement of case definitions and analysis of clinical signs and symptoms.

One specific area where an expanded spectrum of clinical presentations has been noted is in pregnant women with EVD. While most present with typical EVD symptoms and signs, more atypical presentations have recently been documented. In Liberia a pregnant women near term presented with ruptured membranes accompanied by mild lower abdominal pain and sparse contractions but was afebrile (60). Routine testing performed at the time revealed her to be PCR-positive for Ebola virus RNA, with a high viral load. Three days after admission she developed symptoms of EVD and ultimately succumbed to disease with the baby *in utero*. It is hypothesized that in this case the immune tolerance of pregnancy dampened the initial inflammatory clinical manifestations. How frequently this occurs is unknown, although anecdotal reports exist of similar atypical presentations, with obvious challenging implications for case identification and implementation of proper IPC procedures, especially when emergency invasive obstetric procedures are indicated during an outbreak.

CLINICAL MANAGEMENT

Once thought futile or too dangerous to implement, efforts to provide and enhance the quality of clinical care for patients with EVD have gradually increased over the years (61). Treatment guidelines for EVD have been developed by WHO (62) and interim guidelines by MSF. The level of care provided during West Africa 2013 varied widely by the phase of the outbreak and ETU. After being overrun in the early phases, and consequently offering essentially no or minimal care (often only oral rehydration and oral acetaminophen), most ETUs gradually scaled up to at least standard practices of intravenous fluid and electrolyte management. A few in West Africa and virtually all in the United States and Europe provided full-service intensive care, including mechanical ventilation and renal replacement when indicated.

CFRs were consistently higher for patients at the extremes of age (45, 46), but it unfortunately remains difficult to assess the impact of level of care on patient outcome. Reported CFRs from West Africa 2013 vary widely (31 to 76%) by phase of the outbreak and ETU (63, 64), without obvious associations between level of care provided and CFR. This likely reflects patient selection and survival bias from the extremely varied levels of case finding across time and place. In some areas the sickest patients presented to ETUs, while in other areas they hid or absconded. Although caution is in order, since the findings are anecdotal and uncontrolled, it is perhaps illustrative to note that the CFR of the 27 cases who received care in the United States and Europe was only 18.5% (65). It is unknown whether this outcome relates to better fluid and electrolyte monitoring, organ support (including mechanical ventilation and renal replacement therapy), the use of experimental therapies, genetic predisposition, and/or diminished comorbidities relative to the West African population.

After the major struggle to implement the quantity of medical care necessary in West Africa 2013, the outbreak rightly brought up the issue of quality of care. Implicit in this is a just rejection of a perhaps long-held but implicit acceptance of disparate qualities of care between patients in LMICs and resource-rich countries, an archaic notion whose time must now be passed. Regardless of country of origin or personal wealth, patients should have the right to HCWs with the right training for their condition and who implement evidence-based standards of care. Of course, this gap between rich and poor cannot be closed overnight. There is much work to be done with regard to both scientific research to generate the best evidence and advocacy and organization to ensure thorough and equitable implementation.

SEQUELAE, VIRUS PERSISTENCE, AND RECRUDESCENCE

Although a host of both short- and long-term sequelae after EVD have been noted dating back to the first recognized outbreak in the Democratic Republic of the Congo in 1976, little attention was typically afforded to survivors, in part due to the limited infrastructure for study in the outbreak areas (66). Only two controlled studies have been reported (67–69), neither incorporating the detailed microbiological and physical examination (especially ocular, audiometric, and mental health exams) required for a thorough understanding of the sequelae and associated pathogenesis. However, the estimated over 10,000 EVD survivors in West Africa have created both a moral imperative to provide clinical care and an opportunity for greater scientific understanding. In addition, survivors among the 20 medically evacuated cases to the United States and Europe have generally been seen in advanced medical settings that allow more detailed clinical observation and laboratory analysis than is typically possible in West Africa (70–73). WHO has developed clinical care guidelines for EVD survivors (74), and various studies on EVD sequelae are underway. In particular, PREVAIL III, a large multiyear controlled cohort study of EVD sequelae and virus persistence being undertaken in Liberia promises to eventually yield a wealth of information (75).

As preliminary data begin to roll in, it is clear that the full scope of the medical and psychosocial challenges faced by EVD survivors has been underappreciated. Persistent arthralgia, ocular complications (including potentially sight-threatening uveitis that may result in early cataract formation), abdominal pain, extreme fatigue, and anorexia are very frequent, as are mental health sequelae, including sleep and memory disturbances, anxiety disorders, depression, posttraumatic stress disorder, and survivors' guilt in not only survivors, but also other family and community members (53, 66–68, 71, 72, 76–92).

The underlying pathogenesis of EVD sequelae is not well understood, but anecdotal observations increasingly suggest that at least some relate to persistent virus in selected immunologically protected tissue compartments and fluids, including the testes/semen, chambers of the eye, central nervous system, and the fetus, placenta, and amniotic sac/fluid of women infected during pregnancy (53, 67, 71, 86, 87, 93–95). Anecdotal evidence from previous outbreaks of virus in the semen detected by PCR up to 101 days after disease onset and by cell culture up to 82 days (94) are now being complemented by much larger and more systematic investigations in West Africa. Albeit in low copy numbers and in a small minority of EVD survivors, viral RNA has been detected in the semen up to a year or more after acute disease (95). In most cases cell culture data are not yet available, but virus has been cultured from the semen of an EVD survivor in the United States 70 days after disease onset (96). Tests of semen years after recovery from acute EVD have consistently been negative, indicating that the virus is eventually cleared (94).

Although sexual transmission still appears to be rare (97), male-to-female sexual transmission in Liberia 6 months after resolution of acute EVD was well-documented with both classic epidemiologic evidence and a molecular sequence match between the virus found in the man's semen and woman's blood) (86, 87). Interestingly, although PCR-positive for RNA, virus could not be isolated on cell culture from the semen sample, which was taken 20 days after the suspected transmission event. Sexual transmission is also suspected to be behind a flare of EVD in Guinea in an area where the disease had not been seen for over a year. These cases illustrate the need for continued surveillance even after the immediate threat of EVD from more common modes of transmission has been extinguished, and also call into question the norm of calling an EVD outbreak "over" once 42 days (twice the longest incubation period) have passed.

Two recent cases of prolonged virus persistence associated with recrudescence have been noted. In a medically evacuated U.S. HCW with uveitis, Ebola virus was detected by PCR and cell culture from the aqueous humor 14 weeks after disease onset and 9 weeks after clearance from the blood, which remained negative during the episode of uveitis (71). Sequence data from the aqueous humor isolate revealed five point mutations compared to the virus obtained from the blood months earlier during the initial acute EVD, suggesting persistent viral replication in the eye during convalescence. In the United Kingdom, Ebola virus was noted by reverse-transcription PCR in both the cerebrospinal fluid (CSF) and blood in a medically evacuated HCW who developed severe meningitis with seizures nine months after resolution of acute disease (M. Jacobs, personal communication). The RNA copy number was lower in the blood than in the CSF, and virus could be isolated in cell culture only from the CSF, leading to the conclusion that the viremia was due to reseeding of the blood from the central nervous system. Sequencing of viruses obtained from the blood during the initial bout of EVD and the blood and CSF 9 months later showed

greater than 99% homogeneity, again suggesting persistence of virus since initial infection. No obvious underlying immunosuppressive condition or trigger for virus reactivation could be identified in these cases.

A low index of suspicion, and limited diagnostic capacity, may have allowed similar recrudescent EVD with fever, systemic symptoms, and viremia to go undetected or misattributed to malaria and other typical causes in prior outbreaks. An alternative explanation is that these recrudescent cases follow severe initial EVD that previously would have been fatal without intensive medical care and are the consequence of high viremia (true for both cases) that seeds the immune-privileged sites. Nevertheless, recent anecdotal reports of recrudescent disease and viremia exist in West Africa, in some cases thought to be related to underlying HIV infection, although this association remains to be validated (53).

CFRs for pregnant women with EVD and their offspring are extremely high, with fetal loss approaching 100% due to spontaneous abortion, stillbirth, and neonatal death in the first three weeks of life (60, 98–102). However, in West Africa 2013 a few cases have been noted in which women infected with Ebola virus during pregnancy, possibly with no or atypically mild disease, have recovered and remained pregnant, only to spontaneously abort a macerated and nonviable fetus in subsequent weeks or months (101, 107). Although the mothers' blood remained free of virus at the time of delivery, swabs of the fetus, placenta, and amniotic fluid in some cases have tested positive for Ebola virus RNA by reverse-transcription PCR, although cell culture results are not yet available (98, 100, 101, 103). The underlying pathogenesis is yet to be determined but is presumed to be due to delayed virus clearance from the immunologically protected gravid uterus.

In addition to the semen, CSF, and products of conception, Ebola virus RNA has been found in various other body fluids and compartments, including urine (49), skin swabs/sweat (49), vaginal secretions (93), rectal swabs/stool (94), saliva (90), and breast milk (104), for weeks or even months after disease onset and after virus has been cleared from the blood (Fig. 5). However, the significance of these findings is unknown; in most cases infectious virus could not be isolated by cell culture a few weeks after disease onset. With the exception of sexual transmission, no cases of secondary transmission resulting from EVD survivors have been suspected. Nevertheless, nonstigmatizing but heightened surveillance and research are warranted to document the duration of virus persistence in EVD survivors, the implicated cellular reservoirs, and the nature and frequency of recrudescent disease and risk of secondary transmission. Full genome sequencing of Ebola viruses identified during acute infection and recrudescence may help shed light on the mechanisms of these events, especially the possibility of escape mutants.

HCW INFECTIONS AND IPC

IPC for EVD entails diverse measures, including adequate numbers of trained staff with supervision, clear operational protocols (especially for triage), appropriate design for safe workspace flow of patient and staff, water-sanitation measures, disinfection procedures, and the availability and appropriate use and removal of PPE. Unfortunately, many of the measures were lacking during the early chaos of the outbreak in West Africa, during which almost 900 HCWs contracted EVD, with over 500 deaths (14). In addition, three HCWs contracted EVD in the United States and Spain while caring for patients there. Although the high number of HCW infections has engendered speculation that the Makona virus variant of Ebola virus is more transmissible than other variants, no data are available. Most of the focus has turned instead to the issue of appropriate IPC, especially PPE. Although PPE is but one component of IPC, it tends to garner the

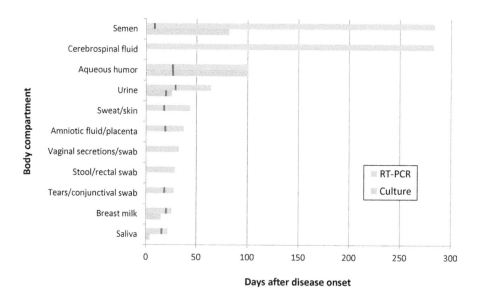

FIGURE 5 Virus persistence after the day of disease onset in various body compartments in survivors of Ebola virus disease as detected by reverse-transcription polymerase chain reaction (RT-PCR, green) and cell culture (blue). Red bars represent the day of the first negative RT-PCR detection in the patient's blood, when available. Reprinted with permission from reference 66.

most attention due to its visibility and the general tendency to focus on commodities rather than HCW competencies and the organization of health care facilities.

Although HCW infections have occurred in virtually every EVD outbreak to date (Table 1), prior to West Africa 2013, they were relatively uncommon once international support and resources arrived to assist with establishing ETUs with appropriate IPC measures. Indeed, implementation of IPC measures was attributed to the abrupt halt of HCW infections in the EVD outbreak in Kikwit, Democratic Republic of the Congo, in 1995 (25). Specific IPC and PPE guidelines were subsequently laid out in a manual coproduced by WHO and the CDC in 1998 (105). These guidelines were employed during the Gulu 2000 outbreak, in which, similar to the Kikwit experience, very few HCW infections occurred once the ETUs and accompanying IPC measures were implemented. However, the death due to EVD of Matthew Lukwiya, the hospital superintendent managing the ETU at St. Mary's Hospital Lacor in Gulu and the person who first recognized that Ebola virus could be circulating in the region, was one very high-profile exception and a tragic reminder that the IPC measures were not foolproof.

After Gulu 2000, different points of view evolved among the principal international organizations involved in EVD outbreaks regarding what constitutes appropriate PPE; MSF took a more conservative approach, requiring all skin to be covered and the use of impermeable but heavy suits originally designed for protection against chemical hazards (Tychem by DuPont Co., USA). In contrast, WHO and the CDC, until recently, emphasized only the use of gloves, an impermeable gown, a waterproof apron, and facial protection (either face shield or mask with goggles) (106) (Fig. 6). The difference in these approaches is very significant with regard to comfort, potentially dangerous heat stress (and thus the duration

that an HCW can work in an ETU), cost, and most importantly, ability to deliver quality clinical care. In April 2014, MSF, WHO, and other key stakeholders agreed to address these issues in a systematic way through a WHO-established process of evidence-based interim guideline development. However, a rapid systematic review concluded that there was insufficient comparative evidence regarding the effectiveness or harm of PPE (107). Although guidelines were nevertheless produced, which for the first time included technical specifications for PPE, the lack of evidence precluded a consensus on the most effective PPE to be used (107). The lack of consensus often generated confusion and posed a significant challenge in training HCWs, with different organizations simultaneously providing training that was not standardized or uniform with regard to PPE (108). The unlikely specter of Ebola virus mutation to enable airborne spread further obfuscated the picture. The CDC chose to offer training on the use of the PPE advocated by both MSF and WHO.

The many HCW infections that occurred during West Africa 2013 have unfortunately shed little light on the common modes of HCW infection and therefore the best IPC practices or most efficacious PPE. First, it is not clear that the attack rate for HCWs living and working in ETUs is consistently higher than that of the general population. Local HCWs are members of the communities where Ebola virus is circulating and thus may share many of the same risks. There are also many anecdotal reports of HCWs seeing patients in their homes, where the use of full PPE and other IPC measures are unlikely to be adequate (109, 110). One might expect the source of exposure for the expatriates infected during West Africa 2013 to be clearer, since this group generally lodged in hotels or the dedicated residence of the sponsoring organization, with less contact in the community at large, and was less likely to engage in informal medical consultation outside the ETU. Nevertheless, for national and expatri-

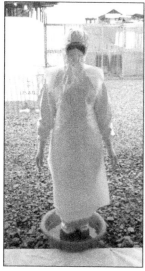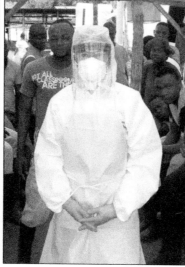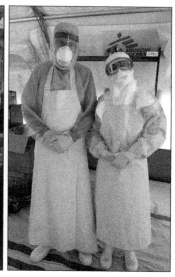

FIGURE 6 Examples of various types of personal protective equipment used during the care of patients with Ebola virus disease during the 2013–2016 outbreak in West Africa. The equipment shown is for demonstration only and should not be construed as advocating or confirming the efficacy of any specific equipment. Photos by Thomas Fletcher and Frederique Jacquerioz.

ate HCWs alike, and regardless of type of PPE worn, the specific route of infection remains unknown in the vast majority of HCW infections during any EVD outbreak, including West Africa 2013. Discrete recognizable exposures, such as needle sticks and blood splashes to mucous membranes, are rare. The procedure for doffing contaminated PPE, often considered confusing and a vulnerable point for infection, is logically a focus of attention, but again, no data are available.

More in-depth investigations are needed, and indeed are ongoing, to reveal vulnerable points for HCW infection in the care of EVD patients. Meanwhile, various initiatives have been taken to encourage innovative approaches to enhance HCW safety while optimizing patient care in ETUs, including various types of redesigned suits that simplify doffing and disinfection and minimize heat stress, aided by the addition of cooling vests and temperature monitors, decontamination chambers and other chemical approaches to inactivation of virus on physical surfaces,

rapidly deployable portable ETUs, and infusion monitors and vital sign sensors to minimize the need for close contact between HCWs and infected body fluids from patients. Although promising, most of these innovative products are still in the pilot phases and have generally come too late to be applied during West Africa 2013. It remains to be seen whether both political will and commercial viability will endure to make them widely available in the future.

EXPERIMENTAL THERAPEUTICS

Before West Africa 2013, the funding for development of EVD therapeutics and vaccines was largely driven by governmental defense departments, which were concerned about the potential use of Ebola virus as a bioweapon. While this development pipeline was far from robust, it is reasonable to suggest that, compared to other emerging infectious diseases with analogous case numbers, the scientific agenda for EVD was not languishing. Numerous therapeutic candidates were under development in cell culture and animal models. As the gravity of the situation in West Africa rose, the global community felt increasingly compelled to consider the use of various experimental therapeutics and vaccines being developed. In August 2014, WHO convened a meeting in Geneva, Switzerland, of the diverse stakeholders, including representatives from ministries of health, pharmaceutical companies, drug regulatory agencies, nongovernmental organizations providing clinical care, and experts in virology and medical ethics. Indeed, one of the first questions to be addressed was whether the use of these experimental compounds, which had varied safety and efficacy profiles, was ethical given the extreme suffering in West Africa, to which the committee unanimously replied in the affirmative. WHO created a scientific and technical advisory committee for Ebola experimental interventions to guide the process. One of their first objectives was to identify the most promising therapeutics among a long list of proposed candidates, including many of dubious quality. This process required consideration not only of the evidence for safety and efficacy, but the anticipated feasibility and utility of conducting a clinical trial in a setting of limited production capacities or intermittent drug availability.

The first therapeutic approach that received priority classification from WHO was convalescent whole blood and plasma (Table 3). This approach has been successful for a number of severe viral infections and was considered feasible in the most affected countries, especially in the context of a growing number of survivors who could serve as donors. Convalescent whole blood was used with apparent success (CFR 12.5%) in eight patients with EVD during the 1995 outbreak in Kikwit (111). However, interpretation of the outcome is confounded by the improved level of general supportive care provided to the patients relative to those seen

earlier in the outbreak (associated with a much higher CFR) and the fact that the transfusions often took place after the mean time to death for EVD during the outbreak and after many of the patients had already produced IgG antibody, suggesting that the recipients may have been likely to survive regardless. Studies of convalescent plasma have met with mixed results in nonhuman primate (NHP) models of EVD (112).

A clinical trial was conducted in Guinea in which two transfusions of convalescent plasma were administered to 84 patients with EVD in a single-arm design (113). No significant survival benefit was noted compared with historical controls. However, due to the lack of a biosafety level 4 (BSL-4) laboratory in Guinea, which is necessary to assess the neutralizing antibody titers in the transfused plasma, this crucial information has not yet been available. Interpretation of the results will therefore be somewhat clouded until these tests can be performed at an overseas BSL-4 laboratory. While convalescent plasma was well tolerated in the trial, a suspected transfusion-related case of acute lung injury was reported in a medically evacuated patient who received convalescent plasma on a compassionate use basis (90).

Monoclonal antibody therapies were considered among the most promising approaches prior to West Africa 2013 and then received significant attention from both the scientific community and the public following compassionate use in medically evacuated HCWs early during the outbreak. Enthusiasm for ZMapp, a cocktail of three monoclonal antibodies, was perhaps highest, based on *in vitro* and NHP data. It provided 100% protection in NHPs when given up to 5 days following a lethal Ebola virus challenge, at which time animals are routinely viremic and symptomatic (114). However, the drug was initially in short supply due to a time-consuming production method reliant on growth in genetically modified tobacco plants. Production was eventually scaled up to allow a multicenter randomized controlled

TABLE 3 Registered clinical trials of experimental therapeutics for Ebola virus disease during the West Africa 2013 outbreak[a]

Agent under investigation	Trial sponsor	Trial objective	Trial design	Registered status (as of April 2016)	Outcome
ZMapp	National Institute of Allergy and Infectious Diseases, USA	Evaluate efficacy on survival at day 28 post-EVD onset (with potential inclusion of other experimental agents)	Open label RCT with adaptive design, with comparison to optimized care alone (including favipiravir in Guinea)	Ongoing analysis but not recruiting	Interim report showed no definitive conclusion but targeted statistical endpoints not yet met 115
TKM 130803	University of Oxford, UK	Evaluate efficacy on survival at day 14 post-EVD onset	Open label, single arm with historical controls, as part of a multistage approach	Completed	No overall survival benefit 119
Favipiravir	Institut National de la Sante et de la Recherche Medicale, France	Evaluate efficacy on survival at day 14 post-EVD onset	Open label, single arm with historical controls	Completed	No overall survival benefit 156
Convalescent plasma	Institute of Tropical Medicine, Belgium	Evaluate efficacy on survival at day 14 post-EVD onset	Open label, single arm with historical controls	Completed	No overall survival benefit 113
Convalescent plasma	Clinical Research Management, Inc., USA	Evaluate efficacy on reducing viral load	Open label, single arm	Recruiting	None reported
Convalescent plasma	Cerus Corporation, USA	Evaluate safety and efficacy on survival at 1 year post-EVD onset	Open label, single arm	Recruiting	None reported
Brincidofovir	University of Oxford, UK	Evaluate efficacy on reducing viral load at day 14 post-EVD onset	Open label, single arm with historical controls, as part of a multistage approach	Recruitment suspended	None reported
Azithromycin, sunitinib, erlotinib, atorvastatin, and irbesartan	Clinical Research Management, Inc., USA	Evaluate efficacy of multiple therapeutic agents on reducing viral load at day 14 post-EVD onset	Multiarm RCT with adaptive design. Initial comparison arms are azithromycin versus sunitinib and erlotinib versus atorvastatin and irbesartan versus intravenous fluids and laboratory testing alone	Not yet open for recruitment	None reported
Amiodarone	Emergency, Italy	Evaluate efficacy on reducing viral load at day 10 post-EVD onset	Open label RCT with comparison to best supportive care	Withdrawn	None reported

[a]Abbreviations: EVD, Ebola virus disease; RCT, randomized controlled trial.

trial in West Africa and the United States. Although patient recruitment to the trial was insufficient to reach targeted statistical endpoints indicating conclusive benefit, preliminary analysis of existing efficacy data look promising (115). Efforts to produce an agent equivalent to ZMapp with a more scalable production method led to the development of the monoclonal antibody formulation MIL-77. Unpublished data suggest efficacy of MIL-77 in NHPs, and the drug has also been given to HCWs with EVD on a compassionate use basis, for which no firm conclusions of efficacy can be drawn. One concern with monoclonal antibody therapies is the development of drug resistance through rapid virus mutation resulting in escape mutants, which have been noted in NHPs treated with a related antibody cocktail, MB-003 (116).

Of the various antiviral drugs proposed, TKM130803, a small interfering RNA compound encapsulated in a lipid nanoparticle formulation, was arguably the front-running candidate. TKM130803 had demonstrated efficacy in NHPs (117), but phase I trials were on partial hold due to concerns of induction of a cytokine release syndrome. These were eventually addressed and, in addition, the drug composition was adjusted to improve specificity to the Makona variant of Ebola virus. Although a small study ($n = 3$) demonstrated 100% efficacy in NHPs (118), a phase II single-arm study completed in June 2015 in Sierra Leone concluded that TKM130803 did not improve survival in patients with severe EVD when compared with historical controls (119).

Several existing broad-spectrum antivirals were also investigated. Of particular interest was favipiravir (T-705), an RNA polymerase inhibitor that showed efficacy against Ebola virus in small animal models (120) and was already licensed in Japan for emergency use in pandemic influenza. A clinical trial conducted in Guinea reported no efficacy in patients with a high viral load (cycle threshold [Ct] < 20), with some suggestion of an effect in patients with less severe disease (Ct ≥ 20), although this remains to be substantiated (121). A clinical trial of brincidofovir, an initially promising broad-spectrum antiviral drug, was abruptly stopped when the drug company withdrew support for use in EVD. No specific reason was given and results have not yet been published. A clinical trial of interferon in Guinea was similarly halted, with no further information available to date.

Alongside these clinical trials, many of the short-listed compounds were used under compassionate use settings, particularly for patients seen in the United States and Europe, of whom 85% received one or more experimental therapies (65). Because of the uncontrolled nature of their use in these settings and variable composition of supportive care received, no conclusions on efficacy can be made. Nevertheless, some intriguing and perhaps promising observations are worthy of mention: the only known neonate with EVD born to a mother who was viremic at birth received the broad-spectrum antiviral GS-5734, as well as ZMapp (66). Lastly, when MSF's supply of the routine antimalarial artemether-lumefantrine given empirically to all patients admitted to the ETU ran out, they replaced it with artesunate-amodiaquine and subsequently noted improved survival (122). More formal clinical trials are necessary to assess efficacy, although it is reasonable to make artesunate-amodiaquine the drug of choice for empiric treatment of malaria coinfection in EVD.

While there is disappointment that clinical trials during West Africa 2013 have not produced definitive evidence of an efficacious drug for EVD, the experience cannot be considered futile. There is no doubt that the many complex scientific, logistical, and sociocultural challenges ultimately could not be met quickly enough to take full advantage of the large case numbers potentially affording statistical power early in the outbreak. There was also an opportunity missed to enroll more patients in clinical trials in resource-rich settings. Many difficult lessons were learned regarding the challenges of inconsistent reproducibility of *in vitro* experiments, poorly predictive animal models, and the operational demands of conducting trials overseas in an ETU during an outbreak without any pre-existing research infrastructure. Rigorous debate continues regarding the scientific and ethical merit of the various clinical trial designs used in this outbreak. Nevertheless, numerous drug candidates progressed through phase I, II, and III clinical trials at an unprecedented pace, and the recognition that some agents are ineffective, along with promising interim results for others, provides a starting point for prioritization in future outbreaks. However, much work remains to be done to capitalize on the lessons learned from West Africa 2013 and make the accelerated pace of clinical trials during outbreaks the norm, including prioritizing drug candidates, working out trial designs, prepositioning protocols and ethics committee reviews, and setting logistical frameworks for rapid operationalization. In addition, we must not forget the importance of the upstream pipeline, recognizing that the potential for clinical trials during West Africa 2013 was heavily bolstered by decades of basic science and preclinical research to provide at least some viable candidates to test in the field. Lastly, it would be naive to think that profit-driven market forces will not retain a major influence on what drugs are developed, or not, for EVD and other emerging infectious diseases.

EXPERIMENTAL VACCINES

As with therapeutics, the urgency of West Africa 2013 thrust vaccines for EVD from a conventional protracted research and development timeline into high gear, with an unprecedented rapid mobilization of researchers, vaccine manufacturers, and coordinating agencies to expedite clinical trials and vaccine deployment. Since the start of West Africa 2013, at least 40 clinical trials are underway with more than eight filovirus vaccine candidates. Resource-rich countries' concerns over Ebola virus as a bioweapon again resulted in having numerous candidates, with at least 15 vaccines under development in North America, Europe, Russia, and China (123). The candidates in the most advanced stages were a replication-competent recombinant vesicular stomatitis virus-vectored vaccine (rVSV-ZEBOV) (124–126) and a replication-incompetent recombinant chimpanzee adenovirus-3-vectored vaccine (ChAd3-EBO-Z) (127), both expressing the Zaire Ebola virus surface glycoprotein.

rVSV-ZEBOV is the only vaccine for which efficacy data exist. Preclinical data had been available for some years showing impressive preventive and postexposure prophylactic efficacy in NHPs, but the vaccine awaited an interested pharmaceutical partner to take it forward into clinical trials. West Africa 2013 finally provided such an initiative. Rapid phase I and II clinical trials were undertaken at various sites in the United States, Europe, and Africa (outside the EVD epidemic zone) with generally favorable results. A large phase III trial was then implemented in Guinea with a ring vaccination approach in which close contacts of newly diagnosed EVD cases were randomized to receive either immediate or 21-day delayed vaccination (124). The trial design is indicative of the unique circumstances and sensitivities of West Africa 2013, in which inclusion of a placebo group was considered to be unacceptable. Preliminary results show 100% efficacy (no infections in those immediately vaccinated, compared with 16 who received delayed vaccination). Given the favorable results, the vaccine was employed in the later stages of the outbreak to help stem the spread from reintroduced virus from sexual transmission. However, the clinical trials also engendered considerable safety concerns, with vaccine-induced arthritis, dermatitis, and vasculitis (124, 130). Further investigation is necessary to determine the cause of these adverse events and the optimal dose to achieve maximal immunogenicity with minimal toxicity.

ChAd3-EBOZ also had undergone promising preclinical testing prior to West Africa 2013. Phase I and II trials were again expedited, with overall favorable safety results, as one might expect from a nonreplicating vaccine (128). However, preliminary data suggest that while a single dose of ChAd3-EBOZ may be sufficient for short-term protection, boosting with a modified vaccinia virus Ankara vaccine (MVA-BN-Filo) is necessary to achieve long-lasting immunity (127, 129), a requirement that would add complexity and expense. The optimal dose of ChAd3-EBOZ may also be quite high—up to 10^{11} particle units. Lastly, the immune response to primary adenovirus vaccination appears to reduce uptake of subsequent vaccinations with the same virus, meaning that subsequent vaccines would be required to use a heterologous adenovirus vector. Thus, although overall ChAd3-EBOZ appears to be a safe and efficacious vaccine, the various logistical complications threaten to reduce its utility during outbreaks. However, it may have a favorable profile for more stable settings, such as vaccination of HCWs or members of the military, or even inclusion in routine Expanded Program on Immunization (EPI) vaccination schedules.

As with the therapeutics, West Africa 2013 prompted significant but incomplete advances in vaccines for EVD, with many lessons on how to conduct vaccine research during complex humanitarian disasters. But many scientific, economic, and logistical questions remain: How do the safety and efficacy profiles of rVSV-ZEBOV and ChAd3-EBOZ compare? The ongoing PREVAIL I trial in Liberia should provide answers by directly comparing the two vaccines. Although designed as a safety and immunogenicity study, it is designed to upgrade to an efficacy trail if EVD were to reemerge in the area. What are the ideal doses of these vaccines that provide the best balance of long-term immunity and minimal toxicity? Are the existing data on rVSV-ZEBOV sufficient to allow full licensure? If so, will rVSV-ZEBOV or any vaccine for EVD be considered sufficiently economically viable to the pharmaceutical industry to ensure production and availability? And if available, how would an EVD vaccine be used—incorporated into the routine vaccine schedule in sub-Saharan Africa, given to all HCWs, or reserved for ring vaccination or mass vaccination campaigns once an outbreak of EVD is confirmed?

NEW DIAGNOSTIC METHODS

The nonspecific clinical presentation of EVD has always posed a challenge for both early detection of outbreaks and identification of individual cases. Furthermore, since most cases that initially appear to be EVD turn out to be other diseases, laboratory diagnosis is imperative. It is a required first step in initiating the international response that has almost always been necessary to control outbreaks and for case identification in the subsequent outbreak response. Unfortunately, very few established laboratories in sub-Saharan Africa had diagnostic capacity for EVD, usually necessitating diagnostic samples to be sent to one of the very few BSL-4 laboratories that specialize in viral hemorrhagic fevers. This has usually resulted in delays of weeks to months between virus introduction and the first cases and laboratory confirmation (6, 18). The first laboratory confirmation of EVD in West Africa in early 2014 was performed by the Institut Pasteur at the Jean Mérieux-INSERM Laboratory in Lyon, France, over 3 months after the retrospectively identified first case in Guinea.

Since the first recognized EVD outbreak in 1976, the capacity for diagnostic laboratory support during outbreaks has gradually increased. For many years, laboratory diagnosis was only available retrospectively. Samples were taken from people who met the EVD case definition and were eventually sent to one of the few overseas laboratories that could perform the diagnostic testing. Enzyme-linked immunosorbent assay with back-up cell culture were the predominant diagnostic modalities (130, 131). In the Gulu 2000 outbreak, for the first time, a laboratory was established on site by the CDC to provide near real-time diagnostics by both PCR and enzyme-linked immunosorbent assay (132). This then became the norm, with one or two diagnostic laboratories on site for virtually all EVD outbreaks since then.

In recent years, PCR has become the platform of choice due to the increasing availability of reagents and thermocyclers and streamlined methods for their use at ever diminishing cost. The incredible number and widespread distribution of cases in West Africa 2013 necessitated a vast laboratory network, a challenge to which the international community responded by establishing over 50 EVD diagnostic laboratories, most providing reliable diagnostic results within 24 hours after receipt of a specimen. This could be considered one of the success stories of the outbreak response. However, a major question now is how much of this capacity will be retained once the outbreak in West Africa has been extinguished. Indeed, most of these laboratories closed, and the staying power of those that remain is yet to be determined. It is imperative that the efforts to establish EVD laboratory diagnostics during the outbreak transition to long-term capacity—perhaps a reference laboratory in each country or, at a minimum, a central laboratory for the region.

Despite its utility, the widespread availability of PCR for EVD has also created some challenges; the laboratories established in the West Africa outbreak did not constitute a coordinated network. Rather, each operated independently with varied PCR platforms and protocols, including criteria for calling a sample positive. Informal quality control efforts performed in Sierra Leone through analysis of a common serum panel did fortunately indicate that most laboratories were rendering comparable results (Gary Kobinger, personal communication). Nevertheless, significant discrepancies have been occasionally noted, especially for samples near the margins of the threshold for being considered positive.

A major challenge throughout the outbreak has been that of interpreting PCR results. The relative availability and ease of the PCR platform has resulted in the technique largely replacing cell culture—a technique that requires not only a BSL-4 laboratory but also overcoming the ever-increasing regulatory hurdles for shipment of biological samples. While cell culture directly demonstrates the presence of infectious virus, interpretation of PCR relies mainly on the Ct, a parameter that varies inversely to viral load (i.e., a low Ct represents a high viral load). Because of the extreme amplification capacity of PCR, very small quantities of viral RNA may result in a positive test, often with a high Ct near the limits of the threshold for a positive test. In these cases, there is considerable confusion about whether the result represents the presence of infectious virus or simply residual RNA in recovering patients. Furthermore, the interpretation of the result has come to have major significance for both individual patients and the overall outbreak response. Despite the lack of evidence-based algorithms for their use, PCR results have been widely incorporated into patient discharge criteria, at times resulting in the perhaps unnecessary retention of patients who have clinically recovered but have persistence "positive PCRs," usually with high Cts. This has even at times resulted in blocking beds in ETUs that are desperately needed for newly diagnosed and highly infectious cases with patients who have largely clinically recovered and likely pose minimal risk of infection (133).

The difficulty in interpreting PCR results is also a reminder of the trade-off of the

United States and other resource-rich countries' research priorities over the past few decades, which have relatively narrowly targeted the development of specific countermeasure products—i.e., diagnostic assays, therapeutics, and vaccines. The program can be considered a success in that regard, having produced numerous products sufficiently advanced in their preclinical development to enable clinical trials when EVD hit West Africa. However, the down side of this approach is that few funds were available for studies oriented toward a deeper understanding of the basic modes of virus transmission or EVD pathogenesis—knowledge gaps that have posed significant challenges both in mounting outbreak response operations in the field and setting public policy. More research regarding the natural history of EVD and virus shedding and the relationship of Ct to the presence of infectious virus as well as standardized PCR reagents and platforms is needed to produce evidence-based patient management and discharge algorithms. Optimal utility will likely only be achieved by incorporating both laboratory and clinical data.

While the widespread availability of PCR diagnostics generally represents a great step forward, the limitations of any technique requiring a fixed laboratory (need for sophisticated equipment and trained laboratory staff, requirements for safe phlebotomy and specimen delivery to the laboratory, and 24-hour turn-around time for results) have brought about great interest in point-of-care rapid tests for EVD. Such tests have a particular attraction given the remote terrain often involved. Suspected cases requiring a rapid decision on the need for isolation and treatment might be seen at sites at a day's drive over rugged terrain from the diagnostic laboratory. In response to this need, numerous rapid diagnostic tests for EVD have been developed and received emergency use approval from WHO (134). However, concerns over moderate sensitivity and specificity, with potentially grave consequences of both

false-positive and -negative results, have brought about considerable hesitation to field implementation, resulting in very limited use to date. Enhancing and validating the sensitivity and specificity of these tests, perhaps in diagnostic algorithms combining clinical and epidemiologic data, could perhaps render a tool that could drastically change the landscape with regard to both initial detection of EVD outbreaks as well as patient management and outbreak control across sub-Saharan Africa.

Lastly, genetic sequencing technology was increasingly employed during West Africa 2013 to give a better understanding of the molecular epidemiology. Whole-genome sequencing was performed on hundreds of samples, a far larger number than had been sequenced before, to give a rapid understanding of the virus evolution and geographic provenance during the outbreak (135, 136). The bulk of this work was done through shipment of samples to overseas laboratories. However, by the end of the outbreak sequencing capability was also being built in West Africa (137). In the future, if real-time sequencing technology can be routinely folded into the repertoire of existing laboratories in sub-Saharan Africa and/or mobile laboratories established during EVD outbreaks, we can envision sequence data becoming an integral and invaluable part of field operations, with real-time transmission of sequence and epidemiological data linked to surveillance teams to provide leads in contact tracing. Sequence data are especially valuable toward the tail end of outbreaks or when cases pop up in new areas with no clear epidemiological link. Indeed, sequence data have been key in helping to pinpoint the probable origins of late EVD flares in Liberia and Guinea (87, 137). In addition to its utility in field surveillance, mutations identified by sequence monitoring could provide early warning of developing drug resistance (especially with monoclonal antibody and sequence-based therapies, such as small interfering RNAs) (138) and primer mismatches that could inhibit sensitivity of sequence-based assays, including PCR.

INFORMATION TECHNOLOGY TO IMPROVE FIELD SURVEILLANCE AND CASE MANAGEMENT

Increasing convergence of the fields of medicine, epidemiology, and information technology holds enormous potential to enhance field surveillance and case management. The incredible dissemination of cell phone technology even to the farthest reaches of sub-Saharan Africa in the past few decades holds the potential for real-time digital sharing that could never have been imagined 20 years ago. Myriad uses can be envisioned.

Digital data sharing and tracking technology through cell phones and simple SMS text messaging could be used to streamline and largely replace the logistically cumbersome, expensive, and slow processes of physical contact tracing, especially for contacts living in remote locations. Instead of relying on physical meetings of surveillance teams, the day could start with cell phone teleconferences to receive the key information from the night before and lay out the day's surveillance priorities, perhaps with set check-ins twice daily to provide and receive updates from the field and relevant laboratory data. The movement of field teams could be monitored with the GPS systems routinely incorporated into smart phones. Daily physical visits to contacts could be replaced by daily time-stamped SMS texts, reserving in-person visits for those who report symptoms. Digital photos could also be taken and sent for verification purposes or for inquiries to expert clinicians. Although somewhat more complex, systems for on-site data entry and immediate download to a central server could provide real-time actionable information to surveillance coordinators as well as improve the quality of data, since such systems have controls to ensure that key

variables are not skipped and are answered within allowed parameters. These data could be augmented by scanning reports of social media programs, such as the popular WhatsApp, to glean informal surveillance chatter, providing early leads to areas of possible new transmission.

Digital technology could also be used to streamline and enhance the quality of case management, enabling patients and their data to be tracked throughout the process. For example, a bar-coded scannable and washable plastic wrist-band could be placed on the patient upon presentation to the ETU or pick-up in their village by the field team. Daily scanning with a simple bar-code reader would allow tracking of the patient from ambulance pick up through admission, stay, and discharge from the ETU. Inside the ETUs, digital data transfer can (and already has been in some ETUs) used to transfer clinical data from the "red zone" to the outside for real-time analysis.

Although the aforementioned applications of information technology, and undoubtedly many more, are certainly possible, most of them remained at the "idea stage" during West Africa 2013. There are also logistical issues about power and connectivity to be considered, although as mentioned above, simple SMS messaging is now possible, and indeed already used, in nearly every community in Africa. Perhaps more challenging as information technology is increasingly relied upon to collect and share data, are ethical issues regarding patient confidentiality and data ownership. Advanced planning to work out these nontrivial issues and allow rapid implementation of these new and powerful tools in future outbreaks will be the challenge now.

CONCLUSIONS AND FUTURE CHALLENGES

Albeit unwelcome, the magnitude of West Africa 2013 provided a unique opportunity and obligation to better understand the biology and epidemiology of EVD and, equally as important, the many scientific, economic, social, political, ethical, and logistical challenges in confronting emerging diseases in the modern era. As the global population surges and becomes more interconnected, the risk of such outbreaks is destined to increase. In the absence of redoubled efforts to build capacity for surveillance and response, outbreaks such as West Africa 2013 threaten to become the "new norm." One need not look much further for the proof than to the Zika virus outbreak that, at this writing, is riffling through the Caribbean and Latin America.

But despite the tragedy of West Africa 2013, the outbreak also provided us with a notion of how we can and must respond better. The pressure is, rightly, on to capitalize on these glimpses of innovation and research progress to create a new norm of comprehensive surveillance and organized response. Much of the pressure rightly falls on WHO to revamp and restructure its operations, but WHO cannot do it alone or in the absence of sufficient funding. Lastly, let us remember that, while important, scientific and technological advancement alone will never be sufficient; poverty and a lack of the fundamental human right to health consistently underlie outbreaks of emerging pathogens (139). EVD is but the proverbial "canary in the coal mine," indicative of the world's most vulnerable populations. We must advocate for and work toward restitution of the right to health in LMICs. This will entail much more than simply building a laboratory or conducting a research project. Local educational institutions must be strengthened and career opportunities created to stop the "brain drain" of HCWs to high-income countries and produce future "home-grown" leaders in the health sciences. Novel and technology-appropriate approaches to local problems must be sought, as well as the funding mechanisms that enable their execution. Responsibility falls also on LMICs to create strong and transparent governmental and public health administrative frameworks that are capable of capitalizing on international collaboration and support. Long after West Africa 2013 is over, these will be our true measures of success.

ACKNOWLEDGMENTS

The authors thank Ian Crozier, Frederique Jacquerioz, Lina Moses, Mikiko Senga, Nahoko Shindo, Armand Sprecher, and Constanza Vallenas for input on the manuscript's content and Lara Schwarz for assistance with its preparation.

DEDICATION

This article is dedicated to the many health care workers who sacrificed their time, energy, and all too often, their lives to combat the Ebola virus disease outbreak in West Africa (140).

CITATION

Bausch DG, Rojek A. 2016. West Africa 2013: Re-examining Ebola. Microbiol Spectrum 4(3):EI10-0022-2016.

REFERENCES

1. **Incident Management System Ebola Epidemiology Team, CDC,Guinea Interministerial Committee for Response Against the Ebola Virus, World Health Organization, CDC Guinea Response Team, Liberia Ministry of Health and Social Welfare, CDC Liberia Response Team, Sierra Leone Ministry of Health and Sanitation, CDC Sierra Leone Response Team, Viral Special Pathogens Branch, National Center for Emerging and Zoonotic Infectious Diseases, CDC.** 2014. Update: ebola virus disease epidemic--West Africa, November 2014. *MMWR Morb Mortal Wkly Rep* **63:**1064–1066.

2. **WHO.** 2015. *Ebola Situation Report - 2 December 2015.* http://apps.who.int/ebola/current-situation/ebola-situation-report-2-december-2015.

3. **Elston JW, Moosa AJ, Moses F, Walker G, Dotta N, Waldman RJ, Wright J.** 2015. Impact of the Ebola outbreak on health systems and population health in Sierra Leone. *J Public Health* (Oxf). [Epub ahead of print.] doi:10.1093/pubmed/fdv158.

4. **Bausch DG, Schwarz L.** 2014. Outbreak of Ebola virus disease in Guinea: where ecology meets economy. *PLoS Negl Trop Dis* **8**:e3056. doi:10.1371/journal.pntd.0003056.

5. **Bausch D.** 2001. Of sickness unknown: death, and health, in Africa. *UN Chron* **38**:5–13.

6. **Bausch D, Rollin P.** 2004. Responding to epidemics of Ebola hemorrhagic fever: progress and lessons learned from recent outbreaks in Uganda, Gabon, and Congo, p 35–57. *In* Scheld W, Murray B, Hughes J (ed), *Emerging Infections 6*. ASM Press, Washington, DC.

7. **Allan R, Mandell S, Ladbury R, Pearce E, Skinner K.** 1998. The progression from endemic to epidemic Lassa fever in war-torn West Africa. p 197. *In* Saluzzo JF, Dodet B (ed), *Emergence and Control of Rodent-borne Diseases: Hantaviral and Arenal Diseases*. Elsevier, Philadelphia.

8. **Bertherat E, Talarmin A, Zeller H, International Committee of Technical and Scientific Coordination of the Durba Epidemic.** 1999. Democratic Republic of the Congo: between civil war and the Marburg virus. International Committee of Technical and Scientific Coordination of the Durba Epidemic. *Med Trop (Mars)* **59**:201–204. (In French.)

9. **Bausch DG, Clougherty MM.** 2015. Ebola virus: sensationalism, science, and human rights. *J Infect Dis* **212**(Suppl 2):S79–S83.

10. **WHO.** 2014. Ground zero in Guinea: the Ebola outbreak smoulders – undetected – for more than 3 months. http://www.who.int/csr/disease/ebola/ebola-6-months/guinea/en/.

11. **Baize S, Pannetier D, Oestereich L, Rieger T, Koivogui L, Magassouba N, Soropogui B, Sow MS, Keïta S, De Clerck H, Tiffany A, Dominguez G, Loua M, Traoré A, Kolié M, Malano ER, Heleze E, Bocquin A, Mély S, Raoul H, Caro V, Cadar D, Gabriel M, Pahlmann M, Tappe D, Schmidt-Chanasit J, Impouma B, Diallo AK, Formenty P, Van Herp M, Günther S.** 2014. Emergence of Zaire Ebola virus disease in Guinea. *N Engl J Med* **371**:1418–1425.

12. **WHO.** 2014. Ebola virus disease in Guinea. http://www.afro.who.int/en/clusters-a-programmes/dpc/epidemic-a-pandemic-alert-and-response/outbreak-news/4063-ebola-hemorrhagic-fever-in-guinea.html.

13. **WHO.** 2015. Ebola virus disease (EVD) in West Africa: an extraordinary epidemic. *Wkly Epidemiol Rec* **90**:89–96.

14. **WHO.** 2015. Ebola situation report - 4 November 2015. http://apps.who.int/ebola/current-situation/ebola-situation-report-4-november-2015.

15. **Forrester JD, Hunter JC, Pillai SK, Arwady MA, Ayscue P, Matanock A, Monroe B, Schafer IJ, Nyenswah TG, De Cock KM, Centers for Disease Control and Prevention (CDC).** 2014. Cluster of Ebola cases among Liberian and U.S. health care workers in an Ebola treatment unit and adjacent hospital: Liberia, 2014. *MMWR Morb Mortal Wkly Rep* **63**:925–929.

16. **Matanock A, Arwady MA, Ayscue P, Forrester JD, Gaddis B, Hunter JC, Monroe B, Pillai SK, Reed C, Schafer IJ, Massaquoi M, Dahn B, De Cock KM, Centers for Disease Control and Prevention (CDC).** 2014. Ebola virus disease cases among health care workers not working in Ebola treatment units: Liberia, June-August, 2014. *MMWR Morb Mortal Wkly Rep* **63**:1077–1081.

17. **Olu O, Kargbo B, Kamara S, Wurie AH, Amone J, Ganda L, Ntsama B, Poy A, Kuti-George F, Engedashet E, Worku N, Cormican M, Okot C, Yoti Z, Kamara KB, Chitala K, Chimbaru A, Kasolo F.** 2015. Epidemiology of Ebola virus disease transmission among health care workers in Sierra Leone, May to December 2014: a retrospective descriptive study. *BMC Infect Dis* **15**:416.

18. **Bausch DG.** 2015. The year that Ebola virus took over west Africa: missed opportunities for prevention. *Am J Trop Med Hyg* **92**:229–232.

19. **Moon S, Sridhar D, Pate MA, Jha AK, Clinton C, Delaunay S, Edwin V, Fallah M, Fidler DP, Garrett L, Goosby E, Gostin LO, Heymann DL, Lee K, Leung GM, Morrison JS, Saavedra J, Tanner M, Leigh JA, Hawkins B, Woskie LR, Piot P.** 2015. Will Ebola change the game? Ten essential reforms before the next pandemic. The report of the Harvard-LSHTM Independent Panel on the Global Response to Ebola. *Lancet* **386**:2204–2221.

20. **Meltzer MI, Atkins CY, Santibanez S, Knust B, Petersen BW, Ervin ED, Nichol ST, Damon IK, Washington ML, Centers for Disease Control and Prevention.** 2014. Estimating the future number of cases in the Ebola epidemic: Liberia and Sierra Leone, 2014-2015. *MMWR Suppl* **63**:1–14.

21. **Bevilacqua N, Nicastri E, Chinello P, Puro V, Petrosillo N, Di Caro A, Capobianchi MR, Lanini S, Vairo F, Pletschette M, Zumla A, Ippolito G, Team IE, INMI Ebola Team.** 2015. Criteria for discharge of patients with Ebola virus diseases in high-income countries. *Lancet Glob Health* **3**:e739–e740.

22. **WHO.** 2016. A review of the role of training in WHO Ebola emergency response. *Wkly Epidemiol Rec* **91:**181–186.

23. **WHO.** 1978. Ebola haemorrhagic fever in Sudan, 1976. *Bull World Health Organ* **56:** 247–270.

24. **WHO.** 1978. Ebola haemorrhagic fever in Zaire, 1976. *Bull World Health Organ* **56:**271–293.

25. **Khan AS, Tshioko FK, Heymann DL, Le Guenno B, Nabeth P, Kerstiëns B, Fleerackers Y, Kilmarx PH, Rodier GR, Nkuku O, Rollin PE, Sanchez A, Zaki SR, Swanepoel R, Tomori O, Nichol ST, Peters CJ, Muyembe-Tamfum JJ, Ksiazek TG.** 1999. The reemergence of Ebola hemorrhagic fever, Democratic Republic of the Congo, 1995. Commission de Lutte contre les Epidémies à Kikwit. *J Infect Dis* **179**(Suppl 1): S76–S86.

26. **WHO.** 2001. Outbreak of Ebola haemorrhagic fever, Uganda, August 2000-January 2001. *Wkly Epidemiol Rec* **76:**41–46.

27. **Formenty P, Libama F, Epelboin A, Allarangar Y, Leroy E, Moudzeo H, Tarangonia P, Molamou A, Lenzi M, Ait-Ikhlef K, Hewlett B, Roth C, Grein T.** 2003. Outbreak of Ebola hemorrhagic fever in the Republic of the Congo, 2003: a new strategy?. *Med Trop (Mars)* **63:**291–295. (In French.)

28. **Anonymous.** 2007. Outbreak news. Ebola virus haemorrhagic fever, Democratic Republic of the Congo: update. *Wkly Epidemiol Rec* **82:**345–346.

29. **Wamala JF, Lukwago L, Malimbo M, Nguku P, Yoti Z, Musenero M, Amone J, Mbabazi W, Nanyunja M, Zaramba S, Opio A, Lutwama JJ, Talisuna AO, Okware SI.** 2010. Ebola hemorrhagic fever associated with novel virus strain, Uganda, 2007-2008. *Emerg Infect Dis* **16:**1087–1092.

30. **WHO.** 2014. Ebola situation report - 31 December 2014. http://apps.who.int/ebola/en/status-outbreak/situation-reports/ebola-situation-report-31-december-2014.

31. **Parra JM, Salmerón OJ, Velasco M.** 2014. The first case of Ebola virus disease acquired outside Africa. *N Engl J Med* **371:**2439–2440.

32. **Lopaz MA, Amela C, Ordobas M, Dominguez-Berjon MF, Alvarez C, Martinez M, Sierra MJ, Simon F, Jansa JM, Plachouras D, Astray J, Working Group of Ebola Outbreak Investigation Team of Madrid.** 2015. First secondary case of Ebola outside Africa: epidemiological characteristics and contact monitoring, Spain, September to November 2014. *Euro Surveill* **20:**20. http://www.eurosurveillance.org/ViewArticle.aspx?ArticleId=21003.

33. **Abdoulaye B, Moussa S, Daye K, Boubakar BS, Cor SS, Idrissa T, Mamadou NH, Oumar BI, Tidiane NC, Selly LM, Tacko DC, Amadou DP, Mandiaye L, Mbaye D, Marie CS.** 2015. Experience on the management of the first imported Ebola virus disease case in Senegal. *Pan Afr Med J* **22**(Suppl 1):6.

34. **Musa EO, Adedire E, Adeoye O, Adewuyi P, Waziri N, Nguku P, Nanjuya M, Adebayo B, Fatiregun A, Enya B, Ohuabunwo C, Sabitu K, Shuaib F, Okoh A, Oguntimehin O, Onyekwere N, Nasidi A, Olayinka A.** 2015. Epidemiological profile of the Ebola virus disease outbreak in Nigeria, July-September 2014. *Pan Afr Med J* **21:**331.

35. **Yacisin K, Balter S, Fine A, Weiss D, Ackelsberg J, Prezant D, Wilson R, Starr D, Rakeman J, Raphael M, Quinn C, Toprani A, Clark N, Link N, Daskalakis D, Maybank A, Layton M, Varma JK, Centers for Disease Control and Prevention (CDC).** 2015. Ebola virus disease in a humanitarian aid worker: New York City, October 2014. *MMWR Morb Mortal Wkly Rep* **64:**321–323.

36. **WHO.** 2014. *Mali: details of the additional cases of Ebola virus disease.* http://www.who.int/mediacentre/news/ebola/20-november-2014-mali/en/.

37. **Chevalier MS, Chung W, Smith J, Weil LM, Hughes SM, Joyner SN, Hall E, Srinath D, Ritch J, Thathiah P, Threadgill H, Cervantes D, Lakey DL, Centers for Disease Control and Prevention (CDC).** 2014. Ebola virus disease cluster in the United States: Dallas County, Texas, 2014. *MMWR Morb Mortal Wkly Rep* **63:**1087–1088.

38. **McCarty CL, Basler C, Karwowski M, Erme M, Nixon G, Kippes C, Allan T, Parrilla T, DiOrio M, de Fijter S, Stone ND, Yost DA, Lippold SA, Regan JJ, Honein MA, Knust B, Braden C, Centers for Disease Control and Prevention (CDC).** 2014. Response to importation of a case of Ebola virus disease: Ohio, October 2014. *MMWR Morb Mortal Wkly Rep* **63:**1089–1091.

39. **Thiam S, Delamou A, Camara S, Carter J, Lama EK, Ndiaye B, Nyagero J, Nduba J, Ngom M.** 2015. Challenges in controlling the Ebola outbreak in two prefectures in Guinea: why did communities continue to resist? *Pan Afr Med J* **22**(Suppl 1):22.

40. **Buli BG, Mayigane LN, Oketta JF, Soumouk A, Sandouno TE, Camara B, Toure MS, Conde A.** 2015. Misconceptions about Ebola seriously affect the prevention efforts: KAP related to Ebola prevention and treatment in Kouroussa Prefecture, Guinea. *Pan Afr Med J* **22**(Suppl 1):11.

41. Nielsen CF, Kidd S, Sillah AR, Davis E, Mermin J, Kilmarx PH, Centers for Disease Control and Prevention. 2015. Improving burial practices and cemetery management during an Ebola virus disease epidemic: Sierra Leone, 2014. *MMWR Morb Mortal Wkly Rep* **64:**20–27.

42. Institute for Health Metrics and Evaluation. 2015. Financing. *Global Health* 2014: *Shifts in Funding as the MDG Era Closes.* Institute for Health Metrics and Evaluation, Seattle, WA.

43. World Health Organization. 2015. *Investing in the World's Health Organization.* World Health Organization, Geneva, Switzerland.

44. Tomori O. 2015. Pre-meeting course: re-defining preparedness, response and recovery to global pandemics: the experience of Ebola in West Africa. Abstr, 64th Annual Meeting of the American Society of Tropical Medicine and Hygiene, Philadelphia, PA, October 25, 2015. American Society of Tropical Medicine and Hygiene.

45. Bah EI, Lamah MC, Fletcher T, Jacob ST, Brett-Major DM, Sall AA, Shindo N, Fischer WA II, Lamontagne F, Saliou SM, Bausch DG, Moumié B, Jagatic T, Sprecher A, Lawler JV, Mayet T, Jacquerioz FA, Méndez Baggi MF, Vallenas C, Clement C, Mardel S, Faye O, Faye O, Soropogui B, Magassouba N, Koivogui L, Pinto R, Fowler RA. 2015. Clinical presentation of patients with Ebola virus disease in Conakry, Guinea. *N Engl J Med* **372:**40–47.

46. Schieffelin JS, Shaffer JG, Goba A, Gbakie M, Gire SK, Colubri A, Sealfon RS, Kanneh L, Moigboi A, Momoh M, Fullah M, Moses LM, Brown BL, Andersen KG, Winnicki S, Schaffner SF, Park DJ, Yozwiak NL, Jiang PP, Kargbo D, Jalloh S, Fonnie M, Sinnah V, French I, Kovoma A, Kamara FK, Tucker V, Konuwa E, Sellu J, Mustapha I, Foday M, Yillah M, Kanneh F, Saffa S, Massally JL, Boisen ML, Branco LM, Vandi MA, Grant DS, Happi C, Gevao SM, Fletcher TE, Fowler RA, Bausch DG, Sabeti PC, Khan SH, Garry RF, KGH Lassa Fever Program, Viral Hemorrhagic Fever Consortium, WHO Clinical Response Team. 2014. Clinical illness and outcomes in patients with Ebola in Sierra Leone. *N Engl J Med* **371:**2092–2100.

47. Fowler RA, Fletcher T, Fischer WA II, Lamontagne F, Jacob S, Brett-Major D, Lawler JV, Jacquerioz FA, Houlihan C, O'Dempsey T, Ferri M, Adachi T, Lamah MC, Bah EI, Mayet T, Schieffelin J, McLellan SL, Senga M, Kato Y, Clement C, Mardel S, Vallenas Bejar De Villar RC, Shindo N, Bausch D. 2014. Caring for critically ill patients with ebola virus disease.

Perspectives from West Africa. *Am J Respir Crit Care Med* **190:**733–737.

48. Chertow DS, Kleine C, Edwards JK, Scaini R, Giuliani R, Sprecher A. 2014. Ebola virus disease in West Africa: clinical manifestations and management. *N Engl J Med* **371:**2054–2057.

49. Kreuels B, Wichmann D, Emmerich P, Schmidt-Chanasit J, de Heer G, Kluge S, Sow A, Renné T, Günther S, Lohse AW, Addo MM, Schmiedel S. 2014. A case of severe Ebola virus infection complicated by Gram-negative septicemia. *N Engl J Med* **371:**2394–2401.

50. Sueblinvong V, Johnson DW, Weinstein GL, Connor MJ Jr, Crozier I, Liddell AM, Franch HA, Wall BR, Kalil AC, Feldman M, Lisco SJ, Sevransky JE. 2015. Critical care for multiple organ failure secondary to Ebola virus disease in the United States. *Crit Care Med* **43:**2066–2075.

51. Wolf T, Kann G, Becker S, Stephan C, Brodt HR, de Leuw P, Grünewald T, Vogl T, Kempf VA, Keppler OT, Zacharowski K. 2015. Severe Ebola virus disease with vascular leakage and multiorgan failure: treatment of a patient in intensive care. *Lancet* **385:**1428–1435.

52. Chertow DS, Nath A, Suffredini AF, Danner RL, Reich DS, Bishop RJ, Childs RW, Arai AE, Palmore TN, Lane HC, Fauci AS, Davey RT. 2016. Severe meningoencephalitis in a case of Ebola virus disease: a case report. *Ann Intern Med.* [Epub ahead of print.] doi:10.7326/M15-3066.

53. Howlett P, Brown C, Helderman T, Brooks T, Lisk D, Deen G, Solbrig M, Lado M. 2016. Ebola virus disease complicated by late-onset encephalitis and polyarthritis, Sierra Leone [letter]. *Emerg Infect Dis* **22:**150–152.

54. Dhillon P, McCarthy S, Gibbs M. 2015. Surviving stroke in an Ebola treatment centre. *BMJ Case Rep* **2015.**

55. Wilson AJ, Martin DS, Maddox V, Rattenbury S, Bland D, Bhagani S, Cropley I, Hopkins S, Mepham S, Rodger A, Warren S, Chowdary P, Jacobs M. 2016. Thromboelastography in the management of coagulopathy associated with Ebola virus disease. *Clin Infect Dis* **62:**610–612.

56. WHO. 2014. *Case definition recommendations for Ebola or Marburg virus diseases.* http://www.who.int/csr/resources/publications/ebola/ebola-case-definition-contact-en.pdf?ua=1&ua=1.

57. Lado M, Walker NF, Baker P, Haroon S, Brown CS, Youkee D, Studd N, Kessete Q, Maini R, Boyles T, Hanciles E, Wurie A, Kamara TB, Johnson O, Leather AJ. 2015. Clinical features of patients isolated for

suspected Ebola virus disease at Connaught Hospital, Freetown, Sierra Leone: a retrospective cohort study. *Lancet Infect Dis* **15:**1024–1033.

58. Zachariah R, Harries AD. 2015. The WHO clinical case definition for suspected cases of Ebola virus disease arriving at Ebola holding units: reason to worry? *Lancet Infect Dis* **15:**989–990.

59. ISARIC. 2014. Case record form: Ebola. *Virus disease.* http://isaric.tghn.org/site_media/media/medialibrary/2014/11/ISARIC_WHO_EVD_CRF_O5OCT14_Instructions.pdf.

60. Akerlund E, Prescott J, Tampellini L. 2015. Shedding of Ebola virus in an asymptomatic pregnant woman. *N Engl J Med* **372:**2467–2469.

61. Bausch DG, Feldmann H, Geisbert TW, Bray M, Sprecher AG, Boumandouki P, Rollin PE, Roth C, Winnipeg Filovirus Clinical Working Group. 2007. Outbreaks of filovirus hemorrhagic fever: time to refocus on the patient. *J Infect Dis* **196**(Suppl 2)**:**S136–S141.

62. WHO. 2014. *Clinical Management of Patients with Viral Haemorrhagic Fever: A Pocket Guide for the Front-Line Health Worker.* WHO, Geneva, Switzerland. http://www.who.int/csr/resources/publications/clinical-management-patients/en/.

63. Ansumana R, Jacobsen KH, Sahr F, Idris M, Bangura H, Boie-Jalloh M, Lamin JM, Sesay S. 2015. Ebola in Freetown area, Sierra Leone: a case study of 581 patients. *N Engl J Med* **372:**587–588.

64. Agua-Agum J, Ariyarajah A, Aylward B, Blake IM, Brennan R, Cori A, Donnelly CA, Dorigatti I, Dye C, Eckmanns T, Ferguson NM, Formenty P, Fraser C, Garcia E, Garske T, Hinsley W, Holmes D, Hugonnet S, Iyengar S, Jombart T, Krishnan R, Meijers S, Mills HL, Mohamed Y, Nedjati-Gilani G, Newton E, Nouvellet P, Pelletier L, Perkins D, Riley S, Sagrado M, Schnitzler J, Schumacher D, Shah A, Van Kerkhove MD, Varsaneux O, Wijekoon Kannangarage N, WHO Ebola Response Team. 2015. West African Ebola epidemic after one year: slowing but not yet under control. *N Engl J Med* **372:**584–587.

65. Uyeki TM, Mehta AK, Davey RT Jr, Liddell AM, Wolf T, Vetter P, Schmiedel S, Grünewald T, Jacobs M, Arribas JR, Evans L, Hewlett AL, Brantsaeter AB, Ippolito G, Rapp C, Hoepelman AI, Gutman J, Working Group of the US–European Clinical Network on Clinical Management of Ebola Virus Disease Patients in the US and Europe. 2016. Clinical management of Ebola virus disease in the United States and Europe. *N Engl J Med* **374:**636–646.

66. Vetter P, Kaiser L, Schibler M, Ciglenecki I, Bausch DG. 2016. Sequelae of Ebola virus disease: the emergency within the emergency. *Lancet Infect Dis.* [Epub ahead of print.] doi:10.1016/S1473-3099(16)00077-3.

67. Rowe AK, Bertolli J, Khan AS, Mukunu R, Muyembe-Tamfum JJ, Bressler D, Williams AJ, Peters CJ, Rodriguez L, Feldmann H, Nichol ST, Rollin PE, Ksiazek TG. 1999. Clinical, virologic, and immunologic follow-up of convalescent Ebola hemorrhagic fever patients and their household contacts, Kikwit, Democratic Republic of the Congo. Commission de Lutte contre les Epidémies à Kikwit. *J Infect Dis* **179**(Suppl 1)**:**S28–S35.

68. Clark DV, Kibuuka H, Millard M, Wakabi S, Lukwago L, Taylor A, Eller MA, Eller LA, Michael NL, Honko AN, Olinger GG Jr, Schoepp RJ, Hepburn MJ, Hensley LE, Robb ML. 2015. Long-term sequelae after Ebola virus disease in Bundibugyo, Uganda: a retrospective cohort study. *Lancet Infect Dis* **15:**905–912.

69. Bausch DG. 2015. Sequelae after Ebola virus disease: even when it's over it's not over. *Lancet Infect Dis* **15:**865–866.

70. Chancellor JR, Padmanabhan SP, Greenough TC, Sacra R, Ellison RT III, Madoff LC, Droms RJ, Hinkle DM, Asdourian GK, Finberg RW, Stroher U, Uyeki TM, Cerón OM. 2016. Uveitis and systemic inflammatory markers in convalescent phase of Ebola virus disease. *Emerg Infect Dis* **22:**295–297.

71. Varkey JB, Shantha JG, Crozier I, Kraft CS, Lyon GM, Mehta AK, Kumar G, Smith JR, Kainulainen MH, Whitmer S, Ströher U, Uyeki TM, Ribner BS, Yeh S. 2015. Persistence of Ebola virus in ocular fluid during convalescence. *N Engl J Med* **372:**2423–2427.

72. Epstein L, Wong KK, Kallen AJ, Uyeki TM. 2015. Post-Ebola signs and symptoms in U.S. survivors. *N Engl J Med* **373:**2484–2486.

73. Lyon GM, Mehta AK, Varkey JB, Brantly K, Plyler L, McElroy AK, Kraft CS, Towner JS, Spiropoulou C, Ströher U, Uyeki TM, Ribner BS, Emory Serious Communicable Diseases Unit. 2014. Clinical care of two patients with Ebola virus disease in the United States. *N Engl J Med* **371:**2402–2409.

74. WHO. 2016. *Clinical care for survivors of Ebola virus disease. Interim guidance.* http://apps.who.int/csr/resources/publications/ebola/guidance-survivors/en/index.html.

75. NIH. 2015. *Study of Ebola survivors opens in Liberia.* http://www.nih.gov/news-events/news-releases/study-ebola-survivors-opens-liberia.

76. De Roo A, Ado B, Rose B, Guimard Y, Fonck K, Colebunders R. 1998. Survey among survivors of the 1995 Ebola epidemic in Kikwit, Democratic Republic of Congo: their feelings and experiences. *Trop Med Int Health* **3:**883–885.

77. Qureshi AI, Chughtai M, Loua TO, Pe Kolie J, Camara HF, Ishfaq MF, N'Dour CT, Beavogui K. 2015. Study of Ebola virus disease survivors in Guinea. *Clin Infect Dis* **61:**1035–1042.

78. Nanyonga M, Saidu J, Ramsay A, Shindo N, Bausch DG. 2016. Sequelae of Ebola virus disease, Kenema District, Sierra Leone. *Clin Infect Dis* **62:**125–126.

79. Bwaka MA, Bonnet MJ, Calain P, Colebunders R, De Roo A, Guimard Y, Katwiki KR, Kibadi K, Kipasa MA, Kuvula KJ, Mapanda BB, Massamba M, Mupapa KD, Muyembe-Tamfum JJ, Ndaberey E, Peters CJ, Rollin PE, Van den Enden E, Van den Enden E. 1999. Ebola hemorrhagic fever in Kikwit, Democratic Republic of the Congo: clinical observations in 103 patients. *J Infect Dis* **179**(Suppl 1):S1–S7.

80. Kibadi K, Mupapa K, Kuvula K, Massamba M, Ndaberey D, Muyembe-Tamfum JJ, Bwaka MA, De Roo A, Colebunders R. 1999. Late ophthalmologic manifestations in survivors of the 1995 Ebola virus epidemic in Kikwit, Democratic Republic of the Congo. *J Infect Dis* **179**(Suppl 1):S13–S14.

81. Wendo C. 2001. Caring for the survivors of Uganda's Ebola epidemic one year on. *Lancet* **358:**1350.

82. Mohammed A, Sheikh TL, Gidado S, Poggensee G, Nguku P, Olayinka A, Ohuabunwo C, Waziri N, Shuaib F, Adeyemi J, Uzoma O, Ahmed A, Doherty F, Nyanti SB, Nzuki CK, Nasidi A, Oyemakinde A, Oguntimehin O, Abdus-Salam IA, Obiako RO. 2015. An evaluation of psychological distress and social support of survivors and contacts of Ebola virus disease infection and their relatives in Lagos, Nigeria: a cross sectional study: 2014. *BMC Public Health* **15:**824.

83. Mattia JG, Vandy MJ, Chang JC, Platt DE, Dierberg K, Bausch DG, Brooks T, Conteh S, Crozier I, Fowler RA, Kamara AP, Kang C, Mahadevan S, Mansaray Y, Marcell L, McKay G, O'Dempsey T, Parris V, Pinto R, Rangel A, Salam AP, Shantha J, Wolfman V, Yeh S, Chan AK, Mishra S. 2015. Early clinical sequelae of Ebola virus disease in Sierra Leone: a cross-sectional study. *Lancet Infect Dis* **16:**331–338.

84. Emond RT, Evans B, Bowen ET, Lloyd G. 1977. A case of Ebola virus infection. *BMJ* **2:**541–544.

85. Formenty P, Hatz C, Le Guenno B, Stoll A, Rogenmoser P, Widmer A. 1999. Human infection due to Ebola virus, subtype Côte d'Ivoire: clinical and biologic presentation. *J Infect Dis* **179**(Suppl 1):S48–S53.

86. Christie A, Davies-Wayne GJ, Cordier-Lassalle T, Blackley DJ, Laney AS, Williams DE, Shinde SA, Badio M, Lo T, Mate SE, Ladner JT, Wiley MR, Kugelman JR, Palacios G, Holbrook MR, Janosko KB, de Wit E, van Doremalen N, Munster VJ, Pettitt J, Schoepp RJ, Verhenne L, Evlampidou I, Kollie KK, Sieh SB, Gasasira A, Bolay F, Kateh FN, Nyenswah TG, De Cock KM, Centers for Disease Control and Prevention (CDC). 2015. Possible sexual transmission of Ebola virus: Liberia, 2015. *MMWR Morb Mortal Wkly Rep* **64:**479–481.

87. Mate SE, Kugelman JR, Nyenswah TG, Ladner JT, Wiley MR, Cordier-Lassalle T, Christie A, Schroth GP, Gross SM, Davies-Wayne GJ, Shinde SA, Murugan R, Sieh SB, Badio M, Fakoli L, Taweh F, de Wit E, van Doremalen N, Munster VJ, Pettitt J, Prieto K, Humrighouse BW, Ströher U, DiClaro JW, Hensley LE, Schoepp RJ, Safronetz D, Fair J, Kuhn JH, Blackley DJ, Laney AS, Williams DE, Lo T, Gasasira A, Nichol ST, Formenty P, Kateh FN, De Cock KM, Bolay F, Sanchez-Lockhart M, Palacios G. 2015. Molecular evidence of sexual transmission of Ebola virus. *N Engl J Med* **373:**2448–2454.

88. Jampol LM, Ferris FL III, Bishop RJ. 2015. Ebola and the eye. *JAMA Ophthalmol* **133:**1105–1106.

89. Liddell AM, Davey RT Jr, Mehta AK, Varkey JB, Kraft CS, Tseggay GK, Badidi O, Faust AC, Brown KV, Suffredini AF, Barrett K, Wolcott MJ, Marconi VC, Lyon GM III, Weinstein GL, Weinmeister K, Sutton S, Hazbun M, Albariño CG, Reed Z, Cannon D, Ströher U, Feldman M, Ribner BS, Lane HC, Fauci AS, Uyeki TM. 2015. Characteristics and clinical management of a cluster of 3 patients with Ebola virus disease, including the first domestically acquired cases in the United States. *Ann Intern Med* **163:**81–90.

90. Mora-Rillo M, Arsuaga M, Ramírez-Olivencia G, de la Calle F, Borobia AM, Sánchez-Seco P, Lago M, Figueira JC, Fernández-Puntero B, Viejo A, Negredo A, Nuñez C, Flores E, Carcas AJ, Jiménez-Yuste V, Lasala F, García-de-Lorenzo A, Arnalich F, Arribas JR, La Paz-Carlos III University Hospital Isolation Unit. 2015. Acute respiratory distress syndrome after convalescent plasma use: treatment of a patient with Ebola virus disease contracted in Madrid, Spain. *Lancet Respir Med* **3:**554–562.

91. Tomori O, Fabiyi A, Sorungbe A, Smith A, McCormick JB. 1988. Viral hemorrhagic fever

antibodies in Nigerian populations. *Am J Trop Med Hyg* **38**:407–410.

92. **Auperin DD, Esposito JJ, Lange JV, Bauer SP, Knight J, Sasso DR, McCormick JB.** 1988. Construction of a recombinant vaccinia virus expressing the Lassa virus glycoprotein gene and protection of guinea pigs from a lethal Lassa virus infection. *Virus Res* **9**:233–248.

93. **Bausch DG, Towner JS, Dowell SF, Kaducu F, Lukwiya M, Sanchez A, Nichol ST, Ksiazek TG, Rollin PE.** 2007. Assessment of the risk of Ebola virus transmission from bodily fluids and fomites. *J Infect Dis* **196** (Suppl 2):S142–S147.

94. **Rodriguez LL, De Roo A, Guimard Y, Trappier SG, Sanchez A, Bressler D, Williams AJ, Rowe AK, Bertolli J, Khan AS, Ksiazek TG, Peters CJ, Nichol ST.** 1999. Persistence and genetic stability of Ebola virus during the outbreak in Kikwit, Democratic Republic of the Congo, 1995. *J Infect Dis* **179**(Suppl 1):S170–S176.

95. **Deen GF, Knust B, Broutet N, Sesay FR, Formenty P, Ross C, Thorson AE, Massaquoi TA, Marrinan JE, Ervin E, Jambai A, McDonald SL, Bernstein K, Wurie AH, Dumbuya MS, Abad N, Idriss B, Wi T, Bennett SD, Davies T, Ebrahim FK, Meites E, Naidoo D, Smith S, Banerjee A, Erickson BR, Brault A, Durski KN, Winter J, Sealy T, Nichol ST, Lamunu M, Ströher U, Morgan O, Sahr F.** 2015. Ebola RNA persistence in semen of Ebola virus disease survivors: preliminary report. *N Engl J Med.* doi:10.1056/NEJMoa1511410.

96. **Uyeki TM, Erickson BR, Brown S, McElroy AK, Cannon D, Gibbons A, Sealy T, Kainulainen MH, Schuh AJ, Kraft CS, Mehta AK, Lyon GM III, Varkey JB, Ribner BS, Ellison RT III, Carmody E, Nau GJ, Spiropoulou C, Nichol ST, Ströher U.** 2016. Ebola virus persistence in semen of male survivors. *Clin Infect Dis.* [Epub ahead of print.] doi:10.1093/cid/ciw202.

97. **Eggo RM, Watson CH, Camacho A, Kucharski AJ, Funk S, Edmunds WJ.** 2015. Duration of Ebola virus RNA persistence in semen of survivors: population-level estimates and projections. *Euro Surveill* **20**:30083. http://www.eurosurveillance.org/ViewArticle.aspx?ArticleId=21326.

98. **Baggi FM, Taybi A, Kurth A, Van Herp M, Di Caro A, Wölfel R, Günther S, Decroo T, Declerck H, Jonckheere S.** 2014. Management of pregnant women infected with Ebola virus in a treatment centre in Guinea, June 2014. *Euro Surveill* **19**:19. http://www.eurosurveillance.org/ViewArticle.aspx?ArticleId=20983.

99. **Mupapa K, Mukundu W, Bwaka MA, Kipasa M, De Roo A, Kuvula K, Kibadi K, Massamba M, Ndaberey D, Colebunders R, Muyembe-Tamfum JJ.** 1999. Ebola hemorrhagic fever and pregnancy. *J Infect Dis* **179**(Suppl 1):S11–S12.

100. **Oduyebo T, Pineda D, Lamin M, Leung A, Corbett C, Jamieson DJ.** 2015. A pregnant patient with Ebola virus disease. *Obstet Gynecol* **126**:1273–1275.

101. **Bower H, Grass JE, Veltus E, Brault A, Campbell S, Basile AJ, Wang D, Paddock CD, Erickson BR, Salzer JS, Belser J, Chege E, Seneca D, Saffa G, Stroeher U, Decroo T, Caleo GM.** 2015. Delivery of an Ebola virus-positive stillborn infant in a rural community health center, Sierra Leone, January 2015. *Am J Trop Med Hyg* **94**:417–419.

102. **Nelson JM, Griese SE, Goodman AB, Peacock G.** 2015. Live neonates born to mothers with Ebola virus disease: a review of the literature. *J Perinatol.* [Epub ahead of print.] doi:10.1038/jp.2015.189.

103. **Caluwaerts S, Fautsch T, Lagrou D, Moreau M, Modet Camara A, Gunther S, Di Caro A, Borremans B, Raymond Koundouno F, Akoi Bore J, Logue CH, Richter M, Wolfel R, Kuisma E, Kurth A, Thomas S, Burkhardt G, Erland E, Lionetto F, Lledo Weber P, de la Rosa O, Macpherson H, Van Herp M.** 2016. Dilemmas in managing pregnant women with Ebola: 2 case reports. *Clin Infect Dis* **62**:903–905.

104. **Nordenstedt H, Bah EI, de la Vega MA, Barry M, N'Faly M, Barry M, Crahay B, Decroo T, Van Herp M, Ingelbeen B.** 2016. Ebola virus in breast milk in an Ebola virus-positive mother with twin babies, Guinea, 2015. *Emerg Infect Dis* **22**:759–760.

105. **CDC, WHO.** 1998. Infection Control for Viral Haemorrhagic Fevers in the African Health Care Setting. http://www.who.int/csr/resources/publications/ebola/whoemcesr982sec1-4.pdf.

106. **WHO.** 2008. Interim Infection Control Recommendations for Care of Patients with Suspected or Confirmed Filovirus (Ebola, Marburg) Haemorrhagic Fever. WHO, Geneva, Switzerland.

107. **Hersi M, Stevens A, Quach P, Hamel C, Thavorn K, Garritty C, Skidmore B, Vallenas C, Norris SL, Egger M, Eremin S, Ferri M, Shindo N, Moher D.** 2015. Effectiveness of personal protective equipment for healthcare workers caring for patients with filovirus disease: a rapid review. *PLoS One* **10**:e0140290. doi:10.1371/journal.pone.0140290.

108. **Franklin SM.** 2016. A comparison of personal protective standards: caring for patients with Ebola virus. *Clin Nurse Spec* **30**:E1–E8.

109. **Faye O, Boëlle PY, Heleze E, Faye O, Loucoubar C, Magassouba N, Soropogui B, Keita S, Gakou**

T, Bah HI, Koivogui L, Sall AA, Cauchemez S. 2015. Chains of transmission and control of Ebola virus disease in Conakry, Guinea, in 2014: an observational study. *Lancet Infect Dis* **15**:320–326.

110. **Brainard J, Pond K, Hooper L, Edmunds K, Hunter P.** 2016. Presence and persistence of Ebola or Marburg virus in patients and survivors: a rapid systematic review. *PLoS Negl Trop Dis* **10**:e0004475. doi:10.1371/journal.pntd.0004475.

111. **Mupapa K, Massamba M, Kibadi K, Kuvula K, Bwaka A, Kipasa M, Colebunders R, Muyembe-Tamfum JJ, International Scientific and Technical Committee.** 1999. Treatment of Ebola hemorrhagic fever with blood transfusions from convalescent patients. *J Infect Dis* **179**(Suppl 1):S18–S23.

112. **Jahrling PB, Geisbert JB, Swearengen JR, Larsen T, Geisbert TW.** 2007. Ebola hemorrhagic fever: evaluation of passive immunotherapy in nonhuman primates. *J Infect Dis* **196**(Suppl 2):S400–S403.

113. **van Griensven J, Edwards T, de Lamballerie X, Semple MG, Gallian P, Baize S, Horby PW, Raoul H, Magassouba N, Antierens A, Lomas C, Faye O, Sall AA, Fransen K, Buyze J, Ravinetto R, Tiberghien P, Claeys Y, De Crop M, Lynen L, Bah EI, Smith PG, Delamou A, De Weggheleire A, Haba N, Ebola-Tx Consortium.** 2016. Evaluation of convalescent plasma for Ebola virus disease in Guinea. *N Engl J Med* **374**:33–42.

114. **Qiu X, Wong G, Audet J, Bello A, Fernando L, Alimonti JB, Fausther-Bovendo H, Wei H, Aviles J, Hiatt E, Johnson A, Morton J, Swope K, Bohorov O, Bohorova N, Goodman C, Kim D, Pauly MH, Velasco J, Pettitt J, Olinger GG, Whaley K, Xu B, Strong JE, Zeitlin L, Kobinger GP.** 2014. Reversion of advanced Ebola virus disease in nonhuman primates with ZMapp. *Nature* **514**:47–53.

115. **Davey RA.** 2016. Prevail II: a randomized controlled trial of ZMapp in acute Ebola virus infection, abstr 77LB. Conf. Retroviruses and Opportunistic Infections, Boston, MA.

116. **Kugelman JR, Kugelman-Tonos J, Ladner JT, Pettit J, Keeton CM, Nagle ER, Garcia KY, Froude JW, Kuehne AI, Kuhn JH, Bavari S, Zeitlin L, Dye JM, Olinger GG, Sanchez-Lockhart M, Palacios GF.** 2015. Emergence of Ebola virus escape variants in infected nonhuman primates treated with the MB-003 antibody cocktail. *Cell Rep* **12**:2111–2120.

117. **Geisbert TW, Lee AC, Robbins M, Geisbert JB, Honko AN, Sood V, Johnson JC, de Jong S, Tavakoli I, Judge A, Hensley LE, Maclachlan I.** 2010. Postexposure protection of non-human primates against a lethal Ebola

virus challenge with RNA interference: a proof-of-concept study. *Lancet* **375**:1896–1905.

118. **Thi EP, Mire CE, Lee ACH, Geisbert JB, Zhou JZ, Agans KN, Snead NM, Deer DJ, Barnard TR, Fenton KA, MacLachlan I, Geisbert TW.** 2015. Lipid nanoparticle siRNA treatment of Ebola-virus-Makona-infected nonhuman primates. *Nature* **521**:362–365.

119. **Dunning J, Sahr F, Rojek A, Gannon F, Carson G, Idriss B, Massaquoi T, Gandi R, Joseph S, Osman HK, Brooks TJ, Simpson AJ, Goodfellow I, Thorne L, Arias A, Merson L, Castle L, Howell-Jones R, Pardinaz-Solis R, Hope-Gill B, Ferri M, Grove J, Kowalski M, Stepniewska K, Lang T, Whitehead J, Olliaro P, Samai M, Horby PW, RAPIDE-TKM Trial Team.** 2016. Experimental treatment of Ebola virus disease with TKM-130803: a single-arm phase 2 clinical trial. *PLoS Med* **13**:e1001997. doi:10.1371/journal.pmed.1001997.

120. **Oestereich L, Lüdtke A, Wurr S, Rieger T, Muñoz-Fontela C, Günther S.** 2014. Successful treatment of advanced Ebola virus infection with T-705 (favipiravir) in a small animal model. *Antiviral Res* **105**:17–21.

121. **Sissoko D, Folkesson E, Abdoul M, Beavogui A, Gunther S, Shepherd S, Danel C, Mentre F, Anglaret X, Malvy D.** 2015. Favipiravir in patients with Ebola virus disease: early results of the JIKI trial in Guinea, abstr 103-ALB. Conference on Retroviruses and Opportunistic Infections, Seattle, WA.

122. **Gignoux E, Azman AS, de Smet M, Azuma P, Massaquoi M, Job D, Tiffany A, Petrucci R, Sterk E, Potet J, Suzuki M, Kurth A, Cannas A, Bocquin A, Strecker T, Logue C, Pottage T, Yue C, Cabrol JC, Serafini M, Ciglenecki I.** 2016. Effect of artesunate-amodiaquine on mortality related to Ebola virus disease. *N Engl J Med* **374**:23–32.

123. **WHO.** 2015. *Vaccines.* http://www.who.int/medicines/ebola-treatment/emp_ebola_vaccines/en/.

124. **Henao-Restrepo AM, Longini IM, Egger M, Dean NE, Edmunds WJ, Camacho A, Carroll MW, Doumbia M, Draguez B, Duraffour S, Enwere G, Grais R, Gunther S, Hossmann S, Kondé MK, Kone S, Kuisma E, Levine MM, Mandal S, Norheim G, Riveros X, Soumah A, Trelle S, Vicari AS, Watson CH, Kéïta S, Kieny MP, Røttingen JA.** 2015. Efficacy and effectiveness of an rVSV-vectored vaccine expressing Ebola surface glycoprotein: interim results from the Guinea ring vaccination cluster-randomised trial. *Lancet* **386**:857–866.

125. Huttner A, Dayer JA, Yerly S, Combescure C, Auderset F, Desmeules J, Eickmann M, Finckh A, Goncalves AR, Hooper JW, Kaya G, Krähling V, Kwilas S, Lemaître B, Matthey A, Silvera P, Becker S, Fast PE, Moorthy V, Kieny MP, Kaiser L, Siegrist CA, VSV-Ebola Consortium. 2015. The effect of dose on the safety and immunogenicity of the VSV Ebola candidate vaccine: a randomised double-blind, placebo-controlled phase 1/2 trial. *Lancet Infect Dis* **15**:1156–1166.

126. Agnandji ST, Huttner A, Zinser ME, Njuguna P, Dahlke C, Fernandes JF, Yerly S, Dayer J-A, Kraehling V, Kasonta R, Adegnika AA, Altfeld M, Auderset F, Bache EB, Biedenkopf N, Borregaard S, Brosnahan JS, Burrow R, Combescure C, Desmeules J, Eickmann M, Fehling SK, Finckh A, Goncalves AR, Grobusch MP, Hooper J, Jambrecina A, Kabwende AL, Kaya G, Kimani D, Lell B, Lemaître B, Lohse AW, Massinga-Loembe M, Matthey A, Mordmüller B, Nolting A, Ogwang C, Ramharter M, Schmidt-Chanasit J, Schmiedel S, Silvera P, Stahl FR, Staines HM, Strecker T, Stubbe HC, Tsofa B, Zaki S, Fast P, Moorthy V, Kaiser L, Krishna S, Becker S, Kieny MP, Bejon P, Kremsner PG, Addo MM, Siegrist C-A. 2015. Phase 1 trials of rVSV Ebola vaccine in Africa and Europe: preliminary report. *N Engl J Med*. doi:10.1056/NEJMoa1502924.

127. De Santis O, Audran R, Pothin E, Warpelin-Decrausaz L, Vallotton L, Wuerzner G, Cochet C, Estoppey D, Steiner-Monard V, Lonchampt S, Thierry AC, Mayor C, Bailer RT, Mbaya OT, Zhou Y, Ploquin A, Sullivan NJ, Graham BS, Roman F, De Ryck I, Ballou WR, Kieny MP, Moorthy V, Spertini F, Genton B. 2016. Safety and immunogenicity of a chimpanzee adenovirus-vectored Ebola vaccine in healthy adults: a randomised, double-blind, placebo-controlled, dose-finding, phase 1/2a study. *Lancet Infect Dis* **16**:311–320.

128. Bausch DG. 2014. One step closer to an Ebola virus vaccine. *N Engl J Med*. doi:10.1056/NEJMe1414305.

129. Tapia MD, Sow SO, Lyke KE, Haidara FC, Diallo F, Doumbia M, Traore A, Coulibaly F, Kodio M, Onwuchekwa U, Sztein MB, Wahid R, Campbell JD, Kieny MP, Moorthy V, Imoukhuede EB, Rampling T, Roman F, De Ryck I, Bellamy AR, Dally L, Mbaya OT, Ploquin A, Zhou Y, Stanley DA, Bailer R, Koup RA, Roederer M, Ledgerwood J, Hill AV, Ballou WR, Sullivan N, Graham B, Levine MM. 2016. Use of ChAd3-EBO-Z Ebola virus vaccine in Malian and US adults, and boosting of Malian adults with MVA-BN-Filo: a phase 1, single-blind, randomised trial, a

phase 1b, open-label and double-blind, dose-escalation trial, and a nested, randomised, double-blind, placebo-controlled trial. *Lancet Infect Dis* **16**:31–42.

130. Ksiazek TG, Rollin PE, Williams AJ, Bressler DS, Martin ML, Swanepoel R, Burt FJ, Leman PA, Khan AS, Rowe AK, Mukunu R, Sanchez A, Peters CJ. 1999. Clinical virology of Ebola hemorrhagic fever (EHF): virus, virus antigen, and IgG and IgM antibody findings among EHF patients in Kikwit, Democratic Republic of the Congo, 1995. *J Infect Dis* **179** (Suppl 1):S177–S187.

131. Ksiazek TG, West CP, Rollin PE, Jahrling PB, Peters CJ. 1999. ELISA for the detection of antibodies to Ebola viruses. *J Infect Dis* **179** (Suppl 1):S192–S198.

132. Towner JS, Rollin PE, Bausch DG, Sanchez A, Crary SM, Vincent M, Lee WF, Spiropoulou CF, Ksiazek TG, Lukwiya M, Kaducu F, Downing R, Nichol ST. 2004. Rapid diagnosis of Ebola hemorrhagic fever by reverse transcription-PCR in an outbreak setting and assessment of patient viral load as a predictor of outcome. *J Virol* **78**:4330–4341.

133. O'Dempsey T, Khan SH, Bausch DG. 2015. Rethinking the discharge policy for Ebola convalescents in an accelerating epidemic. *Am J Trop Med Hyg* **92**:238–239.

134. Dhillon RS, Srikrishna D, Garry RF, Chowell G. 2015. Ebola control: rapid diagnostic testing. *Lancet Infect Dis* **15**:147–148.

135. Gire SK, Goba A, Andersen KG, Sealfon RS, Park DJ, Kanneh L, Jalloh S, Momoh M, Fullah M, Dudas G, Wohl S, Moses LM, Yozwiak NL, Winnicki S, Matranga CB, Malboeuf CM, Qu J, Gladden AD, Schaffner SF, Yang X, Jiang PP, Nekoui M, Colubri A, Coomber MR, Fonnie M, Moigboi A, Gbakie M, Kamara FK, Tucker V, Konuwa E, Saffa S, Sellu J, Jalloh AA, Kovoma A, Koninga J, Mustapha I, Kargbo K, Foday M, Yillah M, Kanneh F, Robert W, Massally JL, Chapman SB, Bochicchio J, Murphy C, Nusbaum C, Young S, Birren BW, Grant DS, Scheiffelin JS, Lander ES, Happi C, Gevao SM, Gnirke A, Rambaut A, Garry RF, Khan SH, Sabeti PC. 2014. Genomic surveillance elucidates Ebola virus origin and transmission during the 2014 outbreak. *Science* **345**:1369–1372.

136. Park DJ, Dudas G, Wohl S, Goba A, Whitmer SL, Andersen KG, Sealfon RS, Ladner JT, Kugelman JR, Matranga CB, Winnicki SM, Qu J, Gire SK, Gladden-Young A, Jalloh S, Nosamiefan D, Yozwiak NL, Moses LM, Jiang PP, Lin AE, Schaffner SF, Bird B, Towner J, Mamoh M, Gbakie M, Kanneh L,

Kargbo D, Massally JL, Kamara FK, Konuwa E, Sellu J, Jalloh AA, Mustapha I, Foday M, Yillah M, Erickson BR, Sealy T, Blau D, Paddock C, Brault A, Amman B, Basile J, Bearden S, Belser J, Bergeron E, Campbell S, Chakrabarti A, Dodd K, Flint M, Gibbons A, Goodman C, Klena J, McMullan L, Morgan L, Russell B, Salzer J, Sanchez A, Wang D, Jungreis I, Tomkins-Tinch C, Kislyuk A, Lin MF, Chapman S, MacInnis B, Matthews A, Bochicchio J, Hensley LE, Kuhn JH, Nusbaum C, Schieffelin JS, Birren BW, Forget M, Nichol ST, Palacios GF, Ndiaye D, Happi C, Gevao SM, Vandi MA, Kargbo B, Holmes EC, Bedford T, Gnirke A, Ströher U, Rambaut A, Garry RF, Sabeti PC. 2015. Ebola virus epidemiology, transmission, and evolution during seven months in Sierra Leone. *Cell* **161**:1516–1526.

137. Matranga CB, Andersen KG, Winnicki S, Busby M, Gladden AD, Tewhey R, Stremlau M, Berlin A, Gire SK, England E, Moses LM, Mikkelsen TS, Odia I, Ehiane PE, Folarin O, Goba A, Kahn SH, Grant DS, Honko A, Hensley L, Happi C, Garry RF, Malboeuf CM, Birren BW, Gnirke A, Levin JZ, Sabeti PC. 2014. Enhanced methods for unbiased deep sequencing of Lassa and Ebola RNA viruses from clinical and biological samples. *Genome Biol* **15**:519.

138. Kugelman JR, Sanchez-Lockhart M, Andersen KG, Gire S, Park DJ, Sealfon R, Lin AE, Wohl S, Sabeti PC, Kuhn JH, Palacios GF. 2015. Evaluation of the potential impact of Ebola virus genomic drift on the efficacy of sequence-based candidate therapeutics. *MBio* **6**:e02227-14. doi:10.1128/mBio.02227-14.

139. United Nations. 1948. *The Universal Declaration of Human Rights.* http://www.un.org/en/universal-declaration-human-rights/.

140. Bausch DG, Bangura J, Garry RF, Goba A, Grant DS, Jacquerioz FA, McLellan SL, Jalloh S, Moses LM, Schieffelin JS. 2014. A tribute to Sheik Humarr Khan and all the healthcare workers in West Africa who have sacrificed in the fight against Ebola virus disease: mae we hush. *Antiviral Res* **111**:33–35.

141. Rosello A, Mossoko M, Flasche S, Van Hoek AJ, Mbala P, Camacho A, Funk S, Kucharski A, Ilunga BK, Edmunds WJ, Piot P, Baguelin M, Tamfum JJ. 2015. Ebola virus disease in the Democratic Republic of the Congo, 1976-2014. *eLife* **4**:4.

142. Heymann DL, Weisfeld JS, Webb PA, Johnson KM, Cairns T, Berquist H. 1980. Ebola hemorrhagic fever: Tandala, Zaire, 1977-1978. *J Infect Dis* **142**:372–376.

143. Baron RC, McCormick JB, Zubeir OA. 1983. Ebola virus disease in southern Sudan: hospital dissemination and intrafamilial spread. *Bull World Health Organ* **61**:997–1003.

144. Georges AJ, Leroy EM, Renaut AA, Benissan CT, Nabias RJ, Ngoc MT, Obiang PI, Lepage JP, Bertherat EJ, Bénoni DD, Wickings EJ, Amblard JP, Lansoud-Soukate JM, Milleliri JM, Baize S, Georges-Courbot MC. 1999. Ebola hemorrhagic fever outbreaks in Gabon, 1994-1997: epidemiologic and health control issues. *J Infect Dis* **179**(Suppl 1):S65–S75.

145. Le Guenno B, Formenty P, Wyers M, Gounon P, Walker F, Boesch C. 1995. Isolation and partial characterisation of a new strain of Ebola virus. *Lancet* **345**:1271–1274.

146. Richards GA, Murphy S, Jobson R, Mer M, Zinman C, Taylor R, Swanepoel R, Duse A, Sharp G, De La Rey IC, Kassianides C. 2000. Unexpected Ebola virus in a tertiary setting: clinical and epidemiologic aspects. *Crit Care Med* **28**:240–244.

147. Okware SI, Omaswa FG, Zaramba S, Opio A, Lutwama JJ, Kamugisha J, Rwaguma EB, Kagwa P, Lamunu M. 2002. An outbreak of Ebola in Uganda. *Trop Med Int Health* **7**:1068–1075.

148. Anonymous. 2003. Outbreak(s) of Ebola haemorrhagic fever, Congo and Gabon, October 2001-July 2002. *Wkly Epidemiol Rec* **78**:223–228.

149. World Health Organization. 2004. *Ebola haemorrhagic fever in the Republic of the Congo: update 6.* World Health Organization, Geneva, Switzerland. http://www.who.int/csr/don/2004_01_06/en/.

150. Anonymous. 2005. Outbreak of Ebola haemorrhagic fever in Yambio, South Sudan, April - June 2004. *Wkly Epidemiol Rec* **80**:370–375.

151. World Health Organization. 2009. *End of Ebola outbreak in the Democratic Republic of the Congo.* World Health Organization, Geneva, Switzerland. http://www.who.int/csr/don/2009_02_17/en/.

152. Shoemaker T, MacNeil A, Balinandi S, Campbell S, Wamala JF, McMullan LK, Downing R, Lutwama J, Mbidde E, Ströher U, Rollin PE, Nichol ST. 2012. Reemerging Sudan Ebola virus disease in Uganda, 2011. *Emerg Infect Dis* **18**:1480–1483.

153. World Health Organization. 2012. *End of Ebola outbreak in Uganda.* World Health Organization, Geneva, Switzerland. http://www.who.int/csr/don/2012_10_04/en/.

154. Anonymous. 2012. Outbreak news. Ebola haemorrhagic fever, Uganda: update. *Wkly Epidemiol Rec* **87**:493.

155. **World Health Organization.** 2015. *Ebola response roadmap situation report.* World Health Organization, Geneva, Switzerland. http://apps/who.int/ebola/current-situation/ebola-situation-report-4-november-2015.

156. Sissoko D, Laouenan C, Folkesson E, M'Lebing AB, Beavogui AH, Baize S, Camara AM, Maes P, Shepherd S, Danel C, Carazo S, Conde MN, Gala JL, Colin G, Savini H, Bore JA, Le Marcis F, Koundouno FR, Petitjean F, Lamah MC, Diederich S, Tounkara A, Poelart G, Berbain E, Dindart JM, Duraffour S, Lefevre A, Leno T, Peyrouset O, Irenge L, Bangoura N, Palich R, Hinzmann J, Kraus A, Barry TS, Berette S, Bongono A, Camara MS, Chanfreau Munoz V, Doumbouya L, Souley Harouna, Kighoma PM, Koundouno FR, Réné Lolamou, Loua CM, Massala V, Moumouni K, Provost C, Samake N, Sekou C, Soumah A, Arnould I, Komano MS, Gustin L, Berutto C, Camara D, Camara FS, Colpaert J, Delamou L, Jansson L, Kourouma E, Loua M, Malme K, Manfrin E, Maomou A, Milinouno A, Ombelet S, Sidiboun AY, Verreckt I, Yombouno P, Bocquin A, Carbonnelle C, Carmoi T, Frange P, Mely S, Nguyen VK, Pannetier D, Taburet AM, Treluyer JM, Kolie J, Moh R, Gonzalez MC, Kuisma E, Liedigk B, Ngabo D, Rudolf M, Thom R, Kerber R, Gabriel M, Di Caro A, Wölfel R, Badir J, Bentahir M, Deccache Y, Dumont C, Durant JF, El Bakkouri K, Gasasira Uwamahoro M, Smits B, Toufik N, Van Cauwenberghe S, Ezzedine K, Dortenzio E, Pizarro L, Etienne A, Guedj J, Fizet A, Barte de Sainte Fare E, Murgue B, Tran-Minh T, Rapp C, Piguet P, Poncin M, Draguez B, Allaford Duverger T, Barbe S, Baret G, Defourny I, Carroll M, Raoul H, Augier A, Eholie SP, Yazdanpanah Y, Levy-Marchal C, Antierrens A, Van Herp M, Günther S, de Lamballerie X, Keïta S, Mentre F, Anglaret X, Malvy D, JIKI StudyGroup. 2016. Experimental treatment with favipiravir for Ebola virus disease (the JIKI Trial): a historically controlled, single-arm proof-of-concept trial in Guinea. *PLoS Med* **13:** e1001967. doi:10.1371/journal.pmed.1001967.

Preparing for Serious Communicable Diseases in the United States: What the Ebola Virus Epidemic Has Taught Us

2

JAY B. VARKEY[1] and BRUCE S. RIBNER[1]

INTRODUCTION

The largest and deadliest outbreak of Ebola virus disease (EVD) began on 2 December 2013 when a 2-year-old child developed an illness characterized by fever, black stools, and vomiting in a town called Meliandou, Guinea—a remote and sparsely populated village of 31 households approximately 20 miles from the borders of Liberia and Sierra Leone (1). The exact source of infection is unclear but likely involved contact with an infected animal. The child died on the 5th day of his illness (2).

Over the next 3 weeks, the child's 3-year-old sister, mother, and grandmother also died. Two women from a nearby village attended the funeral of the child's grandmother; they died 3 weeks later. A midwife from the child's village was hospitalized and subsequently died. Two health care workers who worked at the hospital where the midwife was admitted also became ill and died. Multiple family members who attended the funerals of the health care workers also became ill and died (2). By then, the illness, initially thought to be cholera, had spread to several surrounding districts as well as the capital of Guinea, Conakry—a city of 2 million people (1).

[1]Emory University School of Medicine, Atlanta, GA 30307.
Emerging Infections 10
Edited by W. Michael Scheld, James M. Hughes and Richard J. Whitley
© 2016 American Society for Microbiology, Washington, DC
doi:10.1128/microbiolspec.EI10-0011-2016

By March 2014, cases were identified in neighboring Liberia, and the disease was identified as being caused by the Ebola virus. In April 2014, cases of EVD were identified in Sierra Leone. Guinea, Liberia, and Sierra Leone had previously never experienced an outbreak of EVD. All previous EVD outbreaks had occurred mostly in rural villages in the central African nations of the Democratic Republic of Congo, Sudan, Gabon, Uganda, and the Republic of the Congo. Prior to 2013, the largest documented EVD outbreak occurred in 2000–2001 in the Gulu District of Uganda and resulted in over 400 cases and over 200 deaths (3). As of December 2015, the West Africa EVD outbreak has resulted in over 28,000 cases and over 11,000 deaths in Guinea, Liberia, and Sierra Leone—more than all previous EVD outbreaks combined (4).

The 42-day waiting period after the last known case of EVD had recovered ended in Sierra Leone on 7 November 2015 and ended in Guinea on 28 December 2015. In Liberia, as of the time of writing this chapter, the 42-day waiting period will end on 14 January 2016 (4). Ending the West Africa EVD outbreak required an unprecedented international response. For the United States, participation in this international response provided an opportunity to learn important lessons in four key domains critical to preparing for future outbreaks of EVD and other serious communicable diseases: (i) safe and effective patient care, (ii) the role of experimental therapeutics and vaccines, (iii) infection control, (iv) hospital and community preparedness.

SAFE AND EFFECTIVE PATIENT CARE

There are no specific therapies approved by the U.S. FDA for the treatment of EVD. Therefore, the primary treatment for EVD is supportive care, specifically fluid replacement and electrolyte management. Prior to the West Africa outbreak, the ability of health care workers to provide aggressive supportive care was often hampered by the resource limitations in many Central African Ebola treatment centers (5). Oral rehydration, though readily available even in resource-limited settings, may have been inadequate given the severe fluid losses (5 to 10 liters per day) caused by EVD-associated gastroenteritis and the intractable nausea and vomiting that frequently accompanies this illness (6, 7). Similarly, the ability to safely provide intravenous fluids for rehydration and correction of electrolyte abnormalities was often limited by inadequate staffing, limited supplies of intravenous fluids, and inadequate or unavailable laboratory testing (5). When laboratory testing was available, as during the 2000 outbreak of *Sudan ebolavirus* in Uganda, it demonstrated that renal failure, liver failure, hypocalcemia, hypoalbuminemia, and an elevated D-dimer were associated with increased mortality (8).

The historic size of this West Africa EVD outbreak required an international response that resulted in both the construction of new Ebola treatment units in Guinea, Liberia, and Sierra Leone, as well as the treatment of 27 individuals in Western Europe and the United States. As a result, the ability of heath care workers to provide aggressive supportive care was enhanced. In Conakry, Guinea, aggressive supportive care may have contributed to a reduced case fatality rate compared to other more resource-limited areas of the country and compared to historical cohorts (6). Among patients evacuated to Western Europe and the United States, the majority had significant electrolyte abnormalities (hyponatriemia, hypokalemia, hypocalcemia, and hypomagnesemia) diagnosed by laboratory monitoring. The patients received multiple different, sometimes overlapping, interventions including supportive care. The case-fatality proportion of patients treated in Western Europe and the United States was 18.5%, which is substantially lower than the mortality seen in West Africa Ebola Treatment Units ETUs (9).

The treatment of EVD patients in resource-enhanced settings such as Western Europe and the United States also allowed patients with EVD-associated multiorgan system failure to receive, for the first time, advanced critical care interventions such as mechanical ventilation and renal replacement therapy (10). Multiorgan system failure in EVD historically, and during the West Africa outbreak, has been associated with poor outcomes (11). However, 11/27 patients treated in Western Europe and the United States required advanced critical care interventions (noninvasive mechanical ventilation, mechanical ventilation, vasopressor or inotropic support, and renal replacement therapy); 6 of the 11 survived (9). In addition, the experience of providing critical care support to patients with EVD demonstrated that invasive interventions such as mechanical ventilation and renal replacement therapy can be performed safely if performed by trained health care workers who strictly adhere to infection control practices (10).

The clinical care of patients with EVD does not end with the resolution of viremia. EVD survivors can develop a diverse array of complications during convalescence. Survivors of the 2007 outbreak of *Bundibugyo ebolavirus* in Uganda developed joint pain, sleep disturbances, and neurological abnormalities including hearing loss, memory loss, and confusion. In addition, ocular complaints including retro-orbital pain and blurred vision were common (12). Ocular complaints including sight-threatening uveitis have also been described in survivors of the 1995 outbreak of *Zaire ebolavirus* in Kikwit, Democratic Republic of Congo (13). In a small survey of 85 EVD survivors of the West Africa outbreak, 40% of participants reported "eye problems" (14). During the current outbreak, one survivor developed severe uveitis during convalescence, and viable Ebola virus was isolated from his anterior eye chamber 9 weeks after clearance of viremia (15).

The pathogenesis of complications that occur during EVD convalescence is unclear but may be multifactorial. It has been hypothesized that some of the complications may be related to postviral autoimmune disease (12). It has also been postulated that complications may be from persistent viral replication in immune-privileged sites (15). Persistent viable Ebola virus has been isolated from semen and aqueous humor of EVD survivors (15, 16). In addition, one survivor developed meningoencephalitis 10 months after she had cleared her viremia, and Ebola virus was isolated from her cerebrospinal fluid (17). It is unclear whether Ebola virus persists in other bodily fluids or tissues that are thought to be immune-privileged (e.g., synovial fluid). Prospective cohort studies are underway in West Africa that will hopefully elucidate the causes of complications that occur in EVD survivors during convalescence.

ROLE OF EXPERIMENTAL THERAPEUTICS

While the key to surviving EVD is aggressive supportive care, it is possible that the discovery of effective therapeutic agents may improve patient outcomes. Unfortunately, disproportionate media attention to unproven therapeutics during the recent Ebola outbreak led to unrealistic expectations and the almost universal compassionate use of experimental therapeutics in patients repatriated to resource-rich centers. Of the 27 patients treated in resource-rich centers, 70% received at least two investigational therapeutics (9), despite the fact that none had human efficacy or safety data; patients experienced a wide range of possible adverse effects. These adverse effects included systemic inflammatory response syndrome, hypotension, elevated transaminase levels, and transfusion-associated acute lung injury. It is of interest to note that two of the agents that were felt to be the most promising at the beginning of the outbreak were ultimately found to offer no survival benefits (see below). The use of therapeutics and vaccines in resource-limited environments will face a number of challenges, including supply and distribution uncertainty, administration difficulties with agents that must be given parenterally or intravenously, and the difficulties of utilizing oral agents in patients with intractable nausea and emesis (18). Above all, it is imperative that the search for a "magic bullet" not detract from a focus on supplying aggressive supportive care to all patients presenting with Ebola virus infection.

Therapeutics currently considered the best candidates for efficacy in patients infected with the Ebola virus fall into two categories: those that boost passive immunity and pharmaceutical antivirals. Recovery from EVD is associated with the production of antibody against the virus (19, 20). It has therefore been hypothesized that boosting passive immunity until the host can produce antibody may be of benefit. In a prior outbreak in 1995, eight patients with Ebola virus infection were given whole blood from outbreak survivors (21). Seven of the eight patients survived, for a mortality rate of 12.5%, which compared with a mortality rate of 80% in patients who did not receive such transfusions. However, due to the small numbers and other confounding factors, this survival difference was not felt to be definitive evidence of efficacy (22). Studies of convalescent serum in nonhuman primates have been inconclusive. While the administration of convalescent whole blood transfusion to rhesus macaques was not found to be protective (23), infected rhesus macaques who received multiple administrations of purified, polyclonal, species-matched IgG from vaccinated animals did appear to be protected (22). In addition to the use of convalescent antibodies, pooled antibodies produced *in vitro* have been studied. ZMapp, a combination of three chimeric human/murine IgG1 monoclonal antibodies produced by a tobacco plant (*Nicotiana benthamiana*) has recently been developed (24). In a nonhuman primate trial, ZMapp was 100% protective against Ebola virus infection even when administered 5 days after the animals were infected. While anecdotal evidence supports the efficacy of this preparation in a few of the patients who survived the current outbreak (25), no randomized controlled studies have been completed to date. A definitive answer as to the role of passive immunity in treating patients with EVD will await more robust trials in humans.

Pharmaceutical antivirals directed against the Ebola virus have fallen into two categories: (i) small-molecule inhibitors of virus entry and endosomal escape and (ii) compounds that block viral replication. In the first category is a product called TKM-100802, a small interfering ribonucleic acid that silences RNA replication by enzymatic cleavage of mRNA. TKM-100802 targets the L polymerase and viral protein VP24 and VP35 (26). In both guinea pig and nonhuman primate challenge studies, this agent was found to offer protection (27, 28). Unfortunately, in one of the few randomized controlled trials in humans to be performed during the current outbreak, this agent was not found to offer a survival advantage in humans, and the trial was halted (29). Favipiravir, a broad-spectrum antiviral that inhibits RNA-dependent RNA polymerase, also showed promise in initial animal studies but again was not found to offer a survival advantage in a randomized trial involving humans. However, a *post hoc* analysis did suggest that favipiravir might be of benefit in patients presenting early in disease with lower viral loads (30). Other agents that have shown promise in *in vitro* or animal studies include GS-5734, BCX4430, and AVI7537 (18, 26). Because these agents have not been evaluated in randomized human trials, their efficacy in humans is yet to be determined.

VACCINES

The high mortality rate associated with Ebola virus infection has added urgency to the search for effective vaccines. Practical difficulties in performing controlled clinical trials for Ebola vaccines are that Ebola outbreaks tend to be unpredictable and sporadic, and the ethical concerns about using a placebo control in the face of exposure to a highly lethal disease. In 2002, the FDA promulgated the "animal rule" as an alternative pathway to license products against highly lethal pathogens such as Ebola (31). The animal rule has four conditions: (i) animal efficacy data (good laboratory practice), (ii) immune correlate establishment and protection in animals, (iii) human safety and immunogenicity data (good clinical practice), and (iv) induction of an immune correlate in humans. It is anticipated that an effective vaccine will need to elicit both humoral and cell-mediated immunity against the Ebola virus. Vaccines for pre-exposure (no identified exposure to the virus) and postexposure (identified exposure to the virus) have slightly different requirements. A vaccine for pre-exposure use would optimally induce protection after one, or at most two, vaccinations. It should protect against multiple strains of the Ebola virus and should have minimal adverse effects. A vaccine for postexposure use should produce rapid induction of immunity. For all vaccines, ability to tolerate suboptimal storage conditions will be important, given the supply chain issues in most parts of the world where the Ebola virus is endemic.

Attenuated and inactivated vaccines have not shown protection in nonhuman primate studies (32), and there have been safety concerns due to the risk of incomplete inactivation. Genetic and subunit vaccines have resulted in incomplete protection (33, 34). The leading candidate vaccines at the present time are vector-based: a live, recombinant vesicular stomatitis virus (VSV) vaccine and a replication-incompetent adenoviral vector vaccine. Both of these vaccines promote immunity to the Ebola virus glycoprotein. The Ebola virus glycoprotein is responsible for attachment and fusion between the viral and host membranes and produces inhibition of host immune responses. In nonhuman primate models, an antiglycoprotein antibody level of 1:3,700 and above allows the animal

to survive subsequent lethal challenges with Ebola virus. The VSV vaccine encodes for the Ebola glycoprotein instead of the VSV glycoprotein. The immunity produced by this vaccine is primarily humoral. In nonhuman primates, one dose of vaccine induces immunity and is 100% protective at 14 months (35). Because the vaccine virus is capable of replication, the majority of volunteers exhibit some adverse events: 90% reported systemic symptoms, including fever, chills, myalgia, and headache (36). Pre-exposure studies with this vaccine are limited. In one postexposure study, 7,651 individuals in Guinea who were contacts of patients with laboratory-confirmed EVD were vaccinated either immediately or 21 days following exposure. In the immediate vaccination group there were no cases of EVD with symptom onset at least 10 days after randomization, whereas in the delayed vaccination group there were 16 cases of EVD from 7 clusters, showing a vaccine efficacy of 100% (37).

The adenovirus vaccine encodes for the Ebola glycoprotein of two Ebola strains: Zaire and Sudan. Unlike the VSV vaccine, it promotes cellular as well as humoral immunity (38). Because pre-existing immunity to the adenovirus is more common than immunity to VSV, alternative immunization strategies such as multiple doses must be utilized. In human volunteers, minor adverse reactions were seen in 70% (fever and transient leukopenia) (39). Human trials in endemic areas are planned.

INFECTION CONTROL

Prior to the West Africa EVD outbreak, there were relatively limited data in the medical literature to help guide infection control practices when caring for patients with EVD in the United States. The literature that was available was based on the experience of caring for patients with EVD in central Africa—a setting markedly different from modern hospitals in the United States (40). As of December 2015,

11 patients with EVD have been treated in the United States; 10 of the 11 patients were treated in specialized biocontainment patient care units at Emory University Hospital, the University of Nebraska Medical Center, and the National Institutes of Health Clinical Center. The 11th was cared for in an isolation unit developed in Bellevue Hospital Center. In these settings, key lessons were learned to guide infection control policies and procedures to safely care for patients with EVD and other serious communicable diseases.

Although biocontainment patient care units are not required to treat a patient with EVD (41), specific features in the design of these facilities make them ideal environments to effectively treat patients with serious communicable diseases while minimizing the risk of transmission to health care workers, other patients, and the public (42). In biocontainment patient care units, including the Serious Communicable Diseases Unit (SCDU) at Emory University Hospital (see Fig. 1), individual patient care rooms are designed to deliver a level of care equivalent to that of a standard ICU, allowing health care workers to provide aggressive supportive care to patients who may be critically ill. To maintain staff safety, the SCDU includes dedicated space for staff changing areas and to store personal protective equipment (PPE). Patient care rooms are constructed with seamless surfaces for walls and floors to facilitate effective surface disinfection. To maintain the safety of other hospitalized patients and health care workers, the SCDU is located in a secured area of Emory University Hospital that is separate from other patient care areas. All entrances and exits in the SCDU are continuously monitored and limited to health care workers and other individuals authorized to be in the unit (43).

The SCDU is also designed to safely care for patients with diseases that, unlike Ebola, can be spread through the airborne route. Specifically, air in the patients' rooms is under net negative pressure relative to the surrounding areas. Air in the patient rooms has laminar air flow across the patient bed, and all air from the patient rooms undergoes high-efficiency particulate air filtration before being 100% exhausted to the outside. The outside exhaust is geographically separate from any hospital air intake locations and is high enough to allow for dilutional disbursement (43).

Independent of the specific design features of the treatment facility, the West African EVD outbreak clearly demonstrated that establishing a trained, competent, interdisciplinary team of providers and emphasizing a culture of safety are critical to effectively care for patients with EVD (44, 45). To staff the SCDU, a core team of nurses, physicians, and other health care workers with expertise in infectious diseases, critical care, and an expressed interest in caring for patients with serious communicable diseases were identified. To be part of the team, all providers were required to demonstrate a commitment to practice and promote a "culture of safety." In a culture of safety, all team members commit to strictly adhere to safe and effective practices outlined in standard operating protocols and are empowered to ask questions and voice concerns as they arise. Team members were also required to meet the following criteria: (i) participate in regularly scheduled drill exercises and (ii) demonstrate competency in infection control practices with specific emphasis on protocols for donning and doffing PPE, specimen handling, and waste management (43). Providers who were unable to demonstrate these competencies were not permitted to provide direct patient care to patients with EVD. Drills, training sessions, and competency verification are performed every 3 to 6 months.

The selection of appropriate PPE for the clinical care team is a critical step to maintaining staff safety when caring for a patient with EVD. The specific type of PPE used by health care workers caring for patients with EVD should include a coverall or surgical gowns with head cover that leave no skin exposed. An apron and shoe covers should be added when there is a high risk of exposure to infectious body fluids. At least two sets of

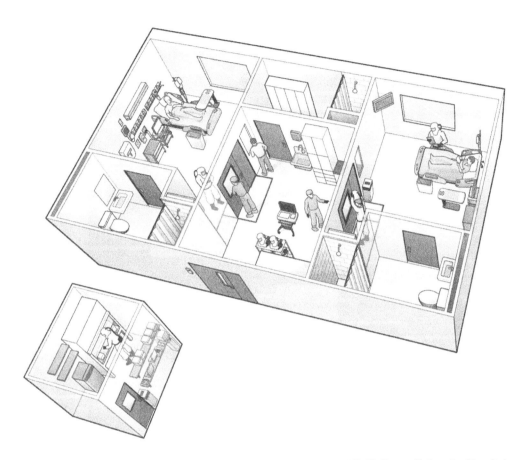

FIGURE 1 Schematic of the Serious Communicable Diseases Unit (SCDU), Emory University Hospital.

gloves should be worn, including an outer glove that has extended cuffs. Although Ebola virus is not transmitted through the air, wearing a powered air purifying respirator or N-95 respirator together with a face shield protects the face and mucus membranes from exposure to infectious fluids and provides additional protection if aerosol-generating procedures are performed (46). Regardless of the specific type of PPE selected, it is imperative that PPE provide adequate protection but remain comfortable for health care workers. It is especially important that direct care providers receive adequate training and demonstrate competency in donning and doffing PPE. Inappropriate donning and doffing of PPE has been identified as a possible risk factor for EVD ac-

quisition among health care workers (47). Therefore, it is imperative that health care workers donning and doffing PPE should always be monitored by partners to ensure strict adherence to proper procedures.

In addition to the core group of nurses and physicians providing direct care to patients with EVD, laboratory technologists are critical members of the interdisciplinary team who need to maintain strict adherence to infection control practices. Patients with EVD have a high viral load that can reach levels of $>10^8$ viral particles/ml of body fluid. Ebola virus is highly infectious, with an infectious dose that has been estimated to be as low as 0.001 ml of blood (48). As a result, it is critical that hospitals that care for patients with EVD develop detailed standard operating protocols to maintain safety during laboratory specimen collection, transport, and processing. Guidelines from the Centers for Disease Control and Prevention (CDC) state that hospital clinical laboratories can safely handle specimens from patients with EVD if risk mitigation strategies (engineering controls, administrative and work controls, use of appropriate PPE) are implemented (49). The American Society for Microbiology has, however, issued guidelines suggesting that specimens from patients with EVD should be limited to point-of-care testing equipment and performed either in the patient's room or in a biological safety cabinet in an isolated area (50). The SCDU at Emory University Hospital established a self-contained point-of-care laboratory and processed all specimens within a 4-foot laminar flow biosafety containment hood (51). All laboratory technologists involved in the transport and processing of specimens containing Ebola virus should receive PPE training and demonstrate competency in donning and doffing.

Hospitals preparing to care for patients with EVD also require a multidisciplinary team to develop standard protocols for the management of regulated medical waste. This team should include environmental services, infection prevention and control, biosafety officers, hospital administration, public health officials, and others with expertise in hazardous waste removal. All waste from patients with EVD is disposed in compliance with local, state, and federal regulations. EVD patient care waste is defined and regulated by the U.S. Department of Transportation as a category A infectious substance. Therefore, all solid medical waste generated in the SCDU during the care of patients with EVD is sterilized in an autoclave that allows the waste to be transported and disposed of safely as regular medical waste. For units that do not have access to an autoclave, contractors who transport and dispose of category A waste have special procedures in place for the packaging of such waste. Although CDC guidelines state that liquid waste may be disposed of without treatment into sanitary sewers, local waste treatment authorities may have different requirements (52). In the Emory University Hospital SCDU, a disinfectant was added to all liquid waste in accordance with manufacturers' directions prior to disposal in the sanitary sewer.

Because of the low infectious dose of Ebola virus, health care workers who care for patients with EVD must develop standard protocols to ensure that environmental surfaces in the direct patient care area, in the laboratory, and in the waste stream receive regular cleaning with an appropriate effective disinfectant. The U.S. Environmental Protection Agency (EPA) has identified EPA-registered disinfectants with a label claim of potency at least equivalent to that for a nonenveloped virus which meet CDC criteria for use against Ebola virus (53, 54). All disinfectants should be used by trained health care workers in accordance with manufacturers' instructions. Strict adherence to regular cleaning significantly reduces the risk of Ebola virus transmission from bodily fluids and fomites in the environment (40). For terminal cleaning of the environment after discharge of a patient with EVD, it is essential that meticulous attention be paid to disinfection of all surfaces. Most units have followed this with a supplemental disinfection modality such as vaporized hydrogen peroxide or a UV generator (55).

HOSPITAL AND COMMUNITY PREPAREDNESS FOR EMERGING INFECTIOUS DISEASES

One of the key lessons that the Ebola outbreak of 2013–2015 has taught us is that the United States and the world were ill prepared to address an outbreak of an emerging infectious disease (56–58). This lesson was particularly jarring given that outbreaks of SARS (severe acute respiratory syndrome), H1N1 influenza, and MERS (Middle East respiratory syndrome) have marked the last decade. Partially due to this lack of preparation, the Ebola outbreak has dwarfed all other outbreaks of EVD in terms of number infected and mortality. On the international front, factors that have been identified as contributing to the unprecedented extent of this outbreak have been identified (Table 1) (58, 59).

In addition to the lack of preparedness for isolating and managing infected patients, the delay in implementing research protocols to evaluate treatment algorithms, therapeutic agents, and vaccines means that many questions regarding these interventions will not be resolved prior to the next outbreak.

In response to this outbreak, many initiatives, both globally and in the United States, have begun. In the international arena, an independent, multinational Commission on a Global Health Risk Framework for the Future has been established to recommend a more effective global architecture for mitigating the threat of epidemic infectious diseases (57, 60). The U.S. National Academy of Medicine is the secretariat for this commission. In addition, an independent panel convened by the WHO has proposed an agenda for change (Table 2) which has been largely accepted by WHO administration (61).

The United States has also witnessed a marked increase in activities focused on emergency preparedness for emerging infectious diseases. In 2015 Congress appropriated $5.48 billion to the effort to control Ebola virus infection (62). These funds will be utilized to address a number of areas that require strengthening to improve the U.S. response to emerging infectious diseases. Under the Hospital Preparedness Program of the Assistant Secretary for Preparedness and Response, funding was distributed to the states and to other grantees to enhance state, local, and health care system preparedness. These funds were also designed to create one regional Ebola and other special pathogen treatment center in each of the 10 Health and Human Services regions (63). In addition, the Centers for Disease Control and Prevention has developed a tiered approach to manage patients with possible or confirmed EVD or infections caused by other serious communicable pathogens (41). Under this strategy, acute health care facilities can serve one of three roles: frontline health care facility, Ebola assessment hospital, or Ebola treatment center. Frontline health care facilities should, in coordination with local and state health authorities, be able to rapidly identify and triage patients who are suspected of being infected with the Ebola virus. Ebola assessment hospitals are facilities prepared to receive and isolate suspect patients and care for the patient until a diagnosis of EVD can be confirmed or ruled out and until discharge or transfer is completed. Ebola treatment centers are facilities that plan to care for and manage a patient with confirmed EVD for the duration of the patient's illness. As the Ebola virus outbreak in West Africa is

---

TABLE 1 Factors contributing to 2013–2015 Ebola outbreak (58, 59)

Failure of member states to implement the core capacities called for under the International Health Regulations (2005)

The implementation of travel bans and other measures that interfered with the response to the outbreak

Delays in the declaration of a public health emergency of international concern (PHEIC) by the WHO

Lack of familiarity with Ebola by health care providers and public health officials in West Africa

The unique introduction of Ebola into an urban setting for the first time as opposed to rural villages

Poor public health infrastructure due to years of civil war

A severe shortage of health care workers exacerbated by the many health care workers who became infected with the Ebola virus early in the outbreak

Closure of health care facilities and departure of foreign health care workers due to perceived danger as the outbreak peaked

High-risk funeral and burial practices in West African countries

Community resistance due to suspicion of the government and lack of familiarity with Ebola

TABLE 2 **WHO's agenda for change (61)**

Strengthen the international health regulations

Identify addition resources to support public health infrastructure in member states

Implement objective measures to assess core capacities of member states

Alter the WHO structure and culture to improve emergency preparedness and response capacity

Develop a global health emergency workforce to respond to outbreaks and emergencies with health consequences

Improve integration of health security and humanitarian systems

Develop a unified WHO program for outbreaks and emergencies

Develop an "R and D blueprint" to accelerate research and development on diagnostics, vaccines, and therapeutics during outbreaks and health emergencies

Establish a WHO contingency fund for emergencies to establish adequate international financing for pandemics and other health emergencies

contained, the focus of this network should gradually shift to other serious communicable diseases, although exactly what these infectious diseases should be is yet to be resolved. The Assistant Secretary for Preparedness and Response has also funded the National Ebola Training and Education Center to develop a robust educational program to improve infectious disease emergency preparedness in the United States. The National Ebola Training and Education Center will be using a multipronged approach including site visits for regional Ebola treatment units, establishment of a web-based learning management system, development of exercise templates for entities to test their state of preparedness, and a research agenda to answer some of the fundamental questions regarding the treatment of patients with EVD and other serious communicable pathogens. The goal of the site visits and exercises is to demonstrate that an institution-wide approach is essential when it comes to managing patients with serious

communicable diseases. Areas of preparedness that will receive targeted attention are listed in (Table 3). One of the most challenging areas for many facilities is to develop a laboratory that can safely evaluate patients for serious communicable pathogens in a timely manner while at the same time testing for other, more common, rapidly fatal diseases such as malaria and typhoid fever.

CONCLUSIONS

The EVD outbreak that began in Guinea in December 2013 has been the largest and deadliest EVD outbreak in human history. The outbreak cruelly demonstrated the significant degree to which developing nations, like those in West Africa, are vulnerable to serious morbidity and mortality caused by the rapid spread of serious communicable diseases like EVD. Paradoxically, the outbreak has also resulted in the largest number of EVD survivors in history. Therefore, it is critical that the unprecedented international response that helped end the EVD outbreak be sustained to build the infrastructure of vulnerable developing nations. Building and maintaining adequate health care infrastructure will be critical to manage the prevalent and poorly understood complications that can occur in EVD survivors as well as to prevent future outbreaks.

The West African EVD outbreak also demonstrated again that emerging infectious diseases have no borders. As such, it is imperative

TABLE 3 **Emergency medical services and emergency department preparedness**

Patient transport

Staffing

Personal protective equipment and donning/doffing procedures

Health care worker (HCW) monitoring and management of exposures

Lab safety and capacity

Environmental infection control

Waste management

Coordinated communication

Management of special populations

that developed nations with advanced health care systems, such as the United States, identify lessons that can be learned from the West African EVD outbreak. Specifically, the key lessons learned in the four domains discussed in this article (safe and effective patient care, experimental therapeutics and vaccines, infection control, and hospital and community preparedness) will hopefully help both the United States and the international community more effectively respond to future outbreaks of EVD and other emerging serious communicable diseases in the future.

ACKNOWLEDGMENTS

This work was funded by NIH National Center for Advancing Translational Sciences (NCATS) grant UL1TR000454.

CITATION

Varkey JB, Ribner BS. 2016. Preparing for serious communicable diseases in the United States: what the Ebola virus epidemic has taught us. Microbiol Spectrum 4(3):EI10-0011-2016.

REFERENCES

1. **World Health Organization.** 2015. *Origins of the 2014 Ebola Epidemic: One Year Into the Ebola Epidemic.* http://www.who.int/csr/disease/ ebola/one-year-report/virus-origin/en/.

2. **Baize S, Pannetier D, Oestereich L, Rieger T, Koivogui L, Magassouba N, Soropogui B, Sow MS, Keïta S, De Clerck H, Tiffany A, Dominguez G, Loua M, Traoré A, Kolié M, Malano ER, Heleze E, Bocquin A, Mély S, Raoul H, Caro V, Cadar D, Gabriel M, Pahlmann M, Tappe D, Schmidt-Chanasit J, Impouma B, Diallo AK, Formenty P, Van Herp M, Günther S.** 2014. Emergence of Zaire Ebola virus disease in Guinea. *N Engl J Med* **371:**1418–1425.

3. **Centers for Disease Control and Prevention.** 2016. *Outbreaks Chronology: Ebola Virus Disease.* http://www.cdc.gov/vhf/ebola/outbreaks/ history/chronology.html.

4. **World Health Organization.** 2016. *Ebola Situation Report: 30 December 2015.* http://apps. who.int/ebola/current-situation/ebola-situation -report-30-december-2015.

5. **Fowler RA, Fletcher T, Fischer WA II, Lamontagne F, Jacob S, Brett-Major D, Lawler JV, Jacquerioz FA, Houlihan C, O'Dempsey T, Ferri M, Adachi T, Lamah MC, Bah EI, Mayet T, Schieffelin J, McLellan SL, Senga M, Kato Y, Clement C, Mardel S, Vallenas Bejar De Villar RC, Shindo N, Bausch D.** 2014. Caring for critically ill patients with Ebola virus disease. Perspectives from West Africa. *Am J Respir Crit Care Med* **190:**733–737.

6. **Bah EI, Lamah MC, Fletcher T, Jacob ST, Brett-Major DM, Sall AA, Shindo N, Fischer WA II, Lamontagne F, Saliou SM, Bausch DG, Moumié B, Jagatic T, Sprecher A, Lawler JV, Mayet T, Jacquerioz FA, Méndez Baggi MF, Vallenas C, Clement C, Mardel S, Faye O, Faye O, Soropogui B, Magassouba N, Koivogui L, Pinto R, Fowler RA.** 2015. Clinical presentation of patients with Ebola virus disease in Conakry, Guinea. *N Engl J Med* **372:**40–47.

7. **Schieffelin JS, Shaffer JG, Goba A, Gbakie M, Gire SK, Colubri A, Sealfon RS, Kanneh L, Moigboi A, Momoh M, Fullah M, Moses LM, Brown BL, Andersen KG, Winnicki S, Schaffner SF, Park DJ, Yozwiak NL, Jiang PP, Kargbo D, Jalloh S, Fonnie M, Sinnah V, French I, Kovoma A, Kamara FK, Tucker V, Konuwa E, Sellu J, Mustapha I, Foday M, Yillah M, Kanneh F, Saffa S, Massally JL, Boisen ML, Branco LM, Vandi MA, Grant DS, Happi C, Gevao SM, Fletcher TE, Fowler RA, Bausch DG, Sabeti PC, Khan SH, Garry RF, KGH Lassa Fever Program, Viral Hemorrhagic Fever Consortium, WHO Clinical Response Team.** 2014. Clinical illness and outcomes in patients with Ebola in Sierra Leone. *N Engl J Med* **371:**2092–2100.

8. **Rollin PE, Bausch DG, Sanchez A.** 2007. Blood chemistry measurements and D-dimer levels associated with fatal and nonfatal outcomes in humans infected with Sudan Ebola virus. *J Infect Dis* **196**(Suppl 2):S364–S371.

9. **Uyeki TM, Mehta AK, Davey RT, Liddell AM, Wolf T, Vetter P, Schmiedel S, Grünewald T, Jacobs M, Arribas JR, Evans L, Hewlett AL, Brantsaeter AB, Ippolito G, Rapp C, Hoepelman AIM, Gutman J, Working Group of the U.S.-European Clinical Network on Clinical Management of Ebola Virus Disease Patients in the U.S. and Europe.** 2016. Clinical management of Ebola virus disease patients in the U.S. and Europe. *N Engl J Med* **374:**636–646.

10. **Connor MJ Jr, Kraft C, Mehta AK, Varkey JB, Lyon GM, Crozier I, Ströher U, Ribner BS, Franch HA.** 2015. Successful delivery of RRT in Ebola virus disease. *J Am Soc Nephrol* **26:**31–37.

11. Sueblinvong V, Johnson DW, Weinstein GL, Connor MJ, Jr, Crozier I, Liddell AM, Franch HA, Wall BR, Kalil AC, Feldman M, Lisco SJ, Sevransky JE. 2015. Critical care for multiple organ failure secondary to Ebola virus disease in the United States. *Crit Care Med* **43**:2066–2075.

12. Clark DV, Kibuuka H, Millard M, Wakabi S, Lukwago L, Taylor A, Eller MA, Eller LA, Michael NL, Honko AN, Olinger GG, Jr, Schoepp RJ, Hepburn MJ, Hensley LE, Robb ML. 2015. Long-term sequelae after Ebola virus disease in Bundibugyo, Uganda: a retrospective cohort study. *Lancet Infect Dis* **15**:905–912.

13. Kibadi K, Mupapa K, Kuvula K, Massamba M, Ndaberey D, Muyembe-Tamfum JJ, Bwaka MA, De Roo A, Colebunders R. 1999. Late ophthalmologic manifestations in survivors of the 1995 Ebola virus epidemic in Kikwit, Democratic Republic of the Congo. *J Infect Dis* **179**(Suppl 1):S13–S14.

14. Trenchard T. 2014. *Survivors cope with new Ebola after-effects.* Al-Jazeera. http://www.aljazeera.com/news/africa/2014/12/survivors-cope-with-new-ebola-after-effects-2014121573521561384.html.

15. Varkey JB, Shantha JG, Crozier I, Kraft CS, Lyon GM, Mehta AK, Kumar G, Smith JR, Kainulainen MH, Whitmer S, Ströher U, Uyeki TM, Ribner BS, Yeh S. 2015. Persistence of Ebola virus in ocular fluid during convalescence. *N Engl J Med* **372**:2423–2427.

16. Mate SE, Kugelman JR, Nyenswah TG, Ladner JT, Wiley MR, Cordier-Lassalle T, Christie A, Schroth GP, Gross SM, Davies-Wayne GJ, Shinde SA, Murugan R, Sieh SB, Badio M, Fakoli L, Taweh F, de Wit E, van Doremalen N, Munster VJ, Pettitt J, Prieto K, Humrighouse BW, Ströher U, DiClaro JW, Hensley LE, Schoepp RJ, Safronetz D, Fair J, Kuhn JH, Blackley DJ, Laney AS, Williams DE, Lo T, Gasasira A, Nichol ST, Formenty P, Kateh FN, De Cock KM, Bolay F, Sanchez-Lockhart M, Palacios G. 2015. Molecular evidence of sexual transmission of Ebola virus. *N Engl J Med* **373**:2448–2454.

17. Fink S. 2015. Ebola survivor from Scotland is critically ill. *New York Times.* http://www.nytimes.com/2015/10/15/world/europe/scottish-nurse-who-had-ebola-is-back-in-hospital-and-critically-ill.html.

18. World Health Organization. 2014. *Potential Ebola Therapies and Vaccines: Interim Guidance.* http://www.who.int/csr/resources/publications/ebola/potential-therapies-vaccines/en/.

19. Kraft CS, Hewlett AL, Koepsell S, Winkler AM, Kratochvil CJ, Larson L, Varkey JB, Mehta AK, Lyon GM III, Friedman-Moraco RJ, Marconi VC, Hill CE, Sullivan JN, Johnson DW, Lisco SJ, Mulligan MJ, Uyeki TM, McElroy AK, Sealy T, Campbell S, Spiropoulou C, Ströher U, Crozier I, Sacra R, Connor MJ, Jr, Sueblinvong V, Franch HA, Smith PW, Ribner BS, Nebraska Biocontainment Unit and the Emory Serious Communicable Diseases Unit. 2015. The use of TKM-100802 and convalescent plasma in 2 patients with Ebola virus disease in the United States. *Clin Infect Dis* **61**:496–502.

20. McElroy AK, Akondy RS, Davis CW, Ellebedy AH, Mehta AK, Kraft CS, Lyon GM, Ribner BS, Varkey J, Sidney J, Sette A, Campbell S, Ströher U, Damon I, Nichol ST, Spiropoulou CF, Ahmed R. 2015. Human Ebola virus infection results in substantial immune activation. *Proc Natl Acad Sci USA* **112**:4719–4724.

21. Mupapa K, Massamba M, Kibadi K, Kuvula K, Bwaka A, Kipasa M, Colebunders R, Muyembe-Tamfum JJ, International Scientific and Technical Committee. 1999. Treatment of Ebola hemorrhagic fever with blood transfusions from convalescent patients. *J Infect Dis* **179**(Suppl 1):S18–S23.

22. Dye JM, Herbert AS, Kuehne AI, Barth JF, Muhammad MA, Zak SE, Ortiz RA, Prugar LI, Pratt WD. 2012. Postexposure antibody prophylaxis protects nonhuman primates from filovirus disease. *Proc Natl Acad Sci USA* **109**:5034–5039.

23. Jahrling PB, Geisbert JB, Swearengen JR, Larsen T, Geisbert TW. 2007. Ebola hemorrhagic fever: evaluation of passive immunotherapy in nonhuman primates. *J Infect Dis* **196**(Suppl 2):S400–S403.

24. Qiu X, Wong G, Audet J, Bello A, Fernando L, Alimonti JB, Fausther-Bovendo H, Wei H, Aviles J, Hiatt E, Johnson A, Morton J, Swope K, Bohorov O, Bohorova N, Goodman C, Kim D, Pauly MH, Velasco J, Pettitt J, Olinger GG, Whaley K, Xu B, Strong JE, Zeitlin L, Kobinger GP. 2014. Reversion of advanced Ebola virus disease in nonhuman primates with ZMapp. *Nature* **514**:47–53.

25. Lyon GM, Mehta AK, Varkey JB, Brantly K, Plyler L, McElroy AK, Kraft CS, Towner JS, Spiropoulou C, Ströher U, Uyeki TM, Ribner BS, Emory Serious Communicable Diseases Unit. 2014. Clinical care of two patients with Ebola virus disease in the United States. *N Engl J Med* **371**:2402–2409.

26. Wong G, Qiu X. 2015. Development of experimental and early investigational drugs for the treatment of Ebola virus infections. *Expert Opin Investig Drugs* **24**:999–1011.

27. **Geisbert TW, Lee AC, Robbins M, Geisbert JB, Honko AN, Sood V, Johnson JC, de Jong S, Tavakoli I, Judge A, Hensley LE, Maclachlan I.** 2010. Postexposure protection of non-human primates against a lethal Ebola virus challenge with RNA interference: a proof-of-concept study. *Lancet* **375:**1896–1905.

28. **Geisbert TW, Hensley LE, Kagan E, Yu EZ, Geisbert JB, Daddario-DiCaprio K, Fritz EA, Jahrling PB, McClintock K, Phelps JR, Lee AC, Judge A, Jeffs LB, MacLachlan I.** 2006. Postexposure protection of guinea pigs against a lethal ebola virus challenge is conferred by RNA interference. *J Infect Dis* **193:**1650–1657.

29. **Pollack A.** 2015. Clinical trial of experimental Ebola drug is halted. *New York Times.* http://www.nytimes.com/2015/06/20/health/clinical-trial-of-experimental-ebola-drug-is-halted.html?_r=0.

30. **Sissoko D, Folkesson E, Abdoul M, Beavogui AH, Gunther S, Shepherd S, Danel C, Mentre F, Anglaret X, Malvy D.** 2015. Favipiravir in patients with Ebola virus disease: early results of the JIKI trial in Guinea. Abstract 103-ALB. Conference on Retroviruses and Opportunistic Infections (CROI), Seattle, WA.

31. **Sullivan NJ, Martin JE, Graham BS, Nabel GJ.** 2009. Correlates of protective immunity for Ebola vaccines: implications for regulatory approval by the animal rule. *Nat Rev Microbiol* **7:**393–400.

32. **Geisbert TW, Pushko P, Anderson K, Smith J, Davis KJ, Jahrling PB.** 2002. Evaluation in nonhuman primates of vaccines against Ebola virus. *Emerg Infect Dis* **8:**503–507.

33. **Reynard O, Mokhonov V, Mokhonova E, Leung J, Page A, Mateo M, Pyankova O, Georges-Courbot MC, Raoul H, Khromykh AA, Volchkov VE.** 2011. Kunjin virus replicon-based vaccines expressing Ebola virus glycoprotein GP protect the guinea pig against lethal Ebola virus infection. *J Infect Dis* **204**(Suppl 3):S1060–S1065.

34. **Hoenen T, Groseth A, Feldmann H.** 2012. Current ebola vaccines. *Expert Opin Biol Ther* **12:**859–872.

35. **Qiu X, Fernando L, Alimonti JB, Melito PL, Feldmann F, Dick D, Ströher U, Feldmann H, Jones SM.** 2009. Mucosal immunization of cynomolgus macaques with the VSVDeltaG/ZEBOVGP vaccine stimulates strong ebola GP-specific immune responses. *PLoS One* **4:**e5547. doi:10.1371/journal.pone.0005547.

36. **Agnandji ST, Huttner A, Zinser ME, Njuguna P, Dahlke C, Fernandes JF, Yerly S, Dayer JA, Kraehling V, Kasonta R, Adegnika AA, Altfeld M, Auderset F, Bache EB, Biedenkopf N, Borregaard S, Brosnahan JS, Burrow R, Combescure C, Desmeules J, Eickmann M, Fehling SK, Finckh A, Goncalves AR, Grobusch MP, Hooper J, Jambrecina A, Kabwende AL, Kaya G, Kimani D, Lell B, Lemaître B, Lohse AW, Massinga-Loembe M, Matthey A, Mordmüller B, Nolting A, Ogwang C, Ramharter M, Schmidt-Chanasit J, Schmiedel S, Silvera P, Stahl FR, Staines HM, Strecker T, Stubbe HC, Tsofa B, Zaki S, Fast P, Moorthy V, Kaiser L, Krishna S, Becker S, Kieny MP, Bejon P, Kremsner PG, Addo MM, Siegrist CA.** 2015. Phase 1 trials of rVSV Ebola vaccine in Africa and Europe: preliminary report. *N Engl J Med.* [Epub ahead of print.] doi:10.1056/NEJMoa1502924.

37. **Henao-Restrepo AM, Longini IM, Egger M, Dean NE, Edmunds WJ, Camacho A, Carroll MW, Doumbia M, Draguez B, Duraffour S, Enwere G, Grais R, Gunther S, Hossmann S, Kondé MK, Kone S, Kuisma E, Levine MM, Mandal S, Norheim G, Riveros X, Soumah A, Trelle S, Vicari AS, Watson CH, Kéïta S, Kieny MP, Røttingen JA.** 2015. Efficacy and effectiveness of an rVSV-vectored vaccine expressing Ebola surface glycoprotein: interim results from the Guinea ring vaccination cluster-randomised trial. *Lancet* **386:**857–866.

38. **Sullivan NJ, Hensley L, Asiedu C, Geisbert TW, Stanley D, Johnson J, Honko A, Olinger G, Bailey M, Geisbert JB, Reimann KA, Bao S, Rao S, Roederer M, Jahrling PB, Koup RA, Nabel GJ.** 2011. CD8+ cellular immunity mediates rAd5 vaccine protection against Ebola virus infection of nonhuman primates. *Nat Med* **17:**1128–1131.

39. **Ledgerwood JE, Costner P, Desai N, Holman L, Enama ME, Yamshchikov G, Mulangu S, Hu Z, Andrews CA, Sheets RA, Koup RA, Roederer M, Bailer R, Mascola JR, Pau MG, Sullivan NJ, Goudsmit J, Nabel GJ, Graham BS, VRC 205 Study Team.** 2010. A replication defective recombinant Ad5 vaccine expressing Ebola virus GP is safe and immunogenic in healthy adults. *Vaccine* **29:**304–313.

40. **Bausch DG, Towner JS, Dowell SF, Kaducu F, Lukwiya M, Sanchez A, Nichol ST, Ksiazek TG, Rollin PE.** 2007. Assessment of the risk of Ebola virus transmission from bodily fluids and fomites. *J Infect Dis* **196**(Suppl 2)**:**S142–S147.

41. **Centers for Disease Control and Prevention.** 2014. *Hospital preparedness: a tiered approach.* http://www.cdc.gov/vhf/ebola/healthcare-us/preparing/treatment-centers.html.

42. **Smith PW, Anderson AO, Christopher GW, Cieslak TJ, Devreede GJ, Fosdick GA, Greiner CB, Hauser JM, Hinrichs SH, Huebner KD,**

Iwen PC, Jourdan DR, Kortepeter MG, Landon VP, Lenaghan PA, Leopold RE, Marklund LA, Martin JW, Medcalf SJ, Mussack RJ, Neal RH, Ribner BS, Richmond JY, Rogge C, Daly LA, Roselle GA, Rupp ME, Sambol AR, Schaefer JE, Sibley J, Streifel AJ, Essen SG, Warfield KL. 2006. Designing a biocontainment unit to care for patients with serious communicable diseases: a consensus statement. *Biosecur Bioterror* **4:**351–365.

43. **Hewlett AL, Varkey JB, Smith PW, Ribner BS.** 2015. Ebola virus disease: preparedness and infection control lessons learned from two biocontainment units. *Curr Opin Infect Dis* **28:** 343–348.

44. **Feistritzer NR, Hill C, Vanairsdale S, Gentry J.** 2014. Care of patients with Ebola virus disease. *J Contin Educ Nurs* **45:**479–481.

45. **Schwedhelm S, Beam EL, Morris RD, Sebastian JG.** 2015. Reflections on interprofessional team-based clinical care in the ebola epidemic: the Nebraska Medicine experience. *Nurs Outlook* **63:**27–29.

46. **Centers for Disease Control and Prevention.** 2015. Guidance on personal protective equipment (PPE) to be used by healthcare workers during management of patients with confirmed Ebola or persons under investigation (PUIs) for Ebola who are clinically unstable or have bleeding, vomiting, or diarrhea in U.S. hospitals, including procedures for donning and doffing PPE. http://www.cdc.gov/vhf/ebola/healthcare-us/ppe/guidance.html.

47. **MacIntyre CR, Chughtai AA, Seale H, Richards GA, Davidson PM.** 2015. Uncertainty, risk analysis and change for Ebola personal protective equipment guidelines. *Int J Nurs Stud* **52:** 899–903.

48. **Iwen PC, Smith PW, Hewlett AL, Kratochvil CJ, Lisco SJ, Sullivan JN, Gibbs SG, Lowe JJ, Fey PD, Herrera VL, Sambol AR, Wisecarver JL, Hinrichs SH.** 2015. Safety considerations in the laboratory testing of specimens suspected or known to contain Ebola virus. *Am J Clin Pathol* **143:**4–5.

49. **Centers for Disease Control and Prevention.** 2015. *Guidance for U.S. laboratories for managing and testing routine clinical specimens when there is a concern about Ebola virus disease.* http://www.cdc.gov/vhf/ebola/healthcare-us/laboratories/safe-specimen-management.html.

50. **American Society for Microbiology.** 2014. *Interim laboratory guidelines for handling/testing specimens from cases or suspected cases of hemorrhagic fever virus (HFV).* https://www.asm.org/images/PSAB/Ebola9-10-14.pdf.

51. **Hill CE, Burd EM, Kraft CS, Ryan EL, Duncan A, Winkler AM, Cardella JC, Ritchie JC,** Parslow TG. 2014. Laboratory test support for Ebola patients within a high-containment facility. *Lab Med* **45:**e109–e111.

52. **Centers for Disease Control and Prevention.** 2014. *Procedures for safe handling and management of Ebola-associated waste.* http://www.cdc.gov/vhf/ebola/healthcare-us/cleaning/handling-waste.html.

53. **Centers for Disease Control and Prevention.** 2015. *Interim guidance for environmental infection control in hospitals for Ebola virus.* http://www.cdc.gov/vhf/ebola/healthcare-us/cleaning/hospitals.html.

54. **United States Environmental Protection Agency.** 2015. *List L: Disinfectants for use against the Ebola virus.* http://www.epa.gov/pesticide-registration/list-l-disinfectants-use-against-ebola-virus.

55. **Lowe JJ, Olinger PL, Gibbs SG, Rengarajan K, Beam EL, Boulter KC, Schwedhelm MM, Hayes AK, Kratochvil CJ, Vanairsdale S, Frislie B, Lewis J, Hewlett AL, Smith PW, Gartland B, Ribner BS.** 2015. Environmental infection control considerations for Ebola. *Am J Infect Control* **43:**747–749.

56. **Gates B.** 2015. The next epidemic: lessons from Ebola. *N Engl J Med* **372:**1381–1384.

57. **Dzau VJ, Rodin J.** 2015. Creating a global health risk framework. *N Engl J Med* **373:**991–993.

58. **World Health Organization.** 2015. *Report of the Ebola interim assessment panel.* http://www.who.int/csr/resources/publications/ebola/ebola-interim-assessment/en/.

59. **World Health Organization.** 2015. *Factors that contributed to undetected spread of the Ebola virus and impeded rapid containment.* http://www.who.int/csr/disease/ebola/one-year-report/factors/en/.

60. **National Academy of Medicine.** 2016. *Global health risk framework.* http://nam.edu/initiatives/global-health-risk-framework/.

61. **World Health Organization.** 2015. *WHO Secretariat response to the report of the Ebola interim assessment panel.* http://www.who.int/csr/resources/publications/ebola/who-response-to-ebola-report.pdf.

62. **Wayne A.** 2014. Congress nearly grants Obama's Ebola wish list with $5.4B. Bloomberg. http://www.bloomberg.com/news/articles/2014-12-10/congress-nearly-grants-obama-s-ebola-wish-list-with-5-4b.

63. **U.S. Department of Health & Human Services.** 2015. *HHS invests in enhancing domestic preparedness efforts for Ebola.* http://www.hhs.gov/about/news/2015/02/20/hhs-invests-in-enhancing-domestic-preparedness-efforts-for-ebola.html.

Ebola Virus Disease: Therapeutic and Potential Preventative Opportunities

3

ROBERT FISHER[1] and LUCIANA BORIO[2]

INTRODUCTION

In mid-1976 an outbreak of hemorrhagic fever was reported in southern Sudan and northern Zaire. Patients with the disease, which appeared first in southern Sudan in June 1976, presented with influenza-like symptoms including headache, fever, and myalgias and rapidly progressed to a more severe illness characterized by diarrhea, vomiting, chest pains, and hemorrhage. The disease was associated with a high mortality rate and was transmitted between close contacts of the severely ill, resulting in a substantial number of cases being linked to a local hospital (1). An outbreak of a disease with similar symptoms was noted in northern Zaire beginning in September 1976, and by 24 October there were 280 deaths out of a total of 318 cases, for a case fatality rate of 88% (2). When samples derived from patients affected by the Sudan and Zaire outbreaks were used to infect Vero cells in culture, guinea pigs, or mice, a filamentous virus similar to Marburg virus was observed (3, 4). Virus particles with a similar morphology were also identified in postmortem liver samples from patients in Zaire (4, 5). Antigenic comparisons of the new virus isolates and Marburg demonstrated that while there was cross-reactivity between the Sudan and Zaire viruses, they were distinct from Marburg virus, and the

[1]Food and Drug Administration, Office of Counterterrorism and Emerging Threats, Silver Spring, MD 20993;
[2]Food and Drug Administration, Office of the Chief Scientist, Silver Spring, MD 20993.
Emerging Infections 10
Edited by W. Michael Scheld, James M. Hughes and Richard J. Whitley
© 2016 American Society for Microbiology, Washington, DC
doi:10.1128/microbiolspec.EI10-0014-2016

new isolates were designated "Ebola virus" (EBOV) after a river near the outbreak site in Zaire (5). Unlike Marburg virus, for which a single species has been described, at least five different species of the *Ebolavirus* genus exist (6). *Zaire ebolavirus* and *Sudan ebolavirus* are the species most frequently associated with human disease (7).

Before the large 2014–2015 epidemic in West Africa, outbreaks of Ebola virus disease (EVD) had occurred with some frequency, but they have been largely limited to Western and Central Africa including Uganda, Sudan, Cote-d'Ivoire, Gabon, the Republic of the Congo, and the Democratic Republic of the Congo, and most involved only a handful of cases (8). After the initial 1976 outbreak and prior to the 2014–2015 epidemic, three outbreaks stood out as exceptional due to high case numbers: the emergence of Ebola virus in Kikwit, Democratic Republic of the Congo, in 1995 (9), of Sudan virus in Uganda during 2000–2001 (10), and again of Ebola virus in the Democratic Republic of the Congo in 2007 (11).

Members of the *Ebolavirus* genus are filamentous, enveloped viruses containing linear, nonsegmented ~19-kb single-stranded RNA genomes that encode seven genes and eight proteins (12, 13); due to RNA editing, the glycoprotein (GP) gene produces separate proteins for the virion envelope GP and a secreted glycoprotein (sGP) (14). While sGP has multiple pathophysiologic and immunomodulatory roles (15), GP is critical for virus binding and fusion, and as the sole surface protein on the intact virion it is an obvious target for vaccine and monoclonal antibody development. Other structural components of the virus such as VP24, VP40, and VP35 also antagonize the innate immune response (16), activities that may be restored by blocking the interaction of the viral proteins with their cellular targets. Finally, as a single-stranded RNA virus, the Ebola virus relies on an RNA-dependent-RNA-polymerase (L) to transcribe the negative strand genome into monocistronic mRNAs for protein synthesis

and a full-length antigenome as a template for replication. As might be expected, the polymerase represents a virus-specific target that can be exploited through the use of nucleoside analogs or knockdown strategies.

MEDICAL COUNTERMEASURE DEVELOPMENT DURING THE 2014–2015 EPIDEMIC

The successful response to any epidemic involving a disease as contagious as Ebola must focus on controlling the spread of disease through the implementation of standard public health measures, such as identifying and isolating infected persons, tracing their contacts to detect secondary infections, protecting contacts and health care workers from exposure, and ensuring the safe burial of the deceased. However, applying these public health measures on a large scale has presented complex challenges because of the limited public health infrastructure within most countries where Ebola outbreaks have occurred, and especially in West Africa when the epidemic emerged in 2014 (17). With 28,598 cases of EVD and 11,299 deaths as of 3 November 2015 (18), the unprecedented scale and speed of the Ebola epidemic in Guinea, Liberia, and Sierra Leone underscored the need for safe, effective, and rapidly deployable medical countermeasures (MCMs). These MCMs include diagnostic tests to assist in disease surveillance and case detection, vaccines to protect health care workers and help interrupt transmission, and drugs to improve outcomes of infected patients.

Significant difficulties in successfully implementing risk communication strategies were encountered, and health care systems and Ebola treatment centers in the affected West African countries rapidly became overwhelmed (19), leading to extremely pessimistic projections on the potential course of the epidemic (20, 21). These projections added to the urgency of conducting properly designed clinical trials to evaluate a number of investigational MCMs still in early stages of development. The sooner one could establish whether an investigational MCM was safe and effective for the treatment or prevention of EVD, the sooner it could be incorporated into the response to the public health emergency (22, 23). One factor limiting the prompt evaluation of some investigational drugs was their availability, since most of the more promising antiviral candidates had been produced only in limited quantities for early development purposes. Convalescent blood and/or plasma was the exception to this rule, but the infrastructure to safely collect, store, and use this resource was not extant in West Africa until November 2014 (24), and the first clinical trials of Ebola therapeutics in West Africa were initiated in December 2014 (25).

Several therapies had been investigated *in vitro* or in animal model systems over the years that preceded the 2014 epidemic. However, at the beginning of the West African epidemic there were no treatments or vaccines that had been shown to be safe or effective for treating or preventing EVD. Clinicaltrials.gov documents only five studies of "Ebola treatments" (as compared to vaccines) prior to March 2014; these were all phase 1 safety studies (26), and of these, one was being developed for postexposure prophylaxis, not treatment. Of the four phase 1 safety studies for drugs with treatment indications, only one was completed, while the others were either withdrawn or terminated. As the epidemic progressed, a number of different compounds, most of which had at least some activity demonstrated in animal models, were selected for evaluation in clinical trials. Product classes considered for treatment of EVD included both biologics (monoclonal antibodies and convalescent plasma) and drugs (small interfering RNAs [siRNAs], nucleoside analogs, and others).

Supportive Care

Supportive care was key to improving patient outcomes and is expected to remain a central component of the care of acutely ill patients, even in the setting of a proven specific treatment. When possible, volume replacement of patients was an important component due to intravascular depletion resulting from emesis, voluminous diarrhea, and fluid shifts within the body that deplete the intravascular space. Antiemetics and antidiarrheals were administered when possible, as were empiric antibiotics because of possible bacteremia from transmigration of Gram-negative bacteria from the gut (27, 28). Antimalarials were also commonly administered because many patients admitted to Ebola treatment units had concomitant malaria infections. Diazepam for sedation and morphine for analgesia (29) were also commonly used. Even when sufficient medication and supplies were available, patient care suffered in the initial months because demand for health care personnel greatly exceeded what was available in affected areas (30, 31). Despite these challenges, there appeared to be an increasing level of care in West Africa over the course of the epidemic (32), with ensuing improved outcomes in the later months of the epidemic.

Supportive care delivered in developed settings, such as Europe and the United States (33, 34) also proved to be demanding. In contrast to the standard of care in West Africa, however, extensive physiological monitoring and aggressive medical interventions were available for patients admitted or evacuated to these facilities (35). A patient treated in Germany for severe EVD required blood products, ventilation, vasopressors, antibiotics and antifungals, and hemodialysis. In addition to general supportive measures, investigational interventions were provided to most patients in Europe and the United States (36), although the effects of these interventions (beneficial or harmful) could not be assessed. Not all patients needed intensive levels of support; some patients, presumably those with less severe disease, rapidly recovered after receiving only minimal support, such as intravenous fluids (37).

Therapeutics

Two American health care workers developed EVD while caring for patients in West Africa and were evacuated to the United States for medical care. In addition to a high level of supportive care, they also received the investigational compound ZMapp (35). Both patients survived, and although no conclusion of safety or efficacy could be drawn from the use of the investigational compound under these circumstances, there were widespread calls for access to early-stage investigational candidates such as ZMapp. An ethics panel advising the WHO indicated that while it was ethical to provide therapies with unproven safety and efficacy profiles, "investigators have a moral duty to evaluate these interventions (for treatment or prevention) in the best possible clinical studies that can be conducted under the circumstances of the epidemic" so that effective therapies could be rapidly identified (38).

Clinical trials for promising treatments were put into place as rapidly as possible, but assembling the infrastructure for conducting trials took some time. In the interim, the use of investigational candidates in the United States, Europe, and West Africa continued on a case-by-case basis under what is colloquially referred to as "compassionate use"; in the United States such use is one type of expanded access that can be permitted under an investigational new drug application (39). This type of use of experimental intervention is not designed to generate conclusions about the safety or efficacy of the investigational drugs being used, given the lack of appropriate comparator groups. Unfortunately, even after clinical trials were established, access to investigational agents outside of clinical trials was advocated for by some organizations as a stop-gap measure, even though this delayed the gathering of interpretable data that would allow the most efficient identification of beneficial treatments or the rapid discontinuation of harmful therapies.

Antibodies

ZMAPP

A series of monoclonal antibodies targeting EBOV GP was developed by researchers at the U.S. Army Medical Research Institute for Infectious Diseases, and several were demonstrated to be protective in mouse models (39). Three of these antibodies (13F6, 13C6, and 6D8) were modified to deimmunize (13F6) and/or chimerize (all three antibodies) through the addition of a human Fc region. The mixture of these three antibodies (MB-003) was found to be effective in a mouse challenge model even when administered as late as 48 hours post-EBOV infection (40, 41). A parallel effort led by the Public Health Agency of Canada also evaluated mixtures of monoclonal antibodies directed against EBOV GP and demonstrated that a combination of three murine monoclonals (1H3, 2G4, and 4G7; ZMAb) were also effective as a postexposure intervention in mice and guinea pigs (42). MB-003 conferred a survival benefit compared to placebo when dosed after the onset of fever in rhesus macaques challenged with EBOV (43), while ZMAb protected cynomolgus macaques from an EBOV challenge when treatment was initiated 48 hours postinfection (44).

The realization that a cooperative effort would benefit both groups led to a collaboration that examined whether an optimized cocktail could be formulated from the individual components of ZMAb and MB-003. As a result, it was demonstrated that a mixture of c13C6 (from MB-003) and c2G4 + c4G7 (humanized versions of two ZMAb components) provided protection even when treatment was delayed to 5 days postinfection in the rhesus macaque EBOV challenge model (45). The combination of c13C6, c2G4, and c4G7 was trademarked as "ZMapp" by MappBio and advanced as a candidate therapy for human EVD in January 2014 (http://mappbio.com/z-mapp/). ZMAb was used in at least two patients in Europe, while ZMapp was used in at least nine EVD patients (46) in the United States, Europe, and West Africa prior to the establishment of a randomized, controlled clinical trial in the United States and West Africa designed to evaluate the safety and efficacy of this investigational product in adults and children infected with EBOV (47). This trial, launched in February 2015 (48), has enrolled approximately 70 research participants at the time of this writing.

Although preliminary results with ZMapp in animal models have been promising and led to its prioritization for evaluation in clinical trials, the plant-based production system created a bottleneck that prevented timely increases in production. Initially, the ability to rapidly move the ZMAb components from a hybridoma platform to one more suitable for preparation of clinical material was considered a major advantage (49), and the use of transgenic *Nicotiana benthamiana* plants improved glycosylation and, thus, antibody-dependent cytotoxicity of the antibodies (41). Unfortunately, only a handful of treatment courses were available at the onset of the West African outbreak, and these were depleted by mid-August 2014 (50). While funding was rapidly made available through the Biomedical Advanced Research and Development Authority (BARDA) (46), the throughput of the facility producing the drug substance was extremely limited and was expected to produce only an additional 10 to 20 treatment courses by the end of 2014 (51).

MIL-77

Produced by a Chinese company, MabWorks, MIL-77 is a cell-derived monoclonal cocktail similar to ZMapp. MIL-77 was developed using the sequence information referenced in the ZMapp patents, raising intellectual property concerns (52). It was first administered to a United Kingdom medic who subsequently recovered from EVD. however, the efficacy could not be attributed to MIL77 (53) in the absence of a properly designed trial, because some patients with EVD re-

cover, especially in the setting of advanced supportive care. According to the WHO, MIL77 is undergoing phase 1 safety trials in China (54).

Convalescent blood and plasma

Largely based on its use during prior outbreaks and the expected availability of suitable donors, in September 2014 the WHO issued a guideline recommending the use of convalescent whole blood or plasma for treatment of patients with early EVD, despite the lack of conclusive evidence of its effectiveness (55) . In their guideline, the WHO noted the lack of a proven treatment for EVD and cited previous use of convalescent material to treat Ebola and other infectious diseases. Interestingly, the collection of convalescent plasma was identified as a priority for the WHO team responding to the first Ebola outbreak in 1976 (1), and units thus collected were administered to at least two patients during the 1976 outbreak (2).

Early administration of convalescent serum or plasma was also documented in a 1976 case involving a researcher at Porton Down who was accidently infected (57). The researcher, who survived, received interferon for 2 weeks plus heat-treated convalescent serum on day 3 and day 6. While there was a decrease in viremia after the first infusion of serum, the decrease cannot be attributed to the serum infusion; viremia decreases in all surviving patients at some time even in the absence of specific treatments. During the 1995 Kikwit outbreak, whole blood from Ebola disease survivors was administered to eight patients (58). There was no clear association between the volume administered or time of administration and survival, and it was noted that a controlled trial would likely be necessary to assess any treatment effect (59).

The results from animal studies evaluating the activity of convalescent plasma or other anti-Ebola hyperimmune material have been variable. An equine IgG preparation was successful in delaying viremia, clinical signs, and death in a postexposure prophylaxis model using 1,000 plaque forming units of Ebola Zaire challenge in cynomolgus macaques but did not confer a survival benefit compared to placebo (60). In contrast, baboons challenged with a lower dose of Ebola Zaire (10 to 30 50% lethal doses) were protected if an equine hyperimmune product similar to the one described above was administered within 60 minutes of infection. No beneficial effect was observed in rhesus macaques receiving whole blood with a high titer of anti-Ebola antibodies (measured by ELISA) immediately after an Ebola Zaire challenge (56). Further complicating the overall interpretation are data indicating that neutralizing antibodies protective in one species may not be efficacious in another (61), and protection may correlate with total anti-Ebola IgG titers and not necessarily with neutralizing antibody titers (62). Antibody-dependent cellular cytotoxicity has been proposed as an important mechanism for efficacy of anti-Ebola monoclonals (41, 63) but has not been investigated in the context of the polyclonal nature of convalescent serum or plasma administered for Ebola disease.

Use of convalescent blood or plasma is not without risks, because it may result in transfusion reactions including transfusion-related acute lung injury (TRALI), hemolytic reactions, anaphylaxis, circulatory overload, and transfusion-transmitted infections. Indeed, acute respiratory distress consistent with TRALI was reported in a patient with EVD who received convalescent plasma and favipiravir on day 10 of her illness (37).

When designing a study to evaluate the efficacy of immune plasma, including a nonimmune control arm in a randomized, controlled trial is important for addressing the question of whether it is the immune component of convalescent plasma or other attributes of infusing plasma such as the hemodynamic support from an infusing fluid and protein and providing clotting factors that is responsible for the observed effects. Another factor to consider is that if immune plasma is collected from vaccine recipients rather than people who have had Ebola infection, the characteristics of the vaccine-generated hyperimmune plasma may differ from plasma collected from people who have recovered from Ebola infection. Further characterization of the similarities and differences in antibodies generated in response to natural infection and vaccination and preclinical studies may provide insights into similarities and differences and the possible clinical implications.

Three phase 2/3 uncontrolled clinical trials were initiated in West Africa with convalescent plasma, one each in Guinea, Liberia, and Sierra Leone (24). The Liberia study was discontinued due to the decline in cases in the country, but as of 19 June 2015, 101 patients had received plasma in the Guinea Ebola-Tx study (54). The investigators for the Guinea convalescent plasma trial, a historically controlled trial, reported that transfusion of convalescent plasma with unknown levels of neutralizing antibodies in 84 patients with confirmed EVD was not associated with a significant improvement in survival (64). The significant limitations of the Guinea convalescent plasma study (a historically controlled trial using plasma with unknown levels of neutralizing antibody) limit the ability to draw any definitive conclusions about the role of convalescent plasma to treat patients with Ebola. Convalescent plasma was also used under an emergency investigational new drug application for several cases of EVD in the United States prior to the establishment of the randomized, controlled clinical trial to evaluate Ebola therapies (65–67).

Small molecules

AVI-7537, AVI-7539, and AVI-6002 (Sarepta)

In 2010 the U.S. Department of Defense's Joint Project Manager Transformational Medical Technologies program awarded a contract to AVI BioPharma (now Sarepta Therapeutics) to advance their antisense-based

PMOplus chemistry for therapeutics against Ebola and Marburg, building upon earlier investments in the company from the Department of Defense's Defense Threat Reduction Agency (68). Antisense-based therapies function by binding a complementary nucleic acid strand to the mRNA encoding for a target viral protein and were first described nearly 40 years ago (69). Affinity, cellular penetration, and stability in the presence of ubiquitous nucleases presented an initial challenge, but the development of chemically modified oligonucleotides made clinical development possible (70). In 2006 phosphorodiamidate morpholino oligomers (PMOs) designed to target EBOV VP24, VP35, and L were demonstrated to provide pre-exposure prophylaxis against an EBOV challenge in rhesus macaques (71); a mixture of VP24 (AVI-7537)– and VP35 (AVI-7539)–directed PMOs (this combination is referred to as AVI-6002) provided protection against EBOV infection in an animal model of postexposure prophylaxis (72). AVI-6002 was advanced into a phase 1 study, where it was found to be well tolerated, albeit with a short plasma half-life (2 to 5 hours) (73). Further research indicated that this mixture of PMOs could be narrowed to a single oligomer (VP-7537) targeting EBOV VP24 and still retain potency in the rhesus challenge model (74). To date, there are no published data on use of AVI-7537, AVI-7539, or AVI-6002 for treatment of EVD in humans, and as of 5 November 2015, further development of these compounds was in question, reportedly due to a lack of funding and intellectual property limitations (75, 76).

BCX4430 (Biocryst)

BCX4430 is a synthetic nucleoside analog of adenosine and has *in vitro* activity against RNA viruses in many families (including *Filoviridae*), as might be expected from its mechanism of action as an RNA chain terminator. This compound is active against EVD and Marburg disease in murine models of pre- and postexposure prophylaxis and protects guinea pigs from Marburg infection when dosed as late as 72 hours postinfection. Similarly, six of six cynomolgus macaques survived a challenge with Marburg when treated with 15 mg/kg BCX4430 twice a day starting at 48 hours postchallenge (77). Biocryst was awarded a 2013 National Institute of Allergy and Infectious Diseases contract to develop BCX4430 for treatment of Marburg disease and to investigate the compound's utility for treating EVD (78). Phase 1 testing started in December 2014 and is ongoing (79); in March 2015 BARDA awarded Biocryst a contract for advanced development including clinical trials and large-scale manufacturing (80).

Favipiravir (T-705; Toyama Chemical)

Favipiravir is a pyrazinecarboxamide derivative that appears to have at least some activity against a number of viruses through the inhibition of RNA-dependent RNA polymerase (81). Approved by the Japanese Ministry of Health, Labor, and Welfare in March 2014 (https://www.toyama-chemical.co.jp/eng/news/news140324e.html), the compound has been stockpiled in Japan for use against pandemic influenza (http://www.fujifilm.com/news/n150722.html). It has demonstrated activity postexposure in animal models of infection against a variety of pathogenic RNA viruses beyond influenza including West Nile virus (82), yellow fever virus (83), Lassa virus (84), and EBOV (85, 86). It has been administered prophylactically (87) to several individuals with EVD (37, 88–90). An open label, historically controlled study of favipiravir in patients with EVD (91) (the JIKI trial; NCT02329054) was sponsored by INSERM in Guinea. Based on an interim analysis of 69 patients, the authors suggest possible benefit in the subset of patients who present to care with lower EBOV viral load (92). However, limitations in the study design as well as improvements in supportive care over the course of the epidemic (32) preclude drawing any meaningful conclusions about its role in the treatment of patients with EVD.

TKM-Ebola (TKM-100802; Tekmira) and TKM-Ebola-Guinea

TKM-Ebola is a lipid-stabilized siRNA targeting EBOV VP35 and polymerase (93), while TKM-Ebola-Guinea is a version of TKM-Ebola modified to remove mismatches in the EBOV Makona variant (http://investor. arbutusbio.com/releasedetail.cfm?rele aseid=907998). The use of nucleic acid–lipid particles, whose development was funded in part by the U.S. Department of Defense, had been demonstrated to be an effective post-exposure therapeutic in guinea pigs and nonhuman primates, although different viral targets were examined in each study: an siRNA against L was used in the guinea pig studies, and a combination of siRNAs against VP24, VP35, and L was used in the nonhuman primate studies (94, 95). TKM-Ebola was used on an infected French Médecins Sans Frontières nurse (96) and administered to two U.S. patients under an emergency investigational new drug application (66). In December 2014 Tekmira partnered with the University of Oxford and the Wellcome Trust to perform a phase 2, single-arm clinical efficacy trial using TKM-Ebola-Guinea in Sierra Leone (http://www.sec.gov/ Archives/edgar/data/1447028/000117184 314006000/newsrelease.htm), but the study reportedly was terminated in June 2015 after reaching a statistical futility boundary (97). Differences in outcomes between animal EVD models and human cases of EVD highlight the difficulty in extrapolating to humans data derived from animal studies. As of August 2015 clinical development work for TKM-Ebola has been terminated (98), and Tekmira Pharmaceuticals has changed its corporate name to Arbutus Biopharma and suspended work on filoviruses to concentrate on chronic hepatitis B (http://investor.arbutusbio.com/releasedetail.cfm?ReleaseID= 925130).

GS-5734 (Gilead)

A late breaker abstract session at the 2015 ID Week Conference described a prodrug of an adenine nucleotide analog that was effective at inhibiting growth of multiple filoviruses in cell culture (99). The presumptive target is the filovirus polymerase; a surrogate RNA polymerase was inhibited by GS-5734 with a 50% inhibitory concentration value of 1 ×M. A survival benefit was demonstrated above that of placebo (50% survival in GS-5734-treated animals versus 0% survival in placebo-treated animals) when GS-5734 was administered to EBOV-infected rhesus macaques with systemic viremia. The compound was administered to a patient with Ebola-related meningitis (100), but the contribution of GS-5734 to her recovery remains unknown.

Vaccines

VSV-ZEBOV

The recovery of recombinant vesicular stomatitis virus (VSV) from cells transfected with DNA plasmids was pioneered by Lawson et al. in 1995 and provided an ideal mechanism for rapidly growing large stocks of high-titer recombinant virus carrying foreign genes that could be used as a vaccine (101). This platform was used to generate VSVΔG/ZEBOVGP, a live-virus vaccine created by substituting EBOV GP for the GP normally present in VSV (102). A single intramuscular injection of VSVΔG/ZEBOVGP vaccine induced both humoral and cellular immunity and was effective at preventing EVD in cynomolgus macaques (103) challenged a month after vaccination. Protection was also observed in cynomolgus macaques challenged with the West African EBOV Makona strain as early as 3 days postvaccination (104). The VSV-based vaccine was effective in postexposure prophylaxis animal models of infection in mice, guinea pigs, and to a lesser degree, rhesus macaques (105). This vaccine, now called VSV-EBOV, has been administered as postexposure prophylaxis to a physician who had a high-risk potential exposure to EBOV as the result of a needlestick (106). VSV-EBOV was also offered as a prophylactic measure to close contacts of the Scottish Ebola patient who experienced a recurrence of symptoms.

VSV-EBOV, originally developed by the Public Health Agency of Canada, was licensed by NewLink Genetics in 2010 and entered advanced development with support from the Department of Defense (http://investors.linkp.com/releasedetail.cfm?ReleaseID=864161) with a phase 1 study initiated in late 2014 (http://investors.linkp.com/releasedetail.cfm?ReleaseID=869082). Responding in part to concerns about scaling up production and overcoming testing delays, NewLink granted exclusive rights to VSV-EBOV to Merck (107), and BARDA provided additional funding to support manufacturing (108). VSV-EBOV elicits neutralizing antibodies and was well tolerated in healthy volunteers (109), and it is currently being evaluated in three ongoing clinical trials in West Africa: the PREVAIL, STRIVE, and *Ebola ça Suffit* trials. The dose of VSV-EBOV used in these trials (2×10^7 plaque forming units) is consistent with that used in the rhesus and cynomolgus macaque challenge studies ($1 - 5 \times 10^7$ plaque forming units [103–105]). PREVAIL is a three-arm, double-blind, randomized phase 2 clinical study to compare the safety and efficacy of VSV-EBOV and ChAd3-EBOZ to placebo in the general population in Liberia (110). STRIVE also seeks to evaluate safety and efficacy, although the target population is composed of health care workers in Sierra Leone. The trial design also differs in that it is unblinded and participants are randomized to immediate vaccination or deferred vaccination (approximately 6 months later [111]). Safety and immunology results are pending for the PREVAIL and STRIVE studies, but the rapid decline in EVD cases in West Africa as the trials were ramping up in early 2015 will require efficacy assessments to be based on immunogenicity instead of disease.

The *Ebola ça Suffit* study utilizes an open-label ring vaccination strategy, where close contacts of Ebola patients are clustered into an epidemiologically defined "ring," and each ring is randomized to either immediate vaccination with VSV-EBOV or to receive vaccination 2 weeks later, with a 1:1 ratio between the study arms (112). This design allows estimation of vaccine efficacy by comparing the hazard ratio between the two groups. As of November 2015 there are promising results from this trial (113), although there are concerns that the interim analysis may overestimate efficacy in the ring vaccination strategy. Specific concerns identified include failing to meet the pre-established statistical test of efficacy between study arms and an analytical bias due to population differences between the study arms (114).

ChAd3-EBOZ

Another approach for recombinant vaccines is based on the use of replication-defective adenovirus (Ad) expressing the antigen of interest. Like VSV, Ad vectors can be grown to high titers and induce a strong immune response, especially when used as the boost component in a heterologous prime-boost system; an EBOV nucleoprotein/glycoprotein (NP/GP) DNA prime/Ad-GP boost vaccine protected cynomolgus macaques against a low-dose EBOV challenge (115). However, this approach required multiple priming immunizations, which presents considerable logistical problems for effective deployment of a vaccine. An accelerated vaccination strategy was investigated, where the DNA prime was abolished and Ad vectors expressing EBOV GP or NP were used concomitantly. A single injection of the Ad-GP/Ad-NP mixture was sufficient for protection against a high-challenge dose of EBOV in the cynomolgus macaque model, and a comparison of the CD4/CD8 response pre- and postchallenge suggests that a CD8 response is important in mediating protection for this vaccine (116). Additional research indicated that the NP component was unnecessary, and Ad-GP alone could provide robust protection in the cynomolgus macaque model (117) and also depended upon CD8 cells (118). To avoid ubiquitous pre-existing immunity to human adenovirus (which had been demonstrated to impact humoral responses to the rAd5 vaccine [119]), the vaccine backbone was changed to a chimpanzee Ad 3 (Ch3Ad). A single immunization with 10^{11} particles of this construct was successful at protecting 50% of cynomolgus macaques when challenged 10 months postvaccination. GlaxoSmithKline (GSK) and the National Institutes of Health partnered to move this vaccine candidate into clinical trials, and a phase 1 study found that while the vaccine was well tolerated, the magnitude of the immune response was less in humans than in the nonhuman primate models (120). As mentioned above, ChAd3-EBOZ is currently being evaluated in the PREVAIL trial, although results will be limited to safety and immunogenicity.

Ad26.ZEBOV (Crucell/Johnson & Johnson) and MVA-BN Filo (Bavarian Nordic)

While EBOV GP expressed in an Ad26 vector rapidly induced a T-cell response and protected against EVD in the cynomolgus macaque model (121), pre-existing immunity and duration of immunity remained a concern for the adenovirus-based vaccines. The heterologous prime-boost approach, where an adenovirus-based EBOV construct was used as the initial vaccine followed by a boost with EBOV GP expressing modified vaccinia Ankara (MVA), was promising since it provided durable immunity (122). The Crucell subsidiary of Johnson & Johnson had developed a monovalent Ebola vaccine using an Ad26 virus vector (Ad26.ZEBOV), while Bavarian Nordic had pursued a multivalent filovirus vaccine (containing the GP from Ebola, Sudan, and Marburg viruses) expressed in an MVA vector (MVA-BN Filo). An interesting collaboration to leverage the heterologous prime-boost strategy was formalized in October 2014 between these two companies (123), and multiple clinical trials are underway (http://id.bavarian-nordic. com/pipeline/filovirus.aspx).

Other vaccines

Several other vaccine candidates are also in the development pipeline. Profectus BioSciences Inc. approached the use of VSV through a different strategy than that utilized by GSK. Instead of replacing VSV G with that of EBOV, Profectus modified the vector by swapping EBOV GP for the VSV N gene, relocating the VSV N gene to a region proximal to VSV G and truncating VSV G. The resulting recombinant had a decreased growth rate *in vitro* and produced lower viremias in vaccinated cynomolgus macaques but was still effective at preventing EVD in this primate model with a single dose of vaccine (124). In contrast to the virally vectored vaccines advanced by Merck, GSK, Crucell, Bavarian Nordic, and Profectus, Novavax is developing a protein-based vaccine to be used with an adjuvant (Matrix-M). A two-dose regimen of the vaccine is effective at preventing EVD in cynomolgus macaques (http://novavax.com/download/ files/presentations/Novavax_EBOV_GP_ Vaccine_2015_07_21_FINAL.pdf), and Novavax initiated a phase 1 study for a recombinant GP protein vaccine in February 2015 (125).

CONCLUSIONS

The development and evaluation of investigational therapies for an emerging infectious disease such as Ebola requires a number of elements to be in place, ranging from the ability to produce or manufacture sufficient quantities of good-quality investigational agents so that clinical trials to evaluate the investigational agents can be conducted, infrastructure to provide care for patients and to support the conduct of clinical trials, engagement of the affected communities in the response effort, information on the disease and its major manifestations, and properly designed clinical trials that have the capacity to draw scientifically valid conclusions and protect patient safety. The epidemic of EVD in West Africa revealed serious weaknesses in international preparedness and response efforts to emerging threats.

The manufacturing or production of sufficient supplies of investigational product to support the conduct of clinical trials was a major challenge in the response to the Ebola epidemic. The reasons for these delays differ for the different types of investigational products that are being developed for Ebola. For example, delays in planning, organizing, and equipping health care providers with the means to collect convalescent serum and blood (identified as one of the highest therapeutic priorities by the WHO [126]) was one factor that impeded the evaluation of these potential therapies. When developing therapies for an emerging infectious disease such as Ebola, it is important to consider the product characteristics, the ability to scale up production, and the time required to deliver adequate supplies in response to an outbreak. For products that are not currently stockpiled, availability and scalability of the production process must be taken into account when prioritizing MCMs or developing contingency plans for their use. These risks can be mitigated in part by ensuring that appropriate mechanisms exist for enlisting additional manufacturing facilities and/or filling lines when necessary.

The characteristics of an investigational product and the setting in which it will be used impact the utility of the product in the response effort. The drugs and vaccines developed by the United States were initially envisioned for use in the context of prophylaxis of military personnel or for a bioterrorist event resulting in cases of EVD, and their use assumed a high degree of coordination between local, state, and federal partners within the United States. Monoclonal antibodies such as ZMapp must be slowly administered over several hours to decrease the risk of infusion-related adverse events. For outbreaks where the ability of health care providers to provide and monitor the admin-

istration of compounds such as ZMapp is compromised, other product classes that can be delivered orally or as an intramuscular injection may be preferable. Likewise, stability can complicate deployment efforts in areas with sporadic electricity and refrigeration. For example, the VSV-EBOV vaccine requires ultra-low (−70°C) storage for long-term stability; experience with polio and smallpox vaccination campaigns demonstrated the importance of a thermally stable vaccine. In the absence of such a stable vaccine, the ability to maintain a cold chain is essential and must be part of contingency planning. This planning should also consider how the vaccines and drugs can be evaluated for safety and efficacy during the outbreak to rapidly identify the safest and most efficacious MCMs.

For therapies against an emerging infectious disease such as Ebola, it is important to consider biological diversity and that the infectious agent may acquire mutations that could alter targets for countermeasures. It would be ideal to have multiple countermeasures with different mechanisms of action in order to have therapies that will remain active in the setting of mutations of the infectious agent or species differences that may impact the activity of some countermeasures. For example, monovalent vaccines developed based on EBOV strains such as Mayinga or Kikwit protect against the Mayinga strain, but had the outbreak been triggered by a separate Ebola virus species (*Sudan ebolavirus* or *Bundibugyo ebolavirus*), cross-neutralization would be unlikely and the vaccines would require modification. Similarly, MCMs that are highly specific to specific strains and species of virus are vulnerable to the emergence of sequence variants. TKM-Ebola was modified to TKM-Ebola-Guinea to more closely match the sequence of the Makona strain of EBOV. Therefore, stockpiles of monovalent MCMs may be less valuable for response than those composed of multivalent vaccines and antivirals with broad activity.

Demonstrating the safety and efficacy of a new drug or vaccine can be a challenging endeavor under normal circumstances. These challenges were amplified by the rapidly evolving Ebola epidemic (a communicable agent causing severe illness with significant mortality), the unprecedented stress on the West African health care system and society in general, and the need to establish infrastructure to support clinical trials to identify beneficial therapies. Properly designed clinical trials are an essential component of the response effort. The findings from such trials can help patients by identifying whether an investigational therapy benefits patients. Conducting clinical trials that are not properly designed can delay the identification of effective therapies, lead to uninterpretable or misleading conclusions, and impede the ability to adequately monitor patient safety. For example, the lack of well-designed clinical trials and information about the characteristics of the convalescent plasma tested have impeded the ability to evaluate the role of convalescent plasma in treating patients with EVD. Fortunately, there were some successful and partially successful efforts during the epidemic. Some well-controlled trials of vaccines and a therapeutic were implemented during the epidemic. While these trials were implemented very quickly compared to the usual time to launch a clinical trial, it is apparent that we need to continue to build on this effort so that the evaluation of countermeasures can be implemented even more rapidly in the response to any future outbreak.

The importance of the advance preparation of protocols to allow the evaluation of safety and efficacy of MCMs in an outbreak setting cannot be overstated. Randomized clinical trials offer advantages in terms of rapidly providing interpretable, robust data on the safety and efficacy of an MCM (127). Careful consideration must be given to inclusion and exclusion criteria, and if need be, flexibility must be introduced into the protocol to allow for adaptation; for example,

the PREVAIL I protocol was modified in November 2015 to include an open-label cluster vaccination component in response to new clusters of EVD in Liberia. The use of a common protocol that allows the flexibility for evaluating multiple unproven MCMs is one potential solution to quickly identify the most effective therapy or prophylactic while weeding out those that actually cause harm, and it can help communicate a standard level of supportive care that is expected for patients (22). If there are debates about how to ethically conduct certain trials, these conversations should take place before an outbreak instead of during the outbreak. Community engagement also has a role to play in trial design. When the purpose for randomized, controlled trials—to evaluate the safety as well as efficacy in untested products—was articulated to local populations by individuals trusted by those in the community, there was acceptance as evidenced by enrollment and high visit compliance in the *Ebola ça Suffit* and PREVAIL vaccine trials (110, 113). In addition, the above-mentioned cluster vaccination component of the PREVAIL I protocol was implemented by the Liberian partners, building on the training they had received for the initial trial.

Sadly, for the first time in history, a sufficient number of EVD cases existed to allow for the collection of data on the natural history of disease in humans. Applied research to address knowledge gaps benefitted from a great deal of collaborative work accomplished through partnerships between nongovernmental organizations, industry, academia, and government agencies. While the data thus generated will be analyzed and subjected to scrutiny and debate for years to come, we do not have the same luxury of time in which to apply the lessons of how the world responded to this unprecedented outbreak. Considering severe acute respiratory syndrome–associated coronavirus, pandemic influenza, and now EVD, we must do more in terms of preparedness and contingency planning for every stage of the MCM product development cycle. Instead of asking "What do we have?" during an outbreak, the question should be reframed to "Which contingency plan is appropriate?" for any given outbreak situation.

ACKNOWLEDGMENTS

This book chapter reflects the views of the authors and should not be construed to represent the FDA's views or policies.

CITATION

Fisher R, Borio L. 2016. Ebola virus disease: therapeutic and potential preventative opportunities. Microbiol Spectrum 4(3):EI10-0014-2016.

REFERENCES

1. **World Health Organization.** 1978. Ebola haemorrhagic fever in Sudan, 1976. *Bull World Health Organ* **56:**247–270.
2. **World Health Organization.** 1978. Ebola haemorrhagic fever in Zaire, 1976. *Bull World Health Organ* **56:**271–293.
3. **Bowen ET, Lloyd G, Harris WJ, Platt GS, Baskerville A, Vella EE.** 1977. Viral haemorrhagic fever in southern Sudan and northern Zaire. Preliminary studies on the aetiological agent. *Lancet* **1:**571–573.
4. **Pattyn S, van der Groen G, Jacob W, Piot P, Courteille G.** 1977. Isolation of Marburg-like virus from a case of haemorrhagic fever in Zaire. *Lancet* **1:**573–574.
5. **Johnson KM, Lange JV, Webb PA, Murphy FA.** 1977. Isolation and partial characterisation of a new virus causing acute haemorrhagic fever in Zaire. *Lancet* **1:**569–571.
6. **Bukreyev AA, Chandran K, Dolnik O, Dye JM, Ebihara H, Leroy EM, Mühlberger E, Netesov SV, Patterson JL, Paweska JT, Saphire EO, Smither SJ, Takada A, Towner JS, Volchkov VE, Warren TK, Kuhn JH.** 2014. Discussions and decisions of the 2012–2014 International Committee on Taxonomy of Viruses (ICTV) Filoviridae Study Group, January 2012–June 2013. *Arch Virol* **159:**821–830.
7. **Weyer J, Grobbelaar A, Blumberg L.** 2015. Ebola virus disease: history, epidemiology and outbreaks. *Curr Infect Dis Rep* **17:**480.
8. **Centers for Disease Control and Prevention.** 2016. Outbreaks Chronology: *Ebola Virus Disease.* http://www.cdc.gov/vhf/ebola/outbreaks/history/chronology.html#one.
9. **Khan AS, Tshioko FK, Heymann DL, Le Guenno B, Nabeth P, Kerstiëns B, Fleerackers Y, Kilmarx PH, Rodier GR, Nkuku O, Rollin PE, Sanchez A, Zaki SR, Swanepoel R, Tomori O, Nichol ST, Peters CJ, Muyembe-Tamfum JJ, Ksiazek TG.** 1999. The reemergence of Ebola hemorrhagic fever, Democratic Republic of the Congo, 1995. Commission de Lutte contre les Epidémies à Kikwit. *J Infect Dis* **179**(Suppl 1):S76–S86.
10. **Centers for Disease Control and Prevention (CDC).** 2001. Outbreak of Ebola hemorrhagic fever Uganda, August 2000-January 2001. *MMWR Morb Mortal Wkly Rep* **50:**73–77.
11. **Leroy EM, Epelboin A, Mondonge V, Pourrut X, Gonzalez J-P, Muyembe-Tamfum J-J, Formenty P.** 2009. Human Ebola outbreak resulting from direct exposure to fruit bats in Luebo, Democratic Republic of Congo, 2007. *Vector Borne Zoonotic Dis* **9:**723–728.
12. **Sanchez A, Kiley MP, Holloway BP, Auperin DD.** 1993. Sequence analysis of the Ebola virus genome: organization, genetic elements, and comparison with the genome of Marburg virus. *Virus Res* **29:**215–240.
13. **Elliott LH, Kiley MP, McCormick JB.** 1985. Descriptive analysis of Ebola virus proteins. *Virology* **147:**169–176.
14. **Sanchez A, Trappier SG, Mahy BW, Peters CJ, Nichol ST.** 1996. The virion glycoproteins of Ebola viruses are encoded in two reading frames and are expressed through transcriptional editing. *Proc Natl Acad Sci USA* **93:**3602–3607.
15. **de La Vega M-A, Wong G, Kobinger GP, Qiu X.** The multiple roles of sGP in Ebola pathogenesis. *Viral Immunol* [Epub ahead of print.] doi:10.1089/vim.2014.0068.
16. **Ramanan P, Shabman RS, Brown CS, Amarasinghe GK, Basler CF, Leung DW.** 2011. Filoviral immune evasion mechanisms. *Viruses* **3:**1634–1649.
17. **Berman M, du Lac JF, Izadi E, Dennis B.** 2014. As Ebola confirmed in U.S., CDC vows: 'We're stopping it in its tracks'. *The Washington Post.* https://www.washingtonpost.com/news/to-your-health/wp/2014/09/30/cdc-confirms-first-case-of-ebola-in-the-u-s/.
18. **World Health Organization.** 2016. Ebola data and statistics. http://apps.who.int/gho/data/view.ebola-sitrep.ebola-summary-latest?lang=en.
19. **Butler D.** 2014. Global Ebola response kicks into gear at last. *Nature* **513:**469–469.

20. Meltzer MI, Atkins CY, Santibanez S, Knust B, Petersen BW, Ervin ED, Nichol ST, Damon IK, Washington ML, Centers for Disease Control and Prevention (CDC). 2014. Estimating the future number of cases in the Ebola epidemic: Liberia and Sierra Leone, 2014-2015. *MMWR Surveill Summ* **63**(Suppl 3):1–14.

21. WHO Ebola Response Team. 2014. Ebola virus disease in West Africa: the first 9 months of the epidemic and forward projections. *N Engl J Med* **371**:1481–1495.

22. Borio L, Cox E, Lurie N. 2015. Combating emerging threats: accelerating the availability of medical therapies. *N Engl J Med* **373**:993–995.

23. Joffe S. 2014. Evaluating novel therapies during the Ebola epidemic. *JAMA* **312**:1299–1300.

24. van Griensven J, Weiggheleire AD, Delamou A, Smith PG, Edwards T, Vandekerckhove P, Bah EI, Colebunders R, Herve I, Lazaygues C, Haba N, Lynen L. 2015. The use of Ebola convalescent plasma to treat Ebola virus disease in resource-constrained settings: a perspective from the field. *Clin Infect Dis* **62**:69–74.

25. Gulland A. 2014. Clinical trials of Ebola therapies to begin in December. *BMJ* **349**:g6827.

26. FDA. 2014. Information for consumers (drugs): the FDA's drug review process: ensuring drugs are safe and effective. http://www.fda.gov/drugs/resourcesforyou/consumers/ucm143534.htm.

27. Chertow DS, Kleine C, Edwards JK, Scaini R, Giuliani R, Sprecher A. 2014. Ebola virus disease in West Africa: clinical manifestations and management. *N Engl J Med* **371**:2054–2057.

28. Boyles T. 2015. Priorities in Ebola research: a view from the field. *Lancet* **385**:23.

29. World Health Organization. 2014. WHO list of essential medicines necessary to treat Ebola cases. http://www.who.int/csr/resources/publications/ebola/ebola-medicines/en/.

30. Lamontagne F, Clément C, Fletcher T, Jacob ST, Fischer WA II, Fowler RA. 2014. Doing today's work superbly well: treating Ebola with current tools. *N Engl J Med* **371**:1565–1566.

31. Fowler RA, Fletcher T, Fischer WA II, Lamontagne F, Jacob S, Brett-Major D, Lawler JV, Jacquerioz FA, Houlihan C, O'Dempsey T, Ferri M, Adachi T, Lamah M-C, Bah EI, Mayet T, Schieffelin J, McLellan SL, Senga M, Kato Y, Clement C, Mardel S, Vallenas Bejar De Villar RC, Shindo N, Bausch D. 2014. Caring for critically ill patients with Ebola virus disease. Perspectives from West Africa. *Am J Respir Crit Care Med* **190**:733–737.

32. Wong KK, Perdue CL, Malia J, Kenney JL, Peng S, Gwathney JK, Raczniak GA, Monrovia Medical Unit. 2015. Supportive care of the first 2 Ebola virus disease patients at the Monrovia Medical Unit. *Clin Infect Dis* **61**:e47–e51.

33. Johnson DW, Sullivan JN, Piquette CA, Hewlett AL, Bailey KL, Smith PW, Kalil AC, Lisco SJ. 2015. Lessons learned: critical care management of patients with Ebola in the United States. *Crit Care Med* **43**:1157–1164.

34. Rodríguez-Caravaca G, Timermans R, Parra-Ramírez JM, Domínguez-Hernández FJ, Algora-Weber A, Delgado-Iribarren A, Hermida-Gutiérrez G, Ebola Virus Management Committee. 2015. Health-care management of an unexpected case of Ebola virus disease at the Alcorcón Foundation University Teaching Hospital. *Enferm Infecc Microbiol Clin* **33**:228–232.

35. Lyon GM, Mehta AK, Varkey JB, Brantly K, Plyler L, McElroy AK, Kraft CS, Towner JS, Spiropoulou C, Ströher U, Uyeki TM, Ribner BS, Emory Serious Communicable Diseases Unit. 2014. Clinical care of two patients with Ebola virus disease in the United States. *N Engl J Med* **371**:2402–2409.

36. Büttner S, Koch B, Dolnik O, Eickmann M, Freiwald T, Rudolf S, Engel J, Becker S, Ronco C, Geiger H. 2014. Extracorporeal virus elimination for the treatment of severe Ebola virus disease: first experience with lectin affinity plasmapheresis. *Blood Purif* **38**:286–291.

37. Mora-Rillo M, Arsuaga M, Ramírez-Olivencia G, de la Calle F, Borobia AM, Sánchez-Seco P, Lago M, Figueira JC, Fernández-Puntero B, Viejo A, Negredo A, Nuñez C, Flores E, Carcas AJ, Jiménez-Yuste V, Lasala F, García-de-Lorenzo A, Arnalich F, Arribas JR, La Paz-Carlos III, University Hospital Isolation Unit. 2015. Acute respiratory distress syndrome after convalescent plasma use: treatment of a patient with Ebola virus disease contracted in Madrid, Spain. *Lancet Respir Med* **3**:554–562.

38. World Health Organization. 2014. Ethical considerations for use of unregistered interventions for Ebola virus disease. http://www.who.int/csr/resources/publications/ebola/ethical-considerations/en/.

39. Food and Drug Administration. 2016. Expanded access (compassionate use). http://www.fda.gov/NewsEvents/PublicHealthFocus/ExpandedAccessCompassionateUse/default.htm.

40. Wilson JA, Hevey M, Bakken R, Guest S, Bray M, Schmaljohn AL, Hart MK. 2000. Epitopes involved in antibody-mediated protection from Ebola virus. *Science* **287**:1664–1666.

41. Zeitlin L, Pettitt J, Scully C, Bohorova N, Kim D, Pauly M, Hiatt A, Ngo L, Steinkellner

H, Whaley KJ, Olinger GG. 2011. Enhanced potency of a fucose-free monoclonal antibody being developed as an Ebola virus immuno-protectant. *Proc Natl Acad Sci USA* **108:** 20690–20694.

42. **Qiu X, Fernando L, Melito PL, Audet J, Feldmann H, Kobinger G, Alimonti JB, Jones SM.** 2012. Ebola GP-specific monoclonal antibodies protect mice and guinea pigs from lethal Ebola virus infection. *PLoS Negl Trop Dis* **6:** e1575. doi:10.1371/journal.pntd.0001575.

43. **Pettitt J, Zeitlin L, Kim DH, Working C, Johnson JC, Bohorov O, Bratcher B, Hiatt E, Hume SD, Johnson AK, Morton J, Pauly MH, Whaley KJ, Ingram MF, Zovanyi A, Heinrich M, Piper A, Zelko J, Olinger GG.** 2013. Therapeutic intervention of Ebola virus infection in rhesus macaques with the MB-003 monoclonal antibody cocktail. *Sci Transl Med* **5:**199ra113.

44. **Qiu X, Audet J, Wong G, Pillet S, Bello A, Cabral T, Strong JE, Plummer F, Corbett CR, Alimonti JB, Kobinger GP.** 2012. Successful treatment of Ebola virus–infected cynomolgus macaques with monoclonal antibodies. *Sci Transl Med* **4:**138ra81.

45. **Qiu X, Wong G, Audet J, Bello A, Fernando L, Alimonti JB, Fausther-Bovendo H, Wei H, Aviles J, Hiatt E, Johnson A, Morton J, Swope K, Bohorov O, Bohorova N, Goodman C, Kim D, Pauly MH, Velasco J, Pettitt J, Olinger GG, Whaley K, Xu B, Strong JE, Zeitlin L, Kobinger GP.** 2014. Reversion of advanced Ebola virus disease in nonhuman primates with ZMapp. *Nature* **514:**47–53.

46. **McCarthyM.** 2014. US signs contract with ZMapp maker to accelerate development of the Ebola drug. *BMJ* **349:**g5488.

47. **Anonymous.** 2015. Putative investigational therapeutics in the treatment of patients with known Ebola infection. https://clinicaltrials.gov/ct2/show/NCT02363322.

48. **National Institute of Allergy and Infectious Diseases.** 2015. Liberia-U.S. clinical research partnership opens trial to test Ebola treatments. http://www.niaid.nih.gov/news/newsreleases/2015/Pages/ZMapp.aspx.

49. **Whaley KJ, Hiatt A, Zeitlin L.** 2011. Emerging antibody products and *Nicotiana* manufacturing. *Hum Vaccin* **7:**349–356.

50. **Bernstein L, Dennis B.** 2014. Ebola test drug's supply "exhausted" after shipments to Africa, U.S. company says. *The Washington Post.* https://www.washingtonpost.com/national/health-science/ebola-test-drugs-supply-exhausted-after-shipments-to-africa-us-company-says/2014/08/11/020cefc0-2199-11e4-958c-268a320a60ce_story.html.

51. **Pollack A.** 2014. U.S. will increase production of the Ebola drug ZMapp, but may not meet demand. *NY Times.* http://www.nytimes.com/2014/10/02/world/us-to-increase-production-of-experimental-drug-but-may-not-meet-demand.html.

52. **Fink S.** 2015. A Chinese Ebola drug raises hopes, and rancor. *NY Times.* http://www.nytimes.com/2015/06/12/world/chinese-ebola-drug-brings-american-objections.html.

53. **Sky News.** 2015. Is MIL-77 the new Ebola-fighting wonder drug? *Sky News.* http://news.sky.com/story/1454079/is-mil-77-the-new-ebola-fighting-wonder-drug.

54. **World Health Organization.** 2015. Ebola vaccines, therapies, and diagnostics. http://www.who.int/medicines/emp_ebola_q_as/en/.

55. **World Health Organization.** 2014. *Use of Convalescent Whole Blood or Plasma Collected from Patients Recovered from Ebola Virus Disease.* WHO, Geneva, Switzerland. http://www.who.int/csr/resources/publications/ebola/convalescent-treatment/en/.

56. **Jahrling PB, Geisbert JB, Swearengen JR, Larsen T, Geisbert TW.** 2007. Ebola hemorrhagic fever: evaluation of passive immunotherapy in nonhuman primates. *J Infect Dis* **196**(Suppl 2):S400–S403.

57. **Emond RT, Evans B, Bowen ET, Lloyd G.** 1977. A case of Ebola virus infection. *BMJ* **2:** 541–544.

58. **Mupapa K, Massamba M, Kibadi K, Kuvula K, Bwaka A, Kipasa M, Colebunders R, Muyembe-Tamfum JJ, International Scientific and Technical Committee.** 1999. Treatment of Ebola hemorrhagic fever with blood transfusions from convalescent patients. *J Infect Dis* **179**(Suppl 1):S18–S23.

59. **Sadek RF, Khan AS, Stevens G, Peters CJ, Ksiazek TG.** 1999. Ebola hemorrhagic fever, Democratic Republic of the Congo, 1995: determinants of survival. *J Infect Dis* **179** (Suppl 1):S24–S27.

60. **Jahrling PB, Geisbert J, Swearengen JR, Jaax GP, Lewis T, Huggins JW, Schmidt JJ, LeDuc JW, Peters CJ.** 1996. Passive immunization of Ebola virus-infected cynomolgus monkeys with immunoglobulin from hyperimmune horses. *Arch Virol Suppl* **11:**135–140.

61. **Oswald WB, Geisbert TW, Davis KJ, Geisbert JB, Sullivan NJ, Jahrling PB, Parren PW, Burton DR.** 2007. Neutralizing antibody fails to impact the course of Ebola virus infection in monkeys. *PLoS Pathog* **3:**e9.

62. **Wong G, Richardson JS, Pillet S, Patel A, Qiu X, Alimonti J, Hogan J, Zhang Y, Takada A, Feldmann H, Kobinger GP.** 2012. Immune

parameters correlate with protection against Ebola virus infection in rodents and nonhuman primates. *Sci Transl Med* **4:**158ra146.

63. **Olinger GG, Pettitt J, Kim D, Working C, Bohorov O, Bratcher B, Hiatt E, Hume SD, Johnson AK, Morton J, Pauly M, Whaley KJ, Lear CM, Biggins JE, Scully C, Hensley L, Zeitlin L.** 2012. Delayed treatment of Ebola virus infection with plant-derived monoclonal antibodies provides protection in rhesus macaques. *Proc Natl Acad Sci USA* **109:**18030–18035.

64. **van Griensven J, Edwards T, de Lamballerie X, Semple MG, Gallian P, Baize S, Horby PW, Raoul H, Magassouba N, Antierens A, Lomas C, Faye O, Sall AA, Fransen K, Buyze J, Ravinetto R, Tiberghien P, Claeys Y, De Crop M, Lynen L, Bah EI, Smith PG, Delamou A, De Weggheleire A, Haba N, Ebola-Tx Consortium.** 2016. Evaluation of convalescent plasma for Ebola virus disease in Guinea. *N Engl J Med* **374:**33–42.

65. **Florescu DF, Kalil AC, Hewlett AL, Schuh AJ, Stroher U, Uyeki TM, Smith PW.** 2015. Administration of brincidofovir and convalescent plasma in a patient with Ebola virus disease. *Clin Infect Dis* **61:**969–973.

66. **Kraft CS, Hewlett AL, Koepsell S, Winkler AM, Kratochvil CJ, Larson L, Varkey JB, Mehta AK, Lyon GM, Friedman-Moraco RJ, Marconi VC, Hill CE, Sullivan JN, Johnson DW, Lisco SJ, Mulligan MJ, Uyeki TM, McElroy AK, Sealy T, Campbell S, Spiropoulou C, Ströher U, Crozier I, Sacra R, Connor MJ, Sueblinvong V, Franch HA, Smith PW, Ribner BS.** 2015. Nebraska Biocontainment Unit and the Emory Serious Communicable Diseases Unit. The use of TKM-100802 and convalescent plasma in 2 patients with Ebola virus disease in the United States. *Clin Infect Dis* **61:**496–502.

67. **Liddell AM, Davey RT Jr, Mehta AK, Varkey JB, Kraft CS, Tseggay GK, Badidi O, Faust AC, Brown KV, Suffredini AF, Barrett K, Wolcott MJ, Marconi VC, Lyon GM III, Weinstein GL, Weinmeister K, Sutton S, Hazbun M, Albariño CG, Reed Z, Cannon D, Ströher U, Feldman M, Ribner BS, Lane HC, Fauci AS, Uyeki TM.** 2015. Characteristics and clinical management of a cluster of 3 patients with Ebola virus disease, including the first domestically acquired cases in the United States. *Ann Intern Med* **163:**81–90.

68. **U.S. Securities and Exchange Commission.** 2010. Biopharma AVI. 10-Q report. http://www.sec.gov/Archives/edgar/data/873303/000110465910043138/a10-12966_110q.htm.

69. **Zamecnik PC, Stephenson ML.** 1978. Inhibition of Rous sarcoma virus replication and cell transformation by a specific oligodeoxynucleotide. *Proc Natl Acad Sci USA* **75:**280–284.

70. **Watts JK, Corey DR.** 2012. Gene silencing by siRNAs and antisense oligonucleotides in the laboratory and the clinic. *J Pathol* **226:**365–379.

71. **Warfield KL, Swenson DL, Olinger GG, Nichols DK, Pratt WD, Blouch R, Stein DA, Aman MJ, Iversen PL, Bavari S.** 2006. Gene-specific countermeasures against Ebola virus based on antisense phosphorodiamidate morpholino oligomers. *PLoS Pathog* **2:**e1. doi:10.1371/journal.ppat.0020001.

72. **Warren TK, Warfield KL, Wells J, Swenson DL, Donner KS, Van Tongeren SA, Garza NL, Dong L, Mourich DV, Crumley S, Nichols DK, Iversen PL, Bavari S.** 2010. Advanced antisense therapies for postexposure protection against lethal filovirus infections. *Nat Med* **16:**991–994.

73. **Heald AE, Iversen PL, Saoud JB, Sazani P, Charleston JS, Axtelle T, Wong M, Smith WB, Vutikullird A, Kaye E.** 2014. Safety and pharmacokinetic profiles of phosphorodiamidate morpholino oligomers with activity against ebola virus and marburg virus: results of two single-ascending-dose studies. *Antimicrob Agents Chemother* **58:**6639–6647.

74. **Warren TK, Whitehouse CA, Wells J, Welch L, Heald AE, Charleston JS, Sazani P, Reid SP, Iversen PL, Bavari S.** 2015. A single phosphorodiamidate morpholino oligomer targeting VP24 protects rhesus monkeys against lethal Ebola virus infection. *mBio* **6:**e02344-14. doi:10.1128/mBio.02344-14.

75. **U.S. Securities and Exchange Commission.** 2015. Sarepta Therapeutics, Inc. 10-Q Report. http://www.sec.gov/Archives/edgar/data/873303/000156459015009495/srpt-10q_20150930.htm.

76. **Calma J.** 2015. Ebola drug killed by congressional inaction less than two years before outbreak. NOVA Next, PBS. http://www.pbs.org/wgbh/nova/next/body/ebola-drug-halted/.

77. **Warren TK, Wells J, Panchal RG, Stuthman KS, Garza NL, Van Tongeren SA, Dong L, Retterer CJ, Eaton BP, Pegoraro G, Honnold S, Bantia S, Kotian P, Chen X, Taubenheim BR, Welch LS, Minning DM, Babu YS, Sheridan WP, Bavari S.** 2014. Protection against filovirus diseases by a novel broad-spectrum nucleoside analogue BCX4430. *Nature* **508:**402–405.

78. **U.S. Securities and Exchange Commission.** 2015. Biocryst Pharmaceuticals. 10-Q report. http://www.sec.gov/Archives/edgar/data/882796/000117184315004473/gfpf10q_080715.htm.

79. **ClinicalTrialsgov.** 2014. A phase 1 study to evaluate the safety, tolerability and pharmacokinetics of BCX4430. https://clinicaltrials.gov/ct2/show/NCT02319772.

80. **U.S. Department of Health and Human Services.** 2015. HHS contracts to develop new Ebola drug. http://www.hhs.gov/news/press/2015pres/03/20150331a.html.

81. **Furuta Y, Takahashi K, Shiraki K, Sakamoto K, Smee DF, Barnard DL, Gowen BB, Julander JG, Morrey JD.** 2009. T-705 (favipiravir) and related compounds: novel broad-spectrum inhibitors of RNA viral infections. *Antiviral Res* **82:**95–102.

82. **Morrey JD, Taro BS, Siddharthan V, Wang H, Smee DF, Christensen AJ, Furuta Y.** 2008. Efficacy of orally administered T-705 pyrazine analog on lethal West Nile virus infection in rodents. *Antiviral Res* **80:**377–379.

83. **Julander JG, Shafer K, Smee DF, Morrey JD, Furuta Y.** 2009. Activity of T-705 in a hamster model of yellow fever virus infection in comparison with that of a chemically related compound, T-1106. *Antimicrob Agents Chemother* **53:**202–209.

84. **Safronetz D, Rosenke K, Westover JB, Martellaro C, Okumura A, Furuta Y, Geisbert J, Saturday G, Komeno T, Geisbert TW, Feldmann H, Gowen BB.** 2015. The broad-spectrum antiviral favipiravir protects guinea pigs from lethal Lassa virus infection post-disease onset. *Sci Rep* **5:**14775. doi:10.1038/srep14775.

85. **Oestereich L, Lüdtke A, Wurr S, Rieger T, Muñoz-Fontela C, Günther S.** 2014. Successful treatment of advanced Ebola virus infection with T-705 (favipiravir) in a small animal model. *Antiviral Res* **105:**17–21.

86. **Smither SJ, Eastaugh LS, Steward JA, Nelson M, Lenk RP, Lever MS.** 2014. Post-exposure efficacy of oral T-705 (Favipiravir) against inhalational Ebola virus infection in a mouse model. *Antiviral Res* **104:**153–155.

87. **Jacobs M, Aarons E, Bhagani S, Buchanan R, Cropley I, Hopkins S, Lester R, Martin D, Marshall N, Mepham S, Warren S, Rodger A.** 2015. Post-exposure prophylaxis against Ebola virus disease with experimental antiviral agents: a case-series of health-care workers. *Lancet Infect Dis* **15:**1300–1304.

88. **Schibler M, Vetter P, Cherpillod P, Petty TJ, Cordey S, Vieille G, Yerly S, Siegrist C-A, Samii K, Dayer J-A, Docquier M, Zdobnov EM, Simpson AJH, Rees PSC, Sarria FB, Gasche Y, Chappuis F, Iten A, Pittet D, Pugin J, Kaiser L.** 2015. Clinical features and viral kinetics in a rapidly cured patient with Ebola virus disease: a case report. *Lancet Infect Dis* **15:**1034–1040.

89. **Petrosillo N, Nicastri E, Lanini S, Capobianchi MR, Di Caro A, Antonini M, Puro V, Lauria FN, Shindo N, Magrini N, Kobinger GP, Ippolito G, INMI EBOV Team.** 2015. Ebola virus disease complicated with viral interstitial pneumonia: a case report. *BMC Infect Dis* **15:**432.

90. **Wolf T, Kann G, Becker S, Stephan C, Brodt H-R, de Leuw P, Grünewald T, Vogl T, Kempf VAJ, Keppler OT, Zacharowski K.** 2015. Severe Ebola virus disease with vascular leakage and multiorgan failure: treatment of a patient in intensive care. *Lancet* **385:**1428–1435.

91. **ClinicalTrialsgov.** 2015. Efficacy of favipiravir against ebola (JIKI). https://clinicaltrials.gov/ct2/show/NCT02329054?term=favipiravir&rank=5.

92. **Sissoko D, Anglaret X, Malvy D, Folkesson E, M'lebing A, Shepherd S, Danel C, Beavogui AH, Gunther S, Mentre F.** 2015. Favipiravir in patients with Ebola virus disease: early results of the JIKI trial in Guinea, abstr 103-ALB. Abstr. Conf Retroviruses and Opportunistic Infections, Int Antiviral Soc, Seattle, WA. http://www.croiconference.org/sessions/favipiravir-patients-ebola-virus-disease-early-results-jiki-trial-guinea.

93. **Thi EP, Mire CE, Lee ACH, Geisbert JB, Zhou JZ, Agans KN, Snead NM, Deer DJ, Barnard TR, Fenton KA, MacLachlan I, Geisbert TW.** 2015. Lipid nanoparticle siRNA treatment of Ebola-virus-Makona-infected nonhuman primates. *Nature* **521:**362–365.

94. **Geisbert TW, Hensley LE, Kagan E, Yu EZ, Geisbert JB, Daddario-DiCaprio K, Fritz EA, Jahrling PB, McClintock K, Phelps JR, Lee ACH, Judge A, Jeffs LB, MacLachlan I.** 2006. Postexposure protection of guinea pigs against a lethal Ebola virus challenge is conferred by RNA interference. *J Infect Dis* **193:**1650–1657.

95. **Geisbert TW, Lee AC, Robbins M, Geisbert JB, Honko AN, Sood V, Johnson JC, de Jong S, Tavakoli I, Judge A, Hensley LE, Maclachlan I.** 2010. Postexposure protection of non-human primates against a lethal Ebola virus challenge with RNA interference: a proof-of-concept study. *Lancet* **375:**1896–1905.

96. **Kroll D.** 2014. Tekmira tempers FDA OK for Ebola drug access. http://www.forbes.com/sites/davidkroll/2014/09/22/tekmira-tempers-fda-ok-for-ebola-drug-access/.

97. **Associated Press.** 2015. Tekmira says Ebola drug unlikely to work in study. *US News World Rep.* http://www.usnews.com/news/business/articles/2015/06/19/tekmira-stops-adding-patients-in-african-study-of-ebola-drug.

98. **ClinicalTrialsgov.** 2015. Safety, tolerability and pharmacokinetic first in human (FIH) study for intravenous (IV) TKM-100802. https://clinicaltrials.gov/ct2/show/NCT02041715.

99. **Warren T.** 2015. Nucleotide prodrug GS-5734 is a broad-spectrum filovirus inhibitor that provides complete therapeutic protection against the development of Ebola virus disease (EVD) in infected non-human primates. Presented at ID Week 2015, San Diego, CA. https://idsa.confex.com/idsa/2015/webprogram/Paper54208.html.

100. **Donnelly L.** 2015. Ebola caused meningitis in nurse Pauline Cafferkey. *The Telegraph.* http://www.telegraph.co.uk/news/health/news/11945802/Ebola-caused-meningitis-in-nurse-Pauline-Cafferkey.html.

101. **Lawson ND, Stillman EA, Whitt MA, Rose JK.** 1995. Recombinant vesicular stomatitis viruses from DNA. *Proc Natl Acad Sci USA* **92:**4477–4481.

102. **Garbutt M, Liebscher R, Wahl-Jensen V, Jones S, Möller P, Wagner R, Volchkov V, Klenk H-D, Feldmann H, Ströher U.** 2004. Properties of replication-competent vesicular stomatitis virus vectors expressing glycoproteins of filoviruses and arenaviruses. *J Virol* **78:**5458–5465.

103. **Jones SM, Feldmann H, Ströher U, Geisbert JB, Fernando L, Grolla A, Klenk HD, Sullivan NJ, Volchkov VE, Fritz EA, Daddario KM, Hensley LE, Jahrling PB, Geisbert TW.** 2005. Live attenuated recombinant vaccine protects nonhuman primates against Ebola and Marburg viruses. *Nat Med* **11:**786–790.

104. **Marzi A, Robertson SJ, Haddock E, Feldmann F, Hanley PW, Scott DP, Strong JE, Kobinger G, Best SM, Feldmann H.** 2015. EBOLA VACCINE. VSV-EBOV rapidly protects macaques against infection with the 2014/15 Ebola virus outbreak strain. *Science* **349:**739–742.

105. **Feldmann H, Jones SM, Daddario-DiCaprio KM, Geisbert JB, Ströher U, Grolla A, Bray M, Fritz EA, Fernando L, Feldmann F, Hensley LE, Geisbert TW.** Effective postexposure treatment of Ebola infection. *PLoS Pathog* **3:**e2. doi:10.1371/journal.ppat.0030002.

106. **Lai L, Davey R, Beck A, Xu Y, Suffredini AF, Palmore T, Kabbani S, Rogers S, Kobinger G, Alimonti J, Link CJ, Jr, Rubinson L, Ströher U, Wolcott M, Dorman W, Uyeki TM, Feldmann H, Lane HC, Mulligan MJ.** 2015. Emergency postexposure vaccination with vesicular stomatitis virus-vectored Ebola vaccine after needlestick. *JAMA* **313:**1249–1255.

107. **Schnirring L.** 2014. *NewLink, Merck deal boosts prospects for Ebola vaccine.* Univ Minn CIDRAP. http://www.cidrap.umn.edu/news-perspective/2014/11/newlink-merck-deal-boosts-prospects-ebola-vaccine.

108. **Genetic Engineering and Biotechnology News.** 2014. BARDA awards $30M toward NewLink-Merck Ebola vaccine candidate. http://www.genengnews.com/gen-news-highlights/barda-awards-30m-toward-newlink-merck-ebola-vaccine-candidate/81250726/.

109. **Agnandji ST, Huttner A, Zinser ME, Njuguna P, Dahlke C, Fernandes JF, Yerly S, Dayer J-A, Kraehling V, Kasonta R, Adegnika AA, Altfeld M, Auderset F, Bache EB, Biedenkopf N, Borregaard S, Brosnahan JS, Burrow R, Combescure C, Desmeules J, Eickmann M, Fehling SK, Finckh A, Goncalves AR, Grobusch MP, Hooper J, Jambrecina S, Kabwende AL, Kaya G, Kimani D, Lell B, Lemaître B, Lohse AW, Massinga-Loembe M, Matthey A, Mordmüller B, Nolting A, Ogwang C, Ramharter M, Schmidt-Chanasit J, Schmiedel S, Silvera P, Stahl FR, Staines HM, Strecker T, Stubbe HC, Tsofa B, Zaki Z, Fast P, Moorthy V, Kaiser L, Krishna S, Stephan Becker S, Kieny M-P, Bejon P, Kremsner PG, Addo MM, Siegrist C-A.** 2015. Phase 1 trials of rVSV Ebola vaccine in Africa and Europe: preliminary report. *N Engl J Med.* doi:10.1056/NEJMoa1502924.

110. **Pierson JF.** 2015. Overview of the Partnership for Research on Ebola Vaccines in Liberia (PREVAIL) Study. Presentation to the Vaccines and Related Biological Products Advisory Committee, Silver Spring, MD. http://www.fda.gov/downloads/AdvisoryCommittees/CommitteesMeetingMaterials/BloodVaccinesandOtherBiologics/VaccinesandRelatedBiologicalProductsAdvisoryCommittee/UCM448001.pdf.

111. **Helfand R.** 2015. Overview of the Sierra Leone Trial to Introduce a Vaccine against Ebola (STRIVE) Study. Presentation to the Vaccines and Related Biological Products Advisory Committee, Silver Spring, MD. http://www.fda.gov/downloads/AdvisoryCommittees/CommitteesMeetingMaterials/BloodVaccinesandOtherBiologics/VaccinesandRelatedBiologicalProductsAdvisoryCommittee/UCM448002.pdf.

112. **Ebola ça Suffit Ring Vaccination Trial Consortium.** 2015. The ring vaccination trial: a novel cluster randomised controlled trial design to evaluate vaccine efficacy and effectiveness during outbreaks, with special reference to Ebola. *BMJ* **351:**h3740.

113. **Henao-Restrepo AM, Longini IM, Egger M, Dean NE, Edmunds WJ, Camacho A, Carroll**

MW, Doumbia M, Draguez B, Duraffour S, Enwere G, Grais R, Gunther S, Hossmann S, Kondé MK, Kone S, Kuisma E, Levine MM, Mandal S, Norheim G, Riveros X, Soumah A, Trelle S, Vicari AS, Watson CH, Kéïta S, Kieny MP, Røttingen J-A. 2015. Efficacy and effectiveness of an rVSV-vectored vaccine expressing Ebola surface glycoprotein: interim results from the Guinea ring vaccination cluster-randomised trial. *Lancet* **386:**857–866.

114. Krause PR. 2015. Interim results from a phase 3 Ebola vaccine study in Guinea. *Lancet* **386:**831–833.

115. Sullivan NJ, Sanchez A, Rollin PE, Yang ZY, Nabel GJ. 2000. Development of a preventive vaccine for Ebola virus infection in primates. *Nature* **408:**605–609.

116. Sullivan NJ, Geisbert TW, Geisbert JB, Xu L, Yang ZY, Roederer M, Koup RA, Jahrling PB, Nabel GJ. 2003. Accelerated vaccination for Ebola virus haemorrhagic fever in non-human primates. *Nature* **424:**681–684.

117. Sullivan NJ, Geisbert TW, Geisbert JB, Shedlock DJ, Xu L, Lamoreaux L, Custers JHHV, Popernack PM, Yang Z-Y, Pau MG, Roederer M, Koup RA, Goudsmit J, Jahrling PB, Nabel GJ. 2006. Immune protection of nonhuman primates against Ebola virus with single low-dose adenovirus vectors encoding modified GPs. *PLoS Med* **3:**e177. doi:10.1371/journal.pmed.0030177.

118. Sullivan NJ, Hensley L, Asiedu C, Geisbert TW, Stanley D, Johnson J, Honko A, Olinger G, Bailey M, Geisbert JB, Reimann KA, Bao S, Rao S, Roederer M, Jahrling PB, Koup RA, Nabel GJ. 2011. CD8+ cellular immunity mediates rAd5 vaccine protection against Ebola virus infection of nonhuman primates. *Nat Med* **17:**1128–1131.

119. Ledgerwood JE, DeZure AD, Stanley DA, Novik L, Enama ME, Berkowitz NM, Hu Z, Joshi G, Ploquin A, Sitar S, Gordon IJ, Plummer SA, Holman LA, Hendel CS, Yamshchikov G, Roman F, Nicosia A, Colloca S, Cortese R, Bailer RT, Schwartz RM, Roederer M, Mascola JR, Koup RA, Sullivan NJ, Graham BS, the VRC 207 Study Team. 2014. Chimpanzee adenovirus vector Ebola vaccine: preliminary report. *N Engl J Med* **373:**775–776.

120. Rampling T, Ewer K, Bowyer G, Wright D, Imoukhuede EB, Payne R, Hartnell F, Gibani M, Bliss C, Minhinnick A, Wilkie M, Venkatraman N, Poulton I, Lella N, Roberts R, Sierra-Davidson K, Krähling V, Berrie E, Roman F, De Ryck I, Nicosia A, Sullivan NJ, Stanley DA, Ledgerwood JE, Schwartz RM, Siani L, Colloca S, Folgori A, Di Marco S, Cortese R, Becker S, Graham BS, Koup RA, Levine MM, Moorthy V, Pollard AJ, Draper SJ, Ballou WR, Lawrie A, Gilbert SC, Hill AVS. 2015. A monovalent chimpanzee adenovirus Ebola vaccine: preliminary report. *N Engl J Med*. [Epub ahead of print.] doi:10.1056/NEJMoa1411627.

121. Geisbert TW, Bailey M, Hensley L, Asiedu C, Geisbert J, Stanley D, Honko A, Johnson J, Mulangu S, Pau MG, Custers J, Vellinga J, Hendriks J, Jahrling P, Roederer M, Goudsmit J, Koup R, Sullivan NJ. 2011. Recombinant adenovirus serotype 26 (Ad26) and Ad35 vaccine vectors bypass immunity to Ad5 and protect nonhuman primates against ebolavirus challenge. *J Virol* **85:**4222–4233.

122. Stanley DA, Honko AN, Asiedu C, Trefry JC, Lau-Kilby AW, Johnson JC, Hensley L, Ammendola V, Abbate A, Grazioli F, Foulds KE, Cheng C, Wang L, Donaldson MM, Colloca S, Folgori A, Roederer M, Nabel GJ, Mascola J, Nicosia A, Cortese R, Koup RA, Sullivan NJ. 2014. Chimpanzee adenovirus vaccine generates acute and durable protective immunity against ebolavirus challenge. *Nat Med* **20:**1126–1129.

123. Genetic Engineering and Biotechnology News. 2014. Janssen, Bavarian Nordic enter Ebola vaccine deal. *GEN News*. http://www.genengnews.com/gen-news-highlights/janssen-bavarian-nordic-enter-ebola-vaccine-deal/81250500/.

124. Mire CE, Geisbert JB, Agans KN, Satterfield BA, Versteeg KM, Fritz EA, Feldmann H, Hensley LE, Geisbert TW. 2014. Durability of a vesicular stomatitis virus-based Marburg virus vaccine in nonhuman primates. *PLoS One* **9:**e94355. doi:10.1371/journal.pone.0094355.

125. Grover N. 2015. Novavax starts Ebola vaccine trial in humans. *Reuters*. http://www.reuters.com/article/us-health-ebola-novavax-idUSKBN0LG1NX20150212.

126. World Health Organization. 2014. *WHO consultation on potential Ebola therapies and vaccines*. WHO, Geneva, Switzerland. http://www.who.int/csr/resources/publications/ebola/ebola-therapies/en/.

127. Cox E, Borio L, Temple R. 2014. Evaluating Ebola therapies: the case for RCTs. *N Engl J Med* **371:**2350–2351.

Middle East Respiratory Syndrome (MERS)

4

SONJA A. RASMUSSEN,[1] AMELIA K. WATSON,[2] and DAVID L. SWERDLOW[1]

INTRODUCTION

The first patient identified with Middle East respiratory syndrome (MERS) was a 60-year-old male who presented in June of 2012 with fever, cough, and shortness of breath in Jeddah, Kingdom of Saudi Arabia (Saudi Arabia). The patient developed acute respiratory distress syndrome and subsequently died of respiratory and renal failure after being hospitalized for 11 days (1). After tests for other more common respiratory viruses were negative, a novel coronavirus was identified, which was initially called HCoV-EMC (human coronavirus-Erasmus Medical Center, referring to where the virologic studies had been performed) and later became known as Middle East respiratory syndrome coronavirus (MERS-CoV) (1). After information about this newly identified coronavirus was posted on the Program for Monitoring Emerging Diseases (ProMED) website by Dr. Ali Mohamed Zaki (2), a second patient with MERS-CoV was identified. This patient was a 49-year-old male with a history of travel to Saudi Arabia who presented to a hospital in Qatar with bilateral pneumonia in September 2012 and was later transported to the United Kingdom for intensive care, where he was determined to have the same novel coronavirus (3). Via genetic analysis, the cases from Saudi Arabia and Qatar were found to be 99.5% identical (4). Later, two deceased patients who

[1]Centers for Disease Control and Prevention, Atlanta, GA 30333; [2]The University of Georgia, Athens, GA 30602
Emerging Infections 10
Edited by W. Michael Scheld, James M. Hughes and Richard J. Whitley
© 2016 American Society for Microbiology, Washington, DC
doi:10.1128/microbiolspec.EI10-0020-2016

TABLE 1 Comparison of characteristics of SARS and MERS[a,b]

Characteristic	SARS	MERS
First patients reported	Guangdong, China, in November 2002	Zarqa, Jordan, in April 2012 Jeddah, Saudi Arabia, in June 2012
Virus	SARS-CoV	MERS-CoV
Type of coronavirus	Lineage b betacoronavirus	Lineage c betacoronavirus
Host cell receptor	Angiotensin converting enzyme 2	Dipeptidyl peptidase 4
Animal hosts	Chinese horseshoe bats, palm civets	Not yet confirmed, but camel is likely host
Incubation period		
Mean (95% CI; days)	4.6 (3.8–5.8)	5.2 (1.9–14.7)
Range (days)	2–14	2–13
Serial interval (days)	8.4	7.6
Basic reproduction number	2–3	<1
Patient characteristics		
Adults	93%	98%
Children	5–7%	2%
Age range (years)	1–91	1–94
Average age (years)	Mean 39.9	Median 50
Sex ratio (M:F)	43%:57%	64.5%:35.5%
Mortality		
Case fatality rate overall	9.6%	40%
Case fatality rate with comorbidities	46%	60%
Time (days) from symptom onset to hospitalization	2–8	0–16
Time (days) from symptom onset to death	21	12
Comorbidities	10–30%	76%
Clinical manifestations		
Fever	99–100%	98%
Chills/rigors	15–73%	87%
Cough	62–100%	83%
Hemoptysis	0–1%	17%
Headache	20–56%	11%
Myalgia	45–61%	32%
Malaise	31–45%	38%
Shortness of breath	40–42%	72%
Nausea	20–35%	21%
Vomiting	20–35%	21%
Diarrhea	20–25%	26%
Sore throat	13–25%	14%
Rhinorrhea	2–24%	6%
Laboratory results		
Radiographic abnormalities	94–100%	90–100%
Leukopenia	25–35%	14%
Lymphopenia	68–85%	32%
Thrombocytopenia	40–45%	36%
Elevated LDH	50–71%	48%
Elevated ALT	20–30%	11%
Elevated AST	20–30%	14%
Respiratory failure requiring mechanical ventilation	14–20%	80%

[a]Modified from references 26, 159, and 160.
[b]Abbreviations: SARS, severe acute respiratory syndrome; MERS, Middle East respiratory syndrome; CoV, coronavirus; LDH, lactate dehydrogenase; ALT, alanine aminotransferase; AST, aspartate transaminase.

were part of a cluster of 13 cases of suspected pneumonia among health care personnel at a hospital in Jordan that had occurred in April 2012 were diagnosed retrospectively as having MERS-CoV infection (5).

Many of the clinical features of MERS were similar to those seen in severe acute respiratory syndrome (SARS), which is caused by another coronavirus, SARS-coronavirus (SARS-CoV) (see Table 1 for characteristics of SARS compared to MERS), and because of these similarities, a high level of concern was raised (6, 7). SARS had caused an epidemic in 2002-2003 after it rapidly spread from China, where it originated, to over 8,000 people in 27 countries, with a case-fatality rate of nearly

TABLE 2 Chronology of key events[a,b]

Date	Key events
April 2012	Cluster of 13 patients in a hospital in Jordan with acute respiratory illness; two deceased patients of this cluster were retrospectively diagnosed (in September 2012) through study of stored specimens with MERS-CoV (5, 90)
13 June 2012	60-year-old man admitted to hospital in Saudi Arabia with a 7-day history of fever, cough, and dyspnea (1)
20 September 2012	Isolation of MERS-CoV from June case in Saudi Arabia reported on Program for Monitoring Emerging Diseases (ProMED) website by Dr. Ali Mohamed Zaki (1, 2)
September 2012	Diagnostic RT-PCR assay for MERS-CoV developed and used by Health Protection Agency in United Kingdom to identify second case of MERS in a patient who had been transferred from Qatar (4, 126)
25 September 2012	WHO releases case definition for MERS (162)
November 2012	Full genome of MERS-CoV characterized by Erasmus Medical Center (25)
February 2013	Definitive evidence of human-to-human transmission observed in family cluster in the United Kingdom (59)
March 2013	Dipeptidyl peptidase 4 determined to be host-cell receptor for MERS-CoV (27)
April 2013	Study in rhesus macaque animal model shows that MERS-CoV fulfills Koch's postulates (115)
April 2013	Largest cluster of MERS to date (as of April 2013) (23 cases) occurs in eastern Saudi Arabia (55)
3 June 2013	CDC activates its Emergency Operations Center to strengthen preparedness for MERS (deactivated on 13 August 2013) (23)
11 June 2013	Interim infection prevention and control recommendations for hospitalized patients with known or suspected MERS-CoV infection for U.S. hospitals issued by CDC (163)
9 and 17 July 2013 25 September 2013 4 December 2013 14 May 2014 17 June 2014 1 October 2014 5 February 2015 17 June 2015 3 September 2015	10 meetings of the International Health Regulations Emergency Health Committee convened by the WHO between July 2013 and December 2015: situation serious and of great concern, but conditions for Public Health Emergency of International Concern not met (http://www.who.int/ihr/ihr_ec_2013/en/)
August 2013	MERS-CoV neutralizing antibodies identified in Omani camels (73)
September 2013	Full genome sequence analysis of 21 MERS-CoV genomes identifies multiple zoonotic introductions, suggesting lower reproduction number (164)
November 2013	MERS-CoV detected in three camels and epidemiologically linked to two human cases (85)
Spring 2014	Rapid increase in the numbers of MERS cases reported in Arabian Peninsula (22)
2 and 11 May 2014	CDC confirms first and second (19) cases of MERS in the United States in Indiana and Florida, respectively. CDC activates its Emergency Operations Center on 2 May to respond to domestic case (deactivated on 12 June 2014)
20 May 2015	First patient with MERS reported in Republic of Korea (64); outbreak affecting >180 people ensues; largest outbreak outside of Saudi Arabia (165)

[a]Adapted in part from reference 161.
[b]Abbreviations: MERS-CoV, Middle East respiratory syndrome coronavirus; RT-PCR, reverse transcription PCR; WHO, World Health Organization.

10% and an estimated cost of tens of billions of dollars (8, 9). Genomic analysis of SARS-CoV showed that the virus evolved early on in the outbreak to become better adapted to humans, which permitted more efficient human-to-human transmission (10–13). The basic reproduction number for SARS (the expected number of secondary infections resulting from one infected person in a susceptible population) was estimated to be 2 to 4 (14, 15). However, SARS was characterized by superspreading events, in which a few cases were responsible for a large number of secondary cases; the majority of SARS cases did not transmit to others. The outbreak was brought under control in July 2003 after implementation of public health interventions, although additional cases related to laboratory or animal market exposures were seen later in 2003 and in 2004 (13). Since 2004, no additional SARS cases have been reported.

Since its discovery in 2012, MERS-CoV has been referred to by several different names, including HCoV-EMC, human betacoronavirus 2c EMC, HCoV-EMC/2012, human betacoronavirus 2c England-Qatar, human betacoronavirus 2C Jordan-N3, betacoronavirus England 1, and novel coronavirus, among others. Because of the confusion that these different names caused in the scientific literature, the Coronavirus Study Group of the International Committee on Taxonomy of Viruses met in 2013 and agreed to name the new coronavirus Middle East respiratory syndrome coronavirus (MERS-CoV) (16).

The outbreak of MERS has continued (see Table 2 for key events in the outbreak). As of 5 February 2016, 1,638 laboratory-confirmed cases (see Fig. 1 for epidemic curve) and 587 (36%) deaths had been reported to the World Health Organization (17). Strong evidence supports the role of the dromedary camel as

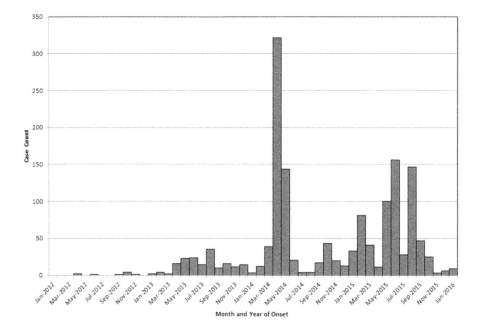

FIGURE 1 Cases of Middle East respiratory syndrome coronavirus, 2012 to 2016, by month and year of onset (total = 1,638 cases), as reported by the World Health Organization (data as of 5 February 2016). The total case counts include 130 cases identified from Saudi Arabia Ministry of Health's retrospective reviews, but these are not depicted in the epidemic curve due to unknown case onset dates.

the animal reservoir for MERS-CoV, but how the virus is transmitted to humans is not well understood (18). The vast majority of cases have been reported from Saudi Arabia, and all cases thus far recognized have direct or indirect links through travel or residence to countries in or near the Arabian Peninsula (Saudi Arabia, United Arab Emirates, Qatar, Oman, Jordan, Kuwait, Iran, Lebanon, and Yemen). Currently, the country with the second highest number of cases is the Republic of Korea, with an outbreak of more than 180 cases in 2015 following introduction into the country by a single patient who had traveled from the Middle East. As of 5 February 2016, 26 countries have reported cases of MERS to the World Health Organization (Fig. 2), with two patients with MERS reported in the United States, one in Indiana and the other in Florida, both in May of 2014 (19). Despite extensive evaluation and testing of contacts of these two patients in their households, communities, and health care settings, no

additional people infected with MERS were identified (20).

The Emergency Committee convened by the World Health Organization Director-General under the International Health Regulations (2005) met 10 times regarding MERS between July 2013 and December 2015, most recently on 2 September 2015. The Committee has continued to state that MERS does not currently constitute a Public Health Emergency of International Concern but noted a continued heightened sense of concern about the overall MERS situation. At the most recent meeting, the Emergency Committee emphasized the following (21):

• National authorities should ensure that all health care facilities have the capacity, knowledge, and training to implement and maintain good practices, especially infection prevention and control measures and early identification of cases.

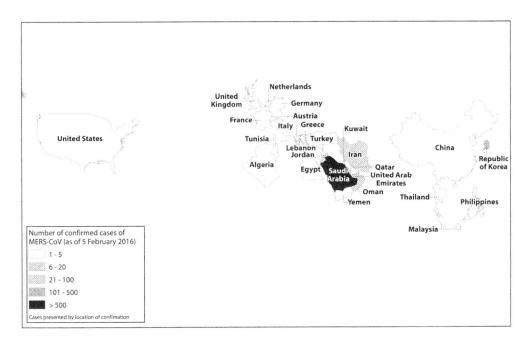

FIGURE 2 Global map of countries with confirmed cases of Middle East respiratory syndrome coronavirus (MERS-CoV), 2012 to 2016, as reported by the World Health Organization (data as of 5 February 2016) (http://www.who.int/emergencies/mers-cov/en/).

- Appropriate authorities should collaboratively address deeper systemic issues that are impeding control of MERS, both in animals and humans.
- National authorities should ensure the rapid and timely sharing of information of public health importance, including epidemiological investigations, viral genetic sequence information, and findings from research studies.
- International collaboration to develop human and animal vaccines and therapeutics should be accelerated.
- In view of the evidence that camels are the main source of community-acquired infections, public health, animal health, and agricultural sectors must improve their collaboration to address the public health risk of MERS.
- National leadership is essential to ensure a flexible, efficient, and well-coordinated whole-of-government response to the challenges posed by MERS.

Although much has been learned about MERS-CoV since its emergence in 2012, many questions remain. Human-to-human transmission occurs, usually in health care settings, but sustained and efficient human-to-human transmission has not been observed. However, vigilance is needed, because MERS-CoV could develop the ability to transmit efficiently from person to person, as was seen with SARS-CoV during the outbreak of 2002-2003. For countries without active transmission of MERS-CoV, such as the United States, preparedness efforts are essential. These include efforts toward prevention of travelers becoming infected with MERS-CoV (by providing information to travelers on avoidance of high-risk settings for MERS transmission), enhancement of the ability to rapidly identify and isolate patients with MERS (by educating clinicians regarding patients that should be tested for MERS-CoV and ensuring laboratory capacity for MERS-CoV diagnostic testing), and prevention of MERS-CoV transmission should an

imported case occur (by developing and disseminating infection control guidelines for prevention of MERS-CoV transmission in health care settings) (22, 23).

MERS-COV

Coronaviruses are large single-stranded, positive-sense RNA viruses capable of infecting humans and many animal species. A high degree of diversity has been observed in coronaviruses, related to their high rate of mutation and the large size of their genomes. Four coronavirus genera have been identified based on genomic and serologic characteristics: *Alpha-*, *Beta-*, *Gamma-*, and *Delta-coronavirus*. A total of six coronaviruses that infect humans have been identified in two of these genera: *Alphacoronavirus* (NL63 and HCoV-229E) and *Betacoronavirus* (HCoV-OC43, HCoV-HKU1, MERS-CoV, and SARS-CoV) (24). MERS-CoV is in lineage c of the genus *Betacoronavirus*; this lineage also includes two bat coronavirus species, *Tylonycteris* bat coronavirus HKU4 and *Pipistrellus* bat coronavirus HKU5 (16). SARS-CoV is a lineage b *Betacoronavirus*. SARS-CoV and MERS-CoV both cause severe respiratory infections in humans, whereas the other coronaviruses that infect humans generally cause mild, self-limited respiratory infections, similar to the common cold.

The MERS-CoV genome is ~30 kb in length and contains at least 10 open reading frames (ORFs) (25). The MERS-CoV genome encodes four structural proteins: the spike (S) protein, the envelope (E) protein, the membrane (M) protein, and the nucleocapsid (N) protein (26). Virions are made up of a core (composed of viral RNA and multiple copies of the N protein) and a viral membrane, made up of the E, M, and S proteins (Fig. 3). The S proteins are distributed throughout the envelope and give the virus a crown-like (corona) appearance (Fig. 4). Dipeptidyl peptidase 4 (DPP4) is the host cell receptor for MERS-CoV (27). DPP4 attaches to the

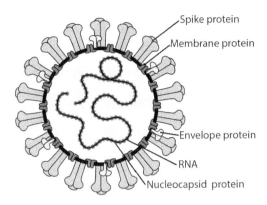

FIGURE 3 Depiction of components of the MERS-coronavirus including the membrane, envelope, and spike proteins that make up the viral membrane and nucleocapsid protein, which is associated with the viral RNA. Image source: CDC, Jennifer Oosthuizen.

receptor binding domain of the MERS-CoV S protein, which results in S protein cleavage, fusion of the virus and host cell, and release of the viral RNA into the cytoplasm (28). The S protein has two subunits: S1 mediates virus binding through the receptor binding domain, and S2 mediates virus entry by fusing the virus and host cell membranes. For membrane fusion to occur, the S protein must be cleaved at the S1/S2 boundary by human proteases. The use of DPP4 as a receptor in MERS is in contrast to SARS-CoV, which uses angiotensin-converting enzyme 2 as its receptor (29). DPP4 is necessary for the virus to enter cells, explaining the ability of MERS-CoV to infect cells from some animals (e.g., nonhuman primates, bats, and camels) but not others (e.g., hamsters, mice, dogs, and cats) (30). DPP4 is also expressed on many types of human tissues, including lung, kidney, small intestine, liver, and prostate (27, 30, 31), and might be responsible for some of the extrapulmonary manifestations (e.g., renal failure) seen in MERS. In the respiratory tract, DPP4 receptors are localized to the alveolar regions, which might explain why MERS is primarily a lower respiratory tract disease. Further, the fact that DPP4 receptors are minimally expressed

in the nasal cavity and conducting airways might explain why efficient human-to-human transmission has not been seen (32).

Recent comparison of the genomic sequences of spike proteins from MERS-CoV, a virus with the ability to enter human cells, to those from a related bat coronavirus HKU4, a virus that is unable to enter human cells, identified two sequence differences that allowed the spike protein to interact with human proteases, genetic changes that gave MERS-CoV the ability to enter human cells (33). The authors suggested that these mutations were critical to the evolution of a bat coronavirus to one that could infect humans, either directly or through an intermediate host.

Whole-genome sequencing of 65 MERS-CoV specimens in 2013 showed the presence of four phylogenetic clades, three of which were no longer circulating. The authors hypothesized that the disappearance of

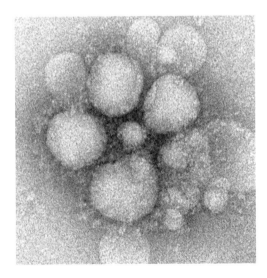

FIGURE 4 Middle East respiratory syndrome coronavirus as seen by electron microscopy. The spike proteins protrude from the viral membrane and give the virus a crown-like (corona) appearance. Image source: CDC's Public Health Image Library (http://www.cdc.gov/coronavirus/mers/photos.html), Cynthia Goldsmith/Maureen Metcalfe/Azaibi Tamin.

these clades could be due to implementation of improved infection control measures, along with a basic reproduction number of less than 1, or possibly to transmission from people who were asymptomatic and undiagnosed (34). The differences observed in the genomic sequences suggested that the infections were not the result of a continuous chain of human-to-human transmission, but were more likely related to the virus being intermittently reintroduced into humans from an animal reservoir. Continued genomic analysis of MERS-CoV is needed to determine if mutations are occurring that allow for better adaptation to humans and more efficient human-to-human transmission.

RISK FACTORS

Risk factors for MERS appear to have changed as the spread of MERS has progressed. Early patients identified with MERS were much more likely to have comorbidities such as diabetes, heart disease, and chronic renal disease (33) and to be older males (10). However, the predominance of males has become less impressive as the outbreak has continued (11), including in the recent outbreak in the Republic of Korea, in which 61% of infected patients were male (35). Several possible reasons for the male predominance have been hypothesized including that males have a higher level of exposure to camels (although this would not explain the male predominance in the Republic of Korea, where all cases were secondary), males are more likely to seek health care (although this seems the opposite of what is typically observed in Korea), males are more likely to be tested for MERS-CoV or reported to the WHO, or males are more susceptible to MERS.

In an analysis of the first 144 laboratory-confirmed and 17 probable MERS-CoV cases reported to the WHO (36), cases were divided into those that were sporadic or index cases and cases that were secondary

(ones with epidemiological links to known MERS-CoV cases). Among the 146 cases that could be classified, 51 (35%) were sporadic or index cases and 95 (65%) were secondary. Sporadic/index cases were more likely to have severe disease (defined as admission to an intensive care unit; use of extracorporeal membrane oxygenation, mechanical ventilation, or vasopressors; reported as "critical" or "severe"; or who died) than secondary cases (90.2% for sporadic/index and 49.5% for secondary). Median age was 59 and 43 years among sporadic/index and secondary cases, respectively. Among the sporadic/index cases, 70.6% were over 50 years of age and 72.6% were male, compared to 37.4% over 50 years of age and 60.0% male in the secondary group of cases. Underlying conditions were reported in 80.9% of sporadic/index cases and 67.2% of secondary cases. These results suggest that sporadic and index cases are more likely to be detected when people are severely ill; as more infections are identified through contact investigations, patients are more likely to be mildly affected or asymptomatic and to be younger and less likely to have underlying conditions.

A case-control study was performed during an outbreak in Saudi Arabia in 2014 to identify risk factors for primary MERS-CoV illness (37). To identify patients with primary MERS-CoV, those with a history of exposure to other MERS-CoV cases or to people with acute respiratory illness of unknown cause or with a history of exposure to health care settings during the 14 days before symptom onset were excluded. Multivariable analysis identified direct exposure to dromedary camels during the 2 weeks before onset of illness, diabetes mellitus, heart disease, and smoking as independent risk factors for primary MERS-CoV illness. Milking dromedary camels was the only specific camel-related exposure that was significantly associated with MERS-CoV illness. However, even among these cases classified as primary, only about a third reported exposure to dromedary camels during the 2 weeks before illness onset. Living in the same household as people who reported working on or visiting a farm with dromedary camels was also a risk factor, suggesting that indirect exposure might be important. A male predominance was noted among the primary case patients; only 1 of 30 primary case patients in this study was female; however, sex was used to match cases and controls and thus could not be analyzed in the case-control study.

In addition to identifying risk factors for becoming ill with MERS-CoV, other studies have analyzed possible risk factors for dying of MERS. Underlying health conditions and older age have been identified as risk factors for death from MERS in several studies (38–42). For example, in a study from the recent outbreak in the Republic of Korea (42), the authors used a multivariate logistic regression model to identify risk factors for death and found that the odds of dying for persons with underlying health conditions were 7 times higher than for persons without underlying conditions. In that study, for every 1-year increase in a patient's age, the odds of dying increased by 12%. Viral load also might play a role; a recent study, which used multiple logistic regression analysis, showed that patients who were older (>60 years of age), who had an underlying condition, and who had a higher viral load of MERS-CoV in the upper respiratory tract were at increased risk of death (43). The length of the incubation period might also play a role in the likelihood of a person dying of MERS. Data from an analysis of cases from the Republic of Korea suggest that a longer incubation period is associated with a lower rate of death (44), similar to what has been seen in SARS (45).

MERS has been diagnosed in children, although it appears to be rare (98% of people infected with MERS-CoV have been adults) (26). In a study of 11 cases in children diagnosed with MERS in Saudi Arabia, 9 were asymptomatic (identified as part of contact investigations) and 2 were symptomatic (46). Both children who were symptomatic had underlying illnesses; one was a 2-year-old

with cystic fibrosis and the other was a 14-year-old with Down syndrome.

We are aware of only one report of a pregnant woman with MERS. This woman was identified as part of a follow-up investigation of the April 2012 outbreak in Jordan conducted in May 2013. The 39-year-old woman reported respiratory symptoms consistent with MERS during the outbreak period and was subsequently positive for MERS-CoV antibody, suggesting that she had been infected during the outbreak (because she was antibody-positive on a single specimen and she had been symptomatic, she met the WHO case definition for "probable MERS"). During her illness, she delivered a stillborn infant at around 5 months gestation (47). Based on only this one report, we are unable to determine the risks to the pregnant woman or her fetus associated with MERS. However, data from SARS suggest that pregnant women with MERS and their fetuses might be at increased risk of adverse pregnancy outcomes (48).

Data suggest that time of year could be a risk factor for MERS; although MERS illnesses appear throughout the year, the first cases of MERS (identified retrospectively) occurred in April of 2012, and significant increases in numbers of cases have occurred in the spring of the following years (2013, 2014, and 2015). The reason for the seasonal pattern is not known; however, links to the timing of the camel calving season have been made (camels are typically born between late October and late February) (49, 50). Some authors have noted an association between the timing of weaning of camel calves and of diarrhea in these calves with increased numbers of MERS cases (50). Others have hypothesized that the seasonal pattern might occur because young camels are more likely to become ill and shed virus than older camels that are already seropositive for MERS-CoV (49, 51). In a recent study of over 800 dromedary camels of different ages (52), acute MERS-CoV infection was seen in calves but not in older camels, supportive of this hypothesis. These authors suggest that camel-to-human transmission of MERS-CoV could be prevented if humans avoided young camels (<2 years of age) (52).

Serologic studies have been used to identify occupational risk factors for MERS-CoV infection; in a recent seroprevalence study, shepherds and slaughterhouse workers (persons with occupational camel exposure) were 15 and 23 times more likely to be seropositive for MERS-CoV antibodies than members of the general population (53). In another study, 10 of 294 people with occupational exposure to camels (slaughterhouse workers, barn workers at a camel racing track, and camel farm workers) were seropositive for MERS-CoV antibody, compared with none of 204 without dromedary camel exposure (54).

TRANSMISSION

Cases of MERS can be categorized as primary (sporadic or index cases in a cluster) or secondary (epidemiologically linked to an index case). Among the first 161 confirmed or likely cases reported to the WHO between September 2012 and October 2013, 95 (59%) were believed to be secondary cases, in which person-to-person transmission had occurred (36). Person-to-person transmission of MERS-CoV has occurred in both household and hospital settings (55–57). Household transmission was first suspected in November of 2012 in a family cluster in Saudi Arabia in which there were three confirmed and one probable case (an elderly male, his two sons, and his grandson) (58). Although person-to-person transmission seemed likely, a common source of infection could not be ruled out. Definitive evidence of person-to-person transmission was observed in February of 2013 in the United Kingdom. Two secondary cases among family members (without history of travel) were identified among contacts of an adult male with MERS who had traveled to the Arabian Peninsula 10 days

before symptom onset. Among the two secondary cases, one was believed to have been infected in the household setting, while the other was believed to be infected while visiting the patient when he was hospitalized. This cluster provided strong evidence for human-to-human transmission, but it appeared that transmission was infrequent: only two cases of MERS were identified among the 135 persons who had been in contact with the patients (59). These data are consistent with later studies of household contacts. In a study of 26 index patients and their 280 household contacts, only 12 cases (4%, 95% CI 2-7) of probable secondary transmission were identified (56). Low likelihood of transmission has also been seen in other situations; for example, in an analysis of 61 contacts of the first patient with MERS in the United States (all those who had a face-to-face contact with the patient or who entered the patient's room without recommended personal protective equipment before airborne and contact precautions were instituted), all had negative test results for MERS-CoV (20).

The majority of secondary cases have been observed in hospital settings (5, 55, 60–62). Among 74 secondary cases reported to the WHO between September 2012 and October 2013 for whom setting of transmission was reported, 13 (18%) had been infected in household settings, 60 (81%) were infected in health care settings, and one was infected in a workplace other than a health care setting. Among those infected in a health care setting, 30 were health care personnel who had treated MERS patients, 19 were patients receiving treatment in hospitals, and 6 were visitors (36).

In the spring of 2014, a large outbreak of MERS occurred in Saudi Arabia, with more cases reported during April and May of 2014 than all cases reported previously. Concern was raised regarding whether the virus had evolved to allow for more efficient human-to-human transmission. In a study from a health care facility in Jeddah, Saudi Arabia, that was involved in the outbreak (62), 255 patients with laboratory-confirmed MERS-CoV infection were identified. Of those, 64 patients (25.1%) were asymptomatic or mildly symptomatic. Among the symptomatic patients, 40 (20.9%) were health care personnel. Of the non–health care personnel who had data that could be assessed, nearly all (109/112 or 97.3%) had an epidemiological link to a health care facility, a person with confirmed MERS-CoV infection, or a person with severe respiratory illness in the 14 days before symptom onset. Only three patients reported no such contacts. Based on these data and subsequent genomic analyses that showed no significant changes in the MERS-CoV genome, it appears that person-to-person spread in the health care setting was the basis for this outbreak (63).

The recent outbreak in the Republic of Korea in which one person with MERS who traveled from the Arabian Peninsula resulted in 186 cases in less than two months is further illustrative of the impact of transmission in health care facilities. In this outbreak, 181 (97%) of the cases had exposures to health care facilities, and 82% of these cases occurred in four hospitals (64). Among the 186 cases, 25 (13.4%) were health care personnel, 82 (44.1%) were patients who were exposed in the health care setting, and 61 (32.8%) were caregivers (65).

This outbreak was fueled in part by superspreading events, in which a single patient transmits infection to a large number of others. Superspreading events were critical for the transmission of SARS (66) but had not been previously described for MERS. However, in the outbreak in Korea, over 80% of transmission events were linked to five patients, and most cases (91.3%) resulted in no transmission. Genomic analysis showed no evidence of mutations in MERS-CoV that might have modified its transmissibility. The patients who transmitted MERS-CoV to the highest numbers of people were ones with a severe cough, but they were otherwise similar to other patients. The reasons hypothe-

sized for the superspreading events seen in this outbreak were a delay in diagnosis and isolation of MERS patients, the fact that many patients sought health care at multiple facilities, frequent transfers between hospitals, significant numbers of paid caregivers in hospitals, and high numbers of contacts (including other patients, paid caregivers, and family members and friends, who typically accompany patients in hospitals in Korea) with MERS patients in large, crowded health care facilities (65).

Based on data from secondary cases, the MERS incubation period is approximately 5 to 6 days, with a range of 2 to 14 days (36, 39, 65). Transmission of MERS is not well understood. Possible transmission routes include (i) droplet (in which droplets >5 ×m in diameter with the ability to travel approximately 6 feet contain infectious virus and make contact with mucous membranes), (ii) airborne (in which droplet nuclei <5 ×m in diameter with the ability to travel >6 feet are inhaled into a susceptible person's respiratory tract), (iii) direct contact transmission (contact without a contaminated intermediate object or person), and (iv) indirect contact transmission (involving transfer through an intermediate contaminated object or person) (http://www.cdc.gov/hicpac/2007IP/2007ip_part1.html). Experimental data show that MERS-CoV is able to survive on contaminated surfaces for 48 hours and to maintain stability when aerosolized, suggesting that aerosol, droplet, and contact (direct and indirect) transmission all might play a role (67).

The most likely source of virus when transmission occurs in health care settings appears to be from the lower respiratory tract. In a study of 37 hospitalized patients with MERS, the highest level of MERS-CoV viral load was in specimens from the lower respiratory tract (average viral load from the lower respiratory tract was 5.0×10^6 copies per ml, compared to 1.9×10^4 copies per ml from the upper respiratory tract) (68). Viral RNA was detected in 33% of sera, 14.6% of stool, and 2.4% of urine specimens. Attempts to isolate infectious virus from sera and stool failed, suggesting that these sources are unlikely to contribute substantially to health care–associated infections.(68)

The basic reproduction number can be used to assess the likelihood that an infectious disease will develop sustained transmission. Several analyses have attempted to estimate the basic reproduction number for MERS. The first, based on data collected before 21 June 2013, estimated a reproduction number ranging from 0.60 to 0.69 (69). In an analysis that used data from human clusters through 8 August 2013, the authors concluded that transmission was not sustained when infection control measures were utilized, but in the absence of these measures, the reproduction number was estimated to be 0.8 to 1.3 (70). The most recent analysis, based on data from two large health care–associated outbreaks in Saudi Arabia in the spring of 2014, estimated much higher reproduction numbers, with a reproduction number of 3.5 to 6.7 for the Jeddah outbreak and 2.0 to 2.8 for the Riyadh outbreak (71). However, these estimates were obtained during specific outbreaks with high levels of transmission and are unlikely to reflect the overall reproduction number.

ANIMAL RESERVOIR

For primary cases (cases without an epidemiologic link to a known MERS case), the source of MERS-CoV is unknown. Some of these primary cases might have been exposed to a person infected with MERS-CoV who was mildly affected or asymptomatic and thus not known to have MERS. Another source might be an animal reservoir for MERS-CoV.

Based on the similarity of MERS-CoV's genetic sequence to those of bat coronaviruses, MERS-CoV is assumed to have a bat-related ancestral origin. Analysis of specimens from bats living in close proximity to the household of a human patient with MERS identified one specimen (from a bat fecal pellet) with 100% genetic identity, based on analysis of a fragment, to the MERS-CoV obtained from the patient, supporting involvement of bats in transmission of MERS to humans (72). However, the lack of exposure to bats for most MERS patients and the finding that MERS-CoV has only rarely been identified in bats (72) suggested that an intermediate host species is likely to be involved.

Several pieces of evidence suggest that dromedary camels are important in the transmission of MERS-CoV. Studies have identified anti-MERS-CoV antibodies in dromedary camels, but not in other animals such as cows, goats, or sheep (73–77). These antibodies were seen in camels from the Middle East, but also from other countries such as Spain, Nigeria, Tunisia, and Ethiopia (73, 75). Stored serum samples from camels from Saudi Arabia from as early as 1992 (78, 79), from the United Arab Emirates in 2003 (80), and from Africa as early as 1983 (81, 82) were positive for MERS-CoV antibodies. This suggests that MERS-CoV has circulated widely in dromedary camel populations for decades. However, transmission to humans appears to be a recent and infrequent phenomenon; MERS-CoV antibodies were not seen in serum samples collected in the fall of 2012 from 130 blood donors and 226 workers in slaughterhouses for camels, cattle, and sheep in Saudi Arabia (83). A more recent cross-sectional serological survey of healthy people over 15 years of age in Saudi Arabia between 1 December 2012 and 1 December 2013 showed a low frequency of MERS-CoV antibody seropositivity (seen in 15 of 10,009 individuals or about 0.15%). However, rates were significantly higher among people with exposure to camels; shepherds were 15 times more likely and slaughterhouse workers were 23 times more likely to be seropositive for MERS-CoV antibodies (53).

In addition to the finding of MERS-CoV antibodies, MERS-CoV viruses have also been found in camels, including ones that are genetically identical (84) or closely related (85, 86) to those identified in patients ill with MERS. For example, MERS-CoV was isolated from nasal swabs from a patient who died of MERS and from one of his nine camels who previously had rhinorrhea and with whom the patient had close contact. Of note, only nasal swabs from the camel tested positive for MERS-CoV; milk, urine, and rectal samples tested negative. Full genome sequencing showed that the MERS-CoV culture isolates from the patient and his camel were 100% identical. Based on serologic analysis, it appeared that the camel had transmitted the virus to his owner; the first serum sample from the camel showed high levels of MERS-CoV antibodies, while the patient's first serum sample was negative for MERS-CoV antibody, with high antibody levels measured in the patient's sample collected two weeks later (84). In addition, MERS-CoV that was identical in sequence to that obtained from the patient and his camel was later identified in an air sample from the camel barn (87).

As discussed previously, a case-control study conducted during the 2014 outbreak in Saudi Arabia (37) evaluated animal exposures as potential risk factors for contracting MERS-CoV infection among patients with primary MERS-CoV infection. No associations were observed between primary MERS-CoV infection and exposures to bats, goats, horses, sheep, or the products of these animals. Direct cattle exposure was more likely among cases than controls (OR 6.00, 95% CI 1.02 to 48.44). No significant differences were noted in exposures to animal products, including uncooked meat, unpasteurized animal milk, or dromedary urine. Direct exposure to dromedary camels within the 2 weeks before onset of illness was significantly associated with primary MERS-CoV infection on multivariable analysis (adjusted OR 7.45, 95% CI 1.57 to 35.28). However, not all case-patients reported direct exposure to dromedary camels during

the 2 weeks before illness onset. Living in a household with a person who had direct contact with dromedary camels was also a risk factor.

Although transmission from dromedary camels to humans appears likely, many patients with MERS-CoV have no history of camel exposure, and the frequency of transmission from infected camels to exposed humans appears to be low (88). Reasons for the lack of exposure to camels among some people with MERS-CoV could be that exposures occurred through consumption of unpasteurized camel milk, undercooked camel meat, or medicinal use of camel urine (50). Viral RNA has been detected in camel milk (74) and can be detected up to 72 hours when stored at 4°C and 22°C (89), suggesting that transmission through consumption of camel milk could be possible. After camel milk spiked with MERS-CoV was heat-treated for 30 minutes, no infectious virus could be recovered (89). However, no epidemiologic data support these other modes of transmission. Another possibility is that some patients might be infected by people with MERS-CoV infection who are asymptomatic and thus not identified as infected (58). When serologic studies were performed in outbreak settings, a significant proportion of people with evidence of past infection with MERS-CoV were not symptomatic (25% in one study) (62).

INFECTION CONTROL RECOMMENDATIONS FOR HEALTH CARE FACILITIES

Infections in health care settings have played a major role in the transmission of MERS-CoV (35, 57, 62, 90). The modality of transmission in health care settings is not fully understood. However, data from SARS (91) and MERS (5) suggest that implementation of health care infection control measures is effective in preventing transmission. An important question with regard to infection control measures is whether airborne precautions are required. MERS-CoV RNA fragments were detected in an air sample from a barn that housed a camel with MERS-CoV that was owned by an infected patient; these fragments were identical to those from the camel and patient, suggesting that airborne transmission might be possible (87). However, questions have been raised about the methods used in this study (92).

Screening and triage procedures to ensure early identification of patients potentially infected with MERS-CoV in health care settings are essential. Once a patient is suspected of having MERS, infection control measures should be immediately implemented. The U.S. Centers for Disease Control and Prevention has provided interim recommendations for infection control when patients are suspected of or confirmed to have MERS-CoV infection. The CDC acknowledged that the modes of transmission of MERS-CoV are incompletely defined, but given the absence of a vaccine or chemoprophylaxis and a possible high rate of morbidity and mortality, the recommendations include adherence to standard, contact, and airborne precautions. Airborne precautions include patient placement in an airborne infection isolation room, when feasible, and use of respiratory protection (e.g., a National Institute for Occupational Safety and Health–certified, fit-tested N95 filtering face-piece respirator) by health care workers entering the care area or room. Eye protection with goggles or a face shield is also recommended. Aerosol-generating procedures (including cough-generating procedures, bronchoscopy, sputum induction, intubation and extubation, cardiopulmonary resuscitation, and open suctioning of airways) appear to present particularly high risk of MERS-CoV transmission to health care workers (61, 63, 93). Thus, the CDC recommends conducting these procedures only when medically necessary and in an airborne infection isolation room if possible, limiting the number of health care personnel present during these procedures to the minimum number needed for patient care, prohibiting health care personnel without appropriate personal protective equipment from entering the room until sufficient time has elapsed for infectious particles to be cleared, and conducting environmental surface cleaning after the procedures are completed. These recommendations will be updated when additional nformation becomes available (http://www.cdc.gov/coronavirus/mers/infection-prevention-control.html).

WHO recommendations for MERS-CoV standard, contact, and droplet precautions are similar to those from the CDC; however, airborne precautions are reserved for situations where aerosol-generating procedures might be performed. The latest infection control guidelines from the WHO can be obtained at http://www.who.int/csr/disease/coronavirus_infections/ipc-mers-cov/en/.

PREVENTION OF TRAVEL-ASSOCIATED TRANSMISSION

All cases identified thus far with MERS-CoV infection have been directly or indirectly linked to the Arabian Peninsula. These include cases associated with travel (94) and with spread of MERS to 17 countries outside those in or near the Arabian Peninsula (http://www.cdc.gov/coronavirus/mers/). Strategies to prevent travel-associated transmission have been recommended by the CDC and the WHO. No travel restrictions to or from the Arabian Peninsula have been recommended. For travelers to the Arabian Peninsula, the CDC currently recommends general hygiene measures, including hand hygiene (frequent hand washing) and avoiding close contact with people who are sick (22, 95). People traveling to the Arabian Peninsula to work as health care workers are directed to become familiar with infection control guidelines for patients with confirmed and suspected MERS. CDC travel recommendations will be updated as additional information becomes available: http://wwwnc.cdc.gov/travel/.

Specific recommendations have also been made by the CDC and WHO regarding exposure to camels, given the increasing evidence that camels play a critical role in transmission in primary cases. Travelers who will be visiting farms, markets, barns, or other settings where they might be in contact with animals, should practice general hygiene measures, including hand-washing before and after touching animals and avoiding contact with ill animals. Eating raw or undercooked animal products should be avoided. The WHO recommends additional precautions for people at risk for developing severe MERS illness (people with diabetes, renal failure, or chronic lung disease and immunocompromised people), including avoiding contact with camels and avoiding consumption of raw camel milk, urine, and undercooked meat, especially camel meat. The latest information from the WHO is available at http://www.who.int/csr/disease/coronavirus_infections/faq/en/ and http://www.who.int/csr/disease/coronavirus_infections/MERS_CoV_RA_20140613.pdf?ua=1.

Travelers to regions with MERS transmission should be instructed that if they develop symptoms of MERS, they should seek medical care. In addition, travelers should make the health care facility aware of their recent travel before presenting for care so that appropriate infection control measures can be put in place (22, 95). Although clinicians caring for patients with signs and symptoms consistent with MERS-CoV following travel to countries affected by MERS need to consider the possibility of MERS, studies have shown that these patients frequently have other (non-MERS) respiratory illnesses, usually influenza (96, 97).

A high level of concern has been raised about transmission during the Hajj, in which more than 2 million Muslim visitors from around the world travel to Saudi Arabia during one week each year as part of a religious pilgrimage (98, 99). In addition to the close contact with other pilgrims, visitors are likely to have contact with animals, including some that might be infected with MERS. However, despite increased surveillance following the Hajj, no Hajj-associated cases of MERS have been confirmed (98, 100–103), but several travel-associated cases have been observed among people returning after Umrah, a Muslim pilgrimage in which ~6 million pilgrims participate in each year; this pilgrimage can occur at any time during the calendar year (104, 105).

ANIMAL MODELS

The availability of animal models for a novel infectious pathogen such as MERS-CoV allows for more rapid advances in research (106). Small animals typically used for experimental studies (e.g., Syrian hamsters, mice, and ferrets) cannot be used as animal models without modification because MERS-CoV is unable to replicate in these species (107–109) due to differences in the DPP4 host cell receptor. Rabbits can be infected with MERS-CoV but are asymptomatic (110); because of this, rabbit models can be used for studies of disease transmission but not for studies of illness or response to therapeutics.

Although mice, which are preferred for experimental studies over larger animals because they are less resource intensive, cannot become naturally infected with MERS-CoV because murine DPP4 does not serve as a receptor, researchers have recently developed mouse models for MERS, either by sensitizing mice to MERS-CoV with an adenovirus that expresses human DPP4 (111) or by creating transgenic mouse lines that express human DPP4 (112–114). Mice that are intranasally inoculated with a human DPP4-expressing adenovirus and then infected with MERS develop pneumonia, similar to that in humans, and can be helpful in studying immune response and to evaluate MERS-CoV therapeutics and vaccines. Transgenic mouse lines that have been modified to express human DPP4 become infected with MERS-CoV and have major effects on the lungs and the brain, often resulting in death, limiting the ability to study host response to the virus; however, severity of disease appears to be related to the dose of virus provided (112–114). These models show promise for the study of the pathogenesis of MERS as well as assessment of potential vaccines and therapeutics.

Two species of nonhuman primates have been used as animal models for MERS-CoV: the rhesus macaque and the common marmoset (106). In these species, inoculation with MERS-CoV results in viral replication and clinical illness. The rhesus macaque was the first animal model to be used for MERS-CoV. Inoculation of these animals with MERS-CoV resulted in transient disease that was mild to moderate in severity, including fever, increased respiratory rate, and decreased appetite. This animal model was used to fulfill Koch's postulates for MERS-CoV, confirming the virus as the causative agent for the clinical illness seen in patients with MERS (115). After studies of the DPP4 receptor showed that the common marmoset's receptor was similar to the human receptor (27), the common marmoset was pursued as an animal model for MERS. Following inoculation with MERS-CoV, the common marmoset develops moderate to severe illness, with increased respiratory rate, loss of appetite, and decreased activity, and severe interstitial pneumonia, sometimes resulting in death. These nonhuman primate models can be seen as complementary, with the macaque developing mild to moderate disease and the marmoset developing disease at the more severe end of the spectrum (116).

Dromedary camels also have been experimentally inoculated with MERS-CoV, and when infected, they develop mild symptoms, including rhinorrhea and temperature elevations, and shed high quantities of virus from the upper respiratory tract (117). These animals could be used to better understand the ecology and transmission of MERS-CoV (106).

CLINICAL FINDINGS

People infected with MERS-CoV can present with a wide range of clinical findings, ranging from asymptomatic to severe illness and death. Cases with mild or no symptoms often have been identified as part of contact investigations (36, 46, 62). People who are asymptomatic or who have only mild symptoms are frequently identified when serologic testing is performed; a quarter of patients with MERS-CoV infection identified in an outbreak at a health care facility in Jeddah, Saudi Arabia, were asymptomatic (62). Clinical manifestations are often nonspecific and indistinguishable from more common illnesses such as influenza; thus, travel and exposure histories are critical.

Most symptomatic patients with MERS have had fever, chills or rigors, cough, and shortness of breath (26, 38, 39, 41, 55). Other findings commonly seen include malaise, myalgia, sore throat, and headache. Gastrointestinal symptoms (nausea, vomiting, and diarrhea) are also often seen (Table 2). The respiratory illness often progresses to pneumonia and subsequently to acute respiratory distress syndrome. Abnormalities on chest radiographs range from minor to interstitial infiltrates to total opacification of lung segments and lobes (39, 55, 60). Abnormal laboratory findings seen in some patients include leukopenia, lymphopenia, thrombocytopenia, and elevated lactate dehydrogenase, alanine aminotransferase, and aspartate aminotransferase (26, 39, 118).

Kidney failure has been described in some patients with MERS. Based on a systematic review performed in 2013, MERS patients developed acute renal failure more often and earlier than patients with SARS (119). Whether this is due to direct infection of the kidney or related to critical illness (68) is unknown. MERS-CoV RNA was detected in a small proportion (2.4%) of urine specimens from infected patients in a recent study (68).

A recent report of three patients with MERS-CoV who developed a severe neurological syndrome has raised the question of whether the central nervous system might be another target of MERS-CoV (120). All three patients had severe neurologic symptoms including altered level of consciousness, ataxia, and focal motor deficit. Brain MRIs showed widespread, bilateral hyperintense lesions within the white matter on T-2 weighted imaging. Cerebrospinal fluid was obtained from two of the three patients and MERS-CoV reverse transcription PCR (RT-PCR) was negative for both; findings were remarkable only for an increased protein level.

Limited information is available on the pathology of MERS, given the rarity of autopsy examinations for cultural and religious reasons among many affected patients (121). Based on data from chest CT scans, respiratory features appear to be consistent with an organizing pneumonia, based on the findings of ground-glass opacities with a distribution in the subpleural and peribronchovascular regions (122). These findings differ from those seen in patients with SARS, in which a bronchiolitis obliterans organizing pneumonia-like pattern and fibrosis tend to occur in late stages of the disease (123). A recent report of an autopsy on a single patient provides additional insight (124): diffuse alveolar damage was observed in the lungs, with localization to type 2 pneumocytes and epithelial syncytial cells. Despite the patient having renal failure requiring dialysis, MERS-CoV antigens were not detected outside of the lungs, including in the kidneys, suggesting that the renal failure was due to factors other than direct MER-CoV infection of the kidney. Additional pathologic examination of materials from autopsies will be needed to confirm these findings.

CASE DEFINITION

Both the CDC and the WHO have developed case definitions for diagnosis of confirmed and probable cases of MERS (Tables 3 and 4).

In addition, the CDC has a case definition for "patients under investigation" to assist health care personnel in determining which patients warrant testing for MERS-CoV (Table 3). As more information is learned about MERS-CoV, these case definitions will be updated. For the latest information, the CDC (http://www.cdc.gov/coronavirus/mers/case-def.html) and WHO (http://www.who.int/csr/disease/coronavirus_infections/case_definition/en/) websites should be consulted.

An important consideration when determining which patients to test for MERS-CoV is that coinfection with other respiratory pathogens has been reported (38, 125). Thus, identification of another respiratory pathogen does not rule out the possibility that a patient has MERS-CoV.

VIROLOGIC DIAGNOSIS

Shortly after description of the first patient with MERS, real-time RT-PCR assays were developed to allow for rapid laboratory diagnosis of MERS (126, 127). These assays targeted regions upstream of the E gene (upE), within open reading frame 1b (ORF1b) and within ORF1a. These authors recommended use of the two highly sensitive assays upE and ORF1a for diagnostic purposes (ORF1b was found to be of lower sensitivity than ORF1a) (127). The authors also described two RT-PCR assays for sequencing, which targeted the RNA-dependent RNA polymerase (RdRp) and nucleocapsid genes (RdRpSeq and NSeq assays, respectively) (127).

The CDC developed an assay that incorporates additional RT-PCR targets focused on the MERS-CoV nucleocapsid gene (N2 and N3); this assay uses upE and N2 targets for screening of specimens and the N3 target for positive test confirmation (128). On 5 June 2013, this CDC Novel Coronavirus 2012 Real-time RT-PCR Assay was approved for use by the U.S. Food and Drug Administration through an emergency use authorization (http://www.fda.gov/MedicalDevices/

TABLE 3 Middle East Respiratory Syndrome Coronavirus (MERS-CoV) definitions from the CDC[a,b]

Clinical features		Epidemiologic risk
Patient under investigation		
Severe illness: Fever[c] and pneumonia or acute respiratory distress syndrome (based on clinical or radiological evidence)	And	A history of travel from countries in or near the Arabian Peninsula[d] within 14 days before symptom onset or close contact[e] with a symptomatic traveler who developed fever[c] and acute respiratory illness (not necessarily pneumonia) within 14 days after traveling from countries in or near the Arabian Peninsula[d]Or A member of a cluster of patients with severe acute respiratory illness (e.g., fever[c] and pneumonia requiring hospitalization) of unknown etiology in which MERS-CoV is being evaluated, in consultation with state and local health departments in the United States
Milder illness: Fever[c] and symptoms of respiratory illness (not necessarily pneumonia; e.g., cough, shortness of breath)	And	A history of being in a health care facility (as a patient, worker, or visitor) within 14 days before symptom onset in a country or territory in or near the Arabian Peninsula[d] in which recent health care–associated cases of MERS have been identified
Fever[c] or symptoms of respiratory illness (not necessarily pneumonia; e.g., cough, shortness of breath)	And	Close contact[e] with a confirmed MERS patient while the patient was ill
Confirmed case		
A person with laboratory confirmation of MERS-CoV infection; confirmatory laboratory testing requires a positive PCR on at least two specific genomic targets or a single positive target with sequencing on a second		
Probable case		
A patient under investigation with absent or inconclusive laboratory results for MERS-CoV infection who is a close contact[e] of a laboratory-confirmed MERS-CoV patient; examples of laboratory results that may be considered inconclusive include a positive test on a single PCR target, a positive test with an assay that has limited performance data available, or a negative test on an inadequate specimen		

[a]From http://www.cdc.gov/coronavirus/mers/case-def.html#modalIdString_CDCTable_0 (see CDC website for up–to–date information).

[b]These criteria serve as guidance for testing; however, patients should be evaluated and discussed with public health departments on a case-by-case basis if their clinical presentation or exposure history is equivocal (e.g., uncertain history of health care exposure).

[c]Fever may not be present in some patients, such as those who are very young, elderly, immunosuppressed, or taking certain medications. Clinical judgment should be used to guide testing of patients in such situations.

[d]Countries considered in the Arabian Peninsula and neighboring include Bahrain; Iraq; Iran; Israel, the West Bank, and Gaza; Jordan; Kuwait; Lebanon; Oman; Qatar; Saudi Arabia; Syria; the United Arab Emirates; and Yemen.

[e]Close contact is defined as (i) being within approximately 6 feet (2 meters) or within the room or care area for a prolonged period of time (e.g., health care personnel, household members) while not wearing recommended personal protective equipment (i.e., gowns, gloves, respirator, eye protection) or (ii) having direct contact with infectious secretions (e.g., being coughed on) while not wearing recommended personal protective equipment (i.e., gowns, gloves, respirator, eye protection). Data to inform the definition of close contact are limited. At this time, brief interactions such as walking by a person are considered low risk and do not constitute close contact.

Safety/EmergencySituations/ucm161496.htm). Reagent kits for this assay were subsequently distributed through the CDC Laboratory Response Network to state health departments as well as to international public health laboratories (128).

The WHO has developed interim guidance for laboratory testing for MERS, most recently updated in June 2015 (129). For the WHO to consider a case of MERS confirmed by RT-PCR, one of the following criteria must be met: (i) a positive RT-PCR result for at least two specific targets on the MERS-CoV genome using a validated assay or (ii) one positive RT-PCR result for a specific target on the MERS-CoV genome and MERS-CoV sequence confirmation from a separate viral genomic target (127). The WHO considers cases with positive RT-PCR results at only a single target but with signs consistent

TABLE 4 Middle East respiratory syndrome coronavirus (MERS-CoV) case definition for reporting to the WHO[a]

Confirmed case

A person with laboratory confirmation of MERS-CoV infection[b], irrespective of clinical signs and symptoms

Probable case

Definition 1:

A febrile acute respiratory illness with clinical, radiological, or histopathological evidence of pulmonary parenchymal disease (e.g., pneumonia or acute respiratory distress syndrome)	And	Direct epidemiologic link[c] with a confirmed MERS-CoV case	And	Testing for MERS-CoV is unavailable, negative on a single inadequate specimen[d], or inconclusive[e]

Definition 2:

A febrile acute respiratory illness with clinical, radiological, or histopathological evidence of pulmonary parenchymal disease (e.g., pneumonia or acute respiratory distress syndrome)	And	The person resides or travelled in the Middle East or in countries where MERS-CoV is known to be circulating in dromedary camels or where human infections have recently occurred	And	Testing for MERS-CoV is inconclusive[e]

Definition 3:

An acute febrile respiratory illness of any severity	And	Direct epidemiologic link[b] with a confirmed MERS-CoV case	And	Testing for MERS-CoV is inconclusive[e]

[a]From http://www.who.int/csr/disease/coronavirus_infections/case_definition/en/ (see WHO website for up-to-date information).

[b]A case may be laboratory confirmed by detection of viral nucleic acid or serology. The presence of viral nucleic acid can be confirmed by either a positive reverse transcription PCR result on at least two specific genomic targets or a single positive target with sequencing of a second target. A case confirmed by serology requires demonstration of seroconversion in two samples, ideally taken at least 14 days apart, by a screening (enzyme-linked immunosorbent assay [ELISA], indirect fluorescent antibody [IFA]), and by a neutralization assay. However, the interim recommendations for laboratory testing for MERS-CoV should be consulted for the most recent standard for laboratory confirmation.

[c]A direct epidemiological link with a confirmed MERS-CoV patient may include (i) health care–associated exposure, including providing direct care for MERS-CoV patients, working with health care workers infected with MERS-CoV, visiting patients, or staying in the same close environment of individuals infected with MERS-CoV; (ii) working in close proximity or sharing the same classroom environment with individuals infected with MERS-CoV; (iii) traveling with individuals infected with MERS-CoV in any kind of conveyance; (iv) living in the same household as individuals infected with MERS-CoV; (v) the epidemiological link may have occurred within a 14-day period before or after the onset of illness in the case under consideration.

[d]An inadequate specimen would include a nasopharyngeal swab without an accompanying lower respiratory specimen, a specimen that has had improper handling, is judged to be of poor quality by the testing laboratory, or was taken too late in the course of illness.

[e]Inconclusive tests may include (i) a positive screening test on a single real-time reverse transcription PCR target without further confirmation and (ii) evidence of sero-reactivity by a single convalescent serum sample, ideally taken at least 14 days after exposure by a screening assay (ELISA or IFA) and a neutralization assay in the absence of molecular confirmation from respiratory specimens.

with MERS and a history of potential exposure as "probable."

Collection of specimens from symptomatic patients can include lower respiratory tract specimens (i.e., sputum, bronchoalveolar lavage, tracheal aspirates), upper respiratory tract specimens (i.e., oropharyngeal swabs, nasopharyngeal swabs, aspirate, or wash), and serum (especially if lower respiratory tract specimens are unavailable) (129). Lower respiratory tract specimens have the highest MERS-CoV viral load (130–132) and thus should be collected whenever possible (129). MERS-CoV has sometimes been detected in lower respiratory tract specimens or in serum when upper respiratory tract specimens previously tested negative (19, 133). MERS-CoV has been detected in serum, urine, and stool, although at lower concentrations than in the lower respiratory tract (68, 134). In cases with confirmed MERS-CoV, WHO guidance recommends sequential sampling of specimens from multiple sites (including urine and stool) to improve understanding of virus shedding and to guide infection control measures (129).

To confirm MERS-CoV clearance in clinically recovered patients, the WHO recommends two consecutive negative PCR results from respiratory specimens collected at least every 2 to 4 days. Samples can be collected daily if a patient's discharge from isolation requires consecutive negative results (129).

Development of serological assays for MERS-CoV has been challenging because of problems with cross-reactivity with other coronaviruses and has been further complicated by the limited availability of MERS-CoV convalescent sera to allow for protocol validation (135). Methods for different types of serological tests for MERS have been published, including enzyme-linked immunosorbent assay (ELISA), indirect fluorescent antibody (IFA), and virus neutralization assays, among others (127, 136–138). Virus neutralization assays are considered the "gold standard" but require live virus and thus must be performed under biosafety lab 3 conditions. Therefore, laboratories often initially use less specific assays (e.g., ELISA) and then when those studies are positive, proceed to more definitive tests such as IFA or virus neutralization assays (56). For example, the CDC used a two-stage approach for detecting MERS-CoV antibodies that included testing using ELISA, followed by confirmation with either an IFA or a microneutralization test (5).

The WHO guidance includes recommendations for the use of serologic testing to make a diagnosis of MERS-CoV infection for reporting to the WHO under international health regulations (129). For a patient to be considered a confirmed case by the WHO, seroconversion must be documented by at least one screening assay (e.g., ELISA, IFA) and confirmed by a neutralization assay. To test for seroconversion, samples should be obtained at least 14 days apart. Based on data from SARS and preliminary data from MERS, a minimum 4-fold increase in titers would be expected with seroconversion (129).

A symptomatic patient with positive results on antibody testing (at least one screening assay—ELISA or IFA—and a positive result for a neutralization assay) on only a single specimen is considered a probable case, in the absence of a positive RT-PCR test for MERS-CoV. A person who is asymptomatic with positive results of antibody testing on a single specimen does not meet WHO criteria for either a confirmed or probable case (129).

IMMUNE RESPONSE

Information on the immune response to MERS-CoV infection is limited. In a recent analysis of 37 hospitalized MERS patients (68), viral load and antibody response were followed longitudinally beginning at the time of diagnosis through the course of their hospitalization. Antibodies were detected in most patients in the second week after diagnosis (estimated to be 2 to 3 weeks after illness onset). An inverse correlation was noted between the level of antibodies and viral load in the sera. In some cases, antibodies to MERS-CoV and viral RNA were detected in the same serum specimens. Even in the presence of neutralizing antibodies, virus was not cleared from the lower respiratory tract, leading the authors to suggest that vaccine strategies should not rely solely on the production of neutralizing antibodies (68).

Limited information is available on the contribution of T-cells to the MERS-CoV immune response (139). Using the mouse model that has been sensitized to MERS-CoV with an adenovirus that expresses human DPP4, mice that were T-cell deficient were compared to control mice following infection with MERS-CoV; the T-cell-deficient mice had viral persistence in the lungs, whereas control mice were able to clear the MERS-CoV from the lungs (111). These data suggest that T-cells are likely to be important in the immune response to MERS-CoV.

CLINICAL MANAGEMENT AND ANTIVIRALS

No specific antiviral treatment for MERS is available. Treatment of severely ill patients is primarily supportive, including mechanical ventilation, lung protective ventilation strategies, extracorporeal membrane oxygenation, inotropic support, antimicrobial therapy for secondary infections, and hemodialysis, as indicated (4, 131, 140).

Screening of potential therapeutics using cell culture has been used to identify treatment options that might be effective against MERS-CoV, including interferons, mycophenolate mofetil, cyclosporine A, ribavirin, nitazoxanide, lopinavir, and monoclonal antibodies (141–146); a few of these have shown anti-coronavirus activity and thus have potential as therapeutic options. In addition, animal models have been used to study possible therapeutics for MERS. Treatment with ribavirin and interferon-α2b was shown to improve clinical outcomes in rhesus macaques (147). Better outcomes were observed in the common marmoset animal model following treatment with lopinavir/ritonavir or interferon-β1b, while animals treated with mycophenolate mofetil had worse outcomes (148).

Based on studies of the utility of convalescent plasma among patients with SARS-CoV or influenza, MERS convalescent plasma has been proposed as a possible treatment for MERS patients (149). A protocol for a study of feasibility, safety, and clinical and laboratory endpoints of treatment with convalescent plasma was recently published, and this study is anticipated as a precursor to a randomized controlled trial (150). A systematic review of treatments used for patients with SARS showed that systemic steroids might be harmful (151); thus, steroids should not be used in MERS patients. Certain medications have been studied in MERS patients; for example, in a small retrospective cohort study (20 treated compared to 24 untreated patients), survival was improved after treatment with ribavirin and interferon-α2a after 14 days, but at 28 days, the results were not statistically significant (30% survival among treated versus 17% among those untreated, $p = 0.54$) (152). Randomized controlled trials will be required to determine whether these therapeutics have clinical benefit.

VACCINES

Currently no vaccine is available to protect humans or animals from developing MERS, but efforts are ongoing to develop a MERS vaccine. Based on the current epidemiology of MERS, in which most illness appears to occur in certain groups, widespread vaccination with a MERS vaccine is unlikely to be recommended. Instead, targeting patients at high risk of infection (those with occupational exposure to camels or people working in health care settings in locations with MERS transmission) or those at high risk of severe illness (people with underlying conditions) might be warranted. Another approach that has been considered is vaccination of camels to prevent illness in humans by decreasing the introduction of the virus into the human population (153).

Much has been learned about coronavirus vaccines as part of the efforts to develop a SARS vaccine, and this information can be used in the development of a safe and effective MERS vaccine. For example, a full-length S-protein-based SARS vaccine has been shown to produce neutralizing antibodies in vaccinated ferrets following infection with SARS-CoV, but inflammation of the liver was also seen, suggesting that enhancement of disease can occur following vaccination (154), which raises concerns about using this vaccine approach for MERS-CoV. As another example, data from SARS suggest that intranasal vaccination might be advantageous compared to other modes of vaccine administration because it can produce a mucosal response, thus blocking viral replication in the respiratory tract, in addition to inducing a systemic humoral response (155). Results from studies of intranasal versus other modes of administration of MERS vaccines are comparable (156).

Several different types of MERS vaccines are under development, including vaccines based on viral vectors, recombinant viral proteins, DNAs, nanoparticles, and recombinant virus (157, 158). These vaccines are currently undergoing testing in cell culture and in animal models (mice, rabbits, camels, and nonhuman primates). Many of these vaccines target part or all of the S protein, its subunit, or the receptor-binding domain, and in some cases immunogenicity has been demonstrated in animal models (31). Clinical trials will be required to test these vaccines in humans, and planning is under way for trials of some of the more promising vaccine candidates (157).

CONCLUSIONS

The first patients with novel coronavirus infection, now known as Middle East respiratory syndrome coronavirus (MERS-CoV), were reported in 2012. In the ensuing years, over 1,600 cases have been reported, as of February 2016. Most of these have occurred in Saudi Arabia or in other countries on or near the Arabian Peninsula, but travel-associated cases have also occurred. In 2015, in the Republic of Korea, a single travel-associated case led to a significant outbreak of over 180 cases. MERS-CoV causes a severe respiratory illness in many patients, although when contacts are investigated, a significant proportion of patients are asymptomatic or only have mild symptoms. The case fatality rate may be as high as 40%, although this estimate is likely to have been based on cases in which mildly affected and asymptomatic cases were missed. At this time, no vaccines or treatments are available. Based on genomic data, MERS-CoV is likely of bat ancestral origin; however, epidemiological and other data suggest that the source of most primary cases is exposure to camels. Person-to-person spread occurs, both in household and health care settings, although sustained and efficient person-to-person transmission has not been observed. Strict adherence to infection control recommendations has been associated with control of previous outbreaks. Based on the experience with SARS, it is recognized that genomic changes in MERS-CoV could result in increased transmissibility; thus, vigilance is needed.

Given the frequency of air travel, all countries are at risk for patients with MERS, and preparedness efforts are critical. These include prevention of travelers becoming infected with MERS-CoV, enhancement of the ability to rapidly identify and isolate patients with MERS, and prevention of MERS-CoV transmission in health care settings should an imported case occur.

ACKNOWLEDGMENTS

The authors would like to thank Jessica Rudd and Huong Pham for assistance with developing Fig. 1 and Michael Wellman and Jacqueline Burkholder for assistance with developing Fig. 2.
The findings and conclusions in this report are those of the authors and do not necessarily represent the official position of the Centers for Disease Control and Prevention. Current affiliation for Dr. Swerdlow is Pfizer, Inc.

CITATION

Rasmussen SA, Watson AK, Swerdlow DL. 2016. Middle East respiratory syndrome (MERS). Microbiol Spectrum 4(3):EI10-0020-2016.

REFERENCES

1. **Zaki AM, van Boheemen S, Bestebroer TM, Osterhaus ADME, Fouchier RAM.** 2012. Isolation of a novel coronavirus from a man

with pneumonia in Saudi Arabia. *N Engl J Med* **367:**1814–1820.

2. **Zaki AM.** 2012. *Novel coronavirus—Saudi Arabia: human isolate. Program for Monitoring Emerging Diseases (ProMED).* http://www.promedmail.org/.

3. **Pebody RG, Chand MA, Thomas HL, Green HK, Boddington NL, Carvalho C, Brown CS, Anderson SR, Rooney C, Crawley-Boevey E, Irwin DJ, Aarons E, Tong C, Newsholme W, Price N, Langrish C, Tucker D, Zhao H, Phin N, Crofts J, Bermingham A, Gilgunn-Jones E, Brown KE, Evans B, Catchpole M, Watson JM.** 2012. The United Kingdom public health response to an imported laboratory confirmed case of a novel coronavirus in September 2012. *Euro Surveill* **17:**20292. http://www.eurosurveillance.org/ViewArticle.aspx?ArticleId=20292.

4. **Bermingham A, Chand MA, Brown CS, Aarons E, Tong C, Langrish C, Hoschler K, Brown K, Galiano M, Myers R, Pebody RG, Green HK, Boddington NL, Gopal R, Price N, Newsholme W, Drosten C, Fouchier RA, Zambon M.** 2012. Severe respiratory illness caused by a novel coronavirus, in a patient transferred to the United Kingdom from the Middle East, September 2012. *Euro Surveill* **17:**20290. http://www.eurosurveillance.org/ViewArticle.aspx?ArticleId=20290.

5. **Al-Abdallat MM, Payne DC, Alqasrawi S, Rha B, Tohme RA, Abedi GR, Al Nsour M, Iblan I, Jarour N, Farag NH, Haddadin A, Al-Sanouri T, Tamin A, Harcourt JL, Kuhar DT, Swerdlow DL, Erdman DD, Pallansch MA, Haynes LM, Gerber SI.** 2014. Hospital-associated outbreak of Middle East respiratory syndrome coronavirus: a serologic, epidemiologic, and clinical description. *Clin Infect Dis* **59:**1225–1233.

6. **Drosten C.** 2013. Is MERS another SARS? *Lancet Infect Dis* **13:**727–728.

7. **Kupferschmidt K.** 2014. Emerging diseases. Soaring MERS cases in Saudi Arabia raise alarms. *Science* **344:**457–458.

8. **World Health Organization.** *Summary of probable SARS cases with onset of illness from 1 November 2002 to 31 July 2003.* http://www.who.int/csr/sars/country/table2004_04_21/en/index.html.

9. **Weinstein RA.** 2004. Planning for epidemics: the lessons of SARS. *N Engl J Med* **350:**2332–2334.

10. **Chinese SARS Molecular Epidemiology Consortium.** 2004. Molecular evolution of the SARS coronavirus during the course of the SARS epidemic in China. *Science* **303:**1666–1669.

11. **Guan Y, Peiris JS, Zheng B, Poon LL, Chan KH, Zeng FY, Chan CW, Chan MN, Chen JD, Chow KY, Hon CC, Hui KH, Li J, Li VY, Wang Y, Leung SW, Yuen KY, Leung FC.** 2004. Molecular epidemiology of the novel coronavirus that causes severe acute respiratory syndrome. *Lancet* **363:**99–104.

12. **Yeh SH, Wang HY, Tsai CY, Kao CL, Yang JY, Liu HW, Su IJ, Tsai SF, Chen DS, Chen PJ, National Taiwan University SARS Research Team.** 2004. Characterization of severe acute respiratory syndrome coronavirus genomes in Taiwan: molecular epidemiology and genome evolution. *Proc Natl Acad Sci USA* **101:**2542–2547.

13. **Peiris JS, Guan Y, Yuen KY.** 2004. Severe acute respiratory syndrome. *Nat Med* **10:**S88–S97.

14. **Lipsitch M, Cohen T, Cooper B, Robins JM, Ma S, James L, Gopalakrishna G, Chew SK, Tan CC, Samore MH, Fisman D, Murray M.** 2003. Transmission dynamics and control of severe acute respiratory syndrome. *Science* **300:**1966–1970.

15. **Riley S, Fraser C, Donnelly CA, Ghani AC, Abu-Raddad LJ, Hedley AJ, Leung GM, Ho LM, Lam TH, Thach TQ, Chau P, Chan KP, Lo SV, Leung PY, Tsang T, Ho W, Lee KH, Lau EM, Ferguson NM, Anderson RM.** 2003. Transmission dynamics of the etiological agent of SARS in Hong Kong: impact of public health interventions. *Science* **300:**1961–1966.

16. **de Groot RJ, Baker SC, Baric RS, Brown CS, Drosten C, Enjuanes L, Fouchier RA, Galiano M, Gorbalenya AE, Memish ZA, Perlman S, Poon LL, Snijder EJ, Stephens GM, Woo PC, Zaki AM, Zambon M, Ziebuhr J.** 2013. Middle East respiratory syndrome coronavirus (MERS-CoV): announcement of the Coronavirus Study Group. *J Virol* **87:**7790–7792.

17. **World Health Organization 2015.** *Middle East Respiratory Syndrome Coronavirus (MERS-CoV): Saudi Arabia.* http://www.who.int/csr/don/29-october-2015-mers-saudi-arabia/en/.

18. **Reusken CB, Raj VS, Koopmans MP, Haagmans BL.** 2016. Cross host transmission in the emergence of MERS coronavirus. *Curr Opin Virol* **16:**55–62.

19. **Bialek SR, Allen D, Alvarado-Ramy F, Arthur R, Balajee A, Bell D, Best S, Blackmore C, Breakwell L, Cannons A, Brown C, Cetron M, Chea N, Chommanard C, Cohen N, Conover C, Crespo A, Creviston J, Curns AT, Dahl R, Dearth S, DeMaria A, Echols F, Erdman DD, Feikin D, Frias M, Gerber SI, Gulati R, Hale C, Haynes LM, Heberlein-Larson L, Holton K, Ijaz K, Kapoor M, Kohl K, Kuhar DT, Kumar AM, Kundich M, Lippold S, Liu L, Lovchik JC, Madoff L, Martell S, Matthews S, Moore J,

Murray LR, Onofrey S, Pallansch MA, Pesik N, Pham H, Pillai S, Pontones P, Poser S, Pringle K, Pritchard S, Rasmussen S, Richards S, Sandoval M, Schneider E, Schuchat S, Sheedy K, Sherin K, Swerdlow DL, Tappero JW, Vernon MO, Watkins S, Watson J. 2014. First confirmed cases of Middle East respiratory syndrome coronavirus (MERS-CoV) infection in the United States, updated information on the epidemiology of MERS-CoV infection, and guidance for the public, clinicians, and public health authorities - May 2014. *MMWR Morb Mortal Wkly Rep* **63**:431–436.

20. Breakwell L, Pringle K, Chea N, Allen D, Allen S, Richards S, Pantones P, Sandoval M, Liu L, Vernon M, Conover C, Chugh R, DeMaria A, Burns R, Smole S, Gerber SI, Cohen NJ, Kuhar D, Haynes LM, Schneider E, Kumar A, Kapoor M, Madrigal M, Swerdlow DL, Feikin DR. 2015. Lack of transmission among close contacts of patient with case of Middle East respiratory syndrome imported into the United States, 2014. *Emerg Infect Dis* **21**:1128–1134.

21. World Health Organization 2015. *WHO statement on the tenth meeting of the IHR Emergency Committee regarding MERS — September 3, 2015.* http://www.who.int/mediacentre/news/statements/2015/ihr-emergency-committee-mers/en/.

22. Rasmussen SA, Gerber SI, Swerdlow DL. 2015. Middle East respiratory syndrome coronavirus: update for clinicians. *Clin Infect Dis* **60**:1686–1689.

23. Williams HA, Dunville RL, Gerber SI, Erdman DD, Pesik N, Kuhar D, Mason KA, Haynes L, Rotz L, St Pierre J, Poser S, Bunga S, Pallansch MA, Swerdlow DL. 2015. CDC's early response to a novel viral disease, Middle East respiratory syndrome coronavirus (MERS-CoV), September 2012-May 2014. *Public Health Rep* **130**:307–317.

24. Lu G, Wang Q, Gao GF. 2015. Bat-to-human: spike features determining 'host jump' of coronaviruses SARS-CoV, MERS-CoV, and beyond. *Trends Microbiol* **23**:468–478.

25. van Boheemen S, de Graaf M, Lauber C, Bestebroer TM, Raj VS, Zaki AM, Osterhaus AD, Haagmans BL, Gorbalenya AE, Snijder EJ, Fouchier RA. 2012. Genomic characterization of a newly discovered coronavirus associated with acute respiratory distress syndrome in humans. *MBio* **3**:e00473-12. doi:10.1128/mBio.00473-12.

26. Zumla A, Hui DS, Perlman S. 2015. Middle East respiratory syndrome. *Lancet* **386**:995–1007.

27. Raj VS, Mou H, Smits SL, Dekkers DH, Muller MA, Dijkman R, Muth D, Demmers JA, Zaki A, Fouchier RA, Thiel V, Drosten C, Rottier PJ, Osterhaus AD, Bosch BJ, Haagmans BL. 2013. Dipeptidyl peptidase 4 is a functional receptor for the emerging human coronavirus-EMC. *Nature* **495**:251–254.

28. Mou H, Raj VS, van Kuppeveld FJ, Rottier PJ, Haagmans BL, Bosch BJ. 2013. The receptor binding domain of the new Middle East respiratory syndrome coronavirus maps to a 231-residue region in the spike protein that efficiently elicits neutralizing antibodies. *J Virol* **87**:9379–9383.

29. Li W, Moore MJ, Vasilieva N, Sui J, Wong SK, Berne MA, Somasundaran M, Sullivan JL, Luzuriaga K, Greenough TC, Choe H, Farzan M. 2003. Angiotensin-converting enzyme 2 is a functional receptor for the SARS coronavirus. *Nature* **426**:450–454.

30. van Doremalen N, Miazgowicz KL, Milne-Price S, Bushmaker T, Robertson S, Scott D, Kinne J, McLellan JS, Zhu J, Munster VJ. 2014. Host species restriction of Middle East respiratory syndrome coronavirus through its receptor, dipeptidyl peptidase 4. *J Virol* **88**:9220–9232.

31. Chan JF, Lau SK, To KK, Cheng VC, Woo PC, Yuen KY. 2015. Middle East respiratory syndrome coronavirus: another zoonotic betacoronavirus causing SARS-like disease. *Clin Microbiol Rev* **28**:465–522.

32. Meyerholz DK, Lambertz AM, McCray PB Jr. 2016. Dipeptidyl peptidase 4 distribution in the human respiratory tract: implications for the Middle East respiratory syndrome. *Am J Pathol* **186**:76–86.

33. Yang Y, Liu C, Du L, Jiang S, Shi Z, Baric RS, Li F. 2015. Two mutations were critical for bat-to-human transmission of Middle East respiratory syndrome coronavirus. *J Virol* **89**:9119–9123.

34. Cotten M, Watson SJ, Zumla AI, Makhdoom HQ, Palser AL, Ong SH, Al Rabeeah AA, Alhakeem RF, Assiri A, Al-Tawfiq JA, Albarrak A, Barry M, Shibl A, Alrabiah FA, Hajjar S, Balkhy HH, Flemban H, Rambaut A, Kellam P, Memish ZA. 2014. Spread, circulation, and evolution of the Middle East respiratory syndrome coronavirus. *MBio* **5**:01062-13. doi:10.1128/mBio.01062-13.

35. Cowling BJ, Park M, Fang VJ, Wu P, Leung GM, Wu JT. 2015. Preliminary epidemiological assessment of MERS-CoV outbreak in South Korea, May to June 2015. *Euro Surveill* **20**:7–13. http://www.eurosurveillance.org/ViewArticle.aspx?ArticleId=21163.

36. WHO MERS-Cov Research Group. 2013. State of knowledge and data gaps of Middle East

respiratory syndrome coronavirus (MERS-CoV) in humans. *PLoS Curr* **5**. doi:10.1371/currents. outbreaks.0bf719e352e7478f8ad85fa30127ddb8.

37. **Alraddadi BM, Watson JT, Almarashi A, Abedi GR, Turkistani A, Sadran M, Housa A, Almazroa MA, Alraihan N, Banjar A, Albalawi E, Alhindi H, Choudhry AJ, Meiman JG, Paczkowski M, Curns A, Mounts A, Feikin DR, Marano N, Swerdlow DL, Gerber SI, Hajjeh R, Madani TA.** 2016. Risk factors for primary Middle East respiratory syndrome coronavirus illness in humans, Saudi Arabia, 2014. *Emerg Infect Dis* **22**:49–55.

38. **Arabi YM, Arifi AA, Balkhy HH, Najm H, Aldawood AS, Ghabashi A, Hawa H, Alothman A, Khaldi A, Al Raiy B.** 2014. Clinical course and outcomes of critically ill patients with Middle East respiratory syndrome coronavirus infection. *Ann Intern Med* **160**:389–397.

39. **Assiri A, Al-Tawfiq JA, Al-Rabeeah AA, Al-Rabiah FA, Al-Hajjar S, Al-Barrak A, Flemban H, Al-Nassir WN, Balkhy HH, Al-Hakeem RF, Makhdoom HQ, Zumla AI, Memish ZA.** 2013. Epidemiological, demographic, and clinical characteristics of 47 cases of Middle East respiratory syndrome coronavirus disease from Saudi Arabia: a descriptive study. *Lancet Infect Dis* **13**:752–761.

40. **Memish ZA, Zumla AI, Al-Hakeem RF, Al-Rabeeah AA, Stephens GM.** 2013. Family cluster of Middle East respiratory syndrome coronavirus infections. *N Engl J Med* **368**:2487–2494. (Erratum **369**:587.)

41. **Saad M, Omrani AS, Baig K, Bahloul A, Elzein F, Matin MA, Selim MA, Al Mutairi M, Al Nakhli D, Al Aidaroos AY, Al Sherbeeni N, Al-Khashan HI, Memish ZA, Albarrak AM.** 2014. Clinical aspects and outcomes of 70 patients with Middle East respiratory syndrome coronavirus infection: a single-center experience in Saudi Arabia. *Int J Infect Dis* **29**:301–306.

42. **Majumder MS, Kluberg SA, Mekaru SR, Brownstein JS.** 2015. Mortality risk factors for Middle East respiratory syndrome outbreak, South Korea, 2015. *Emerg Infect Dis* **21**:2088–2090.

43. **Feikin DR, Alraddadi B, Qutub M, Shabouni O, Curns A, Oboho IK, Tomczyk SM, Wolff B, Watson JT, Madani TA.** 2015. Association of higher MERS-CoV virus load with severe disease and death, Saudi Arabia, 2014. *Emerg Infect Dis* **21**:2029–2035.

44. **Virlogeux V, Park M, Wu JT, Cowling BJ.** 2016. Association between severity of MERS-CoV infection and incubation period. *Emerg Infect Dis* **22**. doi:10.3201/eid2203.151437.

45. **Virlogeux V, Fang VJ, Wu JT, Ho LM, Peiris JS, Leung GM, Cowling BJ.** 2015. Brief report: incubation period duration and severity of clinical disease following severe acute respiratory syndrome coronavirus infection. *Epidemiology* **26**:666–669.

46. **Memish ZA, Al-Tawfiq JA, Assiri A, AlRabiah FA, Al Hajjar S, Albarrak A, Flemban H, Alhakeem RF, Makhdoom HQ, Alsubaie S, Al-Rabeeah AA.** 2014. Middle East respiratory syndrome coronavirus disease in children. *Pediatr Infect Dis J* **33**:904–906.

47. **Payne DC, Iblan I, Alqasrawi S, Al Nsour M, Rha B, Tohme RA, Abedi GR, Farag NH, Haddadin A, Al Sanhouri T, Jarour N, Swerdlow DL, Jamieson DJ, Pallansch MA, Haynes LM, Gerber SI, Al Abdallat MM.** 2014. Stillbirth during infection with Middle East respiratory syndrome coronavirus. *J Infect Dis* **209**:1870–1872.

48. **Wong SF, Chow KM, Leung TN, Ng WF, Ng TK, Shek CC, Ng PC, Lam PW, Ho LC, To WW, Lai ST, Yan WW, Tan PY.** 2004. Pregnancy and perinatal outcomes of women with severe acute respiratory syndrome. *Am J Obstet Gynecol* **191**:292–297.

49. **Hemida MG, Elmoslemany A, Al-Hizab F, Alnaeem A, Almathen F, Faye B, Chu DK, Perera RA, Peiris M.** 2015. Dromedary camels and the transmission of Middle East respiratory syndrome coronavirus (MERS-CoV). *Transbound Emerg Dis*. [Epub ahead of print.] doi:10.1111/tbed.12401.

50. **Gossner C, Danielson N, Gervelmeyer A, Berthe F, Faye B, Kaasik Aaslav K, Adlhoch C, Zeller H, Penttinen P, Coulombier D.** 2016. Human-dromedary camel interactions and the risk of acquiring zoonotic Middle East respiratory syndrome coronavirus infection. *Zoonoses Public Health* **63**:1–9.

51. **Hemida MG, Chu DK, Poon LL, Perera RA, Alhammadi MA, Ng HY, Siu LY, Guan Y, Alnaeem A, Peiris M.** 2014. MERS coronavirus in dromedary camel herd, Saudi Arabia. *Emerg Infect Dis* **20**:1231–1234.

52. **Wernery U, Corman VM, Wong EY, Tsang AK, Muth D, Lau SK, Khazanehdari K, Zirkel F, Ali M, Nagy P, Juhasz J, Wernery R, Joseph S, Syriac G, Elizabeth SK, Patteril NA, Woo PC, Drosten C.** 2015. Acute middle East respiratory syndrome coronavirus infection in livestock dromedaries, Dubai, 2014. *Emerg Infect Dis* **21**:1019–1022.

53. **Muller MA, Meyer B, Corman VM, Al-Masri M, Turkestani A, Ritz D, Sieberg A, Aldabbagh S, Bosch BJ, Lattwein E, Alhakeem RF, Assiri AM, Albarrak AM, Al-Shangiti AM, Al-Tawfiq**

JA, Wikramaratna P, Alrabeeah AA, Drosten C, Memish ZA. 2015. Presence of Middle East respiratory syndrome coronavirus antibodies in Saudi Arabia: a nationwide, cross-sectional, serological study. *Lancet Infect Dis* **15:**559–564.

54. Reusken CB, Farag EA, Haagmans BL, Mohran KA, Godeke G-J, Raj S, Alhajri F, Al-Marri SA, Al-Romaihi HE, Al-Thani M, Bosch BJ, van der Eijk AA, El-Sayed AM, Ibrahim AK, Al-Molawi N, Muller MA, Pasha SK, Drosten C, AlHajri MM, Koopmans MP. 2015. Occupational exposure to dromedaries and risk for MERS-CoV infection, Qatar, 2013-2014. *Emerg Infect Dis* **21:**1422-1425.

55. Assiri A, McGeer A, Perl TM, Price CS, Al Rabeeah AA, Cummings DA, Alabdullatif ZN, Assad M, Almulhim A, Makhdoom H, Madani H, Alhakeem R, Al-Tawfiq JA, Cotten M, Watson SJ, Kellam P, Zumla AI, Memish ZA. 2013. Hospital outbreak of Middle East respiratory syndrome coronavirus. *N Engl J Med* **369:**407–416.

56. Drosten C, Meyer B, Muller MA, Corman VM, Al-Masri M, Hossain R, Madani H, Sieberg A, Bosch BJ, Lattwein E, Alhakeem RF, Assiri AM, Hajomar W, Albarrak AM, Al-Tawfiq JA, Zumla AI, Memish ZA. 2014. Transmission of MERS-coronavirus in household contacts. *N Engl J Med* **371:**828–835.

57. Drosten C, Muth D, Corman VM, Hussain R, Al Masri M, HajOmar W, Landt O, Assiri A, Eckerle I, Al Shangiti A, Al-Tawfiq JA, Albarrak A, Zumla A, Rambaut A, Memish ZA. 2015. An observational, laboratory-based study of outbreaks of middle East respiratory syndrome coronavirus in Jeddah and Riyadh, kingdom of Saudi Arabia, 2014. *Clin Infect Dis* **60:**369–377.

58. Omrani AS, Matin MA, Haddad Q, Al-Nakhli D, Memish ZA, Albarrak AM. 2013. A family cluster of Middle East respiratory syndrome coronavirus infections related to a likely unrecognized asymptomatic or mild case. *Int J Infect Dis* **17:**e668–e672.

59. Health Protection Agency (HPA) UK Novel Coronavirus Investigation team. 2013. Evidence of person-to-person transmission within a family cluster of novel coronavirus infections, United Kingdom, February 2013. *Euro Surveill* **18:**20427. http://www.eurosurveillance.org/ViewArticle.aspx?ArticleId=20427.

60. Al-Tawfiq JA, Hinedi K, Ghandour J, Khairalla H, Musleh S, Ujayli A, Memish ZA. 2014. Middle East respiratory syndrome coronavirus: a case-control study of hospitalized patients. *Clin Infect Dis* **59:**160–165.

61. Memish ZA, Al-Tawfiq JA, Assiri A. 2013. Hospital-associated Middle East respiratory syndrome coronavirus infections. *N Engl J Med* **369:**1761–1762.

62. Oboho IK, Tomczyk SM, Al-Asmari AM, Banjar AA, Al-Mugti H, Aloraini MS, Alkhaldi KZ, Almohammadi EL, Alraddadi BM, Gerber SI, Swerdlow DL, Watson JT, Madani TA. 2015. 2014 MERS-CoV outbreak in Jeddah: a link to health care facilities. *N Engl J Med* **372:**846–854.

63. Zumla A, Hui DS. 2014. Infection control and MERS-CoV in health-care workers. *Lancet* **383:**1869–1871.

64. Oh MD, Choe PG, Oh HS, Park WB, Lee SM, Park J, Lee SK, Song JS, Kim NJ. 2015. Middle East respiratory syndrome coronavirus superspreading event involving 81 persons, Korea 2015. *J Korean Med Sci* **30:**1701–1705.

65. Korea Centers for Disease Control and Prevention. 2015. Middle East respiratory syndrome coronavirus outbreak in the Republic of Korea, 2015. *Osong Public Health Res Perspect* **6:**269–278.

66. Shen Z, Ning F, Zhou W, He X, Lin C, Chin DP, Zhu Z, Schuchat A. 2004. Superspreading SARS events, Beijing, 2003. *Emerg Infect Dis* **10:**256–260.

67. van Doremalen N, Bushmaker T, Munster VJ. 2013. Stability of Middle East respiratory syndrome coronavirus (MERS-CoV) under different environmental conditions. *Euro Surveill* **18:**20590. http://www.eurosurveillance.org/ViewArticle.aspx?ArticleId=20590.

68. Corman VM, Albarrak AM, Omrani AS, Albarrak MM, Farah ME, Almasri M, Muth D, Sieberg A, Meyer B, Assiri AM, Binger T, Steinhagen K, Lattwein E, Al-Tawfiq J, Muller MA, Drosten C, Memish ZA. 2016. Viral shedding and antibody response in 37 patients with MERS-coronavirus infection. *Clin Infect Dis* **62:**477–483.

69. Breban R, Riou J, Fontanet A. 2013. Interhuman transmissibility of Middle East respiratory syndrome coronavirus: estimation of pandemic risk. *Lancet* **382:**694–699.

70. Cauchemez S, Fraser C, Van Kerkhove MD, Donnelly CA, Riley S, Rambaut A, Enouf V, van der Werf S, Ferguson NM. 2014. Middle East respiratory syndrome coronavirus: quantification of the extent of the epidemic, surveillance biases, and transmissibility. *Lancet Infect Dis* **14:**50–56.

71. Majumder MS, Rivers C, Lofgren E, Fisman D. 2014. Estimation of MERS-coronavirus reproductive number and case fatality rate for the spring 2014 Saudi Arabia outbreak: insights from publicly available data. *PLoS Curr* **6**. doi:10.1371/currents.outbreaks.98d2f8f3382d84f390736cd5f5fe133c.

72. Memish ZA, Mishra N, Olival KJ, Fagbo SF, Kapoor V, Epstein JH, Alhakeem R, Durosinloun A, Al Asmari M, Islam A, Kapoor A, Briese T, Daszak P, Al Rabeeah AA, Lipkin WI. 2013. Middle East respiratory syndrome coronavirus in bats, Saudi Arabia. *Emerg Infect Dis* **19:**1819–1823.

73. Reusken CB, Haagmans BL, Muller MA, Gutierrez C, Godeke GJ, Meyer B, Muth D, Raj VS, Smits-De Vries L, Corman VM, Drexler JF, Smits SL, El Tahir YE, De Sousa R, van Beek J, Nowotny N, van Maanen K, Hidalgo-Hermoso E, Bosch BJ, Rottier P, Osterhaus A, Gortazar-Schmidt C, Drosten C, Koopmans MP. 2013. Middle East respiratory syndrome coronavirus neutralising serum antibodies in dromedary camels: a comparative serological study. *Lancet Infect Dis* **13:**859–866.

74. Reusken CB, Farag EA, Jonges M, Godeke GJ, El-Sayed AM, Pas SD, Raj VS, Mohran KA, Moussa HA, Ghobashy H, Alhajri F, Ibrahim AK, Bosch BJ, Pasha SK, Al-Romaihi HE, Al-Thani M, Al-Marri SA, AlHajri MM, Haagmans BL, Koopmans MP. 2014. Middle East respiratory syndrome coronavirus (MERS-CoV) RNA and neutralising antibodies in milk collected according to local customs from dromedary camels, Qatar, April 2014. *Euro Surveill* **19:**20829. http://www.eurosurveillance.org/ViewArticle.aspx?ArticleId=20829.

75. Reusken CB, Messadi L, Feyisa A, Ularamu H, Godeke GJ, Danmarwa A, Dawo F, Jemli M, Melaku S, Shamaki D, Woma Y, Wungak Y, Gebremedhin EZ, Zutt I, Bosch BJ, Haagmans BL, Koopmans MP. 2014. Geographic distribution of MERS coronavirus among dromedary camels, Africa. *Emerg Infect Dis* **20:**1370–1374.

76. Reusken CB, Ababneh M, Raj VS, Meyer B, Eljarah A, Abutarbush S, Godeke GJ, Bestebroer TM, Zutt I, Muller MA, Bosch BJ, Rottier PJ, Osterhaus AD, Drosten C, Haagmans BL, Koopmans MP. 2013. Middle East respiratory syndrome coronavirus (MERS-CoV) serology in major livestock species in an affected region in Jordan, June to September 2013. *Euro Surveill* **18:**20662. http://www.eurosurveillance.org/ViewArticle.aspx?ArticleId=20662.

77. Alexandersen S, Kobinger GP, Soule G, Wernery U. 2014. Middle East respiratory syndrome coronavirus antibody reactors among camels in Dubai, United Arab Emirates, in 2005. *Transbound Emerg Dis* **61:**105–108.

78. Hemida MG, Perera RA, Al Jassim RA, Kayali G, Siu LY, Wang P, Chu KW, Perlman S, Ali MA, Alnaeem A, Guan Y, Poon LL, Saif L,

Peiris M. 2014. Seroepidemiology of Middle East respiratory syndrome (MERS) coronavirus in Saudi Arabia (1993) and Australia (2014) and characterisation of assay specificity. *Euro Surveill* **19:**20828. http://www.eurosurveillance.org/ViewArticle.aspx?ArticleId=20828.

79. Alagaili AN, Briese T, Mishra N, Kapoor V, Sameroff SC, Burbelo PD, de Wit E, Munster VJ, Hensley LE, Zalmout IS, Kapoor A, Epstein JH, Karesh WB, Daszak P, Mohammed OB, Lipkin WI. 2014. Middle East respiratory syndrome coronavirus infection in dromedary camels in Saudi Arabia. *MBio* **5:**e00884-14. doi:10.1128/mBio.00884-14.

80. Meyer B, Muller MA, Corman VM, Reusken CB, Ritz D, Godeke GJ, Lattwein E, Kallies S, Siemens A, van Beek J, Drexler JF, Muth D, Bosch BJ, Wernery U, Koopmans MP, Wernery R, Drosten C. 2014. Antibodies against MERS coronavirus in dromedary camels, United Arab Emirates, 2003 and 2013. *Emerg Infect Dis* **20:**552–559.

81. Corman VM, Jores J, Meyer B, Younan M, Liljander A, Said MY, Gluecks I, Lattwein E, Bosch BJ, Drexler JF, Bornstein S, Drosten C, Muller MA. 2014. Antibodies against MERS coronavirus in dromedary camels, Kenya, 1992–2013. *Emerg Infect Dis* **20:**1319–1322.

82. Muller MA, Corman VM, Jores J, Meyer B, Younan M, Liljander A, Bosch BJ, Lattwein E, Hilali M, Musa BE, Bornstein S, Drosten C. 2014. MERS coronavirus neutralizing antibodies in camels, Eastern Africa, 1983–1997. *Emerg Infect Dis* **20:**2093–2095.

83. Aburizaiza AS, Mattes FM, Azhar EI, Hassan AM, Memish ZA, Muth D, Meyer B, Lattwein E, Muller MA, Drosten C. 2014. Investigation of anti-middle East respiratory syndrome antibodies in blood donors and slaughterhouse workers in Jeddah and Makkah, Saudi Arabia, fall 2012. *J Infect Dis* **209:**243–246.

84. Azhar EI, El-Kafrawy SA, Farraj SA, Hassan AM, Al-Saeed MS, Hashem AM, Madani TA. 2014. Evidence for camel-to-human transmission of MERS coronavirus. *N Engl J Med* **370:**2499–2505.

85. Haagmans BL, Al Dhahiry SH, Reusken CB, Raj VS, Galiano M, Myers R, Godeke GJ, Jonges M, Farag E, Diab A, Ghobashy H, Alhajri F, Al-Thani M, Al-Marri SA, Al Romaihi HE, Al Khal A, Bermingham A, Osterhaus AD, AlHajri MM, Koopmans MP. 2014. Middle East respiratory syndrome coronavirus in dromedary camels: an outbreak investigation. *Lancet Infect Dis* **14:**140–145.

86. Memish ZA, Cotten M, Meyer B, Watson SJ, Alsahafi AJ, Al Rabeeah AA, Corman VM,

Sieberg A, Makhdoom HQ, Assiri A, Al Masri M, Aldabbagh S, Bosch BJ, Beer M, Muller MA, Kellam P, Drosten C. 2014. Human infection with MERS coronavirus after exposure to infected camels, Saudi Arabia, 2013. *Emerg Infect Dis* **20:**1012–1015.

87. Azhar EI, Hashem AM, El-Kafrawy SA, Sohrab SS, Aburizaiza AS, Farraj SA, Hassan AM, Al-Saeed MS, Jamjoom GA, Madani TA. 2014. Detection of the Middle East respiratory syndrome coronavirus genome in an air sample originating from a camel barn owned by an infected patient. *mBio* **5:**e01450-14. doi:10.1128/mBio.01450-14.

88. Hemida MG, Al-Naeem A, Perera RA, Chin AW, Poon LL, Peiris M. 2015. Lack of middle East respiratory syndrome coronavirus transmission from infected camels. *Emerg Infect Dis* **21:**699–701.

89. van Doremalen N, Bushmaker T, Karesh WB, Munster VJ. 2014. Stability of Middle East respiratory syndrome coronavirus in milk. *Emerg Infect Dis* **20:**1263–1264.

90. Hijawi B, Abdallat M, Sayaydeh A, Alqasrawi S, Haddadin A, Jaarour N, Alsheikh S, Alsanouri T. 2013. Novel coronavirus infections in Jordan, April 2012: epidemiological findings from a retrospective investigation. *East Mediterr Health J* **19**(Suppl 1)**:**S12–S18.

91. Cheng VC, Chan JF, To KK, Yuen KY. 2013. Clinical management and infection control of SARS: lessons learned. *Antiviral Res* **100:**407–419.

92. Al-Tawfiq JA, Memish ZA. 2015. Managing MERS-CoV in the healthcare setting. *Hosp Pract* **43:**158–163.

93. Seto WH, Conly JM, Pessoa-Silva CL, Malik M, Eremin S. 2013. Infection prevention and control measures for acute respiratory infections in healthcare settings: an update. *East Mediterr Health J* **19**(Suppl 1)**:**S39–S47.

94. Al-Tawfiq JA, Zumla A, Memish ZA. 2014. Travel implications of emerging coronaviruses: SARS and MERS-CoV. *Travel Med Infect Dis* **12:**422–428.

95. Rha B, Rudd J, Feikin D, Watson J, Curns AT, Swerdlow DL, Pallansch MA, Gerber SI. 2015. Update on the epidemiology of Middle East respiratory syndrome coronavirus (MERS-CoV) infection, and guidance for the public, clinicians, and public health authorities: January 2015. *MMWR Morb Mortal Wkly Rep* **64:**61–62.

96. German M, Olsha R, Kristjanson E, Marchand-Austin A, Peci A, Winter AL, Gubbay JB. 2015. Acute respiratory infections in travelers returning from MERS-CoV-affected areas. *Emerg Infect Dis* **21:**1654–1656.

97. Shahkarami M, Yen C, Glaser C, Xia D, Watt J, Wadford DA. 2015. Laboratory testing for Middle East respiratory syndrome coronavirus, California, USA, 2013-2014. *Emerg Infect Dis* **21:**1664–1666.

98. Public Health England. 2015. *MERS, influenza and respiratory illness in travellers returning from the Hajj.* https://www.gov.uk/government/publications/health-protection-report-volume-9-2015/hpr-volume-9-issue-36-news-9-october#mers-influenza-and-respiratory-illness-in-travellers-returning-from-the-hajj.

99. Khan K, Sears J, Hu VW, Brownstein JS, Hay S, Kossowsky D, Eckhardt R, Chim T, Berry I, Bogoch I, Cetron M. 2013. Potential for the international spread of middle East respiratory syndrome in association with mass gatherings in saudi arabia. *PLoS currents* **5**. doi:10.1371/currents.outbreaks.a7b70897ac2fa4f79b59f90d24c860b8.

100. Rashid H, Azeem MI, Heron L, Haworth E, Booy R, Memish ZA. 2014. Has Hajj-associated Middle East respiratory syndrome coronavirus transmission occurred? The case for effective post-Hajj surveillance for infection. *Clin Microbiol Infect* **20:**273–276.

101. Memish ZA, Assiri A, Almasri M, Alhakeem RF, Turkestani A, Al Rabeeah AA, Al-Tawfiq JA, Alzahrani A, Azhar E, Makhdoom HQ, Hajomar WH, Al-Shangiti AM, Yezli S. 2014. Prevalence of MERS-CoV nasal carriage and compliance with the Saudi health recommendations among pilgrims attending the 2013 Hajj. *J Infect Dis* **210:**1067–1072.

102. Memish ZA, Almasri M, Turkestani A, Al-Shangiti AM, Yezli S. 2014. Etiology of severe community-acquired pneumonia during the 2013 Hajj-part of the MERS-CoV surveillance program. *Int J Infect Dis* **25:**186–190.

103. Waldron G, Doherty L. 2015. Low public health risk of MERS-CoV in people returning from the Hajj. *BMJ* **351:**h5543.

104. Soliman T, Cook AR, Coker RJ. 2015. Pilgrims and MERS-CoV: what's the risk? *Emerg Themes Epidemiol* **12:**3.

105. Sridhar S, Brouqui P, Parola P, Gautret P. 2015. Imported cases of Middle East respiratory syndrome: an update. *Travel Med Infect Dis* **13:**106–109.

106. van Doremalen N, Munster VJ. 2015. Animal models of Middle East respiratory syndrome coronavirus infection. *Antiviral Res* **122:**28–38.

107. Coleman CM, Matthews KL, Goicochea L, Frieman MB. 2014. Wild-type and innate immune-deficient mice are not susceptible to the Middle East respiratory syndrome coronavirus. *J Gen Virol* **95:**408–412.

108. de Wit E, Prescott J, Baseler L, Bushmaker T, Thomas T, Lackemeyer MG, Martellaro C, Milne-Price S, Haddock E, Haagmans BL, Feldmann H, Munster VJ. 2013. The Middle East respiratory syndrome coronavirus (MERS-CoV) does not replicate in Syrian hamsters. *PLoS One* **8:**e69127. doi:10.1371/journal.pone.0069127.

109. Raj VS, Smits SL, Provacia LB, van den Brand JM, Wiersma L, Ouwendijk WJ, Bestebroer TM, Spronken MI, van Amerongen G, Rottier PJ, Fouchier RA, Bosch BJ, Osterhaus AD, Haagmans BL. 2014. Adenosine deaminase acts as a natural antagonist for dipeptidyl peptidase 4-mediated entry of the Middle East respiratory syndrome coronavirus. *J Virol* **88:**1834–1838.

110. Haagmans BL, van den Brand JM, Provacia LB, Raj VS, Stittelaar KJ, Getu S, de Waal L, Bestebroer TM, van Amerongen G, Verjans GM, Fouchier RA, Smits SL, Thijs K, Osterhaus AD. 2015. Asymptomatic Middle East respiratory syndrome coronavirus infection in rabbits. *J Virol* **89:**6131–6135.

111. Zhao J, Li K, Wohlford-Lenane C, Agnihothram SS, Fett C, Zhao J, Gale MJ Jr, Baric RS, Enjuanes L, Gallagher T, McCray PB Jr, Perlman S. 2014. Rapid generation of a mouse model for Middle East respiratory syndrome. *Proc Natl Acad Sci USA* **111:**4970–4975.

112. Tao X, Garron T, Agrawal AS, Algaissi A, Peng BH, Wakamiya M, Chan TS, Lu L, Du L, Jiang S, Couch RB, Tseng CK. 2015. Characterization and demonstration of value of a lethal mouse model of Middle East respiratory syndrome coronavirus infection and disease. *J Virol* **90:**57–67.

113. Agrawal AS, Garron T, Tao X, Peng BH, Wakamiya M, Chan TS, Couch RB, Tseng CT. 2015. Generation of a transgenic mouse model of middle East respiratory syndrome coronavirus infection and disease. *J Virol* **89:**3659–3670.

114. Li K, Wohlford-Lenane C, Perlman S, Zhao J, Jewell AK, Reznikov LR, Gibson-Corley KN, Meyerholz DK, McCray PB Jr. 2016. Middle East respiratory syndrome coronavirus causes multiple organ damage and lethal disease in mice transgenic for human dipeptidyl peptidase 4. *J Infect Dis* **213:**712–722.

115. Munster VJ, de Wit E, Feldmann H. 2013. Pneumonia from human coronavirus in a macaque model. *N Engl J Med* **368:**1560–1562.

116. Falzarano D, de Wit E, Feldmann F, Rasmussen AL, Okumura A, Peng X, Thomas MJ, van Doremalen N, Haddock E, Nagy L, LaCasse R, Liu T, Zhu J, McLellan JS, Scott DP, Katze MG, Feldmann H, Munster VJ. 2014. Infection with MERS-CoV causes lethal pneumonia in the common marmoset. *PLoS Pathog* **10:**e1004250. doi:10.1371/journal.ppat.1004250.

117. Adney DR, van Doremalen N, Brown VR, Bushmaker T, Scott D, de Wit E, Bowen RA, Munster VJ. 2014. Replication and shedding of MERS-CoV in upper respiratory tract of inoculated dromedary camels. *Emerg Infect Dis* **20:**1999–2005.

118. Saad M, Omrani AS, Baig K, Bahloul A, Elzein F, Matin MA, Selim MA, Mutairi MA, Nakhli DA, Aidaroos AY, Sherbeeni NA, Al-Khashan HI, Memish ZA, Albarrak AM. 2014. Clinical aspects and outcomes of 70 patients with Middle East respiratory syndrome coronavirus infection: a single-center experience in Saudi Arabia. *Int J Infect Dis* **29:**301–306.

119. Eckerle I, Muller MA, Kallies S, Gotthardt DN, Drosten C. 2013. *In-vitro* renal epithelial cell infection reveals a viral kidney tropism as a potential mechanism for acute renal failure during Middle East respiratory syndrome (MERS) coronavirus infection. *Virol J* **10:**359.

120. Arabi YM, Harthi A, Hussein J, Bouchama A, Johani S, Hajeer AH, Saeed BT, Wahbi A, Saedy A, AlDabbagh T, Okaili R, Sadat M, Balkhy H. 2015. Severe neurologic syndrome associated with Middle East respiratory syndrome corona virus (MERS-CoV). *Infection* **43:**495–501.

121. van den Brand JM, Smits SL, Haagmans BL. 2015. Pathogenesis of Middle East respiratory syndrome coronavirus. *J Pathol* **235:**175–184.

122. Ajlan AM, Ahyad RA, Jamjoom LG, Alharthy A, Madani TA. 2014. Middle East respiratory syndrome coronavirus (MERS-CoV) infection: chest CT findings. *Am J Roentgenol* **203:**782–787.

123. van den Brand JM, Haagmans BL, van Riel D, Osterhaus AD, Kuiken T. 2014. The pathology and pathogenesis of experimental severe acute respiratory syndrome and influenza in animal models. *J Comp Pathol* **151:**83–112.

124. Ng DL, Al Hosani F, Keating MK, Gerber SI, Jones TL, Metcalfe MG, Tong S, Tao Y, Alami NN, Haynes LM, Mutei MA, Abdel-Wareth L, Uyeki TM, Swerdlow DL, Barakat M, Zaki SR. 2016. Clinicopathologic, immunohistochemical, and ultrastructural findings of a fatal case of Middle East respiratory syndrome coronavirus infection in United Arab Emirates, April 2014. *Am J Pathol* **186:**652–658.

125. Thomas HL, Zhao H, Green HK, Boddington NL, Carvalho CF, Osman HK, Sadler C, Zambon M, Bermingham A, Pebody RG.

2014. Enhanced MERS coronavirus surveillance of travelers from the Middle East to England. *Emerg Infect Dis* **20**:1562–1564.

126. **Corman VM, Eckerle I, Bleicker T, Zaki A, Landt O, Eschbach-Bludau M, van Boheemen S, Gopal R, Ballhause M, Bestebroer TM, Muth D, Muller MA, Drexler JF, Zambon M, Osterhaus AD, Fouchier RM, Drosten C.** 2012. Detection of a novel human coronavirus by real-time reverse-transcription polymerase chain reaction. *Euro Surveill* **17**:20285. http://www.eurosurveillance.org/ViewArticle.aspx?ArticleId=20285.

127. **Corman VM, Muller MA, Costabel U, Timm J, Binger T, Meyer B, Kreher P, Lattwein E, Eschbach-Bludau M, Nitsche A, Bleicker T, Landt O, Schweiger B, Drexler JF, Osterhaus AD, Haagmans BL, Dittmer U, Bonin F, Wolff T, Drosten C.** 2012. Assays for laboratory confirmation of novel human coronavirus (hCoV-EMC) infections. *Euro Surveill* **17**:20334. http://www.eurosurveillance.org/ViewArticle.aspx?ArticleId=20334.

128. **Lu X, Whitaker B, Sakthivel SK, Kamili S, Rose LE, Lowe L, Mohareb E, Elassal EM, Al-sanouri T, Haddadin A, Erdman DD.** 2014. Real-time reverse transcription-PCR assay panel for Middle East respiratory syndrome coronavirus. *J Clin Microbiol* **52**:67–75.

129. **World Health Organization.** 2015. *Laboratory Testing for Middle East Respiratory Syndrome Coronavirus (MERS-CoV) Interim Guidance Updated June 2015.* http://apps.who.int/iris/bitstream/10665/176982/1/WHO_MERS_LAB_15.1_eng.pdf.

130. **Memish ZA, Al-Tawfiq JA, Makhdoom HQ, Assiri A, Alhakeem RF, Albarrak A, Alsubaie S, Al-Rabeeah AA, Hajomar WH, Hussain R, Kheyami AM, Almutairi A, Azhar EI, Drosten C, Watson SJ, Kellam P, Cotten M, Zumla A.** 2014. Respiratory tract samples, viral load, and genome fraction yield in patients with Middle East respiratory syndrome. *J Infect Dis* **210**:1590–1594.

131. **Guery B, Poissy J, el Mansouf L, Sejourne C, Ettahar N, Lemaire X, Vuotto F, Goffard A, Behillil S, Enouf V, Caro V, Mailles A, Che D, Manuguerra JC, Mathieu D, Fontanet A, van der Werf S.** 2013. Clinical features and viral diagnosis of two cases of infection with Middle East respiratory syndrome coronavirus: a report of nosocomial transmission. *Lancet* **381**:2265–2272.

132. **Poissy J, Goffard A, Parmentier-Decrucq E, Favory R, Kauv M, Kipnis E, Mathieu D, Guery B, MERS-CoV Biology Group.** 2014. Kinetics and pattern of viral excretion in biological specimens of two MERS-CoV cases. *J Clin Virol* **61**:275–278.

133. **Kapoor M, Pringle K, Kumar A, Dearth S, Liu L, Lovchik J, Perez O, Pontones P, Richards S, Yeadon-Fagbohun J, Breakwell L, Chea N, Cohen NJ, Schneider E, Erdman D, Haynes L, Pallansch M, Tao Y, Tong S, Gerber S, Swerdlow D, Feikin DR.** 2014. Clinical and laboratory findings of the first imported case of Middle East respiratory syndrome coronavirus to the United States. *Clin Infect Dis* **59**:1511–1518.

134. **Drosten C, Seilmaier M, Corman VM, Hartmann W, Scheible G, Sack S, Guggemos W, Kallies R, Muth D, Junglen S, Muller MA, Haas W, Guberina H, Rohnisch T, Schmid-Wendtner M, Aldabbagh S, Dittmer U, Gold H, Graf P, Bonin F, Rambaut A, Wendtner CM.** 2013. Clinical features and virological analysis of a case of Middle East respiratory syndrome coronavirus infection. *Lancet Infect Dis* **13**:745–751.

135. **Meyer B, Drosten C, Muller MA.** 2014. Serological assays for emerging coronaviruses: challenges and pitfalls. *Virus Res* **194**:175–183.

136. **Perera RA, Wang P, Gomaa MR, El-Shesheny R, Kandeil A, Bagato O, Siu LY, Shehata MM, Kayed AS, Moatasim Y, Li M, Poon LL, Guan Y, Webby RJ, Ali MA, Peiris JS, Kayali G.** 2013. Seroepidemiology for MERS coronavirus using microneutralisation and pseudoparticle virus neutralisation assays reveal a high prevalence of antibody in dromedary camels in Egypt, June 2013. *Euro Surveill* **18**:20574. http://www.eurosurveillance.org/ViewArticle.aspx?ArticleId=20574.

137. **Reusken C, Mou H, Godeke GJ, van der Hoek L, Meyer B, Muller MA, Haagmans B, de Sousa R, Schuurman N, Dittmer U, Rottier P, Osterhaus A, Drosten C, Bosch BJ, Koopmans M.** 2013. Specific serology for emerging human coronaviruses by protein microarray. *Euro Surveill* **18**:20441. http://www.eurosurveillance.org/ViewArticle.aspx?ArticleId=20441.

138. **Zhao G, Du L, Ma C, Li Y, Li L, Poon VK, Wang L, Yu F, Zheng BJ, Jiang S, Zhou Y.** 2013. A safe and convenient pseudovirus-based inhibition assay to detect neutralizing antibodies and screen for viral entry inhibitors against the novel human coronavirus MERS-CoV. *Virol J* **10**:266.

139. **Channappanavar R, Zhao J, Perlman S.** 2014. T cell-mediated immune response to respiratory coronaviruses. *Immunol Res* **59**:118–128.

140. **Madani TA.** 2014. Case definition and management of patients with MERS coronavirus in Saudi Arabia. *Lancet Infect Dis* **14**:911–913.

141. **Hart BJ, Dyall J, Postnikova E, Zhou H, Kindrachuk J, Johnson RF, Olinger GG Jr,**

Frieman MB, Holbrook MR, Jahrling PB, Hensley L. 2014. Interferon-beta and myco-phenolic acid are potent inhibitors of Middle East respiratory syndrome coronavirus in cell-based assays. *J Gen Virol* **95:**571–577.

142. de Wilde AH, Raj VS, Oudshoorn D, Bestebroer TM, van Nieuwkoop S, Limpens RW, Posthuma CC, van der Meer Y, Barcena M, Haagmans BL, Snijder EJ, van den Hoogen BG. 2013. MERS-coronavirus replica-tion induces severe *in vitro* cytopathology and is strongly inhibited by cyclosporin A or interferon-alpha treatment. *J Gen Virol* **94:**1749–1760.

143. Cao J, Forrest JC, Zhang X. 2015. A screen of the NIH Clinical Collection small molecule library identifies potential anti-coronavirus drugs. *Antiviral Res* **114:**1–10.

144. Chan JF, Chan KH, Kao RY, To KK, Zheng BJ, Li CP, Li PT, Dai J, Mok FK, Chen H, Hayden FG, Yuen KY. 2013. Broad-spectrum antivirals for the emerging Middle East respiratory syn-drome coronavirus. *J Infect* **67:**606–616.

145. Dyall J, Coleman CM, Hart BJ, Venkataraman T, Holbrook MR, Kindrachuk J, Johnson RF, Olinger GG Jr, Jahrling PB, Laidlaw M, Johansen LM, Lear-Rooney CM, Glass PJ, Hensley LE, Frieman MB. 2014. Repurposing of clinically developed drugs for treatment of Middle East respiratory syndrome coronavirus infection. *Antimicrob Agents Chemother* **58:**4885–4893.

146. Jiang L, Wang N, Zuo T, Shi X, Poon KM, Wu Y, Gao F, Li D, Wang R, Guo J, Fu L, Yuen KY, Zheng BJ, Wang X, Zhang L. 2014. Potent neutralization of MERS-CoV by human neutralizing monoclonal antibodies to the viral spike glycoprotein. *Sci Transl Med* **6:**234ra259.

147. Falzarano D, de Wit E, Rasmussen AL, Feldmann F, Okumura A, Scott DP, Brining D, Bushmaker T, Martellaro C, Baseler L, Benecke AG, Katze MG, Munster VJ, Feldmann H. 2013. Treatment with interferon-alpha2b and ribavirin improves outcome in MERS-CoV-infected rhesus macaques. *Nat Med* **19:**1313–1317.

148. Chan JF, Yao Y, Yeung ML, Deng W, Bao L, Jia L, Li F, Xiao C, Gao H, Yu P, Cai JP, Chu H, Zhou J, Chen H, Qin C, Yuen KY. 2015. Treatment with lopinavir/ritonavir or inter-feron-beta1b improves outcome of MERS-CoV infection in a nonhuman primate model of common marmoset. *J Infect Dis* **212:**1904–1913.

149. Mair-Jenkins J, Saavedra-Campos M, Baillie JK, Cleary P, Khaw FM, Lim WS, Makki S, Rooney KD, Beck CR, Convalescent Plasma Study Group. 2015. The effectiveness of convalescent plasma and hyperimmune immu-noglobulin for the treatment of severe acute respiratory infections of viral etiology: a systematic review and exploratory meta-anal-ysis. *J Infect Dis* **211:**80–90.

150. Arabi Y, Balkhy H, Hajeer AH, Bouchama A, Hayden FG, Al-Omari A, Al-Hameed FM, Taha Y, Shindo N, Whitehead J, Merson L, AlJohani S, Al-Khairy K, Carson G, Luke TC, Hensley L, Al-Dawood A, Al-Qahtani S, Modjarrad K, Sadat M, Rohde G, Leport C, Fowler R. 2015. Feasibility, safety, clinical, and laboratory effects of convalescent plasma therapy for patients with Middle East respi-ratory syndrome coronavirus infection: a study protocol. *Springerplus* **4:**709.

151. Stockman LJ, Bellamy R, Garner P. 2006. SARS: systematic review of treatment effects. *PLoS Med* **3:**e343. doi:10.1371/journal.pmed.0030343.

152. Omrani AS, Saad MM, Baig K, Bahloul A, Abdul-Matin M, Alaidaroos AY, Almakhlafi GA, Albarrak MM, Memish ZA, Albarrak AM. 2014. Ribavirin and interferon alfa-2a for severe Middle East respiratory syndrome coronavirus infection: a retrospective cohort study. *Lancet Infect Dis* **14:**1090–1095. (Erra-tum **211:**13.)

153. Mackay IM, Arden KE. 2015. Middle East respiratory syndrome: an emerging coronavirus infection tracked by the crowd. *Virus Res* **202:**60–88.

154. Weingartl H, Czub M, Czub S, Neufeld J, Marszal P, Gren J, Smith G, Jones S, Proulx R, Deschambault Y, Grudeski E, Andonov A, He R, Li Y, Copps J, Grolla A, Dick D, Berry J, Ganske S, Manning L, Cao J. 2004. Immuniza-tion with modified vaccinia virus Ankara-based recombinant vaccine against severe acute respi-ratory syndrome is associated with enhanced hepatitis in ferrets. *J Virol* **78:**12672–12676.

155. See RH, Zakhartchouk AN, Petric M, Lawrence DJ, Mok CP, Hogan RJ, Rowe T, Zitzow LA, Karunakaran KP, Hitt MM, Graham FL, Prevec L, Mahony JB, Sharon C, Auperin TC, Rini JM, Tingle AJ, Scheifele DW, Skowronski DM, Patrick DM, Voss TG, Babiuk LA, Gauldie J, Roper RL, Brunham RC, Finlay BB. 2006. Comparative evaluation of two severe acute respiratory syndrome (SARS) vac-cine candidates in mice challenged with SARS coronavirus. *J Gen Virol* **87:**641–650.

156. Ma C, Li Y, Wang L, Zhao G, Tao X, Tseng CT, Zhou Y, Du L, Jiang S. 2014. Intranasal vaccination with recombinant receptor-bind-ing domain of MERS-CoV spike protein induces much stronger local mucosal immune responses than subcutaneous immunization:

implication for designing novel mucosal MERS vaccines. *Vaccine* **32:**2100–2108.

157. **Du L, Jiang S.** 2015. Middle East respiratory syndrome: current status and future prospects for vaccine development. *Expert Opin Biol Ther* **15:**1647–1651.

158. **Wang L, Shi W, Joyce MG, Modjarrad K, Zhang Y, Leung K, Lees CR, Zhou T, Yassine HM, Kanekiyo M, Yang ZY, Chen X, Becker MM, Freeman M, Vogel L, Johnson JC, Olinger G, Todd JP, Bagci U, Solomon J, Mollura DJ, Hensley L, Jahrling P, Denison MR, Rao SS, Subbarao K, Kwong PD, Mascola JR, Kong WP, Graham BS.** 2015. Evaluation of candidate vaccine approaches for MERS-CoV. *Nat Commun* **6:**7712.

159. **Hui DS, Memish ZA, Zumla A.** 2014. Severe acute respiratory syndrome vs. the Middle East respiratory syndrome. *Curr Opin Pulm Med* **20:**233–241.

160. **Banik GR, Khandaker G, Rashid H.** 2015. Middle East respiratory syndrome coronavirus "MERS-CoV": current knowledge gaps. *Paediatr Respir Rev* **16:**197–202.

161. **Milne-Price S, Miazgowicz KL, Munster VJ.** 2014. The emergence of the Middle East respiratory syndrome coronavirus. *Pathog Dis* **71:**121–136.

162. **World Health Organization.** 2012. *Case definition for case finding severe respiratory disease associated with novel coronavirus.* http://www.who.int/csr/disease/coronavirus_infections/case_definition_25_09_2012/en/.

163. **Centers for Disease Control and Prevention.** 2013. Updated information on the epidemiology of Middle East respiratory syndrome coronavirus (MERS-CoV) infection and guidance for the public, clinicians, and public health authorities, 2012-2013. *MMWR Morb Mortal Wkly Rep* **62:**793–796.

164. **Cotten M, Watson SJ, Kellam P, Al-Rabeeah AA, Makhdoom HQ, Assiri A, Al-Tawfiq JA, Alhakeem RF, Madani H, AlRabiah FA, Al Hajjar S, Al-nassir WN, Albarrak A, Flemban H, Balkhy HH, Alsubaie S, Palser AL, Gall A, Bashford-Rogers R, Rambaut A, Zumla AI, Memish ZA.** 2013. Transmission and evolution of the Middle East respiratory syndrome coronavirus in Saudi Arabia: a descriptive genomic study. *Lancet* **382:**1993–2002.

165. **Yang JS, Park S, Kim YJ, Kang HJ, Kim H, Han YW, Lee HS, Kim DW, Kim AR, Heo DR, Kim JA, Kim SJ, Nam JG, Jung HD, Cheong HM, Kim K, Lee JS, Kim SS.** 2015. Middle East respiratory syndrome in 3 persons, South Korea, 2015. *Emerg Infect Dis* **21:**2084–2087.

5

The Emergence of Enterovirus-D68

KEVIN MESSACAR,[1,2] MARK J. ABZUG,[1] and SAMUEL R. DOMINGUEZ[1]

INTRODUCTION

Enteroviruses are some of the most common human viral pathogens. Although infections are often asymptomatic, enteroviruses are capable of causing a wide spectrum of illness. They cause mild and self-limited, often febrile illness, hand-foot-and-mouth disease, herpangina, conjunctivitis, pleurodynia, hepatitis, myocarditis, sepsis, meningitis, encephalitis, and acute flaccid paralysis (1). Disease can be particularly severe in neonates and the immunocompromised (2). Historically, enteroviruses have been uncommonly associated with severe respiratory disease (1).

BIOLOGICAL CHARACTERISTICS AND PATHOGENESIS

Human enteroviruses are members of the *Enterovirus* genus of the *Picornaviridae* family. Like other picornaviruses, enteroviruses are small, positive-sense, single-stranded RNA viruses. Viral RNA is enclosed within an icosahedral capsid composed of four structural proteins: VP1–3, comprising the outer

[1]University of Colorado School of Medicine, Department of Pediatrics, Section of Infectious Disease; [2]Section of Hospital Medicine, Aurora, CO 80045.
Emerging Infections 10
Edited by W. Michael Scheld, James M. Hughes and Richard J. Whitley
© 2016 American Society for Microbiology, Washington, DC
doi:10.1128/microbiolspec.EI10-0018-2016

surface of the capsid, and VP4, which is on the internal surface of the capsid shell. Enteroviruses lack a lipid envelope.

Enteroviruses were originally classified based on biological activity, disease associations, and antigenicity into polioviruses, coxsackie A viruses, coxsackie B viruses, echoviruses, and more newly discovered, numbered enteroviruses. To properly classify the newer enteroviruses in the era of molecular typing, the International Committee on the Taxonomy of Viruses changed the classification scheme in 2005 to group viruses based on genome organization, sequence similarity, and biological properties. Under this new system, the human enteroviruses are now classified into four species: human enterovirus A (HEV-A), HEV-B, HEV-C, and HEV-D. Molecular studies suggest that VP1 nucleotide sequence correlates well with enterovirus serotypes (3). Three rhinoviruses species (rhinovirus A, B, and C) and five animal enterovirus species (enterovirus E, G, F, H, and J) are also grouped within the enterovirus genus (4).

Enterovirus-D68 (EV-D68), a species D enterovirus (along with EV-D70 and EV-D94) (5), is unique among enteroviruses in that it behaves biologically more like human rhinoviruses (6) than enteroviruses. In fact, human rhinovirus 87, discovered in 1963, was subsequently reclassified using molecular analysis as EV-D68 (7, 8). Similar to rhinoviruses, EV-D68 optimally grows at 33°C compared to the 37°C preferred by other enteroviruses, and unlike most enteroviruses, it is both heat and acid labile (6). Transmission of EV-D68, therefore, is thought to occur primarily via the respiratory route, rather than the fecal-oral route, the predominant method of transmission for most other enteroviruses. Mechanisms of spread include inhalation of aerosolized particles, direct inoculation by hand contact with secretions from an infected person, as well as autoinoculation to mucous membranes from contaminated surfaces. Once in the upper respiratory tract, the virus attaches to mucosal epithelial cells and spreads locally. Crystal structure studies demonstrate that EV-D68 binds to sialic acids on respiratory epithelial cells via the "canyon" on the viral capsid VP1 protein (9). This leads to expulsion of a pocket factor which changes the conformational state of the virus to allow entry (9). Glycan binding arrays have demonstrated preferential binding of multiple EV-D68 strains to α2-6-linked sialic acid terminals, commonly found in upper respiratory tract epithelial cells, with minimal affinity for α2-3-linked sialic acids, more commonly found in the lower respiratory tract (10). Older studies have suggested that decay accelerating factor (CD55), a membrane protein involved in regulation of the complement system and known to be a receptor for other enteroviruses, might also be a receptor for EV-D68 (8).

EPIDEMIOLOGY

EV-D68 was first isolated by Schieble et al. in 1962 from respiratory specimens of four children with lower respiratory tract disease (11). The Centers for Disease Control and Prevention (CDC) Passive National Enterovirus Surveillance System identified 26 cases of EV-D68 infection between 1970 and 2005 in the United States, which represented only 0.1% of reported enterovirus infections (12). Small clusters of EV-D68 respiratory illness were reported in North America (United States: Georgia, Pennsylvania, Arizona, New York), Asia (The Philippines, Japan, Cambodia), and Europe (The Netherlands, Italy, France) from 2008 to 2010 (13–19). Between 2010 and 2014, an increasing number of small clusters of EV-D68 respiratory disease were reported in Europe (England, Italy, France, Finland, The Netherlands), Asia (The Philippines, Thailand, China, Japan), Oceania (New Zealand, Australia), and Africa (Gambia, Senegal, South Africa, Kenya) (13, 20–28).

In August 2014, pediatricians at Children's Mercy Hospital (Kansas City, MO) reported an unexpected increase in children with severe respiratory disease and increased detection of rhinoviruses/enteroviruses by multiplex PCR testing of respiratory specimens (29, 30). The CDC identified EV-D68 as the predominant virus via sequencing of rhinovirus/enterovirus-positive samples. Reports of increases in severe respiratory disease from the University of Chicago Comer Children's Hospital and Children's Hospital Colorado followed shortly thereafter, and EV-D68 was similarly identified in a majority of evaluated specimens (31, 32). Hospitals across the United States subsequently reported surges in pediatric patient volumes and resource utilization due to respiratory disease (33, 34).

The CDC reported a total of 1,153 confirmed EV-D68 infections in 49 states and the District of Columbia between August 2014 and January 2015 (35). This is likely a large underestimate of cases, because EV-D68-specific testing to confirm infection was only available through reference laboratories, and CDC testing focused on patients with severe illness. Thus, in the absence of active population-based surveillance during the outbreak, only a fraction of compatible cases had confirmatory microbiologic testing performed. For example, syndromic surveillance demonstrated 1,185 excess emergency department visits, 387 excess hospitalizations, and 96 excess pediatric intensive care unit admissions above expected volumes for respiratory disease at Children's Hospital Colorado from August to September 2014, but only 101 samples had confirmatory EV-D68 testing (36). Similar dramatic increases in emergency room visits, hospitalizations, and pediatric intensive care unit admissions for respiratory illness occurred in northern Illinois and northwest Missouri during this same time frame compared to the previous 2 years, but only a minority of cases were tested for EV-D68 (31). The CDC estimated that millions of cases of milder disease due to EV-D68 probably occurred throughout the United States in the summer and fall of 2014 (35).

The 2014 EV-D68 outbreak was not limited to the United States. Clusters of severe respiratory disease with detection of EV-D68 were also reported from Canada, and the Public Health Agency of Canada identified 268 cases of EV-D68-associated respiratory disease during September 2014 in Ontario, Alberta, and British Columbia through enhanced surveillance (37). Likewise, an increase in emergency department visits in August to September 2014 for influenza-like and respiratory illness compared with 2013 was identified via syndromic surveillance in Alberta, and EV-D68 was the predominant respiratory virus identified (38). Reports of increased detection of EV-D68 soon followed from several European countries, including The Netherlands (25, 39), Germany (40), Denmark (41), Sweden (42), Spain (43), Italy (44), and France (45, 46), as well as from Chile and Brazil (47, 48).

EV-D68-associated respiratory illness during the 2014 North American outbreak was predominantly a pediatric phenomenon. Preschool and school-aged children were most frequently identified; the median age among confirmed cases was 5 years (31). However, the age range was wide (3 days to 92 years), and predominant reporting from children's hospitals likely skewed the data toward a younger age range (31). More than half of children with confirmed EV-D68 infection in the United States had a previous history of asthma, and this group of children more frequently required intensive care (31, 49, 50).

In contrast to the predominance of cases in children in the 2014 North American experience, EV-D68 detection in bio-banked specimens from patients with respiratory symptoms collected for surveillance of influenza-like illness concurrent with a 2010 cluster of EV-D68 disease in The Netherlands demonstrated the highest prevalence of EV-D68 infection in adults aged 40 to 59 (24). Influenza-like illness surveillance in outpatients in Germany in 2014 identified EV-D68 infection in both children (40%) and adults (60%) (40). Severe respiratory disease due to EV-D68 has been reported in adults with underlying hematologic malignancy and those undergoing hematopoietic stem cell and solid organ transplants (51).

Surveillance data suggest that EV-D68 predominantly has a late summer to early fall seasonality. Limited serological data suggest widespread exposure and potential immunity in adults. A small study of seven healthy adults and pooled human serum in Finland demonstrated high neutralizing titer against EV-D68 in all samples (8). A subsequent, larger study in Finland found that 100% of pregnant women tested in 1983, 1993, and 2003 had neutralizing antibodies against EV-D68 (52). Mean antibody levels decreased over time, suggesting possible antigenic drift among circulating EV-D68 strains. Recent analysis of multiple lots of commercially available intravenous immunoglobulin from five manufacturers in the United States and Europe all demonstrated high neutralizing antibody titers against historical and current EV-D68 strains. Differences in neutralization titers against different EV-D68 strains were observed, suggesting subtle antigenic variation among historical and 2014 EV-D68 strains (53).

Molecular epidemiological analyses suggest that EV-D68 has undergone rapid evolution since the mid-1990s. Genetic diversification led to the emergence of three clades (A to C), multiple sublineages, and novel variants (24, 27, 54). Antigenic variation among recently emerged EV-D68 strains, with resultant loss of neutralization by pre-existing antibodies, has been proposed as a potential explanation for the recent emergence of EV-D68 disease (55). Sequencing of EV-D68 strains circulating during the 2014 U.S. outbreak demonstrate that one major lineage (within clade B) predominated (92%), with minor lineages accounting for a small proportion of cases (Fig. 1) (32). Molecular clock analysis of the major clade B lineage indicates that this strain likely emerged around 2010 and is similar to strains circulating in the United States, Europe, and Asia in 2011 to 2012 (32, 56).

CLINICAL FEATURES AND DISEASE ASSOCIATIONS

Respiratory Disease (Table 1)

The full spectrum of disease attributable to EV-D68 is not fully understood due to a lack of comprehensive surveillance and biased testing toward more severe disease. Nevertheless, reports from outbreaks of EV-D68 and selective surveillance have informed our knowledge of its clinical manifestations. EV-D68 has been reported to cause disease ranging from mild upper respiratory tract infections to lower respiratory tract disease and severe asthma exacerbations. In the influenza-like illness sentinel general practice surveillance conducted in The Netherlands, EV-D68-positive patients during a 2010 outbreak were more likely to have cough and dyspnea than EV-D68-negative patients. The most common clinical diagnoses were bronchitis and acute respiratory illness (24). Similar sentinel surveillance in Germany identified EV-D68 in 7.7% of outpatients with influenza-like illness in 2014; predominant symptoms were sudden onset of fever/shivers, cough, and sore throat; most patients had mild disease (40). During a small outbreak of EV-D68 disease in Japan in 2010, 15 children less than 5 years old had confirmed infections. The most common symptoms in these children were fever, wheezing, and cough, and primary clinical diagnoses were pneumonia and asthmatic bronchitis (15). In a study of children in the Philippines from 2008 to 2009 who met the WHO definition of pneumonia and required hospitalization, 2.6% of respiratory samples were positive for EV-D68. The median age of the 21 EV-D68-positive children was 21 months, and the most frequent symptoms/signs were cough, difficulty breathing, wheeze, and chest-in-drawing; 10% of patients died (13). In a prospective study of children hospitalized for radiographically confirmed community-acquired pneumonia in Italy in 2014, 2.3% of patients were positive for EV-D68. Three

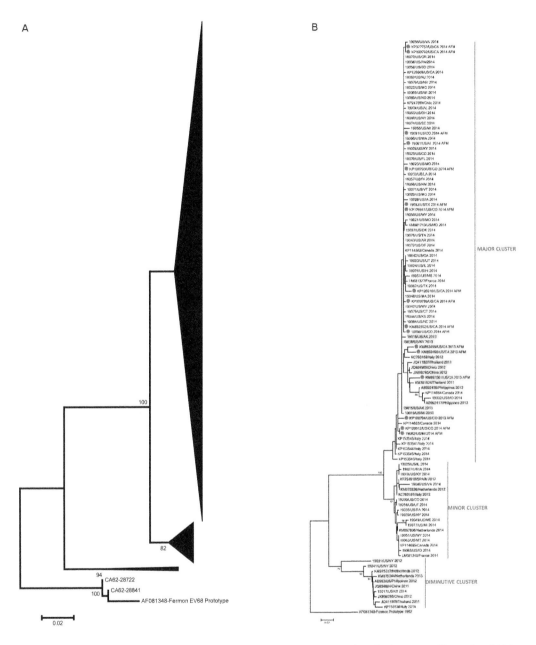

FIGURE 1 (A) Analysis of 606 EV-D68 VP1 sequences from the U.S. outbreak, August to November 2014. Neighbor-joining analysis (MEGA 6.0). (B) Comparison of U.S. 2014 EV-D68 strains with other 2014 strains identified internationally and with EV-D68 strains circulating prior to 2014. Neighbor-joining tree (MEGA 6). Pink shading indicates EV-D68 strains circulating prior to 2014. Red circles indicate strains of EV-D68 identified in respiratory specimens from patients who developed AFM. From Rogers S, Brown B, Nix A, Penaranda S, Lamson D, Chern S-W, Liu H-M, Dybdahl-Sissoko N, Jost H, Vincent A, Maher K, Henderson B, St. George K, Oberste S. Molecular epidemiology of Enterovirus-D68 associated with a nationwide outbreak of severe respiratory illness, United States, 2014. Abstract, 31st Clinical Virology Symposium, 2015, Daytona Beach, FL. Used with permission from the authors at the CDC.

TABLE 1 Enterovirus-D68 respiratory disease: highlights of clinical presentation, diagnosis, and management from the 2014 North American outbreak[a]

Population most affected[b]: School aged children, children with a history of asthma

Presenting symptoms[b]: Acute onset of cough, dyspnea, wheezing; fever in ¼-½

Exam findings[b]: Increased work of breathing, wheezing, decreased breath sounds, hypoxia

Chest radiograph findings[b]: Nonfocal airways disease in most; focal infiltrates in a minority

Diagnostic specimens: Respiratory sample (i.e., nasopharyngeal swab or aspirate); can be found in blood early in course; rare in stool, CSF

Diagnostic testing: Detected as rhinovirus/enterovirus by most commercially available multiplex PCR tests. EV-D68-specific RT-PCR or VP-1 sequencing necessary to identify EV-D68

Management: Respiratory support (supplemental oxygen, noninvasive or invasive ventilatory support) for hypoxia or respiratory failure; bronchodilator and steroid therapy for asthma exacerbation

Prevention: Hand hygiene, decontamination of surfaces, isolation precautions (standard, contact, and droplet), visitation restrictions during periods of high activity, asthma action plans

[a]Reprinted from reference 82, with permission.
[b]Epidemiology and clinical presentation described reflects published, confirmed EV-D68 infections from 2014 outbreak and are not necessarily representative of the full spectrum of EV-D68 disease due to the lack of systematic population-based studies.

of the four patients identified had mild-to-moderate respiratory symptoms and fully recovered. The fourth, a 14-year-old girl with mitochondrial encephalopathy, lactic acidosis, and stroke-like episodes (MELAS syndrome), presented with severe respiratory disease and died 12 days after hospitalization (44).

The large outbreak of EV-D68 in North America in 2014 provided a more extensive picture of the clinical manifestations of EV-D68 disease. Children with confirmed EV-D68 most commonly presented with asthma-like symptoms such as cough, shortness of breath, and wheezing. The most frequent exam findings were increased work of breathing, diminished breath sounds, and hypoxia (32, 49, 50). Notably, fever was present in only 25 to 50% of children with confirmed infection (32, 50). Nonspecific findings of airway disease were frequently present on chest radiographs; focal infiltrates were uncommon (49, 50). White blood cell counts and C-reactive protein levels were normal to mildly elevated (49, 50). Bacterial coinfections were unusual (50).

Most children with severe disease were managed according to standard asthma clinical care guidelines, including treatment with supplemental oxygen, bronchodilators, and corticosteroids. Continuous albuterol and second-line asthma medications including magnesium, terbutaline, aminophylline, and epinephrine were also frequently administered, indicative of the severity of illness observed (49, 50). Consistent with this high acuity, a majority (59%) of children hospitalized in the United States were admitted to intensive care units (32). Disproportionate testing among cases of severe disease and lack of community-based surveillance, however, skew these data; Canadian surveillance found that only 6.8% of hospitalized children with confirmed EV-D68 infection required intensive care (38). Many (44 to 70%) of the children cared for in U.S intensive care units received noninvasive positive pressure ventilation, whereas only a minority (7%) required ventilator support (49, 50). Compared with children infected with 2009 pandemic H1N1 influenza A who were treated in intensive care units, EV-D68-infected children cared for in intensive care units had more rapid presentation and decompensation but faster recovery and fewer complications (49). EV-D68 was detected in 14 U.S. patients who died during the 2014 outbreak; the role of the virus in these deaths is unknown (35).

Potential Association with Neurologic Disease (Table 2)

Beginning in 2012, an increasing number of cases of acute flaccid paralysis associated with spinal cord motor neuron lesions were

TABLE 2 Acute flaccid myelitis potentially associated with enterovirus-D68: highlights of clinical presentation, diagnosis, and management from the 2014 North American outbreak[a]

Population most affected: School aged children (median: 7–11 years)

Presenting symptoms: Acute febrile respiratory prodrome followed by meningeal signs and acute onset of cranial nerve dysfunction (VI, VII, IX, X) and/or acute flaccid paralysis of limbs

Exam findings: Diplopia (CN VI), facial droop (CN VII), bulbar dysfunction (CN IX, X); limp weakness of the arms/legs associated with hyporeflexia and intact sensation

Cerebrospinal fluid findings: Mild pleocytosis with normal to mildly elevated protein, normal glucose

Brain and spinal cord MRI findings: Focal lesions in the brainstem cranial nerve motor nuclei; longitudinally extensive lesions in the spinal cord gray matter (anterior horn predominant). Lesions nonenhancing with gadolinium; best seen on T2 and FLAIR series

Diagnostic specimens: Respiratory specimen (nasopharyngeal swab or aspirate), oropharyngeal swab, stool/rectal samples, blood and cerebrospinal fluid

Diagnostic testing: Evaluate for infectious (e.g., poliovirus and other non-polio-enteroviruses, West Nile virus and other arboviruses, adenovirus, and herpesviruses) and noninfectious causes of acute flaccid paralysis. EV-D68-specific RT-PCR or sequencing of rhinovirus/enterovirus PCR amplicon necessary to identify EV-D68

Management: No antivirals approved for treatment. Supportive care, including intubation and feeding support in cases of loss of bulbar function. Physical and rehabilitation therapies for limb weakness

Prognosis: Long-term prognosis unknown. Mild functional improvements noted in some, though most with residual limb weakness after one year

[a]Reprinted from reference 82, with permission.

reported in the United States. The California Department of Public Health received several requests for poliovirus testing for cases of unexplained sudden paralysis in August 2012 (57). In response, enhanced statewide surveillance was initiated for cases meeting a definition of acute onset flaccid limb weakness with spinal cord gray matter lesions on magnetic resonance imaging (MRI) or electrodiagnostic studies consistent with anterior horn cell damage. From 2012 to 2015, 59 reported cases in California met this case definition (58).

In August 2014, an unusual cluster of children with a similar neurologic syndrome was observed at Children's Hospital Colorado in the midst of the outbreak of EV-D68 respiratory disease (59). Case finding was initiated using a case definition consisting of acute onset focal limb weakness and/or cranial nerve dysfunction associated with MRI findings of predominantly gray matter lesions in the spinal cord and/or brainstem. During August to October 2014, 12 children met the case definition (60).

In response to the California and Colorado experiences, the CDC established a case definition for enhanced nationwide surveillance of acute flaccid myelitis (AFM) in the United

States. This case definition included children less than 21 years old presenting after 1 August 2014 with acute flaccid limb weakness and involvement of predominantly the spinal cord gray matter on MRI, without identified etiology. Between August 2014 and July 2015, 120 children from 34 states were identified (61).

The term "acute flaccid myelitis" has been used to describe these recent cases of acute flaccid limb weakness with evidence of spinal cord gray matter changes on imaging or evidence of spinal motor neuron damage on electrodiagnostic testing. Clinically, AFM cases have been characterized by acute onset of flaccid, asymmetric limb weakness, most often occurring a median of 7 days (range 1 to 16 days) after a prodromal illness characterized by fever, respiratory symptoms, and in some cases, emesis or diarrhea (58). Patients often report household contacts with similar respiratory symptoms (58, 60, 62). Most patients report clinical improvement in their prodromal illness before the return of fever accompanied by meningeal signs (headache, stiff neck, and limb or back pain) around the time of onset of neurologic deficits (58, 60). Progression from full strength to neurologic nadir is rapid, usually occurring over a period of hours. Weakness most profoundly affects proximal muscle groups in the upper extremity (C5 to C7 distribution), although almost half of children have had all four extremities involved (58, 60). Sensation is usually intact, and deep tendon reflexes are decreased or absent. Cranial nerve dysfunction (cranial nerves VI, VII, IX, and X) often accompanies limb weakness, with imaging identifying involvement of cranial nerve motor nuclei in the brainstem, suggesting tropism for motor neurons that is consistent with involvement of the anterior horn of the gray matter seen in the spinal cord. Many children continue to have residual limb weakness at 1-year follow-up, though functional improvements have been seen with rehabilitation therapies.

No infectious agents have been identified in the cerebrospinal fluid (CSF) of any of the AFM cases reported to the CDC in 2014 to 2015, despite extensive microbiologic investigations including next-generation sequencing for novel pathogens in some cases (56, 61). Nearly all patients with AFM reported during this time period received the recommended schedule of inactivated poliovirus vaccines, and poliovirus was not identified in any of these AFM cases. A variety of nonpolio rhinoviruses/enteroviruses were identified in the nasopharynx of children with AFM, with EV-D68 being the predominant organism found (58, 60, 62, 63). EV-D68 was identified in the nasopharynx in 9/41 (22%) cases studied in California (58) and 5/11 (45%) of cases tested in Colorado; these EV-D68 strains were all clade B1 strains, within the predominant circulating lineage during the 2014 respiratory outbreak (59, 60). Similarly, 7/19 (37%) AFM cases identified by CDC surveillance with samples collected within 14 days of onset of prodromal respiratory illness had EV-D68 identified in the nasopharynx (61, 62). Following reports in the United States, cases of AFP associated with EV-D68 have been reported from Canada (64, 65), France (45), Norway (66), Australia (21), and Great Britain (67).

Epidemiologic and virologic evidence supports an association between EV-D68 and AFM cases reported in 2014 to 2015. The increase in AFM cases in the United States both temporally and geographically correlated with the EV-D68 respiratory outbreak (Fig. 2) (58, 60). At Children's Hospital Colorado, the incidence of AFM during August to October 2014 greatly exceeded the incidence in the preceding 4 years ($p = 0.0009$) (59). Furthermore, a case control study comparing the rate of EV-D68 detection in the nasopharynx of AFM cases compared to outpatient controls tested for respiratory pathogens suggested a disproportionate association of EV-D68 recovery with AFM cases (68). The incidence of AFM cases reported in California from August to September 2014, during the EV-D68 outbreak, was also significantly greater than that reported in the preceding 2 years ($p < 0.01$) (58).

The association of other enteroviruses, including poliovirus, EV-A71, and EV-D70, with acute flaccid paralysis syndromes that are clinically, radiographically, and electrophysiologically indistinguishable to recently described AFM cases associated with EV-D68 suggests the plausibility of a common pathophysiology. EV-D68 is genetically most closely related to EV-D70, a cause of epidemic hemorrhagic conjunctivitis that has also been associated with cases of acute flaccid paralysis (69, 70). Previously, EV-D68 has been identified in the CSF of two patients with acute flaccid paralysis (12, 70). In one of these reports, an autopsy demonstrated neuronophagia and cytotoxic T-cell inflammation in motor nuclei of the anterior spinal cord (70). These reports demonstrate that EV-D68 indeed has neuroinvasive potential. Nevertheless, lack of detection of EV-D68 in CSF, and the lack of CNS tissue available for testing from recent AFM cases precludes a definitive conclusion that EV-D68 is the cause of AFM in these cases.

DIAGNOSTICS

EV-D68 can be detected in upper and lower respiratory tract secretions. In contrast to

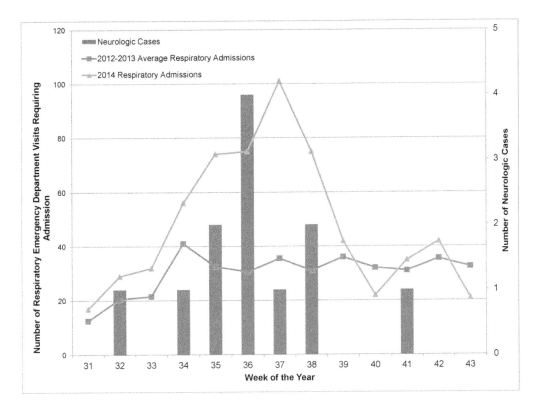

FIGURE 2 **Number of visits for respiratory illness to the Children's Hospital Colorado emergency department requiring hospital admission and the cases of acute flaccid myelitis during the 2014 EV-D68 outbreak. Visits with a chief complaint of respiratory symptoms requiring hospital admission from the week ending 2 August 2014 (week 31) to that ending 25 October 2014 (week 43) compared with the same timeframe for 2012–2013 and the timing of the cases of acute flaccid myelitis. Reprinted from reference 60, with permission.**

other enteroviruses, EV-D68 is less commonly found in stool and rectal specimens, most likely reflecting its acid and heat lability. Virus was detected in the blood of 43% of children with EV-D68 pneumonia in one study, usually in the first 3 days of illness but up to 7 days after onset of illness (71). Detection of EV-D68 in CSF has only rarely been reported (12, 21, 72).

In the past, isolation of virus via inoculation of *in vitro* cell culture systems or suckling mice was the primary method for detection of enteroviruses. Viral culture, however, is rarely available in most clinical laboratories and has generally been replaced by molecular diagnostics. Most currently available commercial multiplex PCR platforms for detection of respiratory viruses detect EV-D68, but

due to genetic similarity, these assays cannot differentiate rhinoviruses and enteroviruses (73). Although time- and labor-intensive, EV-D68 can be definitively identified using seminested PCR amplification and sequencing of VP1 or other gene segments (3). Recently developed EV-D68-specific reverse transcriptase (RT)-PCR assays provide a more rapid and cost-effective method of detecting and confirming EV-D68 and have excellent sensitivity and specificity (74–77).

TREATMENT AND PREVENTION

None of the three antivirals in clinical development for enterovirus or rhinovirus infections (pleconaril, vapendavir/BTA-798, pocapavir/V-073) have consistent *in vitro* activity against the EV-D68 strains that circulated in 2014 (78). Pleconaril inhibited the 1962 Fermon prototype strain of EV-D68, but its activity against 2014 EV-D68 strains was cell-line-specific (no activity in human rhabdomyosarcoma cells but good antiviral activity in HeLa H1 cells) (78–80). DAS181, an agent being developed for aerosol delivery to patients with influenza and parainfluenza virus infections, cleaves α2,6-linked sialic acid moieties (receptors for EV-D68 in addition to influenza and parainfluenza viruses) and strongly inhibits EV-D68 *in vitro* at nanomolar concentrations (78). Fluoxetine is the only FDA-approved medication demonstrated to have significant *in vitro* activity against 2014 EV-D68 isolates (78). This activity involves inhibition of RNA replication via viral protein 2C binding and is independent of selective serotonin reuptake inhibition (81). Clinical efficacy for this indication has not been investigated. Commercially available intravenous immune globulin products contain high levels of neutralizing antibodies against 2014 EV-D68 strains (53) and, therefore, may potentially be useful for prophylaxis and treatment of EV-D68 infections, particularly in patients with antibody deficiencies. There are no available vaccines against EV-D68.

Infection control and prevention strategies are essential to limiting transmission of EV-D68. These include hand-washing, covering the mouth and nose while coughing and sneezing, and cleaning contaminated surfaces. Isolation with standard, contact, and droplet precautions (gown, glove, and mask) in the presence of respiratory symptoms are indicated in the hospital setting. Visitation restriction of symptomatic visitors and school-aged siblings may also be appropriate to limit hospital-acquired infections during periods of high EV-D68 activity (30, 36). Asthma action plans should be enacted during community-wide EV-D68 outbreaks because of the propensity for children with asthma to develop severe disease.

LESSONS LEARNED FROM THE 2014 OUTBREAK

Efficient public health communication was essential to the early recognition of this outbreak and the response to it. Initial communication via an infectious disease listserv from physicians at Mercy Children's Hospital alerted providers throughout the country about an increase in severe respiratory disease in children, ultimately attributed to EV-D68 (31). This allowed rapid recognition of similar surges in patient volumes in Illinois and Colorado, which was promptly communicated to state health departments and the CDC, which in turn quickly demonstrated that EV-D68 was the cause of outbreaks at these sites. In addition, the rapid reporting of a coinciding cluster of acute flaccid paralysis and cranial nerve dysfunction to public health authorities enabled a rigorous national investigation of the possible association of AFM with EV-D68 (59, 60, 62).

Early recognition of the outbreak also allowed proactive public health messaging. Health alerts and media broadcasts provided guidance on when to seek care, both to prevent unnecessary burden on strained emergency services and to ensure appropriate emergent care for respiratory distress. Health care providers were encouraged to implement asthma action plans for children with a known history of wheezing.

Because testing for EV-D68 during the 2014 North American outbreak was limited, surrogate markers of disease burden were utilized to indirectly quantify the impact of the outbreak. Time series seasonal autoregressive integrated moving average modeling was used to estimate the resource utilization burden during the outbreak at Children's Hospital Colorado. This modeling demonstrated that respiratory emergency department visits, hospital admissions, and intensive care unit admissions surged dramatically (36%, 80%, and 79%, respectively) during August to September 2014 compared to expected volumes. Albuterol use increased by

86%, resulting in a critical shortage; second-line asthma medication use also increased, by 101%. Furthermore, demands on respiratory therapy staff and equipment utilization increased to an all-time institutional high (36). These data demonstrate that EV-D68 had a much larger impact than appreciated solely based on virologically proven cases. Providers at Children's Mercy Hospital reported similar findings, including surges in patient volumes and critical shortages of steroids for asthma treatment during the same time frame (29, 30).

The rapid and unexpected increases in patient volumes, medication and supply utilization, and staffing needs due to EV-D68 experienced at Children's Hospital Colorado required effective emergency operational responses. Infection control interventions, bed space allocation, personnel management, and pharmaceutical and equipment supply chain management were critical to preserving operational continuity and assuring safe patient outcomes during the outbreak. To alleviate strain on highly burdened emergency room and critical care units, general inpatient units accepted higher-acuity respiratory patients than typically cared for in these settings, including patients requiring prolonged, continuous bronchodilator therapy and noninvasive positive pressure ventilation. Increased respiratory therapist staffing and use of nursing personnel to deliver inhaled breathing treatments were strategies utilized to meet the demand for supportive respiratory care. Regional shortages of albuterol and corticosteroids and tubing for administration of continuous nebulized medications required splitting of multidose vials of inhaled medications, careful supply chain management, and contingency planning. Antimicrobial stewardship teams helped to limit unnecessary antimicrobial use in patients with viral respiratory disease.

CONCLUSIONS

EV-D68, a previously uncommonly reported enterovirus, has caused increasing numbers of outbreaks of respiratory disease since 2008, most notably an extensive outbreak in North America in 2014 associated with a large clinical burden and considerable morbidity. A possible association with paralytic disease is under investigation. Should EV-D68 continue to have widespread circulation in either an epidemic or endemic manner, development of effective therapies and vaccines will become scientific priorities.

CITATION

Messacar K, Abzug MJ, Dominguez SR. 2016. The emergence of enterovirus D-68. Microbiol Spectrum 4(3):EI10-0018-2016.

REFERENCES

1. **Messacar K, Modlin JF, Abzug MJ.** 2015. Enteroviruses and parechoviruses. *In* Long S, Prober C, Fischer M (ed), *Principles and Practice of Pediatric Infectious Diseases*, 4th ed. Elsevier Saunders, Edinburgh, Scotland.
2. **Pallansch MA, Roos RP.** 2013. Enteroviruses: polioviruses, coxsackievirus, echoviruses, and newer enteroviruses, p 490–530. *In* Knipe DM, Howley PM (ed), *Fields Virology*, Vol. 1, 6th ed. Wolters Kluwer/Lippincott Williams & Wilkins Health, Philadelphia, PA.
3. **Nix WA, Oberste MS, Pallansch MA.** 2006. Sensitive, seminested PCR amplification of VP1 sequences for direct identification of all enterovirus serotypes from original clinical specimens. *J Clin Microbiol* **44:**2698–2704.
4. **Fauquet CM, Fargette D.** 2005. International Committee on Taxonomy of Viruses and the 3,142 unassigned species. *Virol J* **2:**64.
5. **Smura TP, Junttila N, Blomqvist S, Norder H, Kaijalainen S, Paananen A, Magnius LO, Hovi T, Roivainen M.** 2007. Enterovirus 94, a proposed new serotype in human enterovirus species D. *J Gen Virol* **88:**849–858.
6. **Oberste MS, Maher K, Schnurr D, Flemister MR, Lovchik JC, Peters H, Sessions W, Kirk C, Chatterjee N, Fuller S, Hanauer JM, Pallansch MA.** 2004. Enterovirus 68 is associated with respiratory illness and shares biological features with both the enteroviruses and the rhinoviruses. *J Gen Virol* **85:**2577–2584.
7. **Ishiko H, Miura R, Shimada Y, Hayashi A, Nakajima H, Yamazaki S, Takeda N.** 2002. Human rhinovirus 87 identified as human

enterovirus 68 by VP4-based molecular diagnosis. *Intervirology* **45:**136–141.

8. **Blomqvist S, Savolainen C, Råman L, Roivainen M, Hovi T.** 2002. Human rhinovirus 87 and enterovirus 68 represent a unique serotype with rhinovirus and enterovirus features. *J Clin Microbiol* **40:**4218–4223.

9. **Liu Y, Sheng J, Baggen J, Meng G, Xiao C, Thibaut HJ, van Kuppeveld FJ, Rossmann MG.** 2015. Sialic acid-dependent cell entry of human enterovirus D68. *Nat Commun* **6:**8865.

10. **Imamura T, Okamoto M, Nakakita S, Suzuki A, Saito M, Tamaki R, Lupisan S, Roy CN, Hiramatsu H, Sugawara KE, Mizuta K, Matsuzaki Y, Suzuki Y, Oshitani H.** 2014. Antigenic and receptor binding properties of enterovirus 68. *J Virol* **88:**2374–2384.

11. **Schieble JH, Fox VL, Lennette EH.** 1967. A probable new human picornavirus associated with respiratory diseases. *Am J Epidemiol* **85:**297–310.

12. **Khetsuriani N, Lamonte-Fowlkes A, Oberst S, Pallansch MA, Centers for Disease Control and Prevention.** 2006. Enterovirus surveillance: United States, 1970–2005. *MMWR Surveill Summ* **55:**1–20.

13. **Imamura T, Fuji N, Suzuki A, Tamaki R, Saito M, Aniceto R, Galang H, Sombrero L, Lupisan S, Oshitani H.** 2011. Enterovirus 68 among children with severe acute respiratory infection, the Philippines. *Emerg Infect Dis* **17:**1430–1435.

14. **Ikeda T, Mizuta K, Abiko C, Aoki Y, Itagaki T, Katsushima F, Katsushima Y, Matsuzaki Y, Fuji N, Imamura T, Oshitani H, Noda M, Kimura H, Ahiko T.** 2012. Acute respiratory infections due to enterovirus 68 in Yamagata, Japan between 2005 and 2010. *Microbiol Immunol* **56:**139–143.

15. **Kaida A, Kubo H, Sekiguchi J, Kohdera U, Togawa M, Shiomi M, Nishigaki T, Iritani N.** 2011. Enterovirus 68 in children with acute respiratory tract infections, Osaka, Japan. *Emerg Infect Dis* **17:**1494–1497.

16. **Hasegawa S, Hirano R, Okamoto-Nakagawa R, Ichiyama T, Shirabe K.** 2011. Enterovirus 68 infection in children with asthma attacks: virus-induced asthma in Japanese children. *Allergy* **66:**1618–1620.

17. **Rahamat-Langendoen J, Riezebos-Brilman A, Borger R, van der Heide R, Brandenburg A, Schölvinck E, Niesters HG.** 2011. Upsurge of human enterovirus 68 infections in patients with severe respiratory tract infections. *J Clin Virol* **52:**103–106.

18. **Renois F, Bouin A, Andreoletti L.** 2013. Enterovirus 68 in pediatric patients hospitalized for acute airway diseases. *J Clin Microbiol* **51:**640–643.

19. **Centers for Disease Control and Prevention (CDC).** 2011. Clusters of acute respiratory illness associated with human enterovirus 68: Asia, Europe, and United States, 2008–2010. *MMWR Morb Mortal Wkly Rep* **60:**1301–1304.

20. **Opanda SM, Wamunyokoli F, Khamadi S, Coldren R, Bulimo WD.** 2014. Genetic diversity of human enterovirus 68 strains isolated in Kenya using the hypervariable 3′-end of VP1 gene. *PLoS One* **9:**e102866. doi:10.1371/journal.pone.0102866.

21. **Levy A, Roberts J, Lang J, Tempone S, Kesson A, Dofai A, Daley AJ, Thorley B, Speers DJ.** 2015. Enterovirus D68 disease and molecular epidemiology in Australia. *J Clin Virol* **69:**117–121.

22. **Todd AK, Hall RJ, Wang J, Peacey M, McTavish S, Rand CJ, Stanton JA, Taylor S, Huang QS.** 2013. Detection and whole genome sequence analysis of an enterovirus 68 cluster. *Virol J* **10:**103.

23. **Lu QB, Wo Y, Wang HY, Wei MT, Zhang L, Yang H, Liu EM, Li TY, Zhao ZT, Liu W, Cao WC.** 2014. Detection of enterovirus 68 as one of the commonest types of enterovirus found in patients with acute respiratory tract infection in China. *J Med Microbiol* **63:**408–414.

24. **Meijer A, van der Sanden S, Snijders BE, Jaramillo-Gutierrez G, Bont L, van der Ent CK, Overduin P, Jenny SL, Jusic E, van der Avoort HG, Smith GJ, Donker GA, Koopmans MP.** 2012. Emergence and epidemic occurrence of enterovirus 68 respiratory infections in The Netherlands in 2010. *Virology* **423:**49–57.

25. **Meijer A, Benschop KS, Donker GA, van der Avoort HG.** 2014. Continued seasonal circulation of enterovirus D68 in The Netherlands, 2011-2014. *Euro Surveill* **19:**19. http://www.eurosurveillance.org/ViewArticle.aspx?ArticleId=20935.

26. **Piralla A, Girello A, Grignani M, Gozalo-Margüello M, Marchi A, Marseglia G, Baldanti F.** 2014. Phylogenetic characterization of enterovirus 68 strains in patients with respiratory syndromes in Italy. *J Med Virol* **86:**1590–1593.

27. **Tokarz R, Firth C, Madhi SA, Howie SR, Wu W, Sall AA, Haq S, Briese T, Lipkin WI.** 2012. Worldwide emergence of multiple clades of enterovirus 68. *J Gen Virol* **93:**1952–1958.

28. **Furuse Y, Chaimongkol N, Okamoto M, Imamura T, Saito M, Tamaki R, Saito M, Lupisan SP, Oshitani H, Oshitani H, Tohoku-RITM Collaborative Research Team.** 2015. Molecular epidemiology of enterovirus d68 from 2013 to 2014 in Philippines. *J Clin Microbiol* **53:**1015–1018.

29. Oermann CM, Schuster JE, Conners GP, Newland JG, Selvarangan R, Jackson MA. 2015. Enterovirus D68: a focused review and clinical highlights from the 2014 United States outbreak. *Ann Am Thorac Soc* **12:**775–781.

30. Schuster JE, Newland JG. 2015. Management of the 2014 enterovirus 68 outbreak at a pediatric tertiary care center. *Clin Ther* **37:** 2411–2418.

31. Midgley CM, Jackson MA, Selvarangan R, Turabelidze G, Obringer E, Johnson D, Giles BL, Patel A, Echols F, Oberste MS, Nix WA, Watson JT, Gerber SI. 2014. Severe respiratory illness associated with enterovirus D68: Missouri and Illinois, 2014. *MMWR Morb Mortal Wkly Rep* **63:**798–799.

32. Midgley C, Watson J, Nix W, Curns A, Rogers S, Brown B, Conover C, Dominguez S, Feikin D, Gray S, Hassan F, Hoferka S, Jackson M, Johnson D, Leshem E, Miller L, Nichols J, Nyquist A, Obringer E, Patel A, Patel M, Rha B, Schneider E, Schuster J, Selvarangan R, Seward J, Turabelidze G, Oberste M, Pallansch M, Gerber S, EV-D68 Working Group. 2015. Severe respiratory illness associated with a nationwide outbreak of enterovirus D68 in the USA (2014): a descriptive epidemiological evaluation. *Lancet Resp Med* **3:**879–387.

33. Shaw J, Welch TR, Milstone AM. 2014. The role of syndromic surveillance in directing the public health response to the enterovirus D68 epidemic. *JAMA Pediatr* **168:**981–982.

34. Anonymous. 2014. Influx of patients with asthma-like symptoms strains resources in many pediatric EDs. *ED Manag* **26:**121–124.

35. Centers for Disease Control and Prevention. 2015. Enterovirus D68. http://www.cdc.gov/ non-polio-enterovirus/about/EV-D68.html.

36. Messacar K, Hawkins S, Baker J, Pearce K, Tong S, Dominguez SR, Parker SK. 2016. Resource burden during the 2014 enterovirus D68 respiratory disease outbreak at Children's Hospital Colorado: an unexpected strain. *JAMA Pediatr* **170:**294–297.

37. Edwin J, Reyes Domingo F, Booth T, Mersereau T, Skowronski D, Chambers C, Simmonds K, Scott A, Winter A, Peci A, Gubbay J, Drews S, Krajden M, Karnauchow T, Smieja M, Rempel S, Murti M, Pollock S, Gustafson R, Hoyano D, Allison S, Fathima S, Pabbaraju K, Wong S, Tellier R, Tipples G, Gad R, Mukhi S, Jarfari Y, Grudeski E, McDermid A, Wong T. 2015. Surveillance summary of hospitalized pediatric enterovirus D68 cases in Canada, September 2014. *Can Commun Dis Rep* **41**(S1).

38. Drews SJ, Simmonds K, Usman HR, Yee K, Fathima S, Tipples G, Tellier R, Pabbaraju K, Wong S, Talbot J. 2015. Characterization of enterovirus activity, including that of enterovirus D68, in pediatric patients in Alberta, Canada, in 2014. *J Clin Microbiol* **53:**1042–1045.

39. Poelman R, Schölvinck EH, Borger R, Niesters HG, van Leer-Buter C. 2015. The emergence of enterovirus D68 in a Dutch University Medical Center and the necessity for routinely screening for respiratory viruses. *J Clin Virol* **62:**1–5.

40. Reiche J, Böttcher S, Diedrich S, Buchholz U, Buda S, Haas W, Schweiger B, Wolff T. 2015. Low-level circulation of enterovirus D68-associated acute respiratory infections, Germany, 2014. *Emerg Infect Dis* **21:**837–841.

41. Midgley SE, Christiansen CB, Poulsen MW, Hansen CH, Fischer TK. 2015. Emergence of enterovirus D68 in Denmark, June 2014 to February 2015. *Euro Surveill* **20:**20. http:// www.eurosurveillance.org/ViewArticle.aspx? ArticleId=21105.

42. Dyrdak R, Rotzén-Östlund M, Samuelson A, Eriksson M, Albert J. 2015. Coexistence of two clades of enterovirus D68 in pediatric Swedish patients in the summer and fall of 2014. *Infect Dis Lond* **47:**734–738.

43. Gimferrer L, Campins M, Codina MG, Esperalba J, Martin MC, Fuentes F, Pumarola T, Anton A. 2015. First enterovirus D68 (EV-D68) cases detected in hospitalised patients in a tertiary care university hospital in Spain, October 2014. *Enferm Infecc Microbiol Clin* **33:**585–589.

44. Esposito S, Zampiero A, Ruggiero L, Madini B, Niesters H, Principi N. 2015. Enterovirus D68-associated community-acquired pneumonia in children living in Milan, Italy. *J Clin Virol* **68:**94–96.

45. Lang M, Mirand A, Savy N, Henquell C, Maridet S, Perignon R, Labbe A, Peigue-Lafeuille H. 2014. Acute flaccid paralysis following enterovirus D68 associated pneumonia, France, 2014. *Euro Surveill* **19:**19. http://www.eurosurveillance.org/ ViewArticle.aspx?ArticleId=20952.

46. Bal A, Schuffenecker I, Casalegno JS, Josset L, Valette M, Armand N, Dhondt PB, Escuret V, Lina B. 2015. Enterovirus D68 nosocomial outbreak in elderly people, France, 2014. *Clin Microbiol Infect* **21:**e61–e62.

47. Torres JP, Farfan MJ, Izquierdo G, Piemonte P, Henriquez J, O'Ryan ML. 2015. Enterovirus D68 infection, Chile, spring 2014. *Emerg Infect Dis* **21:**728–729.

48. Carney S, Brown D, Siqueira MM, Dias JP, da Silva EE. 2015. Enterovirus D68 detected in

children with severe acute respiratory illness in Brazil. *Emerg Microbes Infect* **4:**e66.

49. Rao S, Messacar K, Torok M, Rick A, Holzberg J, Montano A, Bagdure D, Curtis DJ, Oberste MS, Nix WA, de Masellis G, Robinson C, Dominguez SR. 2015. Enterovirus D68 in critically ill children: a comparison with pandemic H1N1 Influenza. Abstr IDWeek 2015, San Diego, CA.

50. Schuster JE, Miller JO, Selvarangan R, Weddle G, Thompson MT, Hassan F, Rogers SL, Oberste MS, Nix WA, Jackson MA. 2015. Severe enterovirus 68 respiratory illness in children requiring intensive care management. *J Clin Virol* **70:**77–82.

51. Waghmare A, Pergam SA, Jerome KR, Englund JA, Boeckh M, Kuypers J. 2015. Clinical disease due to enterovirus D68 in adult hematologic malignancy patients and hematopoietic cell transplant recipients. *Blood* **125:**1724–1729.

52. Smura T, Ylipaasto P, Klemola P, Kaijalainen S, Kyllönen L, Sordi V, Piemonti L, Roivainen M. 2010. Cellular tropism of human enterovirus D species serotypes EV-94, EV-70, and EV-68 *in vitro*: implications for pathogenesis. *J Med Virol* **82:**1940–1949.

53. Zhang Y, Moore DD, Nix WA, Oberste MS, Weldon WC. 2015. Neutralization of enterovirus D68 isolated from the 2014 US outbreak by commercial intravenous immune globulin products. *J Clin Virol* **69:**172–175.

54. Lauinger IL, Bible JM, Halligan EP, Aarons EJ, MacMahon E, Tong CY. 2012. Lineages, sub-lineages and variants of enterovirus 68 in recent outbreaks. *PLoS One* **7:**e36005. doi:10.1371/journal.pone.0036005.

55. Imamura T, Oshitani H. 2015. Global reemergence of enterovirus D68 as an important pathogen for acute respiratory infections. *Rev Med Virol* **25:**102–114.

56. Greninger AL, Naccache SN, Messacar K, Clayton A, Yu G, Somasekar S, Federman S, Stryke D, Anderson C, Yagi S, Messenger S, Wadford D, Xia D, Watt JP, Van Haren K, Dominguez SR, Glaser C, Aldrovandi G, Chiu CY. 2015. A novel outbreak enterovirus D68 strain associated with acute flaccid myelitis cases in the USA (2012–14): a retrospective cohort study. *Lancet Infect Dis* **15:**671–682.

57. Ayscue P, Van Haren K, Sheriff H, Waubant E, Waldron P, Yagi S, Yen C, Clayton A, Padilla T, Pan C, Reichel J, Harriman K, Watt H, Sejvar J, Nix WA, Feiken D, Glaser C. 2014. Acute flaccid paralysis with anterior myelitis: California, June 2012–June 2014. *MMWRMorb Mortal Wkly Rep* **63:**903–906.

58. Van Haren K, Ayscue P, Waubant E, Clayton A, Sheriff H, Yagi S, Glenn-finer R, Padilla T, Strober JB, Aldrovandi G, Wadford D, Chiu CY, Xia D, Harriman K, Watt JP, Glaser CA. 2015. Acute flaccid myelitis of unknown etiology in California, 2012–2015. *JAMA* **314:**2663–2671.

59. Pastula DM, Aliabadi N, Haynes AK, Messacar K, Schreiner T, Maloney J, Dominguez SR, Davizon ES, Leshem E, Fischer M, Nix WA, Oberste MS, Seward J, Feikin D, Miller L, Centers for Disease Control and Prevention (CDC). 2014. Acute neurologic illness of unknown etiology in children: Colorado, August–September 2014. *MMWR Morb Mortal Wkly Rep* **63:**901–902.

60. Messacar K, Schreiner TL, Maloney JA, Wallace A, Ludke J, Oberste MS, Nix WA, Robinson CC, Glodé MP, Abzug MJ, Dominguez SR. 2015. A cluster of acute flaccid paralysis and cranial nerve dysfunction temporally associated with an outbreak of enterovirus D68 in children in Colorado, USA. *Lancet* **385:**1662–1671.

61. Centers for Disease Control and Prevention. 2014. Investigation of acute neurologic illness with focal limb weakness of unknown etiology in children, fall 2014. http://www.cdc.gov/ncird/investigation/viral/sep2014.html.

62. Division of Viral Diseases National Centers for Immunization and Respiratory Diseases, CDC; Division of Vector-Borne Diseases, Division of High-Consequence Pathogens and Pathology; National Center for Emerging and Zoonotic Infectious Diseases, CDC; Children's Hospital Colorado, Council of State and Territorial Epidemiologists. 2015. Notes from the field: acute flaccid myelitis among persons aged ≤21 years - United States, August 1–November 13, 2014. *MMWR Morb Mortal Wkly Rep* **63:**1243–1244.

63. Horner LM, Poulter MD, Brenton JN, Turner RB. 2015. Acute flaccid paralysis associated with novel enterovirus C105. *Emerg Infect Dis* **21:**1858–1860.

64. Sherwood MDGS, Connolly M, Dobson S. 2014. Acute flaccid paralysis in a child infected with enterovirus D68: a case report. *BC Med J* **56:**495–498.

65. Crone M, Tellier R, Wei XC, Kuhn S, Vanderkooi OG, Kim J, Mah JK, Mineyko A. 2015. Polio-like illness associated with outbreak of upper respiratory tract infection in children. *J Child Neurol* **31:**409–414.

66. Pfeiffer HCBK, Bragstad K, Skram MK, Dahl H, Knudsen PK, Chawla MS, Holberg-Petersen M, Vainio K, Dudman SG, Kran

AM, Rojahn AE. 2015. Two cases of acute severe flaccid myelitis associated with enterovirus D68 infection in children, Norway, autumn 2014. *Euro Surveill* **20:**21062. http://www.eurosurveillance.org/ViewArticle.aspx?ArticleId=21062.

67. **Varghese R, Iyer A, Hunter K, Cargill JS, Cooke RP.** 2015. Sampling the upper respiratory tract for enteroviral infection is important in the investigation of an acute neurological illness in children. *Eur J Paediatr Neurol* **19:**494–495.

68. **Aliabadi N, Messacar K, Pastula DM, Leshem E, Robinson C, Nix WA, Oberste MS, Sejvar J, Feikin D, Dominguez SR.** 2015. A case control study of acute flaccid myelitis (AFM) and enterovirus-D68 (EV-D68), Colorado (CO), 2014. Abstr IDWeek, San Diego, CA.

69. **Anonymous.** 1982. Neurovirulence of enterovirus 70. *Lancet* **1:**373–374.

70. **Parameswari N, Das AK, Mukundan P, John TJ.** 1986. Acute haemorrhagic conjunctivitis & paralytic illness due to enterovirus 70 in 1984. *Indian J Med Res* **83:**349–350.

71. **Imamura T, Suzuki A, Lupisan S, Kamigaki T, Okamoto M, Roy CN, Olveda R, Oshitani H.** 2014. Detection of enterovirus 68 in serum from pediatric patients with pneumonia and their clinical outcomes. *Influenza Other Respir Viruses* **8:**21–24.

72. **Kreuter JD, Barnes A, McCarthy JE, Schwartzman JD, Oberste MS, Rhodes CH, Modlin JF, Wright PF.** 2011. A fatal central nervous system enterovirus 68 infection. *Arch Pathol Lab Med* **135:**793–796.

73. **McAllister SC, Schleiss MR, Arbefeville S, Steiner ME, Hanson RS, Pollock C, Ferrieri P.** 2015. Epidemic 2014 enterovirus D68 cross-reacts with human rhinovirus on a respiratory molecular diagnostic platform. *PLoS One* **10:**e0118529. doi:10.1371/journal.pone.0118529.

74. **Wylie TN, Wylie KM, Buller RS, Cannella M, Storch GA.** 2015. Development and evaluation of an enterovirus D68 real-time reverse transcriptase PCR assay. *J Clin Microbiol* **53:**2641–2647.

75. **Piralla A, Girello A, Premoli M, Baldanti F.** 2015. A new real-time RT-PCR assay for detection of human enterovirus 68 (EV-D68) in respiratory samples. *J Clin Microbiol* **53:**1725–1726.

76. **Centers for Disease Control and Prevention.** 2015. CDC develops a new, faster lab test for enterovirus D68. http://www.cdc.gov/media/releases/2014/p1014-test-enterovirus-d68.html.

77. **Zhuge J, Vail E, Bush JL, Singelakis L, Huang W, Nolan SM, Haas JP, Engel H, Della Posta M, Yoon EC, Fallon JT, Wang G.** 2015. Evaluation of a real-time reverse transcription-PCR assay for detection of enterovirus D68 in clinical samples from an outbreak in New York state in 2014. *J Clin Microbiol* **53:**1915–1920.

78. **Rhoden E, Zhang M, Nix WA, Oberste MS.** 2015. *In vitro* efficacy of antiviral compounds against enterovirus D68. *Antimicrob Agents Chemother* **59:**7779–7781.

79. **Liu Y, Sheng J, Fokine A, Meng G, Shin WH, Long F, Kuhn RJ, Kihara D, Rossmann MG.** 2015. Structure and inhibition of EV-D68, a virus that causes respiratory illness in children. *Science* **347:**71–74.

80. **Sun L, Meijer A, Froeyen M, Zhang L, Thibaut HJ, Baggen J, George S, Vernachio J, van Kuppeveld FJ, Leyssen P, Hilgenfeld R, Neyts J, Delang L.** 2015. Antiviral activity of broad-spectrum and enterovirus-specific inhibitors against clinical isolates of enterovirus D68. *Antimicrob Agents Chemother* **59:**7782–7785.

81. **Ulferts R, van der Linden L, Thibaut HJ, Lanke KH, Leyssen P, Coutard B, De Palma AM, Canard B, Neyts J, van Kuppeveld FJ.** 2013. Selective serotonin reuptake inhibitor fluoxetine inhibits replication of human enteroviruses B and D by targeting viral protein 2C. *Antimicrob Agents Chemother* **57:**1952–1956.

82. **Messacar K, Abzug MJ, Dominguez SR.** 2016. 2014 outbreak of enterovirus D68 in North America. *J Med Virol* [Epub ahead of print.] doi:10.1002/jmv.24410.

The Role of Punctuated Evolution in the Pathogenicity of Influenza Viruses

6

JONATHAN A. McCULLERS[1]

THE PANDEMIC THREAT

Pandemic influenza represents a recurring threat to human health. Several times a century, novel influenza A viruses cross over from the animal reservoirs of the world and establish new, dominant lineages in humans. These newly endemic strains may cocirculate with other established lineages or may replace them. Invariably, zoonotic pandemic influenza viruses are more pathogenic than the better-adapted seasonal strain present upon their emergence. This is partly due to differences in primary viral virulence and partly mediated by an enhanced ability to facilitate bacterial superinfections, such as pneumonia (1). Over time, however, pandemic strains adapt and gradually take on characteristics of seasonal strains with lower virulence and a diminished synergism with bacterial pathogens. Study of this punctuated evolution yields a number of insights into the overall pathogenicity of influenza viruses.

BIOLOGY AND ECOLOGY OF INFLUENZA VIRUSES

Influenza viruses are divided into three types, termed A, B, and C. Influenza B and C viruses diverged evolutionarily from influenza A viruses long ago and

[1]Department of Pediatrics, The University of Tennessee Health Sciences Center, Memphis, TN 38103.
Emerging Infections 10
Edited by W. Michael Scheld, James M. Hughes and Richard J. Whitley
© 2016 American Society for Microbiology, Washington, DC
doi:10.1128/microbiolspec.EI10-0001-2015

are stably adapted to humans. Influenza A viruses are zoonoses that are constantly crossing over from animal reservoirs into humans, causing individual infections and occasionally restricted epidemics (2). Several times a century, one of these zoonotic strains establishes endemicity and circulates for, typically, several decades before being replaced by a new incursion. Human influenza virus lineages do not fully diverge over this evolutionarily short period and frequently cross back over into animals such as swine (3). Although rare interspecies transmission events have been documented with influenza B viruses (e.g., in harbor seals) (4), influenza B and C viruses are predominantly restricted to humans.

Influenza A Virus Biology

Influenza viruses are segmented, negative-strand RNA viruses. Structurally, they take many shapes, from roughly spherical to filamentous to amorphous virions, with a rough size range of 80 to 120 nm. Influenza A viruses have eight gene segments, which code for eight structural proteins, two well-characterized nonstructural proteins, and, variably, several potential accessory proteins (Table 1). These accessory proteins are encoded from alternate open reading frames, alternate in-frame start codons, or early terminal truncation of some gene segments resulting in complex expression patterns and regulation. Although a good deal of work has been done on the accessory protein PB1-F2 (5), the breadth of potential function of other accessory proteins is not clear.

Hemagglutinin (HA) is the primary attachment protein. Binding cell surface sialic acids as a receptor allows internalization by endocytosis (Fig. 1). Matrix protein 2 (M2) protein then acidifies the interior of the virion, triggering HA-mediated fusion of the virus envelope with the endosome and releasing viral RNAs (vRNAs) and the proteins that make up the RNA polymerase complex (PB2, PB1, and PA) into the cytoplasm. These

TABLE 1 Influenza A virus gene functions

Segment	Gene or product	Function
PB2	Basic polymerase 2	Part of transcription and replication complex
PB1	Basic polymerase 1	Part of transcription and replication complex
	PB1-F2	Cell death via mitochondrial targeting
	PB1-N40	Unknown
PA	Acid polymerase	Part of transcription and replication complex
	PA-X	Host shutoff endonuclease
	PA-N155	Unknown
	PA-N182	Unknown
HA	HA	Attachment and fusion
NP	NP	Scaffolding for vRNPs
NA	NA	Sialidase facilitating budding
M	M1	Primary structural protein of virions
	M2	Ion channel
	M42	Alternate form of M2?
NS	Nonstructural gene 1	Multifunctional, including interferon inhibition
	Nonstructural gene 2	Nuclear export
	Nonstructural gene 3	Unknown

move to the nucleus, where transcription of gene segments utilizing a (+)-strand copy RNA intermediate takes place, together with translation to mRNAs. Nascent (−)-strand vRNAs are incorporated with nucleoprotein (NP) into viral ribonucleoproteins (vRNPs) and exported from the nucleus via the nuclear export protein nonstructural protein 2 (NS-2) and matrix protein 1 (M1). mRNAs leave the nucleus and act as templates for synthesis of accessory proteins, structural proteins, and glycoproteins. Structural proteins, primarily M1, congregate at the cell membrane, initiating assembly and preparing for budding. The glycoproteins, HA and the neuraminidase (NA), are shunted through the endoplasmic reticulum (ER) and Golgi

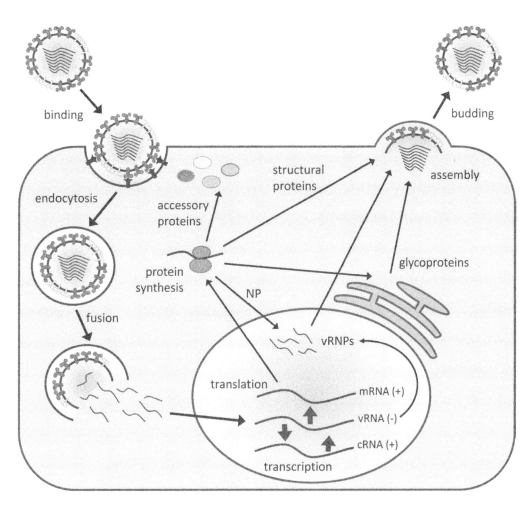

FIGURE 1 Influenza A virus life cycle in cells.

network for folding and posttranslational modification, including addition of glycans, prior to shuttling to the assembly site, where they are inserted into the cell membrane. Nonstructural and accessory proteins are typically not incorporated into the virus. Budding of mature virions is facilitated by the sialidase activity of the NA, which clears cell surface sialic acids from the HAs on the nascent virion (Fig. 1). S-1 has multiple functions within the cell, primarily in countering the antiviral response (6). Full-length PB1-F2, when present, targets mitochondria, inducing cell death and triggering an inflammatory response (7). The functions of multi-ple other accessory proteins are only now being elucidated, but many appear to impact viral and cellular gene regulation (Table 1).

Influenza A Virus Ecology

Influenza A viruses are zoonotic viruses endemic to wild bird populations of the world, particularly migratory waterfowl, such as ducks and shorebirds. There is tremendous diversity in the viruses in these reservoirs, since each of the eight gene segments can be phylogenetically stratified into multiple distinct lineages, and reassortment of segments between different viruses creates an extremely large number of possible combinations. These viruses make constant incursions into other permissive species with which they have contact, most notably domestic poultry (e.g., chickens, turkeys, and ducks) and pigs (Fig. 2). Epidemics of novel viruses in domestic poultry are common, bringing these viruses into close contact with humans (8). Epidemics also occur in swine, with some strains establishing endemic lineages over decades, similar to the process that occurs in humans (3). Reassortment events within epidemics and between epidemic and endemic strains and viruses in other reservoirs are common, increasing the diversity of the extant strains. Viruses in domestic swine and poultry reservoirs frequently cross over to humans, causing individual infections or epidemics, some symptomatic and some inapparent. In rare cases, a virus is able to establish endemicity in humans and cause a pandemic with worldwide spread.

INFLUENZA A VIRUS EVOLUTION AND ADAPTATION IN HUMANS

Pandemics

Influenza A viruses are subtyped by serologic characterization of the two surface glycoproteins, HA and NA. Historically, this nomenclature was adopted because HA and NA are the major antigens of the virus. There have been 18 HA subtypes and 10 NA subtypes identified thus far in nature. Four major lineages have caused pandemics and established themselves as endemic viruses in humans in the last century (Fig. 3). An H1N1 strain caused the most severe pandemic on record in 1918-1919, resulting in more than 50 million deaths. This lineage was maintained in humans until 1956, when it was replaced by a reassortant H2N2 strain with gene segments derived from both the circulating H1N1 strain which it replaced and an avian virus. The H2N2 strain was, in turn,

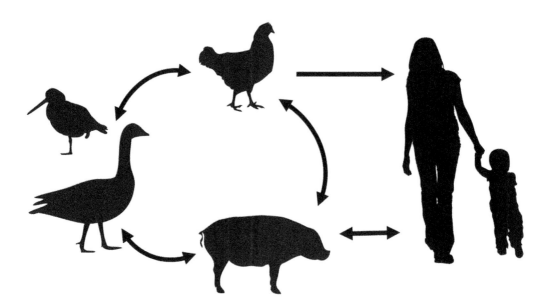

FIGURE 2 Influenza A virus ecology. The wild-bird reservoir is the source of all zoonotic influenza A viruses. These viruses cross over into humans through intermediate species, such as domestic poultry and swine. Farm animal silhouettes by Otutor, used under License CC BY 3.0 (https://creativecommons.org/licenses/by/3.0/us/); oyster catcher silhouette courtesy of Rachison Alexandra; human silhouettes courtesy of Mackey Creations.

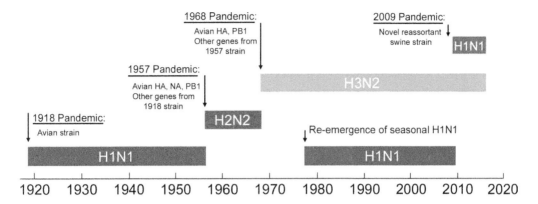

FIGURE 3 Pandemic timeline. Four major lineages of influenza A virus have established endemicity in humans in the last century. The 1957 and 1968 pandemic viruses were reassortants which included genes from the previously circulating viruses which they replaced. The 1918 and 2009 pandemic strains came directly from animal reservoirs. The seasonal H1N1 lineage which circulated early in the 20th century was replaced in 1957 but reemerged in 1976 and cocirculated for 32 years with seasonal H3N2 strains.

replaced by an H3N2 virus, which again was a reassortant of the previously circulating strain. A version of the earlier H1N1 lineage reemerged, likely as a laboratory escape, in 1977 and cocirculated for several decades with the H3N2 viruses. This strain was replaced in 2009 with a novel swine-derived H1N1 strain that currently cocirculates with the H3N2 lineage (Fig. 3).

Adaptation

Variation in the influenza virus genomes results from a high mutation rate, which is an effect of having a low-fidelity polymerase and lacking a proofreading mechanism to correct base pair mismatches. The rapid cycle time and high mutation rate generate a large pool of quasispecies variants that interact together, complementing each other by providing flexibility as environmental conditions change. As a result of this quasispecies-driven diversity, influenza viruses undergo not only positive selection for traits that aid in adaptation but also negative (purifying) selection for disadvantageous traits. These selection events can be at the level of mutation of individual gene segments or via reassortment to acquire completely new gene segments which are a better fit for the present evolutionary pressure. Influenza viruses tend to adapt very rapidly (on a scale of years) to positive selection pressure and more slowly (on a scale of decades) to lose or modify undesirable traits through negative selection.

Rapid Evolution

At least four common scenarios are known to drive evolution of influenza A viruses through positive selection. The most striking is establishing a lineage in a new host through a cross-species jump. In humans, this occurs immediately following the introduction of a new pandemic strain. The virus evolves rapidly for several years, then slows, and eventually (after decades) reaches an equilibrium such that in the absence of other sources of positive selection described below, most genes are not changing except through gradual negative selection for improved fitness in the host (9). As an example, an analysis of swine lineages demonstrated that a recently introduced H3 lineage had a more rapid rate of evolutionary change in each gene than an H1 lineage which had been established for several decades (10).

The most commonly discussed selection pressure is from antibodies induced either by infection or by vaccine campaigns. This largely impacts HA and NA as the primary targets of the immune system. For this reason, HA and NA tend to have higher amino acid substitution rates than the other genes. These common changes are a combination of mutations around the receptor binding site of HA that alter antigenicity and bystander or compensatory structural changes. Interestingly, although changes in glycosylation status have been proposed as evolutionarily advantageous via shielding of antigenic sites from antibodies, one recent analysis suggests that glycosylation sites on HA are not under positive selection in the context of antigenic drift (11).

Antiviral drug use is another commonly encountered selective pressure. Rapid evolution of NA can be seen in sites related to NA activity following introduction of NA inhibitor antivirals into a population (12). Finally, reassortment is a common event, both within human virus populations and between human and animal strains. The presence of gene products from different influenza A virus lineages in a newly reassorted virus causes functional mismatches that drive selection of genes coding for variants of proteins that work better together. A classic example is the need for a balance of HA binding to sialic acids to enable entry and NA sialidase activity to facilitate budding. Reassortment-induced mismatches are corrected by evolutionary change (13).

IMPACT OF ADAPTATION ON PATHOGENICITY

Hemagglutinin

A virus must satisfy three criteria in order to be considered the cause of a pandemic (14). It must have an antigenically novel HA, spread worldwide, and cause disease. The HA gene is therefore the one gene that must adapt after all pandemics, since a change in hosts is required to meet these criteria. Because of its central role in virulence and immunity, the HA of a nascent pandemic strain is under intense positive selection pressure. HAs which have recently emerged from the avian reservoirs typically have residual specificity for α-2,3-sialic acids, the predominant form in birds, while gaining specificity for α-2,6-sialic acids (15), which are the predominant receptor for influenza A viruses in the human respiratory tract. The binding affinity for α-2,3-sialic acids tends to weaken or disappear over time during adaptation. The HA must also adapt to fit any new gene products from segments that reassorted from a different strain, e.g., to maintain functional balance with a new NA. Several stabilizing mutations occur to facilitate growth in the new host, including changes to the pH of fusion specific to replication within the human lung (16).

Over a longer time scale, the HAs of strains which achieve endemicity in humans gain glycans on the head region of the protein (17). N-linked glycosylation is a common post-translational modification of viral glycoproteins (18). Glycans are added during transit of the ER and Golgi apparatus at the glycosylation site motif Asn-X-Ser/Thr, where X may represent any amino acid except proline (19). A diverse repertoire of glycans can result from this process, and these modifications may have substantial effects on the biology of the proteins. Some of these glycosylation sites, primarily in the stalk region, are indispensable to the proper folding and conformation of the HA molecule (20). For many years, the prevailing dogma in the field has been that these glycans serve as an antigenic shield from antibody surveillance in an immune population (21). Although experimental data demonstrate that the presence of glycans on the head of the HA does alter antibody recognition (22), a lack of positive selection (11) suggests that this may not be the dominant effect driving addition of glycans during adaptation. Paradoxically, too much shielding may have harmful consequences to the hosts, as failure to neutralize virus in the setting of T-cell activation during reinfection may enhance immune pathology (22).

More recently, a role for glycosylation in modulation of innate immune surveillance has been recognized. Influenza virus glycoproteins are flagged in the ER as "non-self" when they are poorly glycosylated, triggering the unfolded protein response and ER stress (23). Mediated by IRE1α, signal transduction downstream of the c-Jun N-terminal kinase drives inflammatory responses leading to acute lung injury. As influenza A viruses adapt and gain glycosylation, this innate sensing mechanism no longer recognizes the HA as foreign, the cascade is not activated, and considerably less lung pathology occurs during the infection (23). It is likely that selection of glycosylation variants is therefore an adaptation to avoid innate sensing in the ER, as well as the adaptive immune system in the form of antibodies that recognize epitopes on the head region of the HA. This escape comes at a cost, however, as heavily glycosylated viruses are more easily neutralized by collagenous lectins, such as surfactant protein D (17, 21).

Neuraminidase

The role of NA in virulence is as a complement to HA, facilitating budding by cleaving sialic acids and disrupting sialic acid-HA binding. This requires maintenance of a balance between HA binding affinity and NA activity; viruses with too high NA activity relative to HA affinity have difficulty binding and establishing an infection, while viruses with too little relative NA activity have difficulty budding. Reassortant strains with mismatched HA-NA pairs undergo rapid adaptation, with the NA often evolving to match HA and regain this balance (13). The NA has a major role in secondary bacterial infections such as pneumonia (24). Sialic acid cleavage uncovers receptors for bacteria (25) and releases sialic acids into the extra-

cellular medium, where they can be used as a carbon source, facilitating bacterial growth (26). The strength of the cleavage activity of the NA correlates broadly with the severity of epidemic influenza; circulating viruses with high NA activity map to some of the most severe seasons of the last century (27). It is likely that changes in NA activity either to match HA affinity changes during adaptation or in response to drugs (28) have a downstream impact on pathogenicity through change in support for secondary bacterial infections. Loss of NA activity as a compensatory mechanism to escape NA inhibitors in a population with frequent treatment (29) should diminish pathogenicity in this manner.

PB1-F2

PB1-F2 is a small, multifunctional accessory protein of influenza A viruses which is evolutionarily conserved in avian strains (30). It contributes to pathogenicity by triggering cell death through mitochondrial interactions and through support of secondary bacterial infections (7, 31). Its role in the life cycle of the virus is dispensable in mammalian hosts, as nonfunctional forms are negatively selected over decades during adaptation in both humans and swine. Expressed from an alternate start codon in the +1 reading frame of the PB1 gene segment, PB1-F2 functions in endemic virus lineages are lost through truncation to shorter forms that lack the active sites in the C-terminal portion of the protein (typically to 11 or 56 amino acids, reduced from the full length of 87 to 90 amino acids [30]), or through loss of the start codon itself or mutation of the active site amino acids to a neutral or even antibacterial configuration (32). Strains lacking the cytotoxic functions supported by the C-terminal domain do not support secondary bacterial infections very efficiently, and in the human H3N2 lineage, the antibacterial effect appears to be a form of viral-bacterial warfare supporting the virus in its host niche

(32, 33). Overall, the clear pattern, as seen with changes in HA glycosylation, is evolution away from variants that cause inflammation and immunopathology (7).

Nonstructural Protein 1

NS-1 is another multifunctional nonstructural protein produced by influenza viruses. It performs a number of functions in the life cycle of influenza A viruses (6), chiefly as an antagonist of interferon and the antiviral response. Influenza A virus NS-1 contains three potential src homology binding domains, one SH2bm and two SH3bm, which are conserved in many avian lineages. Most avian strains, excluding H5N1 and H9N2 variants, share a consensus sequence from amino acids 212 to 217 defining an SH3(II)bm (34). This domain allows binding of NS-1 to c-Abl and subsequent inhibition of its functions in lung homeostasis. The end results of this blockade are acute lung injury and greatly increased pathogenicity of viruses that carry the motif (35). The 1918 pandemic strain expressed an avian NS-1 that contained this domain; however, the motif was mutated during adaptation of the H1N1 lineage to humans to a form that could not bind c-Abl and did not enhance acute lung injury (35). As the more pathogenic variant of NS-1 is conserved in many avian lineages, viruses that contain it represent a particularly dangerous pandemic threat. Another SH2bm which is able to bind to the p85 subunit of phosphatidylinositol 3-kinase (PI3K) and activate PI3K signaling with multiple downstream effects on immune function is conserved throughout avian and human influenza viruses (36). The reasons why this src homology domain is not lost during adaptation while the SH3(II)bm was selected against are not clear. However, these adaptive changes in NS-1 reinforce the pattern discussed above of selection for strains that do not activate the immune system or trigger inflammatory responses, as these are likely to be negative for both the virus and the host.

Canonical functions important for virus survival that do not impact inflammatory responses such as inhibition of interferon are preserved.

CONCLUSIONS

The punctuated nature of zoonotic incursions into humans and subsequent establishment of endemicity provide a recurring cycle of high- and low-pathogenicity influenza A viruses. Most pandemic strains express pathogenic variants of multiple difference virulence factors and cause significant morbidity and mortality relative to those caused by seasonal strains (1). These strains adapt over time, consistently modifying or losing virulence factors so that seasonal strains are relatively less pathogenic upon the inevitable emergence of a new pandemic virus. A virus similar to the 1918 pandemic strains possessing multiple such factors, or indeed ones that have not yet been elucidated, could cross over from an animal reservoir at any time. The threat from the avian reservoir appears much more dangerous than that from swine, since adaptation of influenza A viruses in swine parallels that in humans in many ways, with frequent mutation and loss of these pathogenic gene variants. As an example, PB1-F2 of the H1N1 2009 pandemic strain was lost during evolution in swine prior to crossing over to humans, likely reducing the overall virulence of this virus and its ability to support secondary bacterial pneumonia. The underlying reasons for conservation of many of these virulence traits in avian species are unclear but are likely related to competition and survival in the differing host niche in birds, the gut.

Pandemic preparation and surveillance of influenza A viruses in animal reservoirs should focus on strains with these (and potentially other) molecular signatures of virulence, as strains carrying multiple such factors are likely to be the most pathogenic prospects for a severe pandemic. This will allow a more rational, targeted approach to vaccine and antiviral design against the worst-case scenario. In addition, multiple animal coronaviruses and parainfluenza viruses appear capable of making jumps into humans and likely use similar mechanisms to cause disease. Investigation of the virulence of these agents in the context of broad themes related to the pathogenicity of zoonotic agents should be a priority for the research community.

CITATION

McCullers JA. 2016. The role of punctuated evolution in the pathogenicity of influenza viruses. Microbiol Spectrum 4(2):EI10-0001-2015.

REFERENCES

1. **McCullers JA.** 2014. The co-pathogenesis of influenza viruses with bacteria in the lung. *Nat Rev Microbiol* **12**:252–262.

2. **Greenbaum A, Quinn C, Bailer J, Su S, Havers F, Durand LO, Jiang V, Page S, Budd J, Shaw M, Biggerstaff M, de Fijter S, Smith K, Reed C, Epperson S, Brammer L, Feltz D, Sohner K, Ford J, Jain S, Gargiullo P, Weiss E, Burg P, DiOrio M, Fowler B, Finelli L, Jhung MA.** 2015. Investigation of an outbreak of variant influenza A(H3N2) virus infection associated with an agricultural fair—Ohio, August 2012. *J Infect Dis* **2012**:1592–1599.

3. **Vincent A, Awada L, Brown I, Chen H, Claes F, Dauphin G, Donis R, Culhane M, Hamilton K, Lewis N, Mumford E, Nguyen T, Parchariyanon S, Pasick J, Pavade G, Pereda A, Peiris M, Saito T, Swenson S, Van RK, Webby R, Wong F, Ciacci-Zanella J.** 2014. Review of influenza A virus in swine worldwide: a call for increased surveillance and research. *Zoonoses Public Health* **61**:4–17.

4. **Osterhaus AD, Rimmelzwaan GF, Martina BE, Bestebroer TM, Fouchier RA.** 2000. Influenza B virus in seals. *Science* **288**:1051–1053.

5. **Smith AM, McCullers JA.** 2013. Molecular signatures of virulence in the PB1-F2 proteins of H5N1 influenza viruses. *Virus Res* **178**:146–150.

6. **Hale BG, Randall RE, Ortin J, Jackson D.** 2008. The multifunctional NS1 protein of influenza A viruses. *J Gen Virol* **89**:2359–2376.

7. **McAuley JL, Chipuk JE, Boyd KL, Van De Velde N, Green DR, McCullers JA.** 2010. PB1-F2 proteins from H5N1 and 20 century pandemic influenza viruses cause immunopathology. *PLoS Pathog* **6**:e1001014.

8. **Jhung MA, Nelson DI.** 2015. Outbreaks of avian influenza A (H5N2), (H5N8), and (H5N1) among birds—United States, December 2014–January 2015. *MMWR Morb Mortal Wkly Rep* **64**:111.

9. **Wolf YI, Viboud C, Holmes EC, Koonin EV, Lipman DJ.** 2006. Long intervals of stasis punctuated by bursts of positive selection in the seasonal evolution of influenza A virus. *Biol Direct* **1**:34.

10. **Bhatt S, Lam TT, Lycett SJ, Leigh Brown AJ, Bowden TA, Holmes EC, Guan Y, Wood JL, Brown IH, Kellam P, Pybus OG.** 2013. The evolutionary dynamics of influenza A virus adaptation to mammalian hosts. *Philos Trans R Soc Lond B Biol Sci* **368**:20120382.

11. **Koel BF, Burke DF, Bestebroer TM, van d V, Zondag GC, Vervaet G, Skepner E, Lewis NS, Spronken MI, Russell CA, Eropkin MY, Hurt AC, Barr IG, De Jong JC, Rimmelzwaan GF, Osterhaus AD, Fouchier RA, Smith DJ.** 2013. Substitutions near the receptor binding site determine major antigenic change during influenza virus evolution. *Science* **342**:976–979.

12. **Xu J, Davis CT, Christman MC, Rivailler P, Zhong H, Donis RO, Lu G.** 2012. Evolutionary history and phylodynamics of influenza A and B neuraminidase (NA) genes inferred from large-scale sequence analyses. *PLoS One* **7**:e38665.

13. **Ward MJ, Lycett SJ, Avila D, Bollback JP, Leigh Brown AJ.** 2013. Evolutionary interactions between haemagglutinin and neuraminidase in avian influenza. *BMC Evol Biol* **13**:222.

14. **McCullers JA.** 2008. Preparing for the next influenza pandemic. *Pediatr Infect Dis J* **27**:S57–S59.

15. **Elderfield RA, Watson SJ, Godlee A, Adamson WE, Thompson CI, Dunning J, Fernandez-Alonso M, Blumenkrantz D, Hussell T, Zambon M, Openshaw P, Kellam P, Barclay WS.** 2014. Accumulation of human-adapting mutations during circulation of A (H1N1)pdm09 influenza virus in humans in the United Kingdom. *J Virol* **88**:13269–13283.

16. **Castelan-Vega JA, Magana-Hernandez A, Jimenez-Alberto A, Ribas-Aparicio RM.** 2014. The hemagglutinin of the influenza A (H1N1)pdm09 is mutating towards stability. *Adv Appl Bioinform Chem* **7**:37–44.

17. **Vigerust DJ, Ulett KB, Boyd KL, Madsen J, Hawgood S, McCullers JA.** 2007. N-linked glycosylation attenuates H3N2 influenza viruses. *J Virol* **81**:8593–8600.

18. **Marth JD, Grewal PK.** 2008. Mammalian glycosylation in immunity. *Nat Rev Immunol* **8:** 874–887.

19. **Kornfeld R, Kornfeld S.** 1985. Assembly of asparagine-linked oligosaccharides. *Annu Rev Biochem* **54:**631–664.

20. **Daniels R, Kurowski B, Johnson AE, Hebert DN.** 2003. N-linked glycans direct the co-translational folding pathway of influenza hemagglutinin. *Mol Cell* **11:**79–90.

21. **Reading PC, Tate MD, Pickett DL, Brooks AG.** 2007. Glycosylation as a target for recognition of influenza viruses by the innate immune system. *Adv Exp Med Biol* **598:**279–292.

22. **Wanzeck K, Boyd KL, McCullers JA.** 2011. Glycan shielding of the influenza virus hemagglutinin contributes to immunopathology in mice. *Am J Respir Crit Care Med* **183:**767–773.

23. **Hrincius ER, Liedmann S, Finkelstein D, Vogel P, Gansebom S, Samarasinghe AE, You D, Cormier SA, McCullers JA.** 2015. Acute lung injury results from innate sensing of viruses by an ER stress pathway. *Cell Rep* **11:**1591–1603.

24. **Peltola VT, Murti KG, McCullers JA.** 2005. Influenza virus neuraminidase contributes to secondary bacterial pneumonia. *J Infect Dis* **192:** 249–257.

25. **McCullers JA, Bartmess KC.** 2003. Role of neuraminidase in lethal synergism between influenza virus and Streptococcus pneumoniae. *J Infect Dis* **187:**1000–1009.

26. **Siegel SJ, Roche AM, Weiser JN.** 2014. Influenza promotes pneumococcal growth during coinfection by providing host sialylated substrates as a nutrient source. *Cell Host Microbe* **16:**55–67.

27. **Peltola VT, McCullers JA.** 2004. Respiratory viruses predisposing to bacterial infections: role of neuraminidase. *Pediatr Infect Dis J* **23:** S87–S97.

28. **Gubareva LV, Kaiser L, Matrosovich MN, Soo-Hoo Y, Hayden FG.** 2001. Selection of influenza virus mutants in experimentally infected volunteers treated with oseltamivir. *J Infect Dis* **183:**523–531.

29. **Gubareva LV, Nedyalkova MS, Novikov DV, Murti KG, Hoffmann E, Hayden FG.** 2002. A release-competent influenza A virus mutant lacking the coding capacity for the neuraminidase active site. *J Gen Virol* **83:**2683–2692.

30. **Smith AM, McCullers JA.** 2013. Molecular signatures of virulence in the PB1-F2 proteins of H5N1 influenza viruses. *Virus Res* **178:**146–150.

31. **McAuley JL, Hornung F, Boyd KL, Smith AM, McKeon R, Bennink J, Yewdell JW, McCullers JA.** 2007. Expression of the 1918 influenza A virus PB1-F2 enhances the pathogenesis of viral and secondary bacterial pneumonia. *Cell Host Microbe* **2:**240–249.

32. **Alymova IV, Green AM, Van De Velde N, McAuley JL, Boyd KL, Ghoneim HE, McCullers JA.** 2011. Immunopathogenic and antibacterial effects of H3N2 influenza A virus PB1-F2 map to amino acid residues 62, 75, 79, and 82. *J Virol* **85:**12324–12333.

33. **McAuley JL, Hornung F, Boyd KL, Smith AM, McKeon R, Bennink J, Yewdell JW, McCullers JA.** 2007. Expression of the 1918 influenza A virus PB1-F2 enhances the pathogenesis of viral and secondary bacterial pneumonia. *Cell Host Microbe* **2:**240–249.

34. **Hrincius ER, Liedmann S, Anhlan D, Wolff T, Ludwig S, Ehrhardt C.** 2014. Avian influenza viruses inhibit the major cellular signalling integrator c-Abl. *Cell Microbiol* **16:**1854–1874.

35. **Hrincius ER, Liedmann S, Finkelstein D, Vogel P, Gansebom S, Ehrhardt C, Ludwig S, Hains DS, Webby R, McCullers JA.** 2015. Nonstructural protein 1 (NS1)-mediated inhibition of c-Abl results in acute lung injury and priming for bacterial co-infections: insights into 1918 H1N1 pandemic? *J Infect Dis* **211:**1418–1428.

36. **Hrincius ER, Hennecke AK, Gensler L, Nordhoff C, Anhlan D, Vogel P, McCullers JA, Ludwig S, Ehrhardt C.** 2012. A single point mutation (Y89F) within the non-structural protein 1 of influenza A viruses limits epithelial cell tropism and virulence in mice. *Am J Pathol* **180:**2361–2374.

Measles in the United States since the Millennium: Perils and Progress in the Postelimination Era

7

ANNE SCHUCHAT,[1] AMY PARKER FIEBELKORN,[2] and WILLIAM BELLINI[2]

INTRODUCTION

Airborne transmission and population susceptibility make measles one of the most contagious diseases plaguing humans. Prior to the licensure of the measles vaccine in 1963, measles caused millions of deaths around the world and hundreds of thousands of reported cases in the United States each year (Fig. 1) (1). High two-dose vaccination coverage of school-aged children with the measles-mumps-rubella (MMR) vaccine achieved by enforcement of school entry vaccination requirements, systematic case-based surveillance, and rapid case investigations and outbreak responses, as well as better control of measles in the region of the Americas, resulted in the elimination of measles in the United States in 2000 (2). Elimination is the absence of endemic disease transmission (i.e., no epidemiological or virological evidence that measles virus transmission is continuously occurring for ≥12 months in a defined geographical area that has adequate surveillance). Fear associated with caring for a child with measles—whose terribly high fever and extensive rash could progress to pneumonia, encephalitis, or worse—was once universal but has now faded from communal memory. Pediatricians in the United States who

[1]The National Center for Immunization and Respiratory Diseases, Centers for Disease Control and Prevention, Atlanta, GA 30329; [2]Division of Viral Diseases, The National Center for Immunization and Respiratory Diseases, Centers for Disease Control and Prevention, Atlanta, GA 30329.

Emerging Infections 10
Edited by W. Michael Scheld, James M. Hughes and Richard J. Whitley
© 2016 American Society for Microbiology, Washington, DC
doi:10.1128/microbiolspec.EI10-0006-2015

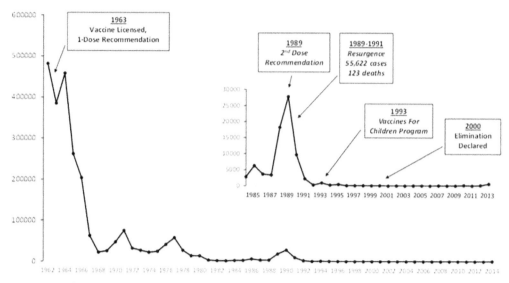

* Provisional total reported cases through Dec 31, 2014

FIGURE 1 Measles, United States, 1962 to 2014. (Adapted from reference 1 with permission.)

began practice in the past 25 years may never have seen a patient with measles. America's success in eliminating measles produced a paradoxical increase in our vulnerability. Attitudes and behaviors that became more prevalent since the beginning of the new millennium have resulted in decreased vaccination coverage in some communities to the point where an imported measles case could lead to very large or prolonged outbreaks. However, in 2015, the nation seemed to reach a tipping point. Public concern in response to a multistate outbreak originating in Disney amusement parks (3, 4) pushed mainstream Americans into more vocal support for vaccination requirements and strengthened confidence in vaccines, which had seemed to be wavering (5–7).

ROAD TO ELIMINATION

Public health funding to address measles outbreaks during the 1970s combined with political and community support to pass and enforce school entry requirements helped to raise immunization coverage across the United States and to lower the numbers of measles cases and deaths (8–11). From 1989 to 1991, measles incidence reemerged, with outbreaks in secondary schools and colleges (12), as well as larger outbreaks among young children in inner cities across the country (13). The resurgence, with 55,000 reported cases and 123 deaths, enhanced political commitment to tackle measles through establishment of a financing system and improved monitoring that would help achieve and then sustain elimination efforts (8, 14).

Investigation of disease outbreaks during this period indicated that two doses of measles vaccine would be needed to ensure sufficiently high and sustained population immunity against measles. In 1989, the Centers for Disease Control and Prevention (CDC)'s Advisory Committee on Immunization Practices (ACIP) recommended a second dose of MMR vaccine for children entering kindergarten (15). Field investigations also revealed that there were large pockets of susceptible young children whose clinicians had missed opportunities to vaccinate them during

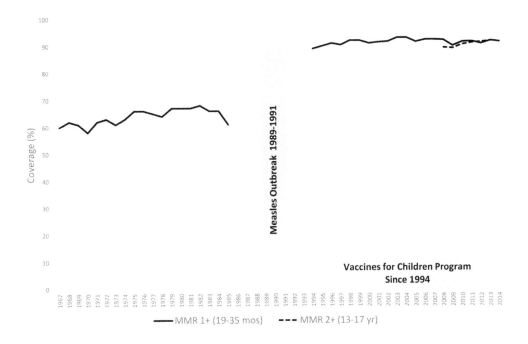

FIGURE 2 Measles virus-containing vaccine coverage among 19- to 35-month-olds (Immunization Information Survey, 1967 to 1985, and National Immunization Survey, 1994 to 2014 [17]) and among 13- to 17-year-olds (NIS-teen), (18) by year. (Adapted from references 17, 18 with permission.)

pediatric care visits (13, 14). Children without insurance were often referred to health departments for vaccination, and many children were not vaccinated when they had mild illnesses, although these visits might be crucial opportunities to administer vaccines. Implementation of the Vaccines for Children (VFC) program in 1994 provided a mechanism for children who were uninsured, Medicaid eligible, American Indian, or Alaska Native to receive free vaccines within the medical home (16). CDC and immunization programs in state and local health departments began providing clinicians participating in the VFC program with ACIP-recommended vaccines and tracking their performance through the Assessment-Feedback-Incentives-eXchange of information (AFIX) system (http://www.cdc.gov/vaccines/programs/afix/index.html) (16). Ongoing monitoring of coverage among 19- to 35-month-olds through the National Immunization Survey permitted programs to track coverage improvements and target low-

performing states for greater support. The National Immunization Survey documented that by 1996, ≥90% of toddlers had been vaccinated with the first dose of MMR (as well as ≥3 doses of polio, diphtheria-tetanus-pertussis, and *Haemophilus influenzae* type b vaccines) (Fig. 2) (17, 18). The United States was certified as having eliminated measles in 2000 (Fig. 1), and in December 2011, an external expert panel verified that the United States sustained elimination of measles from 2001 to 2011 (1, 2, 19).

THE FIRST DECADE FOLLOWING ELIMINATION OF MEASLES IN THE UNITED STATES

Since elimination, virtually all cases of measles in the United States have resulted directly or indirectly from importation of the virus (Fig. 3 and 4) (19–21). Of 507 cases imported between 2001 and 2014, 315 (62%)

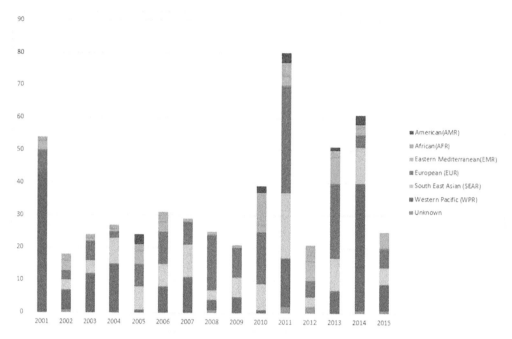

* 2015 data is provisional

FIGURE 3 Reported cases of measles by region of importation, 2001 to 2015. (Adapted from reference 20 with permission.)

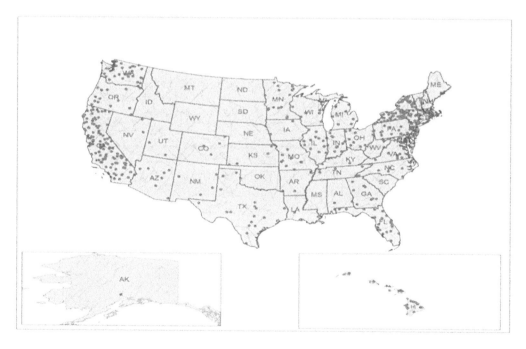

FIGURE 4 Map of imported measles cases, by state, 2001 to 2015. (Source, Division of Viral Diseases, CDC [51].)

occurred among Americans traveling abroad, while 192 (38%) were in international visitors to the United States. Between 2001 and 2008, outbreaks, defined as 3 or more linked cases, were relatively small (median, 5 cases; range, 3 to 34) (20). While importations from Latin America occurred in the 1990s, these became rare following accelerated control in the Pan American Health Organization (PAHO) region and apparent interruption of measles transmission in these countries by 2004 (Fig. 3) (20). There were 232 measles cases imported from 44 countries from 2001 to 2008 (20). From 2001 to 2004, many imported cases derived from the World Health Organization (WHO) Western Pacific region, while from 2005 to 2008, the largest number of cases originated in the WHO's European region (20). The largest outbreak in the United States during this period occurred in a religious community where traditional practice led families to avoid vaccines (22). Many reports described an association with travel related to adoption (23–25). Transmission in the United States occurred in the home, community, religious institutions, health care facilities, schools, child care centers, and the workplace and in association with home schools (20).

In 2008, a startling outbreak in San Diego, CA, garnered national attention after investigators realized that many schools in the affected county had more than 20% of students exempting from required vaccinations (26). The outbreak highlighted a different demographic of parents whose children were unimmunized. In contrast to the 1989-1991 outbreaks, during which clinicians had missed opportunities to vaccinate low-income children, the outbreak in San Diego signaled that more affluent parents were rejecting opportunities for their children to receive MMR vaccine, citing their personal beliefs. Some parents described their behavior as favoring "selective vaccination," and pediatricians reported that many parents were requesting alternative schedules for vaccination of their children (27).

THUNDER IN THE DISTANCE

Concerns about the safety of vaccines have been voiced since the original efforts to immunize against smallpox in the 18th century. Public concern in the past 20 years was amplified in response to fears that vaccines might play a role in autism and related developmental disabilities (28, 29). The hypothesis that MMR vaccine might cause autism was proposed in 1998 in a report in the *Lancet* that has since been retracted (30). In 1999, questions emerged related to the safety of the preservative thimerosal, which was used in multidose vials of some vaccines (31). Numerous studies have now been conducted that fail to identify risk of neurologic developmental disabilities associated with either MMR or thimerosal (32–34), and the Institute of Medicine has updated its review of adverse effects associated with vaccines (28, 35). While the scientific community has redirected research focus to more promising hypotheses to explore factors contributing to risk of autism and autistic spectrum disorder, a belief that there is a link between vaccines and autism has persisted among many (36).

In the United Kingdom, MMR vaccination coverage levels among children 2 years of age fell following the Wakefield report, from 91% during 1997-1998 to 80% during 2003-2004 (37, 38). In 2008, measles transmission in the United Kingdom continued uninterrupted for more than 12 months (39). The United Kingdom reported 1,965 measles cases in 2014 and 5,422 cases in 2013 (https://www.gov.uk/government/publications/measles-confirmed-cases/measles-notifications-and-confirmed-cases-by-quarter-in-england-2013-to-2015).

Research in the United States on attitudes and behaviors related to vaccination suggests that most parents do have some concerns about immunizations, including the number and timing of recommended vaccines and the pain their children appear to experience, but most parents continue to believe that vaccinating their children is important for keeping them healthy (5, 7, 36, 40). Less than 1% of toddlers assessed through the National Immunization Survey has received no vaccines at all (41). Although national statistics and most statewide coverage levels are reassuring, in some communities and schools, a substantial proportion of young children have nonmedical exemptions from the requirement of MMR vaccine for kindergarten attendance (42–44).

CHANGING EPIDEMIOLOGY IN THE UNITED STATES

The San Diego outbreak in 2008 proved to be a harbinger of things to come in the United States. Personal-belief exemptions have been common among unvaccinated people who developed measles over the past 5 years (4, 45–47). Improved methods of tracking school vaccination and exemptions among children entering kindergarten revealed that there were several states where more than 5% of kindergarten students had been granted exemptions from required vaccinations, and within schools in some states, exemption rates were even higher (43, 44, 48–50). Nonetheless, the larger measles outbreaks observed during these years were associated with religious and cultural affiliations, rather than with disease spreading in public schools (21, 45, 46, 51) (Fig. 4). During 2009 to 2014, there were more than twice as many outbreaks annually compared with the numbers during 2001 to 2008 (Tables 1 and 2). The largest outbreak since 2011 occurred in 2014 in Ohio (51). Adult members of an Amish community traveled to the Philippines, where a large outbreak involving tens of thousands of measles case-patients was occurring (52). Upon returning home, they unwittingly introduced measles virus into their own largely unvaccinated community. While 383 measles cases were reported to public health authorities, the virus did not spread to the general population in Ohio or to other Amish communities in

TABLE 1 Characteristics of recent outbreaks of measles in the United States with >20 cases[a]

Yr(s)	No. of cases	Primary state reporting district	Primary setting of outbreak	Median age of case-patients	Source country (genotype)	No. (%) unvaccinated	No. (%) with unknown vaccination status	Philosophical or religious objectors (% of unvaccinated)	No. (%) too young for vaccination
2014	383	Ohio	Household/community	15 yrs	Philippines (D9)	340 (89)	38 (10)	281 (83)	20 (6)
2014-2015	147	California +6 other states	Community	21 yrs	Unknown (B3)	63 (43)	60 (41)	39 (62)	15 (24)
2013	59	New York	Household	4 yrs	United Kingdom (D8)	59 (100)	0 (0)	54 (92)	4 (7)
2014	43	Kansas, Missouri	Household	21 yrs	Federated States of Micronesia (B3)	29 (67)	10 (23)	2 (7)	7 (24)
2014	25	New York	Community	22 yrs	Unknown (B3)	9 (36)	10 (40)	2 (22)	4 (44)
2013	23	North Carolina	Household/community	14 yrs	India (D8)	18 (78)	2 (9)	18 (100)	0 (0)
2013	21	Texas	Church	13 yrs	Indonesia (D9)	18 (86)	1 (5)	17 (94)	1 (6)
2011	21	Minnesota	Shelter	23 mo	Kenya (B3)	17 (81)	4 (19)	7 (41)	7 (41)

[a]Reprinted from reference 65 with permission, with an update to the California outbreak to include data from 2015 (65).

TABLE 2 Comparison of key variables from measles cases reported during 2001 to 2008 versus 2009 to 2014[a]

Characteristic	Value for:		P value[b,c]
	2001–2008 (n = 557)	2009–2014 (n = 1,624)	
Median no. of case-patients reported annually (range)	56 (37–140)	130 (55–667)	0.08
Sex (male) (%)	269 (49)	682/1,252 (55)	**0.02**
Median age (yrs) (range)	15 (0–89)	14 (0–84)	0.53
U.S. resident case-patients (% of total)	438 (79)	1,173 (93)	**<0.0001**
U.S. resident case-patients who were unvaccinated or had unknown vaccination status (% of total)	36 (83)	1,053 (90)	**<0.0001**
U.S. resident case-patients with philosophical or religious objections to vaccination[d]	110 (68)	600/917 (65)	0.54
Preventable case-patients[e]	285 (65)	917 (78)	**<0.01**
Complications	106 (19)	109 (9)	**<0.0001**
Hospitalizations	126 (23)	211 (17)	**0.003**
Median no. of Imported cases annually (range)	26 (18–54)	45 (21–80)	0.32
Median no. of outbreaks annually (range)	4 (2–10)	10 (4–23)	**0.04**
Median no. of outbreak-related case-patients (range)	4 (3–34)[f]	5 (3–383)	0.71
Median outbreak duration, in days (range)	27 (3–79)	17 (3–121)	0.40

[a]Reprinted with permission from reference 65. Data are medians (ranges) for Wilcoxon rank sum results or number/total (percent) for chi-squared results.
[b]Differences in medians were calculated by Wilcoxon rank sums.
[c]Differences in proportions were calculated by Mantel-Haenszel chi-square.
[d]Data on philosophical or religious objections were not routinely collected until 2004. Thus, for earlier postelimination years, the numerator and denominator for this variable reflect data from 2004 to 2008. The denominator includes only vaccine-eligible U.S. resident case-patients.
[e]Case-patients with preventable measles were case-patients for whom vaccination was recommended by the ACIP but who had not received ≥1 dose of measles virus-containing vaccine.
[f]In the previously published summary of measles epidemiological data from 2001 to 2008 (20), the annual median number of outbreak-related case-patients was 5. In that study, there were 3 smaller outbreaks that were recategorized as 1 larger outbreak by the health department after the paper was published. This resulted in a slight shift in the median number of outbreak-related case-patients.

the nearby states. Community and public health efforts were successful in carrying out emergency vaccination clinics and gaining community support for implementing strict quarantine and isolation measures.

On 5 January 2015, California's health department detected multiple cases of measles linked to visits made to Disney amusement parks in Southern California during December (3, 4). A total of 147 cases in California and 6 other states were linked to this outbreak, which also led to exportation of the virus to Mexico and Canada. A measles outbreak in Canada that spread from travelers who had visited a California Disney park eventually caused more than 100 cases in Quebec. Intense follow-up efforts in the United States by state and local public health departments identified susceptible indi-

viduals for appropriate isolation and immunization. In the United States, during 2015 through 21 August, most of the 188 reported measles cases among U.S. residents involved individuals who were unvaccinated (79 [45%]) or did not know their vaccine status (68 [38%]). Of the 79 unvaccinated U.S. resident case-patients reported through 21 August 2015, 40 (51%) reported philosophical, religious, or personal beliefs and 26 (33%) were under the age for vaccination. More than half (107 of 188 [57%]) of the cases reported in 2015 occurred in people 20 years of age or older, many of whom did not know whether they had been appropriately vaccinated. Public health departments facilitated vaccination in the context of the outbreak, and public sector distribution of MMR vaccine for adults during the first quarter of the year increased 3-fold compared with that in the same period in 2014.

IMPLICATIONS OF CURRENT EPIDEMIOLOGICAL CONTEXT

Measles has become so rare that most Americans—clinicians and parents—lack familiarity with its clinical manifestations. Very few clinical specimens are referred to health departments and commercial laboratories in the United States for measles confirmatory testing, and laboratory confirmation of suspected cases can be challenging in a low-incidence, highly vaccinated population. Even when measles is suspected and appropriate specimens are gathered, standard diagnostic test results can be more complicated to interpret in elimination settings where true disease is extremely rare.

Clinical syndromes can be mild or atypical in vaccinated people. Measles is typically confirmed by serology with the detection of IgM antibody. In extremely low-prevalence settings such as the United States, performance of available enzyme-linked immunoassays and other IgM tests is often not sufficient for measles confirmation. The false-positive rate results from multiple factors, including disease prevalence, assay specificity, cross-reacting agents, and interfering substances. To further complicate matters, the IgM response of measles virus-infected, vaccinated persons may be minimal or fleeting, and an absence of IgM does not rule out acute measles virus infection in a vaccinated person.

Real-time RT-PCR (rRT-PCR), a sensitive diagnostic test which detects the presence of the viral genome, has vastly improved detection of cases among previously vaccinated persons, since many (>70%) are PCR positive. However, even the threshold cycle values of the PCR can be increased relative to unvaccinated cases (implying diminished virus production). There are no commercially available rRT-PCR assays for measles diagnosis in the United States. While the CDC's Measles, Mumps, Rubella, and Herpes Virus Laboratory Branch continues to serve as a national referral source for state health departments, in 2013, the CDC worked with the Association of Public Health Laboratories to establish Vaccine Preventable Disease Public Health Laboratory Reference Centers (VPD RCs). In the first two months of 2015, the RCs conducted more than 1,000 rRT-PCR assays to confirm suspected measles cases and about 125 genotyping assays for molecular surveillance. The reference labs are in the state public health laboratories of California, New York, Minnesota, and Wisconsin, and they provide advanced molecular testing and genotype and serotype characterization, diagnostics evaluation, strain banks, and proficiency testing panels for 8 vaccine-preventable diseases (http://www.aphl.org/about aphl/action/pages/vpd-reference-centers. aspx). Nearly all states now have arrangements with one of the VPD-RCs.

Substantial efforts are needed to sustain measles elimination. Public health infrastructure (53) and strong linkages between public health and health care are needed to ensure prompt notification of suspected cases, appropriate laboratory evaluation, identification of contacts, and provision of vaccine or immunoglobulin for susceptible individuals. Enforcement of school laws and maintaining appropriate isolation and infection control practices in medical settings are also important. As the occurrence of measles has become so rare, the rash illness of measles may be misdiagnosed as, for example, Kawasaki's disease or Stevens-Johnson syndrome, and some hospital-associated outbreaks have been exacerbated by delay in recognition of the disease and the patient's need for prompt isolation (54, 55). Outbreak response for nosocomial measles investigations can be challenging when there are incomplete records regarding staff vaccination history and inadequate systems to ensure that health care workers have immunity to measles. Even small outbreaks of measles can require local and state health departments to undertake expensive and labor-intensive response efforts (56).

PUBLIC OPINION AND POLICY CHANGES

Although enforcement of school vaccination requirements reduced measles incidence and increased immunization coverage (8), advocacy groups concerned about vaccine safety and these requirements aimed efforts at promoting state legislative changes to permit philosophical or personal-belief exemptions (50, 57, 58). The frequencies of nonmedical exemptions vary across states and have varied over time. National analyses had been difficult because assessment of school exemptions by states used a variety of methods, such as reviewing records for all schools' complete census versus a small sample of the states' students, and standardization of state surveys is still in progress (44). A recent review of legislative bills about school requirements found that 36 bills were under consideration during 2009 to 2012 (57). Five bills proposed restricting exemptions, while 31 proposed expanding them; none of the attempts to expand exemptions passed, while three states (Washington, California, and Vermont) passed bills that restricted exemptions (57).

Systematic review of immunization requirements suggests that the frequency of exemptions is correlated with the ease with which they can be obtained (42). Other analyses show that school exemption prevalence correlates with risk of outbreaks of measles and pertussis (49, 59, 60). Some recent analyses suggest that after exemption policies become more stringently applied, rates of exemptions decrease (42). These are typically ecologic analyses, and whether policy change leads to differences in behavior or the policy change is itself reflective of changing attitudes and intended behavior is unclear. Bradford and Mandich developed an exemption effectiveness index and found that states with the most effective laws had lower incidences of pertussis (49).

The 2014-2015 outbreak of measles associated with Disney amusement parks in Southern California initiated a change in public dialogue about school requirements. Increased attention to the "innocent bystander"—such as children too young to be vaccinated or unable to be vaccinated because of immunocompromising conditions, like leukemia—appears to have prompted antagonism for those whose personal beliefs were putting others at risk (5, 6, 61–63). A number of state legislatures resumed consideration of tightening school immunization exemption policies. California passed a law eliminating religious and philosophical exemptions (61). Recent public opinion data suggest increased support for vaccine requirements and a significant increase in vaccine acceptance parameters compared with earlier beliefs (5). The durability of these trends bears watching.

CONCLUSION

The story of measles in the United States is closely linked with the establishment and evolution of the nation's immunization program (8). During the 1970s, enforcement of school immunization laws greatly reduced morbidity associated with the virus. By the 1990s, the VFC program was created as a direct result of the resurgence of measles 25 years ago. Since the beginning of the new millennium, wavering confidence in vaccines was partially caused by concerns about MMR and autism, while very recent improvements in the public's confidence in vaccines stem from the 2015 Disney Park-associated measles outbreak, with broadened recognition that routine vaccination protects the most vulnerable in the community, such as babies and those who are immunocompromised and cannot themselves receive the live viral vaccine. Measles continues to circulate in most WHO regions outside the Americas (64), with about 20 million cases estimated each year. Progress toward greater control and eventual elimination of measles from other regions will have the most lasting effect on measles in the United States. Continued assurance that travelers are protected against measles is needed, while support for global immunization improvements can contribute to a future where this disease is finally limited to the history books.

ACKNOWLEDGMENTS

We thank Natarsha Thompson for assistance with preparation of the manuscript and Jane Seward for development of the figures.
The findings and conclusions in this report are those of the authors and do not necessarily represent the views of the Centers for Disease Control and Prevention/the Agency for Toxic Substances and Disease Registry.

CITATION

Schuchat A, Fiebelkorn AP, Bellini W. 2016. Measles in the United States since the millennium: perils and progress in the post-elimination era. Microbiol Spectrum 4(3): EI10-0006-2015.

REFERENCES

1. **Goodson J, Seward J.** 2015. Measles: 50 years after use of measles vaccine. *Infect Dis Clin North Am* **29:**725–743.
2. **Katz S, Hinman A.** 2004. Summary and conclusions: Measles Elimination Meeting, 16–17 March 2000. *J Infect Dis* **189:**S43–S47.
3. **CDC.** 2015. Measles outbreak—California, December 2014–February 2015. *MMWR Morb Mortal Wkly Rep* **64:**153–154.
4. **CDC.** 2015. Measles—United States, January 4–April 2, 2015. *MMWR Morb Mortal Wkly Rep* **64:**373–376.
5. **CS Mott Children's Hospital.** 2015. Safer, with more benefits: parents' vaccines views shifting. *CS Mott Children's Hospital National Poll on Children's Health*, 6 July 2015 ed, **vol 24**. University of Michigan Health System, Ann Arbor, MI.
6. **Funk C, Rainie L.**   2015, posting date. *Americans, politics and science issues.* Pew Research Center, Washington, DC. http://www.pewinternet.org/2015/07/01/Americans-Politics-and-Science-Issues/.
7. **Newport F.**   2015, posting date. *In U.S., percentage saying vaccines are vital dips slightly.* Gallup.com. http://www.gallup.com/poll/181844/percentage-saying-vaccines-vital-dips-slightly.aspx.
8. **Orenstein W.** 2006. The role of measles elimination in development of a national immunization program. *Pediatr Infect Dis J* **25:**1093–1101.
9. **CDC.** 2011. Vaccine-preventable diseases, immunizations, and MMWR—1961–2011. *MMWR Morb Mortal Wkly Rep* **60**(Suppl):49–57.
10. **Orenstein WA, Hinman AR.** 1999. The immunization system in the United States—the role of school immunization laws. *Vaccine* **17**(Suppl 3):S19–S24.
11. **CDC.** 1978. Measles and school immunization requirements—United States, 1978. *MMWR Morb Mortal Wkly Rep* **27:**303–304.
12. **Atkinson WL, Orenstein W, Krugman S.** 1992. The resurgence of measles in the United States, 1989–1990. *Annu Rev Med* **43:**451–463.
13. **Hutchins SS, Escolan J, Markowitz LE, Hawkins C, Kimbler A, Morgan RA, Preblud SR, Orenstein WA.** 1989. Measles outbreak among unvaccinated preschool-aged children: opportunities missed by health care providers to administer measles vaccine. *Pediatrics* **83:**369–374.
14. **NVAC.** 1991. The measles epidemic: the problems, barriers, and recommendations. *JAMA* **266:**1547–1552.
15. **CDC.** 1989. Measles prevention: recommendations of the Immunization Practices Advisory Committee (ACIP). *MMWR Morb Mortal Wkly Rep* **38:**1–18.
16. **Santoli JM, Rodewald LE, Maes EF, Battaglia MP, Coronado VG.** 1999. Vaccines for Children Program, United States, 1997. *Pediatrics* **104:**e15.
17. **CDC.** 2014. Benefits from immunization during the Vaccines for Children Program Era-United States, 1994–2013. *MMWR Morb Mortal Wkly Rep* **63:**352–355.
18. **CDC.** 2015. National, regional, state and selected local area vaccination coverage among adolescents, aged 13–17 years—United States, 2014. *MMWR Morb Mortal Wkly Rep* **64:**784–792.
19. **Papania MJ, Wallace GS, Rota PA, Icenogle JP, Fiebelkorn AP, Armstrong GL, Reef SE, Redd SB, Abernathy ES, Barskey AE, Hao L, McLean Huong Q, Rota J, Bellini WJ,**

Seward JF. 2014. Elimination of endemic measles, rubella, and congenital rubella syndrome from the Western Hemisphere: the U.S. experience. *JAMA Pediatr* **168:**148–155.

20. Parker Fiebelkorn A, Redd SB, Gallagher K, Rota PA, Rota J, Bellini W, Seward J. 2010. Measles in the United States during the postelimination era. *J Infect Dis* **202:**1520–1528.

21. CDC. 2015. *Map of imported cases, by state, 2001 to 2015.* CDC, Atlanta, GA.

22. Parker AA, Staggs W, Dayan GH, Ortega-Sánchez IR, Rota PA, Lowe L, Boardman P, Teclaw R, Graves C, LeBaron CW. 2006. Implications of a 2005 measles outbreak in Indiana for sustained elimination of measles in the United States. *N Engl J Med* **355:**447–455.

23. CDC. 2004. Epidemiology of measles—United States, 2001–2003. *MMWR Morb Mortal Wkly Rep* **53:**713–716.

24. CDC. 2004. Multistate investigation of measles among adoptees from China—April 2004. *MMWR Morb Mortal Wkly Rep* **53:**1–2.

25. CDC. 2007. Measles among adults associated with adoption of children in China—California, Missouri, and Washington, July–August 2006. *MMWR Morb Mortal Wkly Rep* **56:**144–146.

26. Sugerman DE, Barsky AE, Delea MG, Ortega-Sanchez IR, Bi D, Ralston JK, Rota PA, Waters-Montijo K, LeBaron C. 2010. Measles outbreak in a highly vaccinated population, San Diego, 2008: role of the intentionally undervaccinated. *Pediatrics* **125:**747–755.

27. Gust DA, Darling N, Kennedy A, Schwartz B. 2008. Parents with doubts about vaccines: which vaccines and reasons why. *Pediatrics* **122:**718–725.

28. Institute of Medicine. 2011. *Adverse Effects of Vaccines: Evidence and Causality.* The National Academies Press, Washington, DC.

29. Institute of Medicine. 2004. Immunization safety review: vaccines and autism, p 214. *In* The National Academies Press (ed), *Vaccines and Autism.* The National Academies Press, Washington, DC.

30. Godlee F, Smith J, Marcovitch H. 2011. Wakefield's article linking MMR vaccine and autism was fraudulent. *BMJ* **342:**64–66.

31. American Academy of Pediatrics. 1999. Joint statement of the American Academy of Pediatrics (AAP) and the United States Public Health Service (USPHS). *Pediatrics* **104:**568–569.

32. Taylor LE, Swerdfeger AL, Eslick G. 2014. Vaccines are not associated with autism: an evidence-based meta-analysis of case-control and cohort studies. *Vaccine* **32:**3623–3629.

33. Thompson WW, Price C, Goodson B, Shay DK, Benson P, Hinrichsen VL, Lewis E, Eriksen E, Ray P, Marcy SM, Dunn J, Jackson LA, Lieu TA, Black S, Stewart G, Weintraub ES, Davis RL, DeStefano F. 2007. Early thimerosal exposure and neuropsychological outcomes at 7 to 10 years. *N Engl J Med* **357:**1281–1292.

34. Price CS, Thompson WW, Goodson B, Weintraub ES, Croen LA, Hinrichsen VL, Marcy M, Robertson A, Eriksen E, Lewis E, Bernal P, Shay D, Davis RL, DeStefano F. 2010. Prenatal and infant exposure to thimerosal from vaccines and immunoglobulins and risk of autism. *Pediatrics* **126:**656–664.

35. National Vaccine Injury Compensation Program. 2013, posting date. *Vaccine injury table.* Health Resources and Services Administration, Rockville, MD. http://www.hrsa.gov/vaccinecompensation/vaccinetable.html.

36. Kennedy A, LaVail K, Nowak G, Basket M, Landry S. 2011. Confidence about vaccines in the United States: understanding parents' perceptions. *Health Affairs* **30:**1151–1159.

37. Department of Health. 1998, posting date. *NHS immunisation statistics, England: 1997-98.* Department of Health, London, United Kingdom. http://webarchive.nationalarchives.gov.uk/20130107105354/ http://www.dh.gov.uk/prod_consum_dh/groups/dh_digitalassets/@dh/@en/documents/digitalasset/dh_4021496.pdf.

38. Department of Health. 2004, posting date. *NHS immunisation statistics, England: 2003-04.* Department of Health, London, United Kingdom. http://webarchive.nationalarchives.gov.uk/20130107105354/ http://www.dh.gov.uk/prod_consum_dh/groups/dh_digitalassets/@dh/@en/documents/digitalasset/dh_4099577.pdf.

39. Editorial Team. 2008. Measles once again endemic in the United Kingdom. *Euro Surveill* **13**(27)**:**pii=18919.

40. Kennedy A, Basket M, Sheedy K. 2011. Vaccine attitudes, concerns, and information sources reported by parents of young children: results from the 2009 HealthStyles survey. *Pediatrics* **127:**S92–S99.

41. CDC. 2015. National, state, and selected local area vaccination coverage among children aged 19–35 months—United States, 2014. *MMWR Morb Mortal Wkly Rep* **64:**889–896.

42. Wang E, Clymer J, Davis-Hayes C, Buttenheim A. 2014. Nonmedical exemptions from school immunization requirements: a systematic review. *Am J Public Health* **104:**e62–e84.

43. Lieu TA, Ray TG, Klein NP, Chung C, Kulldorff M. 2015. Geographic clusters in underimmunization and vaccine refusal. *Pediatrics* **135:**280–289.

44. CDC. 2015. Vaccination coverage among children in kindergarten—United States, 2014-15 school year. *MMWR Morb Mortal Wkly Rep* **64:**897–904.

45. **CDC.** 2013. Notes from the field: measles outbreak associated with a traveler returning from India—North Carolina, April–May 2013. *MMWR Morb Mortal Wkly Rep* **62:**753.

46. **CDC.** 2013. Notes from the field: measles outbreak among members of a religious community—Brooklyn, New York, March–June 2013. *MMWR Morb Mortal Wkly Rep* **62:**752–753.

47. **CDC.** 2013. Notes from the field: measles—United States, January 1–August 24, 2013. *MMWR Morb Mortal Wkly Rep* **62:**741–743.

48. **Omer SB, Enger KS, Moulton LH, Halsey NA, Stokley S, Salmon DA.** 2008. Geographic clustering of nonmedical exemptions to school immunization requirements and associations with geographic clustering of pertussis. *Am J Epidemiol* **168:**1389–1396.

49. **Bradford WD, Mandich A.** 2015. Some state vaccination laws contribute to greater exemption rates and disease outbreaks in the United States. *Health Affairs* **34:**1383–1390.

50. **Omer SB, Richards JL, Ward M, Bednarczyk R.** 2012. Vaccination policies and rates of exemption from immunization, 2005–2011. *N Engl J Med* **367:**1170–1171.

51. **CDC.** 2014. Measles—United States, January 1–May 23, 2014. *MMWR Morb Mortal Wkly Rep* **63:**496–499.

52. **CDC.** 2015. Progress toward measles elimination—Philippines, 1998–2014. *MMWR Morb Mortal Wkly Rep* **64:**357–362.

53. **NVAC.** 2013. Protecting the public's health: critical functions of the Section 317 Immunization Program—a report of the National Vaccine Advisory Committee. *Public Health Rep* **128:**78–95.

54. **Fiebelkorn AP, Redd SB, Kuhar DT.** 2015. Measles in healthcare facilities in the United States during the postelimination era, 2001–2014. *Clin Infect Dis* **61:**615–618.

55. **Fiebelkorn AP, Seward JF, Orenstein WA.** 2014. A global perspective of vaccination of healthcare personnel against measles: systematic review. *Vaccine* **32:**4823–4839.

56. **Ortega-Sanchez IR, Vijayaraghavan M, Barskey AE, Wallace G.** 2014. The economic burden of sixteen measles outbreaks on United States public health departments in 2011. *Vaccine* **32:**1311–1317.

57. **Omer SB, Peterson D, Curran EA, Hinman A, Orenstein W.** 2014. Legislative challenges to school immunization mandates, 2009–2012. *JAMA* **311:**620–621.

58. **Yang Y, Silverman R.** 2015. Legislative prescriptions for controlling nonmedical vaccine exemptions. *JAMA* **313:**247–248.

59. **Feikin DR, Lezotte DC, Hamman RF, Salmon DA, Chen RT, Hoffman RE.** 2000. Individual and community risks of measles and pertussis associated with personal exemptions to immunization. *JAMA* **284:**3145–3150.

60. **Omer SB, Pan WY, Halsey NA, Stokley S, Moulton LH, Navar AM, Pierce M, Salmon DA.** 2006. Nonmedical exemptions to school immunization requirements: secular trends and association of state policies with pertussis incidence. *JAMA* **296:**1757–1763.

61. **Mello MM, Studdert DM, Parmet WE.** 2015. Shifting vaccination politics—the end of personal-belief exemptions in California. *N Engl J Med* **373:**785–787.

62. **McCoy C.** 2015. Why are vaccination rates dropping in America? *New Republic* http://www.newrepublic.com/article/122367/why-are-vaccination-rates-dropping-america.

63. **Gostin LO.** 2015. Law, ethics, and public health in the vaccination debates: politics of the measles outbreak. *JAMA* **313:**1099–1100.

64. **CDC.** 2014. Progress toward regional measles elimination—worldwide, 2000–2013. *MMWR Morb Mortal Wkly Rep* **63:**1034–1038.

65. **Fiebelkorn AP, Redd SB, Gastañaduy PA, Clemmons N, Rota PA, Rota JS, Bellini WJ, Wallace GS.** 2015. A comparison of post-elimination measles epidemiology in the United States, 2009–2014 versus 2001–2008. *J Pediatr Infect Dis Soc* pii:piv080. [Epub ahead of print] PMID:2666559.

Chikungunya Virus: Current Perspectives on a Reemerging Virus

8

CLAYTON R. MORRISON,[1] KENNETH S. PLANTE,[1] and MARK T. HEISE[1]

CHIKUNGUNYA VIRUS EMERGENCE AND REEMERGENCE

Chikungunya virus (CHIKV) is believed to have originated in Africa and currently exists as three independent virus genotypes: West African, East/Central/South African (ECSA), and Asian. The first described incidence of human disease that was clearly attributable to CHIKV occurred on the Makonde Plateau of Tanzania (formerly Tanganyika) from October of 1952 until April of 1953 (1). The virus responsible for this first outbreak was isolated from the serum of a febrile patient and belonged to what was ultimately designated the ECSA genotype. While this is the first documented incidence of CHIKV, phylogenetic and retrospective analyses of clinical data suggest that the virus may have been present and causing disease much earlier. Many researchers believe that Chikungunya fever (CHIK) may have been incorrectly identified as dengue fever, due to some overlapping symptomatology, in multiple areas throughout Southeast Asia as early as the start of the 18th century (2, 3).

During the initial outbreak in Tanzania, Lumsden noted appreciable numbers of *Aedes aegypti* mosquitoes in the huts of afflicted individuals, thereby providing initial evidence that the virus was vectored by mosquitoes (1). Subsequent studies suggested that in Africa CHIKV is maintained through

[1]Department of Genetics, The University of North Carolina, Chapel Hill, NC 27599.
Emerging Infections 10
Edited by W. Michael Scheld, James M. Hughes and Richard J. Whitley
© 2016 American Society for Microbiology, Washington, DC
doi:10.1128/microbiolspec.EI10-0017-2016

an enzootic (sylvatic cycle) involving nonhuman primates and arboreal *Aedes* mosquitoes (4, 5). Spillover events occur when these CHIKV-infected, arboreal *Aedes* mosquitoes feed on naive humans and transmit the virus. If these infected individuals become viremic and are fed upon by urban *A. aegypti* mosquitoes, an urban transmission cycle involving human-to-mosquito-to-human transmission can be initiated, which can lead to significant disease outbreaks. Since the initial outbreak in Tanzania, sporadic outbreaks of CHIK disease have continued to occur throughout Africa, including in Uganda, Malawi, and Nigeria (4, 5).

In 1958, a CHIKV outbreak was recognized in Bangkok, Thailand (6). Phylogenetic analysis of that outbreak virus demonstrated that the virus was distinct from the virus identified in Tanzania, and it was ultimately designated a separate Asian genotype, which is now endemic in Southeast Asia. Sporadic outbreaks of Asian genotype CHIKV have continued to occur throughout the region, including countries such as India, Vietnam, and Malaysia (7, 8). Unlike in Africa, evidence is lacking to support an enzootic cycle maintaining the Asian genotype virus in nature. Instead, Asian genotype CHIKV is believed to be maintained in an urban cycle between *Aedes* mosquitoes and naive human hosts (9).

While cases of CHIK have been reported in Africa throughout the 20th century, a new strain of virus classified as Indian Ocean Lineage (IOL) reemerged in coastal Kenya in 2004 (10). The IOL strain of the virus quickly spread to Comoros and the Seychelles Islands before jumping to major population centers in the Indian Ocean region, including the Indian Subcontinent, where the virus was estimated to have caused over 1.5 million cases, and Sri Lanka (11–13).

Whole-genome and partial E1 sequences of numerous clinical isolates suggest that the IOL strain most likely evolved from a closely related ECSA strain (14). An important distinction was a single amino acid substitution in the E1 protein, A226V, which was found in the IOL virus isolates compared to ECSA CHIKV. Subsequent *in vivo* studies demonstrated that this change was necessary and sufficient for the virus to adapt to and efficiently utilize *Aedes albopictus* mosquitoes as a major vector of transmission (15). *Aedes aegypti* mosquitoes have historically been the primary vector for CHIKV transmission during other major outbreaks. However, the adaptation of IOL CHIKV to *Aedes albopictus* mosquitoes is viewed as a major factor which allowed the virus to reach epidemic levels in the Indian Ocean region, especially in areas where *A. albopictus* mosquitos were the dominant mosquito species. Importantly, this expanded vector range also had implications for CHIKV's subsequent introduction and spread into temperate areas, such as Italy, where *A. albopictus* was the vector responsible for local transmission (16, 17).

Historically, CHIKV has been a public health threat contained to the Eastern Hemisphere. However, the rapid spread of CHIKV throughout the Indian Ocean region, as well as its emergence in Italy and France, combined with the broad distribution of *Aedes* mosquitoes in both North and South America, raised concern that CHIKV might emerge in the Western Hemisphere (16, 17). Despite frequent incidents of CHIKV-infected individuals traveling into the Western Hemisphere, including a number of viremic travelers entering the United States (reviewed in reference 18), there were no documented cases of localized CHIKV transmission in the Americas during the height of the CHIKV outbreak in the Indian Ocean region (18). However, thoughts that CHIKV might not be capable of establishing infection in the Americas were disproved by an outbreak of CHIKV disease in late 2013, when the first reported cases of human-to-human transmission of CHIKV-induced disease appeared in the French region of the island of St. Martin in the Caribbean (19). These marked the first documented occurrence of non-traveler-associated CHIKV in the Western Hemisphere. Molecular and phylogenetic studies of viruses isolated from the outbreak have identified them as of the Asian genotype, most closely related to those circulating in the Philippines, China, and Micronesia prior to the Caribbean outbreak (20, 21). The Caribbean strain of CHIKV quickly disseminated from St. Martin to other island nations of the Greater and Lesser Antilles, including the Virgin Islands, Aruba, and Barbados (22). By early 2014, cases of the virus were detected in mainland South America in French Guiana, where local spread occurred there and into neighboring Guyana. Furthermore, limited localized transmission also occurred in Florida, with 12 reported cases of localized transmission (CDC ArboNet) (23). The Caribbean outbreak CHIKV has since caused local disease in Puerto Rico, the Dominican Republic, Colombia, and Mexico (Pan American Health Organization), with well over 1 million cases of CHIKV-induced disease occurring in the America's since CHIKV's introduction in 2013 (Pan American Health Organization). Importantly, CHIKV continues to cause disease in countries throughout South and Central America and therefore still has the ability to move into new areas, including the United States.

The recent CHIKV outbreaks in the Indian Ocean region, Southeast Asia, the South Pacific, and the Americas illustrate the importance of several factors in promoting CHIKV transmission. One of the major factors is the increased level of air travel, which almost certainly promotes the spread of CHIKV into new areas. During the height of the Indian Ocean outbreak, a number of CHIKV-infected travelers, who were documented to be viremic and thereby capable of transmitting the virus to permissive mosquitoes, entered the United States (18), and while no outbreak within the United States can be attributed to these individuals, it is likely that much, if not all, of the spread of CHIKV into other areas of the world was mediated by infected travelers (18). Furthermore, the localized transmission of the Caribbean strain of CHIKV observed in Florida in

2014 likely resulted from introduction of the virus by an infected traveler. A second major factor is the distribution of permissive mosquito vectors. Both *A. aegypti* and *A. albopictus* are capable of transmitting CHIKV, and the broad distribution of these mosquito vectors has certainly contributed to the expansion of CHIKV outbreaks in a manner similar to the global circulation of dengue virus and the more recent introduction and spread of Zika virus (24, 25). Lastly, changes in the virus itself have also contributed to the virus's ability to cause widespread outbreaks. As noted above, a mutation in the IOL strain of CHIKV resulted in an expansion of the virus's host range to *A. albopictus* mosquitoes, an event which allowed the virus to be spread in more temperate areas where *A. aegypti* mosquitoes are not found (26). Importantly, unlike the ECSA CHIKV strains, viruses of the Asian CHIKV genotype, which is the type that was introduced into the Caribbean, are less able to adopt the enhanced transmission phenotype in the *A. albopictus* mosquito vector (24, 27). *In vivo* studies of *A. albopictus* mosquitoes infected with engineered mutants of Asian CHIKV indicated that two independent amino acid changes (T98A and E226V in E1), which have yet to be observed in Asian genotype viruses found in nature, are required for the virus to efficiently adapt to use *A. albopictus* mosquitoes (27). Further findings from this study suggest that the acquisition of these separate mutations by Asian genotype viruses is unlikely due to intrinsic evolutionary constraints. This makes it less likely that the Caribbean strain of CHIKV will be capable of efficiently adapting to *A. albopictus* mosquitos, which might limit the virus's ability to be spread in temperate areas within the United States or other parts of the Americas. However, this might be complicated by the fact that in 2014, a strain of CHIKV belonging to the ECSA genotype reemerged in Brazil and has caused significant disease in numerous regions of the country (28). This outbreak marks the first time an ECSA genotype strain of CHIKV has been found in the Western Hemisphere associated with documented cases of local transmission. Abundant *A. aegypti* mosquitoes present in this environment have most likely fueled the outbreak, and currently, there is no evidence to suggest that this virus has mutated to adapt to *A. albopictus* mosquitoes, similar to what was observed with IOL CHIKV. Nevertheless, this virus still has the potential to gain a single adaptive mutation which could ultimately lead to vector expansion and movement of the virus into new regions of the world, including the United States.

CHIKV DISEASE

Most patients suffering from acute CHIKV disease present with high fever and arthralgia, as illustrated by a study by Thiberville et al. in which 100% of outpatients suffering from acute CHIKV infection during the Reunion Island epidemic presented with high fever and arthralgia (29). CHIKV-induced arthritides are often debilitating, and the name chikungunya, which is derived from the Makonde language, translates as "that which bends up," describing the posture taken by persons suffering from CHIKV-induced disease (1). Acute CHIKV-induced arthralgia resolves over a period of several days to weeks; however, arthralgia can persist in some individuals for months to years. In addition to fever and arthralgia, common symptoms of acute CHIKV infection include asthenia, myalgia, and headache (reviewed in reference 30), while other symptoms, such as maculopapular rash and nausea, are also frequently observed in CHIKV patients. Patients frequently present with lymphopenia, while elevated C-reactive protein, elevated liver enzymes, and signs of thrombocytopenia are also observed in a subset of patients with acute CHIKV infection (30). Although the case fatality rate for CHIKV is extremely low, the recent outbreaks have seen a rise in atypical disease manifestations, including encephalitis in infants and multiorgan failure and mortality in elderly individuals or persons with underlying medical conditions (reviewed in reference 30).

CHIKV-Induced Joint and Muscle Disease

Polyarthralgia and myalgia are common attributes of many viral infections; however, severe incapacitating arthralgia is the most prominent feature of acute CHIKV infection (reviewed in reference 30). Following CHIKV infection, patients often rapidly present with sudden onset of severe fever, arthralgia, and myalgia (29, 31). However, while other symptoms, such as fever, resolve within a few days, arthralgia resolves over a longer period, a disease attribute that distinguishes CHIKV-induced arthralgia from that induced by viruses such as dengue virus. This is illustrated by a study by Thiberville et al. in which CHIKV-induced fever had resolved by day 7 after their first medical visit in 100% of patients ($n = 54$), while approximately 65% of patients still reported joint pain 25 days after their initial doctor's visit (29). Furthermore, as noted below, a significant fraction of individuals complain of persistent arthralgia for months to sometimes years after onset (32). During the acute phase of the disease, arthralgia is usually symmetrical and affects multiple joints, commonly the joints of the toes, fingers, ankles, wrists, knees, and elbows (29, 31, 33). Although overt signs of inflammatory cell infiltration are evident in a small subset of affected individuals, acute CHIKV-induced joint disease is generally not erosive, and swelling around the joints is a common feature of acute CHIKV disease (34); however, previously damaged joints may predispose individuals to increased risk of prolonged arthralgia (35).

As noted above, debilitating acute arthralgia is the defining symptom of CHIKV-induced disease, and although CHIKV-induced joint pain is generally most severe at early times post onset, resolution of acute arthralgia can often occur over a period of several weeks. In a subset of infected individuals, symptoms fail to resolve for periods ranging from several months to years after the initial onset of disease, and this joint pain and stiffness can have a significant impact on quality of life (32, 35). The fraction of persons suffering from persistent CHIKV was historically considered to be low, as illustrated by a study by Brighton and Simson that found that 12% of CHIKV patients had persistent symptoms up to 3 years postonset (36). However, during the recent outbreak on Reunion Island, chronic disease appeared to be more prevalent, with 57% of subjects reporting persistence or episodes of recurrence in one study (37), while a second study found 26% of patients reporting residual arthralgia in multiple joints at day 300 after disease onset (29). Furthermore, although recurrent joint stiffness and pain appear to be the major manifestations of chronic CHIKV arthralgia, there have been reports of more severe joint disease in persons suffering from persistent CHIKV-induced arthritides, including erosive arthritis (32, 36, 38). Although the factors that contribute to chronic CHIKV-induced arthralgia are poorly understood, it is clear that increased age, higher viral loads, and the severity of the acute phase of infection are major risk factor for developing persistent disease. Several studies have found that people over the age of 45 are more likely to develop long-term joint pain and stiffness (29, 32, 37, 39), while Thiberville et al. found that persons with ongoing joint pain at 300 days postinfection presented with a higher number of affected joints during the acute stage of the disease (29).

The pathogenesis of acute and chronic CHIKV-induced arthralgia is not completely understood; however, there is strong evidence of CHIKV replication in affected tissues. Furthermore, a growing body of evidence suggests that viral replication within joint tissues elicits an overactive host inflammatory response, which then drives the development of joint pathology and arthralgia. Biopsy results from patients suffering from CHIKV-induced myositis provided evidence that CHIKV can replicate in muscle cells, and this was further confirmed in primary culture studies demonstrating that muscle satellite cells are capable of supporting CHIKV replication (40). Although there is little direct evidence for CHIKV replication within the joints of affected patients due to a lack of synovial biopsy samples from patients with acute CHIKV infection, CHIKV has been shown to replicate efficiently in human synovial fibroblasts (41), and studies from mouse and nonhuman primate models have demonstrated that synovial joints are a major target of CHIKV replication *in vivo* (42–45). There is also evidence suggesting that persistent viral replication may contribute to chronic CHIKV disease. One study, by Hoarau et al., found evidence for persistent CHIKV replication in a single patient suffering from chronic CHIKV arthralgia (46); however, considering the limited sample size in this study, additional studies are needed to confirm these results.

Given the difficulty in obtaining synovial biopsies that span the acute to chronic disease stages from CHIKV-infected humans, a number of groups have turned to animal models to study chronic CHIVK disease. Studies with cynomolgus macaques found that replication was detectable in lymphoid tissues for up to 3 months postinfection (47). Likewise, experiments with mouse models have found detectable levels of CHIKV RNA in joint tissues for up to 4 months postinfection (48), although infectious virus has not yet been detected in these systems. These results all suggest that CHIKV can persist in individuals for long periods, even in the face of a potent antiviral immune response. However, the nature of this persistence and whether persistent viral replication drives long-term chronic joint disease in humans remain to be determined.

Although direct viral replication within joint tissues is thought to contribute to acute CHIKV-induced joint disease, and possibly chronic disease, there is also evidence suggesting that aspects of the host inflammatory response contribute to disease pathogenesis. While components of the innate and adaptive immune response, such as the type I interferon (IFN) system and antiviral antibody, contribute to CHIKV control and clearance (reviewed in reference 49), a significant body of evidence suggests that overactive inflammatory responses clearly contribute to the pathogenesis of acute CHIKV-induced arthralgia and swelling. The severity of CHIKV-induced arthralgia is associated with increased levels of a number of proinflammatory cytokines within the serum of infected humans (50, 51), and inflammatory cell infiltration into joint tissues is a prominent feature in CHIKV-infected mice and nonhuman primates (42, 44, 45, 52), which suggests that aspects of the host inflammatory response contribute to CHIKV-induced joint disease. This is further supported by mouse studies in which depletion of monocytes reduced the severity of CHIKV-induced arthritis (44). Mouse studies also suggest that components of the adaptive immune response modulate the severity of CHIKV-induced arthritis, with CD4 T cells contributing to CHIKV-induced joint swelling (53). Therefore, careful targeting of specific immune components that promote disease may represent a therapeutic avenue in the treatment of CHIKV-induced disease.

Neurologic Involvement

Unlike in the case of encephalitic alphaviruses, such as Eastern and Venezuelan equine encephalitis viruses, neurologic disease is not usually associated with CHIKV. However, a small subset of adult patients requiring hospitalization exhibited signs of syndromes such as acute flaccid paralysis, Guillain-Barré syndrome, and encephalopathy (54–56). This is illustrated by a study during the Reunion Island CHIKV epidemic in which 25% of patients with atypical CHIKV infection reported neurologic involvement, including malaise and meningo-

encephalitis (57). Children are also at risk of developing neurologic complications, where vertical mother-to-child transmission puts newborns at significant risk of developing encephalopathy that can result in lifelong neurologic consequences (58–60).

Mortality Associated with CHIKV Infection

CHIKV-induced mortality, although rare, does occur, with an approximate case fatality rate of 1 in 1,000 (reviewed in reference 30). Very young (e.g., neonates) and elderly individuals, as well as people with underlying medical conditions, comprise the majority of these cases, with causes of death ranging from encephalitis to hepatitis and multiple-organ failure (30).

Other Clinical Manifestations

A transient maculopapular rash on the thorax and the medial aspects of the limbs during CHIKV disease is common; however, a small subset of individuals do develop more severe skin manifestations, including ulcers and vasculitis (reviewed in reference 30). Although the pathogenesis of CHIKV-induced skin disease is poorly understood, active viral replication within the skin might contribute to CHIKV-induced skin disease. Other rare but potentially serious manifestations of CHIKV disease include ocular disease, including uveitis (61). Lastly, fatigue is a common complaint associated with CHIKV infection and may persist for months to years in some individuals (62).

CHIKV VACCINES AND THERAPEUTICS

The reemergence of CHIKV, with subsequent spread in the Indian Ocean region and its introduction into the South Pacific and the Americas, has rekindled interest in the development of vaccines for the prevention of CHIKV infection and therapeutics for treating acute and chronic CHIKV-induced disease. Unfortunately, there are currently no approved CHIKV vaccines or therapies, and despite the scope of the current CHIKV epidemic, treatment options for CHIKV-induced disease are generally limited to palliative care using nonsteroidal anti-inflammatory drugs (NSAIDs) and hydration. Given the scope of the recent CHIKV outbreaks and the limited treatment and prevention options available, significant effort has been put into developing new vaccine and therapeutic pipelines for CHIKV, and we briefly summarize current progress in both of these areas.

CHIKV Vaccines

Although CHIKV is a threat to spread within developed countries, such as the United States and European countries, developing countries have borne the brunt of CHIKV-induced disease over the past 10 years and are at greatest risk of continued CHIKV spread. Therefore, for a CHIKV vaccine to be useful in these areas, it would need to be relatively inexpensive to manufacture and administer and preferably be highly immunogenic after a single dose, while having no to minimal side effects. Furthermore, since older individuals are at increased risk of developing chronic CHIKV-induced arthralgia and for severe CHIKV-induced disease (29, 32, 37, 39), a successful vaccine would ideally be safe and

immunogenic in this population. While multiple vaccine strategies have been explored in preclinical studies (reviewed in depth in reference 63), to date, four vaccines have entered human trials and many vaccines are in differing stages of preclinical testing (Table 1). For the purposes of this review, we focus on vaccines that have entered into clinical trials while briefly discussing other vaccine strategies.

CHIKV vaccine research dates back 40 years, with much of the early CHIKV vaccine work focusing on traditional inactivated and or cell culture-adapted live attenuated vaccines. Initial attempts at generating a CHIKV vaccine focused on using formalin-inactivated virus derived from the African 167 CHIKV strain, which was produced from green monkey kidney cells, chicken embryo cells, or concentrated suspension cultures (64). This inactivated vaccine was initially tested by intraperitoneal inoculation into 3- to 4-week-old Swiss Bragg mice with a prime-boost, 2-dose schedule, followed by intracerebral challenge. The vaccine exhibited good efficacy in the mouse model and was later tested for efficacy in humans, in whom it was found to elicit a neutralizing antibody response with no adverse events (65).

The second vaccine that was tested in humans was developed at the Walter Reed Army Institute of Research, where Levitt et al. set out to increase the efficacy of the

TABLE 1 CHIKV vaccine strategies

Vaccine	Platform	Dosing scheme	Stage of development	Year of original description	Reference(s)
167, inactivated	Inactivated	Multidose	Phase I	1971	64, 65
181/25	Live attenuated	Single dose	Phase II	1986	66–68, 70, 71
Consensus capsid DNA	DNA	Multidose	Preclinical	2008	86
ECSA based, inactivated	Inactivated	Multidose	Preclinical	2009	83
VSV/CHIKV VLP	VLP	Multidose	Phase I	2010	79, 80
Structural gene DNA	DNA	Multidose	Preclinical	2011	87
Adenovirus chimera	Chimeric	Single dose	Preclinical	2011	85
Insect cell VLP	VLP	Single dose	Preclinical	2011	89, 90
CHIKV/IRES	Live attenuated	Single dose	Preclinical	2011	74–78
Alphavirus chimera	Chimeric	Single dose	Preclinical	2011	84
E2 protein	Subunit	Multidose	Preclinical	2012	88
MV/CHIKV VLP	VLP	Multidose	Phase I	2013	81, 82

green monkey kidney-based inactivated vaccine by generating a live attenuated vaccine. A human CHIKV isolate from a 1962 Thai outbreak, strain 15561, was plaque purified and passaged 18 times in human embryonic lung MRC-5 cells (66). On the 18th passage, three plaque-purified clones, clones 25 to 27, which exhibited a uniform plaque morphology, underwent safety testing by intracranial inoculation into neonatal (1- to 3-day-old) mice. In contrast to the parental virus, which caused 61% mortality, none of the three passaged viral isolates caused mortality. In subsequent efficacy studies, clone 25 exhibited 100% protection against lethal CHIKV challenge in weanling mice, and this virus was designated 181/25. Following the successful testing in mice, the 181/25 vaccine was then taken forward for additional evaluation in nonhuman primates (66). In a dose escalation experiment in which the vaccine was administered at doses ranging from 3.5 to 5.5 $\log_{10}$ PFU, vaccinated animals exhibited complete protection from CHIKV viremia following challenge (66).

Following the mouse and nonhuman primate studies, the 181/25 vaccine was tested for virulence in humans in a phase I clinical trial. In this trial, involving 15 people, there were no adverse events reported and no conclusive evidence of a difference between the naive group receiving either the 181/25 vaccine or a mock vaccination (67). Therefore, 181/25 was considered avirulent in humans and proceeded to phase II trials, where the 181/25 vaccine (now called TSI-GSD-218) was evaluated in a double-blind 73-person efficacy trial (68). Following intramuscular injection with 0.5 $\log_{10}$ PFU of vaccine (n = 59) or a mock vaccine (n = 14), subjects were interviewed to discuss symptoms on days 1 to 4, 10, 14, and 28 postvaccination. The group that received the vaccine developed neutralizing antibodies in 98.3% of cases by 28 days postvaccination, with 85% of the vaccinees remaining seropositive 1 year later (68). Some members of both the experimental and control groups experienced symptoms at the site of inoculation and flu-like symptoms, with no statistically significant difference between the groups. However, 5 of the 59 patients that received the vaccine developed transient unilateral arthralgia in 1 or 2 of their joints, compared to 0 cases in the control group, which led the TSI-GSD-218 vaccine to be abandoned following the phase II trial (68).

Although development of the 181/25 vaccine was halted in phase II trials, with the reemergence of CHIKV and subsequent large-scale epidemics, there has been some interest in revisiting this vaccine (69). However, recent work has illustrated potential pitfalls associated with this vaccine, including spread into mosquito species and reversion to virulence. The 181/25 vaccine strain was evaluated for transmission competence in *Aedes albopictus* and *Aedes aegypti* mosquitoes by Turell and Malinoski, and while the 181/25 virus was found to infect and transmit less effectively than the parental 15561 virus, it was still able to be spread by mosquitoes (70). Additionally, Gorchakov et al. found that the attenuation of the 181/25 vaccine was attributed to two point mutations in the E2 protein (71), with a mutation located at position 82 that is associated with heparin sulfate binding believed to be the major attenuating determinant within the virus (72, 73). The capacity for 181/25 to rapidly revert to virulence was further described by Plante et al., who discovered that the 181/25 vaccine could revert to a virulent phenotype after 5 serial mouse brain passages in neonatal type I IFN receptor$^{-/-}$ (IFNAR$^{-/-}$) mice. This reversion to virulence was caused by both direct revertants of the previously identified residue 82 mutation and by other loss of positive-charge, surface-exposed mutations near residue 82 of the E2 protein (74). This work strongly suggested that more stable attenuation strategies were needed for developing safe live attenuated CHIKV vaccines.

Another promising live attenuated vaccine that has been extensively studied in the preclinical stage is the CHIKV/IRES vaccine produced by Plante et al. (75). By utilizing an encephalomyocarditis virus internal ribosomal entry site (IRES) that is incapable of translation in arthropod cells, they were able to produce an immunogenic and attenuated vaccine which was incapable of growing in the mosquito vector. This vaccine was found to be efficacious and safe in multiple mouse models and nonhuman primates (75, 76). The CHIKV/IRES vaccine was further tested for safety and stability by trying to mutate the virus in a worse-case-scenario serial mouse brain passage experiment. The IRES-based vaccine remained attenuated, while the 181/25 vaccine, which was run in parallel as a control, became neurovirulent, leading to fatal outcomes in (IFNAR$^{-/-}$) mice (74). The vaccine was also successfully tested for its ability to protect against a closely related virus in the Semliki Forest clade, o'nyong-nyong virus (77). It was further shown that the neutralizing antibody response elicited by CHIKV/IRES in mice was significant and sufficient to elicit full protection against a lethal challenge (78).

After CHIKV's reemergence, the first new vaccine strategy to go forward for testing in humans was a virus-like particle (VLP) vaccine produced and tested by Akahata et al. (79). The VLPs were produced in HEK293T cells using CHIKV glycoproteins derived from the 37997 CHIKV strain in a lentiviral vector along with the vesicular stomatitis virus G protein. A three-dose vaccination regimen in nonhuman primates elicited neutralizing antibodies which when passively transferred to mice were protective against lethal CHIKV challenge (79). The vaccine has been evaluated in a phase I dose escalation trial (80) in which three different doses, 10 ×g, 20 ×g, and 40 ×g, were administered three times over a period of 20 weeks in cohorts of 5, 10, and 8 people. All three doses elicited a strong neutralizing antibody response and were well tolerated by the subjects (80).

The most recent vaccine candidate to have been evaluated in human trials is a measles virus (MV)-vectored VLP produced by Brandler et al. (81). This vaccine uses a live attenuated Schwarz MV as a vector for CHIKV structural proteins from the La Reunion (OPY2006) strain. This recombinant virus (MV-CHIKV) was tested in type I IFN receptor-deficient (IFNAR$^{-/-}$) mice transgenic for the human CD46 MV receptor that are capable of supporting MV replication. Three doses (3 log$_{10}$ PFU, 4 log$_{10}$ PFU, and 5 log$_{10}$ PFU) were tested by inoculating mice twice over a 1-month interval. All three doses elicited neutralizing anti-CHIKV antibody responses; the low dose was found to be 80% efficacious, and the higher two doses were 100% protective against a lethal challenge. This vaccine was then subjected to a randomized, double-blind, placebo-controlled, phase I clinical trial (82). Doses of either 1.5×10^4 PFU, 7.5×10^4 PFU, or 3.0×10^5 PFU were administered to 12 subjects of each cohort, and a negative control cohort of 6 people received a Priorix measles-mumps-rubella vaccine, with each cohort receiving a total of three inoculations on days 0, 28, and 90. The vaccine did elicit neutralizing antibody in a dose-dependent manner, and importantly, previous measles vaccination did not adversely affect the vaccine's ability to elicit CHIKV-specific immune responses. The vaccine was also relatively well tolerated at the lower two doses, with most adverse events being classified as mild or moderate. However, 58% of the individuals in the cohort with 3.0×10^5 PFU did exhibit adverse events, including flu-like illness, pain at the site of injection, and dispersed but transient myalgia (82).

A multitude of other CHIKV vaccine candidates have been produced and are in different stages of preclinical testing. An inactivated vaccine was produced and tested by Tiwari et al., utilizing a Vero cell-adapted ECSA strain of CHIKV, and proved capable of producing neutralizing antibodies (83). Several chimeric viruses were tested, utilizing the either alphavirus or adenovirus vectors with the structural genes of CHIKV (84, 85). These vaccines were capable of eliciting a neutralizing antibody response and protecting mice from a virulent challenge. Two DNA-based vaccines were also produced and were also found to protect mice and, in nonhuman primates, were found to induce a robust immune response (86, 87). Other vaccine strategies were attempted, such as a series of subunit vaccines (88, 89) and a VLP-based vaccine produced from insect cells (90). These strategies also were found to have their strengths.

As previously stated, a vaccine for CHIKV should exhibit multiple traits for effective use. These traits would be slightly different for a traveler's vaccine compared to one intended for implementation in the regions where this virus is endemic. A traveler's vaccine could be a multidose and expensive and convey only short-lived protection. However, since this virus disproportionately affects equatorial developing countries, cost and efficacy take on added weight when considering utility. The vaccine would have to be manufactured quickly, and at low cost, to be implemented in the large and relatively poor populations most at risk. The vaccine should elicit a strong and long-lived immune response and do so with a single dose. A multidose vaccine may prove ineffective if the patient either chooses not to return or is incapable of coming in for subsequent booster vaccinations. The vaccine would have to be safe and easy to administer due to the lack of advanced health care in some of the regions where the virus is endemic. Another important trait of any live attenuated vaccine is that it proves stable in its non-virulent phenotype and is not going to be accidentally spread by the mosquito vectors. Though this is not an issue in other vaccine platforms, the live attenuated vaccine strategy is thought to be the best option for a virus that so heavily impacts developing countries.

Antivirals against CHIKV

As noted above, although there are multiple CHIKV vaccines in various stages of preclinical and clinical development, there are currently no vaccines approved for use in humans. The situation with antiviral therapies is similar, in that while a number of antiviral strategies are being pursued, currently approved treatments for acute CHIKV infection are limited to NSAIDs. However, given that CHIKV outbreaks can afflict hundreds of thousands or even millions of individuals with severe incapacitating arthralgia, which can have significant impact on an individual's quality of life (30), and a major fraction of these individuals (>1 million) (32) suffer from long-term rheumatologic complaints, there is a significant need for new therapies treating for CHIKV disease. With this in mind, a number of different therapeutic strategies are in development, and these efforts have identified promising pharmacological and biological strategies that have the potential to limit the scope and severity of disease in humans infected with CHIKV. Therefore, this section provides an overview of some of the major therapeutic approaches that are being evaluated as treatments for acute and chronic CHIKV-induced disease (Table 2).

Treatment of acute CHIKV disease

Therapeutic strategies for treating acute CHIKV disease can be roughly broken down into antiviral therapies, which target the virus to reduce viral loads, or host-targeted therapies, which can either inhibit host processes

TABLE 2 CHIKV antivirals

Antiviral	Target	FDA approval no.[a]	Reference(s)
Ribavirin	Virus	018859	92, 93
Mycophenolic acid	Virus	050791	94
6-Azauridine	Virus		93
Homoharringtonine (omacetaxine mepesuccinate)	Virus	203585	97
Polyclonal antibodies	Virus		79, 98
Mabs	Virus		43, 99, 100, 104
Chloroquine	Host	006002	36, 106, 108, 109
Bindarit	Host		112, 115

[a]Reflects approval for applications other than CHIKV. All numbers reflect NDAs.

that are required for viral infection, thereby reducing viral loads, or interfere with components of the host inflammatory response that promote CHIKV-induced disease.

Virus-targeted antivirals

One of the earliest candidate antivirals for treating acute CHIKV disease was ribavirin, a synthetic guanosine nucleoside analogue that exhibits broad-spectrum antiviral activity and which received FDA approval for the treatment of respiratory syncytial virus and hepatitis C virus infections in 1985 (FDA new drug application [NDA] 018859). While the direct antiviral mechanism(s) of ribavirin has yet to be completely elucidated, it has been suggested that the drug largely acts by depleting cellular pools of GTP through the inhibition of the cellular inosine monophosphate dehydrogenase enzyme (91). The depletion of GTP is also postulated to indirectly result in the incorporation of deleterious mutations in various RNA and DNA virus genomes. Notably, ribavirin has been shown to have antiviral activity against CHIKV both *in vitro* and in a small clinical study (92, 93), which suggests that ribavirin may have utility in treating CHIKV cases.

Several other promising antiviral compounds include mycophenolic acid, 6-azauridine, and harringtonine. Similar to ribavirin, mycophenolic acid acts to inhibit inosine monophosphate dehydrogenase, reduces cellular GTP pools, and therefore exhibits broad-spectrum antiviral activity. *In vitro* studies have shown that mycophenolic acid protects cells against CHIKV-induced apoptosis and reduces viral yields from treated cells (94). The compound 6-azauridine is a uridine nucleoside analogue which inhibits the enzyme orotidine monophosphate decarboxylase, required for the synthesis of pyrimidines. Inhibition of pyrimidine synthesis leads to reduced UTP levels, and therefore, 6-azauridine has antiviral activity against a number of DNA and RNA viruses, including CHIKV, with which the drug shows strong inhibition of replica-

tion *in vitro* (93). Harringtonine and its derivative homoharringtonine are natural plant alkaloids which inhibit protein synthesis in eukaryotic cells. Synthetic homoharringtonine, renamed omacetaxine mepesuccinate, received FDA approval for the treatment of chronic myelogenous leukemia (FDA NDA 203585). It is believed to function by stalling host translation by competing with tRNAs at the ribosome and can also halt the cell cycle (95, 96). Recently, harringtonine has been shown to effectively inhibit CHIKV protein synthesis *in vitro* at low 50% effective concentrations (97); however, it has not been tested for efficacy *in vivo*.

Antibody therapies

Anti-CHIKV antibody has long been known to be a correlate of CHIKV vaccine-mediated protection, and a number of passive-immunization studies have shown that CHIKV-specific neutralizing antibodies can protect animals from CHIKV replication and disease (79, 98). Therefore, CHIKV antibodies have been evaluated as both prophylactic and postexposure therapies for the treatment of acute CHIKV disease in patient populations, and a number of antibody formulations are at various stages of preclinical development. Couderc et al. were able to demonstrate protection against CHIKV disease in both neonatal and IFN receptor knockout mice (IFNAR$^{-/-}$) through passive transfer of human donor convalescent-phase plasma (98). In this study, protection from disease was achieved when antibodies were administered within the first 24 h of infection. Akahata et al. have also found that nonhuman primate polyclonal antibodies directed against CHIKV VLPs protected (IFNAR$^{-/-}$) mice against disease (79).

In addition to polyclonal-antibody studies, both human and murine monoclonal antibodies (MAbs) directed at the E1 and E2 structural glycoproteins have also been identified that neutralize virus *in vitro* and are protective in mice (99, 100). Many of the E2 antibodies target diverse regions of the protein to neutralize virus. Generally, clinical improvements in mice are observed when MAb treatment is started within the first 24 h following infection (101–103). In addition to single-MAb therapies, other investigators have developed combinatorial-MAb therapies to help prevent against neutralization escape variants (43). Pal et al. recently demonstrated that genetically engineered escape mutants of CHIKV with resistance to neutralization by two independent MAbs were mildly attenuated in mice and failed to revert to wild type in both mosquitoes and mice (104). The combination of studies on polyclonal antibody and MAb therapies against CHIKV suggest that they have strong potential for use in humans at higher risk for disease, when treated early in infection. However, it remains unclear whether antibody therapy would be useful in general populations during CHIKV outbreaks due to costs and logistical concerns around antibody delivery. However, anti-CHIKV antibody therapies might be very useful in specific at-risk populations, such as laboratory workers suffering from known virus exposures, immunosuppressed individuals, or CHIKV-infected women during the late stage of pregnancy (60, 105). Of particular note, given that mother-to-child CHIKV transmission during childbirth puts infants at increased risk of developing CHIKV-induced neurologic disease, which can result in sequelae with lifelong consequences, anti-CHIKV antibodies represent a promising approach for protecting this population. This could take the form of administering antibodies to women in the latter stages of pregnancy who have active CHIKV infections or reside in an active outbreak locality, as a means of reducing CHIKV viremia and thereby limiting chances of transmission to the infant, or by direct administration of antibody to the neonate.

Host-targeted antivirals
Clinical trials with host targeted antivirals have focused on chloroquine, a class of 4-aminoquinolone drug discovered in 1934 and which was originally used as an antimalarial drug (FDA NDA 006002). Chloroquine has also been demonstrated to have potent antiviral activity against CHIKV *in vitro*. Mechanistic studies suggest that the drug increases endosomal pH, thus preventing the low-pH fusion of the E1 protein during early entry of the virus (106). While Khan et al. were able to demonstrate efficacy of the drug when used preinfection, during infection, and postinfection at micromolar concentrations *in vitro*, it was shown to be ineffective when used greater than 3 h postinfection. An early report from Brighton found that chloroquine treatment improved chronic CHIKV-associated joint symptoms in 50% of a cohort of patients (107). However, this was an open study with a small number of patients. Importantly, in follow-up studies, chloroquine was found to be ineffective during two separate human clinical trials conducted in India and Reunion Island (108, 109). In a study conducted by de Lamballerie et al., patients who received chloroquine complained of more frequent arthralgia than those that received placebo by day 200 of treatment (109). The early mode of action of chloroquine coupled with its ineffectiveness in several clinical studies suggests that it may have limited potential for treatment of acute human CHIK disease.

As noted above, there is a significant body of evidence which suggests that the host inflammatory response contributes to the pathogenesis of CHIKV-induced arthritides. Therefore, therapies that inhibit aspects of the host inflammatory response also hold promise in the treatment of CHIKV-induced disease. Bindarit, a small-molecule inhibitor of monocyte chemotactic protein 1 (MCP-1) synthesis, has shown potent anti-inflammatory actions against cancer-induced inflammation and autoimmune inflammation in several rodent models (110, 111). In mouse models of CHIKV pathogenesis, macrophage numbers and MCP-1 levels have been tightly associated with joint inflammation, arthritis, and myositis. Chen et al. demonstrated that intraperitoneal administration of bindarit twice a day from the day of infection resulted in significant reductions in symptoms and the duration of disease in mice, which was independent of viral loads in affected tissues (112). However, Poo et al. have recently shown that mice deficient for the cognate receptor of MCP-1, CCR2, have prolonged and more severe symptoms and inflammation than wild-type mice challenged with CHIKV (113). Notably, cellular inflammation in $CCR2^{-/-}$ mice is dominated by neutrophils and, later, eosinophils, as opposed to the classical monocyte/macrophage response seen in wild-type mice. Based upon these conflicting results, the use of bindarit to treat CHIKV in humans would require additional small-animal model studies to clarify the mode of action of the drug, while additional the safety and efficacy tests in other models, such as nonhuman primate models of CHIKV infection, are likely warranted.

Therapies for chronic CHIKV disease

As noted above, a significant fraction of CHIKV-infected individuals suffer from chronic joint pain and stiffness for months or even years postinfection. Given the duration of these symptoms and the fact that they cause a significant decrease in quality of life (30), there is a clear need for effective therapies for treating chronic CHIKV-associated joint pain. Unfortunately, the development of effective therapies is hampered by the fact that the pathogenesis of chronic CHIKV-associated joint pain is poorly understood. For example, although there are limited data suggesting that the CHIKV persistence within joints may contribute to chronic disease (46), it is unclear whether drugs that inhibit CHIKV replication will have any benefit if administered during the chronic stage of disease. Furthermore, there is evidence for ongoing inflammation in the joints of at least a subset of individuals suffering from the most severe aspects of chronic CHIKV-induced arthralgia, and

evidence suggests that these individuals are likely to be helped by treatment with NSAIDs, as well as disease-modifying antirheumatic drugs, such as methotrexate (32, 114). However, it is unknown whether broad application of stronger anti-inflammatory and immunosuppressive therapies will be of benefit in treating chronic CHIKV disease, at which point in the disease process these strategies should be applied, or whether more specific anti-inflammatory drugs that target specific host pathways will be of benefit. Therefore, the development of more effective therapies or even approaches for safely using existing treatments, such as methotrexate, for treating chronic CHIKV disease is likely to require a much better understanding of the viral and host factors that drive disease pathogenesis.

CONCLUSIONS

The reemergence of CHIKV and its subsequent global spread illustrate how a combination of rapid global transit, broad mosquito vector distribution, and a lack strategies for treating or controlling emerging pathogens can significantly impact public health, a scenario that is now be repeated with the emergence and spread of Zika virus in the Americas. In the case of CHIKV, the response to outbreaks over the past 12 years has provided important new insights into the pathogenesis of CHIKV disease, as well as strategies for developing new vaccines and therapies for treating acute and chronic CHIKV. However, additional work is needed in all of these areas both to deal with the ongoing CHIKV epidemic in the Americas and to prepare for future CHIKV outbreaks.

ACKNOWLEDGMENTS

Funding was provided by NIH grant U19 AI 109680 to M.T.H. and C.R.M. and by grant T32-AI007151 to K.S.P.

CITATION

Morrison CR, Plante KS, Heise MT. 2016. Chikungunya virus: current perspectives on a reemerging virus. Microbiol Spectrum 4(3):EI10-0017-2016.

REFERENCES

1. **Lumsden WH.** 1955. An epidemic of virus disease in Southern Province, Tanganyika Territory, in 1952-53. II. General description and epidemiology. *Trans R Soc Trop Med Hyg* **49:**33–57.

2. **Kuno G.** 2015. A re-examination of the history of etiologic confusion between dengue and Chikungunya. *PLoS Negl Trop Dis* **9:**e0004101.

3. **Carey DE.** 1971. Chikungunya and dengue: a case of mistaken identity? *J Hist Med Allied Sci* **26:**243–262.

4. **McIntosh BM, Harwin RM, Paterson HE, Westwater ML.** 1963. An epidemic of Chikungunya in South-Eastern Southern Rhodesia. *Cent Afr J Med* **43:**351–359.

5. **Muyembe-Tamfum JJ, Peyrefitte CN, Yogolelo R, Mathina Basisya E, Koyange D, Pukuta E, Mashako M, Tolou H, Durand JP.** 2003. Epidemic of Chikungunya virus in 1999 and 200 in the Democratic Republic of the Congo. *Med Trop (Mars)* **63:**637–638. (In French.)

6. **Hammon WM, Rudnick A, Sather GE.** 1960. Viruses associated with epidemic hemorrhagic fevers of the Philippines and Thailand. *Science* **131:**1102–1103.

7. **Lam SK, Chua KB, Hooi PS, Rahimah MA, Kumari S, Tharmaratnam M, Chuah SK, Smith DW, Sampson IA.** 2001. Chikungunya infection—an emerging disease in Malaysia. *Southeast Asian J Trop Med Public Health* **32:**447–451.

8. **Deller JJ Jr, Russell PK.** 1967. An analysis of fevers of unknown origin in American soldiers in Vietnam. *Ann Intern Med* **66:**1129–1143.

9. **Thiboutot MM, Kannan S, Kawalekar OU, Shedlock DJ, Khan AS, Sarangan G, Srikanth P, Weiner DB, Muthumani K.** 2010. Chikungunya: a potentially emerging epidemic? *PLoS Negl Trop Dis* **4:**e623.

10. **Chretien JP, Anyamba A, Bedno SA, Breiman RF, Sang R, Sergon K, Powers AM, Onyango CO, Small J, Tucker CJ, Linthicum KJ.** 2007. Drought-associated chikungunya emergence along coastal East Africa. *Am J Trop Med Hyg* **76:**405–407.

11. **Kariuki Njenga M, Nderitu L, Ledermann JP, Ndirangu A, Logue CH, Kelly CH, Sang R, Sergon K, Breiman R, Powers AM.** 2008. Tracking epidemic Chikungunya virus into the Indian Ocean from East Africa. *J Gen Virol* **89:**2754–2760.

12. **Paquet C, Quatresous I, Solet JL, Sissoko D, Renault P, Pierre V, Cordel H, Lassalle C, Thiria J, Zeller H, Schuffnecker I.** 2006. Chikungunya outbreak in Réunion: epidemiology and surveillance, 2005 to early January 2006. *Euro Surveill* **11:**E060202.3.

13. **Mavalankar D, Shastri P, Raman P.** 2007. Chikungunya epidemic in India: a major public-health disaster. *Lancet Infect Dis* **7:**306–307.

14. **Schuffenecker I, Iteman I, Michault A, Murri S, Frangeul L, Vaney MC, Lavenir R, Pardigon N, Reynes JM, Pettinelli F, Biscornet L, Diancourt L, Michel S, Duquerroy S, Guigon G, Frenkiel MP, Brehin AC, Cubito N, Despres P, Kunst F, Rey FA, Zeller H, Brisse S.** 2006. Genome microevolution of chikungunya viruses causing the Indian Ocean outbreak. *PLoS Med* **3:**e263.

15. **Tsetsarkin KA, Vanlandingham DL, McGee CE, Higgs S.** 2007. A single mutation in chikungunya virus affects vector specificity and epidemic potential. *PLoS Pathog* **3:**e201.

16. **Rezza G, Nicoletti L, Angelini R, Romi R, Finarelli AC, Panning M, Cordioli P, Fortuna C, Boros S, Magurano F, Silvi G, Angelini P, Dottori M, Ciufolini MG, Majori GC, Cassone A, CHIKV Study Group.** 2007. Infection with chikungunya virus in Italy: an outbreak in a temperate region. *Lancet* **370:**1840–1846.

17. **Grandadam M, Caro V, Plumet S, Thiberge JM, Souares Y, Failloux AB, Tolou HJ, Budelot M, Cosserat D, Leparc-Goffart I, Despres P.** 2011. Chikungunya virus, southeastern France. *Emerg Infect Dis* **17:**910–913.

18. **Gibney KB, Fischer M, Prince HE, Kramer LD, St George K, Kosoy OL, Laven JJ, Staples JE.** 2011. Chikungunya fever in the United States: a fifteen year review of cases. *Clin Infect Dis* **52:**e121–e126.

19. **Khan K, Bogoch I, Brownstein JS, Miniota J, Nicolucci A, Hu W, Nsoesie EO, Cetron M, Creatore MI, German M, Wilder-Smith A.** 2014. Assessing the origin of and potential for international spread of chikungunya virus from the Caribbean. *PLoS Curr* doi:10.1371/currents.outbreaks.2134a0a7bf37fd8d388181539fea2da5.

20. **Nhan TX, Claverie A, Roche C, Teissier A, Colleuil M, Baudet JM, Cao-Lormeau VM, Musso D.** 2014. Chikungunya virus imported into French Polynesia, 2014. *Emerg Infect Dis* **20:**1773–1774.

21. **Tan KK, Sy AK, Tandoc AO, Khoo JJ, Sulaiman S, Chang LY, AbuBakar S.** 2015.

Independent emergence of the cosmopolitan Asian Chikungunya virus, Philippines 2012. *Sci Rep* **5**:12279.

22. **Van Bortel W, Dorleans F, Rosine J, Blateau A, Rousset D, Matheus S, Leparc-Goffart I, Flusin O, Prat C, Cesaire R, Najioullah F, Ardillon V, Balleydier E, Carvalho L, Lemaitre A, Noel H, Servas V, Six C, Zurbaran M, Leon L, Guinard A, van den Kerkhof J, Henry M, Fanoy E, Braks M, Reimerink J, Swaan C, Georges R, Brooks L, Freedman J, Sudre B, Zeller H.** 2014. Chikungunya outbreak in the Caribbean region, December 2013 to March 2014, and the significance for Europe. *Euro Surveill* **19**(13):pii=20759.

23. **Kendrick K, Stanek D, Blackmore C, Centers for Disease Control and Prevention.** 2014. Notes from the field: transmission of chikungunya virus in the continental United States—Florida, 2014. *MMWR Morb Mortal Wkly Rep* **63**:1137.

24. **Vega-Rua A, Zouache K, Girod R, Failloux AB, Lourenco-de-Oliveira R.** 2014. High level of vector competence of *Aedes aegypti* and *Aedes albopictus* from ten American countries as a crucial factor in the spread of Chikungunya virus. *J Virol* **88**:6294–6306.

25. **Marcondes CB, Ximenes MF.** 2015. Zika virus in Brazil and the danger of infestation by Aedes (Stegomyia) mosquitoes. *Rev Soc Bras Med Trop* doi:10.1590/0037-8682-0220-2015.

26. **Vega-Rua A, Zouache K, Caro V, Diancourt L, Delaunay P, Grandadam M, Failloux AB.** 2013. High efficiency of temperate *Aedes albopictus* to transmit chikungunya and dengue viruses in the Southeast of France. *PLoS One* **8**:e59716.

27. **Tsetsarkin KA, Chen R, Leal G, Forrester N, Higgs S, Huang J, Weaver SC.** 2011. Chikungunya virus emergence is constrained in Asia by lineage-specific adaptive landscapes. *Proc Natl Acad Sci U S A* **108**:7872–7877.

28. **Teixeira MG, Andrade AM, Costa Mda C, Castro JN, Oliveira FL, Goes CS, Maia M, Santana EB, Nunes BT, Vasconcelos PF.** 2015. East/Central/South African genotype chikungunya virus, Brazil, 2014. *Emerg Infect Dis* **21**:906–907.

29. **Thiberville SD, Boisson V, Gaudart J, Simon F, Flahault A, de Lamballerie X.** 2013. Chikungunya fever: a clinical and virological investigation of outpatients on Reunion Island, South-West Indian Ocean. *PLoS Negl Trop Dis* **7**:e2004.

30. **Thiberville SD, Moyen N, Dupuis-Maguiraga L, Nougairede A, Gould EA, Roques P, de Lamballerie X.** 2013. Chikungunya fever: epidemiology, clinical syndrome, pathogenesis and therapy. *Antiviral Res* **99**:345–370.

31. **Sissoko D, Ezzedine K, Moendandze A, Giry C, Renault P, Malvy D.** 2010. Field evaluation of clinical features during chikungunya outbreak in Mayotte, 2005-2006. *Trop Med Int Health* **15**:600–607.

32. **Javelle E, Ribera A, Degasne I, Gauzere BA, Marimoutou C, Simon F.** 2015. Specific management of post-chikungunya rheumatic disorders: a retrospective study of 159 cases in Reunion Island from 2006–2012. *PLoS Negl Trop Dis* **9**:e0003603.

33. **Simon F, Parola P, Grandadam M, Fourcade S, Oliver M, Brouqui P, Hance P, Kraemer P, Ali Mohamed A, de Lamballerie X, Charrel R, Tolou H.** 2007. Chikungunya infection: an emerging rheumatism among travelers returned from Indian Ocean islands. Report of 47 cases. *Medicine* (Baltimore) **86**:123–137.

34. **Borgherini G, Poubeau P, Staikowsky F, Lory M, Le Moullec N, Becquart JP, Wengling C, Michault A, Paganin F.** 2007. Outbreak of chikungunya on Reunion Island: early clinical and laboratory features in 157 adult patients. *Clin Infect Dis* **44**:1401–1407.

35. **Borgherini G, Poubeau P, Jossaume A, Gouix A, Cotte L, Michault A, Arvin-Berod C, Paganin F.** 2008. Persistent arthralgia associated with chikungunya virus: a study of 88 adult patients on Reunion Island. *Clin Infect Dis* **47**:469–475.

36. **Brighton SW, Simson IW.** 1984. A destructive arthropathy following Chikungunya virus arthritis—a possible association. *Clin Rheumatol* **3**:253–258.

37. **Sissoko D, Malvy D, Ezzedine K, Renault P, Moscetti F, Ledrans M, Pierre V.** 2009. Post-epidemic Chikungunya disease on Reunion Island: course of rheumatic manifestations and associated factors over a 15-month period. *PLoS Negl Trop Dis* **3**:e389.

38. **Chaaithanya IK, Muruganandam N, Raghuraj U, Sugunan AP, Rajesh R, Anwesh M, Rai SK, Vijayachari P.** 2014. Chronic inflammatory arthritis with persisting bony erosions in patients following chikungunya infection. *Indian J Med Res* **140**:142–145.

39. **Manimunda SP, Vijayachari P, Uppoor R, Sugunan AP, Singh SS, Rai SK, Sudeep AB, Muruganandam N, Chaitanya IK, Guruprasad DR.** 2010. Clinical progression of chikungunya fever during acute and chronic arthritic stages and the changes in joint morphology as revealed by imaging. *Trans R Soc Trop Med Hyg* **104**:392–399.

40. **Ozden S, Huerre M, Riviere JP, Coffey LL, Afonso PV, Mouly V, de Monredon J, Roger**

JC, El Amrani M, Yvin JL, Jaffar MC, Frenkiel MP, Sourisseau M, Schwartz O, Butler-Browne G, Despres P, Gessain A, Ceccaldi PE. 2007. Human muscle satellite cells as targets of Chikungunya virus infection. *PLoS One* **2:**e527.

41. Phuklia W, Kasisith J, Modhiran N, Rodpai E, Thannagith M, Thongsakulprasert T, Smith DR, Ubol S. 2013. Osteoclastogenesis induced by CHIKV-infected fibroblast-like synoviocytes: a possible interplay between synoviocytes and monocytes/macrophages in CHIKV-induced arthralgia/arthritis. *Virus Res* **177:**179–188.

42. Morrison TE, Oko L, Montgomery SA, Whitmore AC, Lotstein AR, Gunn BM, Elmore SA, Heise MT. 2011. A mouse model of chikungunya virus-induced musculoskeletal inflammatory disease: evidence of arthritis, tenosynovitis, myositis, and persistence. *Am J Pathol* **178:**32–40.

43. Pal P, Dowd KA, Brien JD, Edeling MA, Gorlatov S, Johnson S, Lee I, Akahata W, Nabel GJ, Richter MK, Smit JM, Fremont DH, Pierson TC, Heise MT, Diamond MS. 2013. Development of a highly protective combination monoclonal antibody therapy against Chikungunya virus. *PLoS Pathog* **9:**e1003312.

44. Gardner J, Anraku I, Le TT, Larcher T, Major L, Roques P, Schroder WA, Higgs S, Suhrbier A. 2010. Chikungunya virus arthritis in adult wild-type mice. *J Virol* **84:**8021–8032.

45. Messaoudi I, Vomaske J, Totonchy T, Kreklywich CN, Haberthur K, Springgay L, Brien JD, Diamond MS, Defilippis VR, Streblow DN. 2013. Chikungunya virus infection results in higher and persistent viral replication in aged rhesus macaques due to defects in anti-viral immunity. *PLoS Negl Trop Dis* **7:**e2343.

46. Hoarau JJ, Jaffar Bandjee MC, Krejbich Trotot P, Das T, Li-Pat-Yuen G, Dassa B, Denizot M, Guichard E, Ribera A, Henni T, Tallet F, Moiton MP, Gauzere BA, Bruniquet S, Jaffar Bandjee Z, Morbidelli P, Martigny G, Jolivet M, Gay F, Grandadam M, Tolou H, Vieillard V, Debre P, Autran B, Gasque P. 2010. Persistent chronic inflammation and infection by Chikungunya arthritogenic alphavirus in spite of a robust host immune response. *J Immunol* **184:**5914–5927.

47. Labadie K, Larcher T, Joubert C, Mannioui A, Delache B, Brochard P, Guigand L, Dubreil L, Lebon P, Verrier B, de Lamballerie X, Suhrbier A, Cherel Y, Le Grand R, Roques P. 2010. Chikungunya disease in nonhuman primates involves long-term viral persistence in macrophages. *J Clin Invest* **120:**894–906.

48. Hawman DW, Stoermer KA, Montgomery SA, Pal P, Oko L, Diamond MS, Morrison TE. 2013. Chronic joint disease caused by persistent Chikungunya virus infection is controlled by the adaptive immune response. *J Virol* **87:**13878–13888.

49. Long KM, Heise MT. 2015. Protective and pathogenic responses to Chikungunya virus infection. *Curr Trop Med Rep* **2:**13–21.

50. Chow A, Her Z, Ong EK, Chen JM, Dimatatac F, Kwek DJ, Barkham T, Yang H, Renia L, Leo YS, Ng LF. 2011. Persistent arthralgia induced by Chikungunya virus infection is associated with interleukin-6 and granulocyte macrophage colony-stimulating factor. *J Infect Dis* **203:**149–157.

51. Ng LF, Chow A, Sun YJ, Kwek DJ, Lim PL, Dimatatac F, Ng LC, Ooi EE, Choo KH, Her Z, Kourilsky P, Leo YS. 2009. IL-1beta, IL-6, and RANTES as biomarkers of Chikungunya severity. *PLoS One* **4:**e4261.

52. Long KM, Ferris MT, Whitmore AC, Montgomery SA, Thurlow LR, McGee CE, Rodriguez CA, Lim JK, Heise MT. 2016. γδ T cells play a protective role in Chikungunya virus-induced disease. *J Virol* **90:**433–443.

53. Teo TH, Lum FM, Claser C, Lulla V, Lulla A, Merits A, Renia L, Ng LF. 2013. A pathogenic role for CD4+ T cells during Chikungunya virus infection in mice. *J Immunol* **190:**259–269.

54. Rampal, Sharda M, Meena H. 2007. Neurological complications in Chikungunya fever. *J Assoc Physicians India* **55:**765–769.

55. Wielanek AC, Monredon JD, Amrani ME, Roger JC, Serveaux JP. 2007. Guillain-Barre syndrome complicating a Chikungunya virus infection. *Neurology* **69:**2105–2107.

56. Singh SS, Manimunda SP, Sugunan AP, Sahina, Vijayachari P. 2008. Four cases of acute flaccid paralysis associated with chikungunya virus infection. *Epidemiol Infect* **136:**1277–1280.

57. Economopoulou A, Dominguez M, Helynck B, Sissoko D, Wichmann O, Quenel P, Germonneau P, Quatresous I. 2009. Atypical Chikungunya virus infections: clinical manifestations, mortality and risk factors for severe disease during the 2005-2006 outbreak on Reunion. *Epidemiol Infect* **137:**534–541.

58. Gerardin P, Couderc T, Bintner M, Tournebize P, Renouil M, Lemant J, Boisson V, Borgherini G, Staikowsky F, Schramm F, Lecuit M, Michault A, Encephalchik Study Group. 2016. Chikungunya virus-associated encephalitis: a cohort study on La Reunion Island, 2005–2009. *Neurology* **86:**94–102.

59. Fritel X, Rollot O, Gerardin P, Gauzere BA, Bideault J, Lagarde L, Dhuime B, Orvain E,

Cuillier F, Ramful D, Samperiz S, Jaffar-Bandjee MC, Michault A, Cotte L, Kaminski M, Fourmaintraux A, Chikungunya-Mere-Enfant T. 2010. Chikungunya virus infection during pregnancy, Reunion, France, 2006. *Emerg Infect Dis* **16**:418–425.

60. Gerardin P, Barau G, Michault A, Bintner M, Randrianaivo H, Choker G, Lenglet Y, Touret Y, Bouveret A, Grivard P, Le Roux K, Blanc S, Schuffenecker I, Couderc T, Arenzana-Seisdedos F, Lecuit M, Robillard PY. 2008. Multidisciplinary prospective study of mother-to-child chikungunya virus infections on the island of La Reunion. *PLoS Med* **5**:e60.

61. Mahendradas P, Ranganna SK, Shetty R, Balu R, Narayana KM, Babu RB, Shetty BK. 2008. Ocular manifestations associated with chikungunya. *Ophthalmology* **115**:287–291.

62. Soumahoro MK, Gerardin P, Boelle PY, Perrau J, Fianu A, Pouchot J, Malvy D, Flahault A, Favier F, Hanslik T. 2009. Impact of Chikungunya virus infection on health status and quality of life: a retrospective cohort study. *PLoS One* **4**:e7800.

63. Weaver SC, Osorio JE, Livengood JA, Chen R, Stinchcomb DT. 2012. Chikungunya virus and prospects for a vaccine. *Expert Rev Vaccines* **11**:1087–1101.

64. White A, Berman S, Lowenthal JP. 1972. Comparative immunogenicities of Chikungunya vaccines propagated in monkey kidney monolayers and chick embryo suspension cultures. *Appl Microbiol* **23**:951–952.

65. Harrison VR, Eckels KH, Bartelloni PJ, Hampton C. 1971. Production and evaluation of a formalin-killed Chikungunya vaccine. *J Immunol* **107**:643–647.

66. Levitt NH, Ramsburg HH, Hasty SE, Repik PM, Cole FE, Lupton HW. 1986. Development of an attenuated strain of chikungunya virus for use in vaccine production. *Vaccine* **4**:157–162.

67. McClain DJ, Pittman PR, Ramsburg HH, Nelson GO, Rossi CA, Mangiafico JA, Schmaljohn AL, Malinoski FJ. 1998. Immunologic interference from sequential administration of live attenuated alphavirus vaccines. *J Infect Dis* **177**:634–641.

68. Edelman R, Tacket CO, Wasserman SS, Bodison SA, Perry JG, Mangiafico JA. 2000. Phase II safety and immunogenicity study of live chikungunya virus vaccine TSI-GSD-218. *Am J Trop Med Hyg* **62**:681–685.

69. Enserink M. 2006. Infectious diseases. Massive outbreak draws fresh attention to little-known virus. *Science* **311**:1085.

70. Turell MJ, Malinoski FJ. 1992. Limited potential for mosquito transmission of a live, attenuated chikungunya virus vaccine. *Am J Trop Med Hyg* **47**:98–103.

71. Gorchakov R, Wang E, Leal G, Forrester NL, Plante K, Rossi SL, Partidos CD, Adams AP, Seymour RL, Weger J, Borland EM, Sherman MB, Powers AM, Osorio JE, Weaver SC. 2012. Attenuation of Chikungunya virus vaccine strain 181/clone 25 is determined by two amino acid substitutions in the E2 envelope glycoprotein. *J Virol* **86**:6084–6096.

72. Silva LA, Khomandiak S, Ashbrook AW, Weller R, Heise MT, Morrison TE, Dermody TS. 2014. A single-amino-acid polymorphism in Chikungunya virus E2 glycoprotein influences glycosaminoglycan utilization. *J Virol* **88**:2385–2397.

73. Ashbrook AW, Burrack KS, Silva LA, Montgomery SA, Heise MT, Morrison TE, Dermody TS. 2014. Residue 82 of the Chikungunya virus E2 attachment protein modulates viral dissemination and arthritis in mice. *J Virol* **88**:12180–12192.

74. Plante KS, Rossi SL, Bergren NA, Seymour RL, Weaver SC. 2015. Extended preclinical safety, efficacy and stability testing of a live-attenuated chikungunya vaccine candidate. *PLoS Negl Trop Dis* **9**:e0004007.

75. Plante K, Wang E, Partidos CD, Weger J, Gorchakov R, Tsetsarkin K, Borland EM, Powers AM, Seymour R, Stinchcomb DT, Osorio JE, Frolov I, Weaver SC. 2011. Novel chikungunya vaccine candidate with an IRES-based attenuation and host range alteration mechanism. *PLoS Pathog* **7**:e1002142.

76. Roy CJ, Adams AP, Wang E, Plante K, Gorchakov R, Seymour RL, Vinet-Oliphant H, Weaver SC. 2014. Chikungunya vaccine candidate is highly attenuated and protects nonhuman primates against telemetrically monitored disease following a single dose. *J Infect Dis* doi:10.1093/infdis/jiu014.

77. Partidos CD, Paykel J, Weger J, Borland EM, Powers AM, Seymour R, Weaver SC, Stinchcomb DT, Osorio JE. 2012. Cross-protective immunity against o'nyong-nyong virus afforded by a novel recombinant chikungunya vaccine. *Vaccine* **30**:4638–4643.

78. Partidos CD, Weger J, Brewoo J, Seymour R, Borland EM, Ledermann JP, Powers AM, Weaver SC, Stinchcomb DT, Osorio JE. 2011. Probing the attenuation and protective efficacy of a candidate chikungunya virus vaccine in mice with compromised interferon (IFN) signaling. *Vaccine* **29**:3067–3073.

79. Akahata W, Yang ZY, Andersen H, Sun S, Holdaway HA, Kong WP, Lewis MG, Higgs S, Rossmann MG, Rao S, Nabel GJ. 2010. A virus-

like particle vaccine for epidemic Chikungunya virus protects nonhuman primates against infection. *Nat Med* **16:**334–338.

80. Chang LJ, Dowd KA, Mendoza FH, Saunders JG, Sitar S, Plummer SH, Yamshchikov G, Sarwar UN, Hu Z, Enama ME, Bailer RT, Koup RA, Schwartz RM, Akahata W, Nabel GJ, Mascola JR, Pierson TC, Graham BS, Ledgerwood JE, Team VS. 2014. Safety and tolerability of chikungunya virus-like particle vaccine in healthy adults: a phase 1 dose-escalation trial. *Lancet* **384:**2046–2052.

81. Brandler S, Ruffie C, Combredet C, Brault JB, Najburg V, Prevost MC, Habel A, Tauber E, Despres P, Tangy F. 2013. A recombinant measles vaccine expressing chikungunya virus-like particles is strongly immunogenic and protects mice from lethal challenge with chikungunya virus. *Vaccine* **31:**3718–3725.

82. Ramsauer K, Schwameis M, Firbas C, Mullner M, Putnak RJ, Thomas SJ, Despres P, Tauber E, Jilma B, Tangy F. 2015. Immunogenicity, safety, and tolerability of a recombinant measles-virus-based chikungunya vaccine: a randomised, double-blind, placebo-controlled, active-comparator, first-in-man trial. *Lancet Infect Dis* **15:**519–527.

83. Tiwari M, Parida M, Santhosh SR, Khan M, Dash PK, Rao PV. 2009. Assessment of immunogenic potential of Vero adapted formalin inactivated vaccine derived from novel ECSA genotype of Chikungunya virus. *Vaccine* **27:**2513–2522.

84. Wang E, Kim DY, Weaver SC, Frolov I. 2011. Chimeric Chikungunya viruses are nonpathogenic in highly sensitive mouse models but efficiently induce a protective immune response. *J Virol* **85:**9249–9252.

85. Wang D, Suhrbier A, Penn-Nicholson A, Woraratanadharm J, Gardner J, Luo M, Le TT, Anraku I, Sakalian M, Einfeld D, Dong JY. 2011. A complex adenovirus vaccine against chikungunya virus provides complete protection against viraemia and arthritis. *Vaccine* **29:**2803–2809.

86. Muthumani K, Lankaraman KM, Laddy DJ, Sundaram SG, Chung CW, Sako E, Wu L, Khan A, Sardesai N, Kim JJ, Vijayachari P, Weiner DB. 2008. Immunogenicity of novel consensus-based DNA vaccines against Chikungunya virus. *Vaccine* **26:**5128.

87. Mallilankaraman K, Shedlock DJ, Bao H, Kawalekar OU, Fagone P, Ramanathan AA, Ferraro B, Stabenow J, Vijayachari P, Sundaram SG, Muruganandam N, Sarangan G, Srikanth P, Khan AS, Lewis MG, Kim JJ, Sardesai NY, Muthumani K, Weiner DB.

2011. A DNA vaccine against chikungunya virus is protective in mice and induces neutralizing antibodies in mice and nonhuman primates. *PLoS Negl Trop Dis* **5:**e928.

88. Kumar M, Sudeep AB, Arankalle VA. 2012. Evaluation of recombinant E2 protein-based and whole-virus inactivated candidate vaccines against chikungunya virus. *Vaccine* **30:**6142–6149.

89. Metz SW, Geertsema C, Martina BE, Andrade P, Heldens JG, van Oers MM, Goldbach RW, Vlak JM, Pijlman GP. 2011. Functional processing and secretion of Chikungunya virus E1 and E2 glycoproteins in insect cells. *Virol J* **8:**353.

90. Metz SW, Gardner J, Geertsema C, Le TT, Goh L, Vlak JM, Suhrbier A, Pijlman GP. 2013. Effective chikungunya virus-like particle vaccine produced in insect cells. *PLoS Negl Trop Dis* **7:**e2124.

91. Graci JD, Cameron CE. 2006. Mechanisms of action of ribavirin against distinct viruses. *Rev Med Virol* **16:**37–48.

92. Ravichandran R, Manian M. 2008. Ribavirin therapy for Chikungunya arthritis. *J Infect Dev Ctries* **2:**140–142.

93. Briolant S, Garin D, Scaramozzino N, Jouan A, Crance JM. 2004. In vitro inhibition of Chikungunya and Semliki Forest viruses replication by antiviral compounds: synergistic effect of interferon-alpha and ribavirin combination. *Antiviral Res* **61:**111–117.

94. Khan M, Dhanwani R, Patro IK, Rao PV, Parida MM. 2011. Cellular IMPDH enzyme activity is a potential target for the inhibition of Chikungunya virus replication and virus induced apoptosis in cultured mammalian cells. *Antiviral Res* **89:**1–8.

95. Fresno M, Jimenez A, Vazquez D. 1977. Inhibition of translation in eukaryotic systems by harringtonine. *Eur J Biochem* **72:**323–330.

96. Fan IJ, Han R. 1979. The effect of harringtonine on the cell cycle of L-1210 cells and the bone marrow stem cells in mice. *Yao Xue Xue Bao* **14:**467–473. (Author's translation).

97. Kaur P, Thiruchelvan M, Lee RC, Chen H, Chen KC, Ng ML, Chu JJ. 2013. Inhibition of chikungunya virus replication by harringtonine, a novel antiviral that suppresses viral protein expression. *Antimicrob Agents Chemother* **57:**155–167.

98. Couderc T, Khandoudi N, Grandadam M, Visse C, Gangneux N, Bagot S, Prost JF, Lecuit M. 2009. Prophylaxis and therapy for Chikungunya virus infection. *J Infect Dis* **200:**516–523.

99. Warter L, Lee CY, Thiagarajan R, Grandadam M, Lebecque S, Lin RT, Bertin-Maghit S, Ng LF, Abastado JP, Despres P, Wang CI, Nardin

A. 2011. Chikungunya virus envelope-specific human monoclonal antibodies with broad neutralization potency. *J Immunol* **186**:3258–3264.

100. Goh LY, Hobson-Peters J, Prow NA, Gardner J, Bielefeldt-Ohmann H, Pyke AT, Suhrbier A, Hall RA. 2013. Neutralizing monoclonal antibodies to the E2 protein of chikungunya virus protects against disease in a mouse model. *Clin Immunol* **149**:487–497.

101. Selvarajah S, Sexton NR, Kahle KM, Fong RH, Mattia KA, Gardner J, Lu K, Liss NM, Salvador B, Tucker DF, Barnes T, Mabila M, Zhou X, Rossini G, Rucker JB, Sanders DA, Suhrbier A, Sambri V, Michault A, Muench MO, Doranz BJ, Simmons G. 2013. A neutralizing monoclonal antibody targeting the acid-sensitive region in chikungunya virus E2 protects from disease. *PLoS Negl Trop Dis* **7**:e2423.

102. Jin J, Liss NM, Chen DH, Liao M, Fox JM, Shimak RM, Fong RH, Chafets D, Bakkour S, Keating S, Fomin ME, Muench MO, Sherman MB, Doranz BJ, Diamond MS, Simmons G. 2015. Neutralizing monoclonal antibodies block Chikungunya virus entry and release by targeting an epitope critical to viral pathogenesis. *Cell Rep* **13**:2553–2564.

103. Smith SA, Silva LA, Fox JM, Flyak AI, Kose N, Sapparapu G, Khomandiak S, Ashbrook AW, Kahle KM, Fong RH, Swayne S, Doranz BJ, McGee CE, Heise MT, Pal P, Brien JD, Austin SK, Diamond MS, Dermody TS, Crowe JE Jr. 2015. Isolation and characterization of broad and ultrapotent human monoclonal antibodies with therapeutic activity against Chikungunya virus. *Cell Host Microbe* **18**:86–95.

104. Pal P, Fox JM, Hawman DW, Huang YJ, Messaoudi I, Kreklywich C, Denton M, Legasse AW, Smith PP, Johnson S, Axthelm MK, Vanlandingham DL, Streblow DN, Higgs S, Morrison TE, Diamond MS. 2014. Chikungunya viruses that escape monoclonal antibody therapy are clinically attenuated, stable, and not purified in mosquitoes. *J Virol* **88**:8213–8226.

105. Ramful D, Carbonnier M, Pasquet M, Bouhmani B, Ghazouani J, Noormahomed T, Beullier G, Attali T, Samperiz S, Fourmaintraux A, Alessandri JL. 2007. Mother-to-child transmission of Chikungunya virus infection. *Pediatr Infect Dis J* **26**:811–815.

106. Khan M, Santhosh SR, Tiwari M, Lakshmana Rao PV, Parida M. 2010. Assessment of in vitro prophylactic and therapeutic efficacy of chloroquine against Chikungunya virus in Vero cells. *J Med Virol* **82**:817–824.

107. Brighton SW. 1984. Chloroquine phosphate treatment of chronic Chikungunya arthritis. An open pilot study. *S Afr Med J* **66**:217–218.

108. Chopra A, Saluja M, Venugopalan A. 2014. Effectiveness of chloroquine and inflammatory cytokine response in patients with early persistent musculoskeletal pain and arthritis following chikungunya virus infection. *Arthritis Rheumatol* **66**:319–326.

109. de Lamballerie X, Boisson V, Reynier J-C, Enault S, Charrel RN, Flahault A, Roques P, Le Grand R. 2008. Vector-borne and zoonotic diseases. *Infect Disord Drug Targets* **8**:837–840 doi:10.1089/vbz.2008.0049.

110. Mirolo M, Fabbri M, Sironi M, Vecchi A, Guglielmotti A, Mangano G, Biondi G, Locati M, Mantovani A. 2008. Impact of the anti-inflammatory agent bindarit on the chemokinome: selective inhibition of the monocyte chemotactic proteins. *Eur Cytokine Netw* **19**:119–122.

111. Zoja C, Corna D, Benedetti G, Morigi M, Donadelli R, Guglielmotti A, Pinza M, Bertani T, Remuzzi G. 1998. Bindarit retards renal disease and prolongs survival in murine lupus autoimmune disease. *Kidney Int* **53**:726–734.

112. Chen W, Foo SS, Taylor A, Lulla A, Merits A, Hueston L, Forwood MR, Walsh NC, Sims NA, Herrero LJ, Mahalingam S. 2015. Bindarit, an inhibitor of monocyte chemotactic protein synthesis, protects against bone loss induced by chikungunya virus infection. *J Virol* **89**:581–593.

113. Poo YS, Nakaya H, Gardner J, Larcher T, Schroder WA, Le TT, Major LD, Suhrbier A. 2014. CCR2 deficiency promotes exacerbated chronic erosive neutrophil-dominated chikungunya virus arthritis. *J Virol* **88**:6862–6872.

114. Ganu MA, Ganu AS. 2011. Post-chikungunya chronic arthritis—our experience with DMARDs over two year follow up. *J Assoc Physicians India* **59**:83–86.

115. Rulli NE, Rolph MS, Srikiatkhachorn A, Anantapreecha S, Guglielmotti A, Mahalingam S. 2011. Protection from arthritis and myositis in a mouse model of acute chikungunya virus disease by bindarit, an inhibitor of monocyte chemotactic protein-1 synthesis. *J Infect Dis* **204**:1026–1030 doi:10.1093/infdis/jir470.

Zika Virus Disease

9

WERNER SLENCZKA[1]

ZIKA VIRUS DISEASE

Zika virus, a flavivirus, is an example of an emerging virus infection (1–6). The virus was first isolated in the Zika Forest, Uganda, in 1947 during a program on yellow fever research. Rhesus monkeys were housed as sentinel animals in cages in the rain forest. When one of the animals developed fever, a filterable and mouse-pathogenic flavivirus, closely related to the yellow fever virus but not identical, was isolated from its blood. Mosquitoes (*Aedes* [*Stegomyia*] *africana*) trapped in the area were found to carry the virus. In tests with experimentally infected mosquitoes feeding on mice and on a monkey, Zika virus was successfully transmitted (2, 7, 8). Zika virus infection is endemic in many regions of sub-Saharan Africa and in South Asia (9–20). Jungle, or sylvatic, transmission cycles serve as the virus reservoir (12, 13, 17, 20). Infections with Zika virus are asymptomatic in approximately 80% of cases and cause only mild illness, if any, in endemic regions (10–12, 18, 20, 21). Upon importation to the Americas, where Zika virus had not been previously reported, the virus caused outbreaks of mostly asymptomatic mild illness, as in Africa and Asia (3, 4, 22). The difference between "endemic" transmission in the Old World and "epidemic" transmission in Brazil is the occurrence of

[1]Philipps-University Marburg, Institute of Virology, 35037 Marburg, Germany.
Emerging Infections 10
Edited by W. Michael Scheld, James M. Hughes and Richard J. Whitley
© 2016 American Society for Microbiology, Washington, DC
doi:10.1128/microbiolspec.EI10-0019-2016

prenatal infections with serious malformations in cases when the mother had Zika virus disease during the first trimester of gestation (3).

ETIOLOGY

Zika virus is a flavivirus, closely related to yellow fever virus and classified as a member of the Spondweni group (23). Flaviviruses are enveloped viruses of about 50 nm in diameter. They have single-stranded nonsegmented RNA genomes of positive polarity. In contrast to alphaviruses, translation of flavivirus RNA does not include formation of a subgenomic RNA; instead, a polycistronic polyprotein is made, which is cleaved by specific proteases to yield three structural and seven nonstructural polypeptides. The C-protein is the capsid protein. PrM (precursor of M) and E-proteins forming a heterodimer constitute the envelope of immature viruses, which are released by budding from endoplasmatic vesicles. During a "ripening" process prM is split by cellular proteases of the furin type into M-protein, and this process results in a smooth virus surface which is compared with a golf ball. E-protein is the receptor-binding protein, and in addition it functions as a fusion protein (type 2 of fusion proteins) (24). The E-protein contains a group-specific domain (A), a complex-specific domain (B), and a subtype-specific domain (C) (24, 25). These domains induce cross-reactive antibodies that are able to react with antigens from other flaviviruses. Therefore, serologic tests for antibody against any flavivirus may show broad reactivity against other flaviviruses, especially shortly after infection. Anamnestic responses from previous flavivirus infections can produce enhancing antibodies against consecutive flavivirus infections, ergo potentially enhance disease (25). The pathogenesis of any flavivirus disease is determined by these anamnestic responses resulting from previous infections or from vaccination.

OCCURRENCE OF ZIKA VIRUS INFECTION

There are only limited data on the seroprevalence of Zika virus in human populations (10–20). Zika virus has been endemic in Africa and probably in South Asia for a long time before it was introduced into the New World, and that endemicity is based on the existence of rural transmission cycles (9, 12). Prior to its emergence as a new pathogen in South America, Zika virus activity was detected in several African and South Asian countries by virus isolation and seroepidemiologic studies on volunteers using neutralization assays. Zika virus antibody was found in human sera from Uganda, Tanzania, Ethiopia, Central African Republic, Gabon, Sierra Leone, Republic of Nigeria, and in several Asian countries (10–16, 19). Seroepidemiologic studies were performed in Nigeria between 1964 and 1970 (12, 14). In one of these studies neutralizing antibody against Zika virus was found in 40% of the sera (14). In the course of these studies Zika virus was isolated from four febrile children aged 10 months to 3 years. Additional symptoms of Zika virus disease were not noted in these children. In another case the virus was isolated from a 10-year-old boy who had fever, headache, and generalized malaise (11, 14). This is probably the first case in which Zika virus was associated with specific symptoms. In addition, Zika virus was isolated from human serum in Senegal and from a mosquito in Côte d'Ivoire (18).

In South Asia Zika virus activity was established by seroepidemiologic studies in India, Indonesia, Malaysia, Thailand, Vietnam, and the Philippines (18, 19). Seven cases of clinically apparent Zika virus disease were diagnosed serologically, indicating recent infections (18). A subsequent seroepidemiologic study was performed on human volunteers in Lombok, Indonesia, and showed that 13% were positive (18). In 2007 an outbreak of Zika virus occurred in Micronesia. Yap Island has approximately 6,300 inhabitants distributed in 10 municipalities.

There were 49 confirmed and 59 probable cases of Zika virus fever in 9 out of 10 municipalities. It was estimated that 73% of the inhabitants had been recently infected with Zika virus (5, 6).

The first cases of locally transmitted Zika virus infections in Brazil were reported in 2015 (4). In December the Brazilian Ministry of Health estimated that 440,000 to 1,300,000 cases of Zika virus disease had occurred in Brazil by the end of 2015 (26). By 20 January 2016 locally transmitted Zika virus disease had been reported to the Pan American Health Organization from 20 countries or territories in the Americas (26). These included Barbados (3 cases), Bolivia (4 cases), Brazil (1.5 million cases) Columbia (20,000 cases), Ecuador (33 cases), El Salvador (2,500 cases), French Guyana (15 cases), Guadeloupe (1 case), Guatemala (68 cases), Guyana (1 case), Haiti (125 cases), Honduras (3,649 cases), Martinique (47 cases), Mexico (37 cases), Panama (50 cases), Puerto Rico (22 cases), Saint Martin (1 case), Suriname (6 cases), and Venezuela (4,700 cases). In the United States (80 confirmed cases) as well as in several other countries of the northern hemisphere importation of Zika virus infection in returning travelers has been reported (27–29).

TRANSMISSION

According to vector usage, flaviviruses are subdivided into three major groups: tick-borne viruses with more than 10 members, mosquito-borne viruses comprising about 130 members, and a third group of 20 viruses in which vectors were not identified. It is important to know that the host range of arthropod-borne viruses is determined not only by viral surface proteins but also by adaptation of the arthropods to their specific vertebrate hosts. Vector usage has a significant impact on arbovirus epidemiology. The difference between urban and rural infectious cycles is due to different species of vectors,

adapted either to urban or jungle habitats. Most flaviviruses, including yellow fever, Dengue, West Nile fever, and Zika virus, are transmitted by *Aedes* vectors; however, only a quarter of *Aedes* species bite humans. All RNA viruses have a high mutation rate since they lack proofreading mechanisms. New variants can therefore adapt not only to new hosts but also to new vectors. Changes in host or vector specificity can result in the emergence of "new" human pathogenic viruses.

A critical element in the epidemiology of arboviruses is the mechanism by which arthropods are infected. The female arthropod requires blood meals from vertebrates and if, by chance, the vertebrate is viremic the virus can infect the arthropod, which will transmit the infection to another vertebrate host. In rural transmission cycles, animals may be hosts, but in urban cycles humans are the hosts.

If vertical infection in the arthropod can be excluded, only blood meals on vertebrate hosts that have a high virus titer can infect the arthropod. When viremia is absent or exists only at a low titer, the infection chain is aborted. Another prerequisite is that the host animals should lack neutralizing antibodies. To replicate in different hosts, such as in vertebrates and in arthropods, the potential for adaptation to both different host cells and body temperatures is needed. Thus, only a few DNA viruses are among the arboviruses.

The details of the epidemiology of Zika virus remain to be elucidated. The virus may be transmitted by several species of mosquitoes, mainly *Aedes* spp. *Aedes aegypti* is the principal vector, at least in urban cycles. Zika virus has produced only sporadic cases during a period of 60 years. Perhaps the virus was mainly propagated in rural cycles between canopy-dwelling mosquitoes and wild-living vertebrates, and the sporadic occurrence of human cases resulted as an overspill from the jungle cycles. Additionally, asymptomatic infections of humans are frequent, and therefore a high proportion of the population may have acquired immunity.

Thus, in endemic regions Zika virus disease is more or less a childhood illness, being included in the differential diagnosis of several other exanthemas (measles, rubella, Chikungunya, or Dengue). In a mild course of a clinical disease no physician would have ordered virological diagnostic investigations. Notably, flaviviruses are less pathogenic for children than adults.

Zika virus is endemic in Africa and in South Asian countries such as India, Indonesia, Thailand, Vietnam, and Malaysia. Differences exist between African and Asian strains of Zika virus and can be detected by RNA sequencing. In respect to biological behavior and pathogenicity, there are no differences between African and Asian strains. Undeniably, in South America as well as some Pacific atolls, Zika virus has occurred in populations which had no previous exposure to this virus. Thus, presumably, rural infectious cycles have not pre-existed in South America. However, rural transmission cycles of Zika virus are established in tropical and subtropical zones of the Americas. The consequence is that Zika virus will be endemic in the New World in the same way as has happened before with other arboviruses, such as yellow fever, Dengue, and Chikungunya.

No data exist as to whether or not ornithophilic mosquitoes and birds might be involved in the spread of Zika virus. Considering that the virus took 60 years to travel to South America and travelled west and not north, it is unlikely that migrating birds have transported the virus. It is much more likely to assume that Zika virus traveled to South America in the body of an infected tourist or in a mosquito as a passenger in an airplane.

A new development in Zika virus epidemiology is the observation of vertical transmission and of transmission in semen results in human infections (30, 31). Prenatal infections are known to occur with several flavivirus infections such as Dengue, West Nile fever, and yellow fever, but systematic studies are lacking. Often the consequence is spontaneous abortion or preterm delivery. In the case of prenatal infections with yellow fever, mother and child have little chance of survival. With Dengue the mother and the newborn have severe hemorrhagic complications. Historically, serious malformations as in prenatal Zika virus infections have not been observed. Vertical transmission of Zika virus from mother to fetus has been proven in many cases. Sexual transmission (30, 31), intrauterine transmission resulting in congenital infection (32–36), intrapartum transmission from a viremic mother to her child, blood transfusion (37), and laboratory exposure (21, 34) are known routes of infection in addition to mosquito bites. Retrospectively, it will not be possible to confirm to what extent sexual transmission might have contributed to the spread of Zika virus in the Brazilian population.

Although Zika virus has been detected in breast milk, transmission by breast feeding has not yet been reported. There is concern about the possibility that transmission might occur through organ transplantation, since many cases are asymptomatic.

Intrauterine transmission of infection to the fetus is a new manifestation of Zika virus disease. Likely, it would have to be explained either by emergence of a new virus variant or by accepting that in Africa and in South Asia most women are immunized by asymptomatic infections during childhood. An additional possibility is that in many countries malformations are not registered and children with serious malformations would either be aborted or be killed after birth. Notably, enhancing antibodies resulting from previous exposure to flaviviruses increases pathogenicity. Since an individual's previous exposure to other flaviviruses is not known in Zika virus patients, it can only be speculated that differences in the gravity of symptoms might be influenced by enhancing antibodies. Coinfection with Dengue and Zika virus occurs and might also increase the pathogenicity of Zika virus infection (38). Coinfection is relevant not only in South America but also in Asia and in Africa.

Sexual transmission has only recently been identified. The first example of sexual transmission was with Marburg virus disease (39). During the acute phase of disease some male patients suffered from orchitis. One of these patients infected his wife 4 months after the acute phase of his disease. At this time he was no longer viremic, and in the absence of another possibility, intercourse had to be assumed as the route of infection of his wife, who fell ill with Marburg virus disease within 5 days after a single event of intercourse. Virus was detected by injecting undiluted seminal fluid into the peritoneal cavity of guinea pigs. One of the animals fell ill with fever, and Marburg virus was found in the liver and spleen; the other animal remained healthy and did not produce antibody. This means that the probe contained less than one infective dose. Seminal specimens taken from the other male convalescents were negative.

Three female convalescents became pregnant and gave birth to children between 1 and 2 years after their disease. The children had transplacental IgG antibodies at birth, which were catabolized in the course of several months.

With Ebola as in Marburg virus seminal virus excretion is not necessarily combined with viremia and is probably due to virus persisting in the testes. Sexual transmission of filoviruses from viremic people at the end of incubation and before onset of symptoms is possible.

As to the sexual transmission of Zika virus, some of the male partners have had only mild or asymptomatic infections. The possibility exists that clinical disease may be preceded by viremia and seminal shedding of virus. There is at present not enough information to determine if the donors were viremic at the time of the intercourse or had any symptoms of orchitis. It is not known whether Zika virus can be transmitted from the female partner to the male.

Since vertical virus transmission and sexual transmission of Zika virus can occur in people who are not aware of their infection even with clinical mild or asymptomatic illnesses, likely, viremic blood donors can transmit Zika virus by transfusion (40).

Up to this time viral isolates have been obtained from the following mosquitoes: *A. africanus*, *Aedes apicoargenteus*, *Aedes luteocephalus*, *A. aegypti*, *Aedes vittatus*, and *Aedes furcifer* (2, 12, 20).

CLINICAL MANIFESTATIONS

Zika virus disease is characterized as an influenza-like illness. The outbreak of Zika virus disease in Yap Island in 2007 was the first outbreak which had occurred at that time and was characterized by rash, fever, conjunctivitis, and arthralgia. In some patients myalgia, headache, retro-orbital pain, edema, and vomiting were noted. None of the patients required hospitalization, and no deaths resulted (1, 3, 5). Before this event only 14 cases of the disease had been confirmed by viral diagnostic techniques in Africa and in South Asia. The best-confirmed case was an occupationally acquired illness that was described by the patient himself (21). The disease began with mild headache followed the next day by a maculopapular rash covering the face, neck, trunk, and palms and soles. At the same time the patient had fever and suffered from malaise and back pain. The general symptoms lasted for only 2 days. By the 2nd day of disease the patient was afebrile. The rash disappeared 2 days later. Zika virus was isolated from his serum, which was obtained while febrile. Another case was a laboratory-acquired infection (37). This patient developed acute onset of fever, headache, and joint pain but did not develop a rash. Zika virus was isolated from his serum on the first day of his illness. About a week after onset of the symptoms the illness had resolved.

Seven patients were observed in Indonesia (18). All of them had fever, anorexia, diarrhea, constipation, abdominal pain, and dizziness. None of the patients had rash; conjunctivitis was found in one case only. As noted, most Zika virus infections remain clinically inapparent, and the majority of clinically apparent infections are characterized by a mild course and short duration. Zika virus disease in South America remains predominantly asymptomatic (80%) (3–5). Clinically apparent courses had only a mild form of disease. The malformations observed upon intrauterine Zika virus infection include microcephaly and severe ocular changes. Previously, intrauterine infections had not been noted in regions of Africa and South Asia or on Yap Island (6) in spite of sexual transmission (3, 30, 31).

The dramatic increase in pathogenicity, which is observed in Brazil, would have to be explained either by emergence of new virus variants or by special features of the epidemic situation, e.g., changes in vector usage or absence of previous immunologic experience with the new virus. Virus transmission via the sexual route shortly before, during, or after the time of conception might be a conditioning factor of fetal infection. Enhancing antibodies resulting from previous infections with flaviviruses or coinfection with either Dengue or Chikungunya might also play a role in the pathogenesis (38). These questions will have to be elucidated in the future.

COMPLICATIONS OF THE DISEASE

The most serious complications result from prenatal infection of the fetus during the first trimester of pregnancy. Microcephaly and eye defects are described and were confirmed by viral diagnostic tests in about 1% of suspected cases. In a well-documented case a European woman became pregnant during a stay in Natal, the capital of the Rio Grande del Norte state (32). In her 13th week of gestation she fell ill with high fever, musculoskeletal and retro-orbital pain, and a generalized maculopapular rash. Ultrasonography revealed a normal fetus at 14 and at 20 weeks. Ultrasonography performed at 32 weeks of gestation revealed a placenta with numerous calcifications and a fetus with microcephaly with numerous intracranial calcifications. The pregnancy was terminated at this time and the fetus was autopsied. Macroscopic inspection of the brain revealed microcephaly, widely open sylvan fissures, a small cerebellum and brain stem, and almost complete agyria.

Histopathological findings included multifocal collections of filamentous, granular, and neuron-shaped calcifications in the cortex, the subcortical nuclei, and the subcortical white matter with focal involvement of the cortical ribbon. Diffuse astrogliosis was present with focal astrocytic outburst into the subarachnoidal space. Activated microglia cells and macrophages were present throughout the gray and white matter. Scattered perivascular infiltrates of T-cells and some B-cells were present. The cerebellum, brain stem, and spinal cord revealed neither inflammation nor dystrophic calcifications. However, the brain stem and spinal cord showed Wallerian degeneration of the lateral corticospinal tract, whereas ascending dorsal cords were well preserved. Immunofluorescence revealed intracytoplasmic reaction in destroyed neuronal structures. By electron microscopic examination, clusters of dense virus-like particles of 50-nm size were found in damaged cytoplasmic vesicles. Positive results for Zika virus RNA were obtained only in the fetal brain, with 6.5×10^7 copies per milligram of brain tissue. PCR assays for other flaviviruses (Dengue, yellow fever, West Nile fever, and Central European encephalitis [CEE]) and other viruses (Chikungunya, lymphocytic choriomeningitis, cytomegalovirus, rubella, varicella zoster, herpes simplex, and parvovirus B19) and for *Toxoplasma gondii* were negative. A complete genome sequence was recovered from brain tissue and showed identity with a Zika virus strain isolated in Cambodia (98.3%) and with a strain from the outbreak in Micronesia (98.0%).

Ophthalmopathological defects are mostly associated with microcephaly in children with prenatal Zika virus infection (34–36). They include macular alterations (pigment mottling, and/or chorioretinal atrophy) and optic nerve abnormalities (hypoplasia with double-ring sign and/or increased cup-to-disk ratio).

In some cases Zika virus disease is followed immediately by Guillain-Barré syndrome. In a well-documented case a female patient, 40 years old with a history of rheumatoid arthritis, succumbed following an influenza-like illness with paresthesia and tetraplegia, diffuse myalgia, and peripheral facial palsy (41). Deep tendon reflexes were absent. The patient developed chest pain with sustained ventricular tachycardia and orthostatic hypotension. Electrocardiography did not reveal signs of myocarditis or pericarditis. Treatment with polyvalent immunoglobulin resulted in improvement. The patient survived and was discharged on day 13. Blood samples taken on day 8 after disease onset were negative in a Zika virus PCR test. Serological analysis revealed IgG antibodies against Dengue 1–4 antigens and IgM antibodies against Zika virus antigen.

PATHOGENESIS

It is thought that mosquito-borne flaviviruses replicate immediately after infection in dendritic cells near the site of inoculation and spread to the lymph nodes and the bloodstream, where they cause microangiopathy and rash (25). Invasion of the brain is believed to result from infection of microglial cells, which serve as a "Trojan horse" (42). The pathogenesis of developmental retardation and organ defects is not clear. Hypoxia due to microvasculitis and thrombosis may also be involved. With rubella embryopathy is a direct effect of virus replication, virus-induced apoptosis of noninfected cells, and inhibition of mitosis. Maternal antiviral immune reactions, specific and innate, may play a role. IFN-1, binding to cellular receptors, mediates downregulation of the enzyme superoxide dismutase, the most powerful intracellular antioxidant. With respect to flavivirus-caused embryopathy, there is a deficit in knowledge (43).

The dramatic change in the pathogenesis of Zika virus disease observed after its importation to Brazil remains an enigma (3, 32–36). While Zika virus infected an immunologically naïve population, fetal malformations were not noted in other previously uninfected populations (3, 5). Zika virus could have been spread both by mosquitoes and by sexual transmission, facilitating transmission to the fetus.

DIAGNOSIS

Flavivirus serology is complicated by group-specific, complex-specific, and subtype-specific cross-reactivities associated with domains A, B, and C of the viral E-protein. Neutralization tests are believed to be the most specific tests, but even in these tests, antigenically related viruses should be included as controls. All seroepidemiological results in which other flavivirus antigens are not included are at least subject to criticism.

Virus can be isolated in mosquito cells, but reverse transcription PCR (RT-PCR) is the technique of choice for detection of the virus (44, 45). A real-time RT-PCR for amplification of the NS5 coding regions is recommended (44). Primers are designed from conserved regions, and for identification the amplification product must be sequenced and compared with GenBank. Quantitative analysis allows determination of the titer of viremia. A problem is the cocirculation with other flaviviruses, which may result in coinfection with another virus (38).

DIFFERENTIAL DIAGNOSIS

Zika virus infection should be considered in cases with influenza-like disease with acute onset of fever, maculopapular rash, arthralgia, and/or conjunctivitis, especially when the patient has traveled to areas with ongoing Zika virus transmission in the 14 days preceding onset of the illness. Dengue and Chikungunya viruses share the same geographic prevalence with Zika virus, and they produce clinical pictures resembling Zika virus disease. Therefore, Dengue and Chikungunya are differential diagnostic considerations. Coinfection of Zika virus with Dengue or with Chikungunya may occur, confounding diagnosis (38). Other diseases to be considered are malaria, rubella, measles, parvovirus B19, adenovirus, enterovirus, leptospirosis, rickettsiae, and group A streptococcal infections.

THERAPY

Specific antiviral therapeutics are not yet available for flavivirus infections. Principally, there is no need for antiviral therapy, since most patients have mild courses of illness. Supportive treatment should include rest and fluids. Analgesics and antipyretics may be allowed, but aspirin or other nonsteroidal anti-inflammatory drugs (NSAIDs) should be avoided until Dengue can be ruled out to reduce the risk of hemorrhagic disease. For febrile pregnant women acetaminophen is recommended. Patients with Zika virus, Chikungunya, Dengue, or other arboviral disease must be protected from mosquitoes to avoid transmission to other people (3).

PROPHYLAXIS

A vaccine against Zika virus is not available. In flavivirus infections, the value of antiviral immunoglobulins for therapy or prophylaxis is controversial. In some reports it was judged to be helpful, while other reports suggest an unfavorable outcome. Specific experience with immunoglobulins in Zika virus disease does not exist. The best way to avoid Zika virus infection is to prevent mosquito bites by using air conditioning, closed windows, or window and door screens when indoors. For outdoor activities it is recommendable to wear long sleeves and pants and permethrin-treated clothing and to use insect repellents (3, 46, 47). Most repellents, including N,N-diethyl-m-toluamide (DEET), which is registered by the Environmental Protection Agency (EPA), are safe and can be used on children >2 months old. When used according to the product label, EPA-registered repellents are also safe for pregnant and lactating women. All travelers, and especially pregnant women, should take measures to avoid insect bites and arboviral infections (3, 47, 48). Zika virus–infected people may appear healthy and asymptomatic although they have viremia and may shed the virus (49). To avoid transmission of Zika virus via blood donations, blood banks will have to explore the travel anamnesis of their donors (49).

Assuming that sexual transmission might be relevant in the epidemiology and to prevent fetal infection, protection by using condoms is recommended. Application of vaginal rings shedding an antiviral substance such as Dapivirine could be useful but is not yet approved for this purpose (50).

In addition, public health measures should control the reservoirs of drinking water to destroy mosquitoes' breeding places (51).

CONCLUSIONS

Zika virus, a flavivirus of African origin was introduced to the Americas about 70 years after its discovery. Control of this new emerging pathogen will require new strategies to prevent sexual transmission, prenatal infections with serious malformations, and Guillain Barré syndrome in addition to measures against its arthropod vectors *Aedes aegypti* and *Aedes albopictus*. Since antiviral therapeutics and a vaccine are not yet available, the population can only be protected by individual prophylaxis and by elimination of the larvae in the breeding places.

CITATION

Slenczka W. 2016. Zika virus disease. Microbiol Spectrum 4(3):EI10-0019-2016.

REFERENCES

1. **Lanciotti RS, Kosoy OL, Laven JJ, Velez JO, Lambert AJ, Johnson AJ, Stanfield SM, Duffy MR.** 2008. Genetic and serologic properties of Zika virus associated with an epidemic, Yap State, Micronesia, 2007. *Emerg Infect Dis* **14:** 1232–1239.
2. **Hayes EB.** 2009. Zika virus outside Africa. *Emerg Infect Dis* **15:**1347–1350.
3. **Hennessey M, Fischer M, Staples JE.** 2016. Zika virus spreads to new areas: region of the Americas, May 2015–January 2016. *MMWR Morb Mortal Wkly Rep* **65:**55–58.
4. **Zanluca C, de Melo VC, Mosimann AL, Dos Santos GI, Dos Santos CN, Luz K.** 2015. First report of autochthonous transmission of Zika virus in Brazil. *Mem Inst Oswaldo Cruz* **110:**569–572.
5. **Musso D, Nilles EJ, Cao-Lormeau VM.** 2014. Rapid spread of emerging Zika virus in the Pacific area. *Clin Microbiol Infect* **20:**O595–O596.
6. **Duffy MR, Chen TH, Hancock WT, Powers AM, Kool JL, Lanciotti RS, Pretrick M, Marfel M, Holzbauer S, Dubray C, Guillaumot L, Griggs A, Bel M, Lambert AJ, Laven J, Kosoy O, Panella A, Biggerstaff BJ, Fischer M, Hayes EB.** 2009. Zika virus outbreak on Yap Island, Federated States of Micronesia. *N Engl J Med* **360:**2536–2543.
7. **Dick GW, Kitchen SF, Haddow AJ.** 1952. Zika virus. I. Isolations and serological specificity. *Trans R Soc Trop Med Hyg* **46:**509–520.
8. **Dick GW.** 1952. Zika virus. II. Pathogenicity and physical properties. *Trans R Soc Trop Med Hyg* **46:**521–534.
9. **MacNamara FN.** 1954. Zika virus: a report on three cases of human infection during an epidemic of jaundice in Nigeria. *Trans R Soc Trop Med Hyg* **48:**139–145.
10. **Fagbami A.** 1977. Epidemiological investigations on arbovirus infections at Igbo-Ora, Nigeria. *Trop Geogr Med* **29:**187–191.
11. **Fagbami AH.** 1979. Zika virus infections in Nigeria: virological and seroepidemiological investigations in Oyo State. *J Hyg (Lond)* **83:**213–219.
12. **McCrae AW, Kirya BG.** 1982. Yellow fever and Zika virus epizootics and enzootics in Uganda. *Trans R Soc Trop Med Hyg* **76:**552–562.
13. **Haddow AJ, Williams MC, Woodall JP, Simpson DI, Goma LK.** 1964. Twelve isolations of Zika virus from *Aedes* (*Stegomyia*) *africanus* (*theobald*) taken in and above a Ugandan forest. *Bull World Health Organ* **31:**57–69.
14. **Moore DL, Causey OR, Carey DE, Reddy S, Cooke AR, Akinkugbe FM, David-West TS, Kemp GE.** 1975. Arthropod-borne viral infections of man in Nigeria, 1964–1970. *Ann Trop Med Parasitol* **69:**49–64.
15. **Jan C, Languillat G, Renaudet J, Robin Y.** 1978. A serological survey of arboviruses in Gabon. *Bull Soc Pathol Exot* **71:**140–146. [In French.]
16. **Saluzzo JF, Gonzales JP, Hervé JP, Georges AJ.** 1981. Serological survey for the prevalence of arboviruses in the human population of the south-east area of Central African Republic. *Bull Soc Pathol Exot* **74:**490–499. [In French.]
17. **Monlun E, Zeller H, Le Guenno B, Traoré-Lamizana M, Hervy JP, Adam F, Ferrara L, Fontenille D, Sylla R, Mondo M.** 1993. Surveillance of the circulation of arbovirus of medical interest in the region of eastern Senegal. *Bull Soc Pathol Exot* **86:**21–28. [In French.]
18. **Olson JG, Ksiazek TG, Gubler DJ, Lubis SI, Simanjuntak G, Lee VH, Nalim S, Juslis K, See R.** 1983. A survey for arboviral antibodies in sera of humans and animals in Lombok, Republic of Indonesia. *Ann Trop Med Parasitol* **77:**131–137.
19. **Darwish MA, Hoogstraal H, Roberts TJ, Ahmed IP, Omar F.** 1983. A sero-epidemiological survey for certain arboviruses (*Togaviridae*) in Pakistan. *Trans R Soc Trop Med Hyg* **77:**442–445.
20. **Marchette NJ, Garcia R, Rudnick A.** 1969. Isolation of Zika virus from *Aedes aegypti* mosquitoes in Malaysia. *Am J Trop Med Hyg* **18:**411–415.
21. **Simpson DI.** 1964. Zika virus infection in man. *Trans R Soc Trop Med Hyg* **58:**335–338.
22. **Cardoso CW, Paploski IAD, Kikuti M, Rodrigues MS, Silva MM, Campos GS, Sardi SI, Kitron U, Reis MG, Ribeiro GS.** 2015. Outbreak of exanthematous illness associated with Zika, Chikungunya, and Dengue virus, Salvador, Brazil. *Emerg Infect Dis* **21:**2274–2276.
23. **Cook S, Holmes EC.** 2006. A multigene analysis of the phylogenetic relationships among the flaviviruses (family: *Flaviviridae*) and the evolution of vector transmission. *Arch Virol* **151:**309–325.
24. **Lindenbach BD, Thiel HJ.** 2007. *Flaviviridae*: the viruses and their replication, pp. 1101–1152.

In Knipe DM, Howley PM, Griffin DE (ed), *Fields Virology*, 5th ed. Lippincott, Williams, and Wilkins, Philadelphia, PA.

25. **Gubler D, Goro K, Markoff L.** 2007. Flaviviruses, pp. 1153–1252. *In* Knipe DM, Howley PM, Griffin DE (ed), *Fields Virology*, 5th ed. Lippincott, Williams, and Wilkins, Philadelphia, PA.

26. **World Health Organization/PAN American Health Organization.** 2016. Zika virus microcephaly and Guillain-Barré syndrome: situation report. http://who.int/emergencies/zika-virus/situation-report/26-february-2016/en/.

27. **Zammarchi L, Tappe D, Fortuna C, Remoli ME, Günther S, Venturi G, Bartoloni A, Schmidt-Chanasit J.** 2015. Zika virus infection in a traveller returning to Europe from Brazil, March 2015. *Euro Surveill* 20:21153. http://www.eurosurveillance.org/ViewArticle.aspx?ArticleId=21153.

28. **Fonseca K, Meatherall B, Zarra D, Drebot M, MacDonald J, Pabbaraju K, Wong S, Webster P, Lingsay R, Tellier R.** 2014. First case of Zika virus infection in a returning Canadian traveller. *Am J Trop Med Hyg* 91:1035–1038.

29. **Leung GH, Baird RW, Druce J, Anstey NM.** 2015. Zika virus infection in Australia following a monkey bite in Indonesia. *Southeast Asian J Trop Med Public Health* 46:460–464.

30. **Musso D, Roche C, Robin E, Nhan T, Teissier A, Cao-Lormeau VM, Cao-Lormeau VM.** 2015. Potential sexual transmission of Zika virus. *Emerg Infect Dis* 21:359–361.

31. **Centers for Disease Control and Prevention.** 2016. *Update: interim guidelines for prevention of sexual transmission of Zika virus – United States, 2016.* http://emergency.cdc.gov/han/han00388.asp.

32. **Mlakar J, Korva M, Tul N, Popović M, Poljšak-Prijatlj M, Mraz J, Kolenc M, Resman Rus K, Vesnaver Vipolnik T, Vodusek VF, Vizjak A, Pizem J, Petrovec M, Avsic Zupanc T.** 2016. Zika virus associated with microcephaly. *N Engl J Med* 374:951–958.

33. **Calvet G, Aguiar RS, Melo AS, Sampaio SA, de Filippis I, Fabri A, Araújo ES, de Sequeira PC, de Mendonca MC, de Oliveira L, Tschoeke DA, Schrago CG, Thompson FL, Brasil P, Dos Santos FB, Noqueira RM, Tanuri A, de Filippis AM.** 2016. Detection and sequencing of Zika virus from amniotic fluid of fetuses with microcephaly in Brazil: a case study. *Lancet Infect Dis.* [Epub ahead of print.] doi:10.1016/S1473-3099(16)00095-5.

34. **Martines RB, Bhatnagar J, Keating MK, Silva-Flannery L, Muehlenbachs A, Gary J, Goldsmith C, Hale G, Ritter J, Rollin D, Shieh WJ,** Luz KG, Ramos AM, Davi HP, Kleber de Oliveria W, Lanciotti R, Lambert A, Zaki S. 2016. Notes from the field: evidence of Zika virus infection in brain and placental tissues from two congenitally infected newborns and two fetal losses: Brazil 2015. *MMWR Morb Mortal Wkly Rep* 65:159–160.

35. **Ventura CV, Maia M, Ventura BV, Linden VV, Araújo EB, Ramos RC, Rocha MAW, Carvalho MD, Belfort R Jr, Ventura LO, Ventura LO.** 2016. Ophthalmological findings in infants with microcephaly and presumable intra-uterus Zika virus infection. *Arq Bras Oftalmol* 79:1–3.

36. **Da Paula Freitas B, de Oliveira Dias JR, Prazeres J, Sacramento GA, Ko AI, Maia M, Belfort R.** 2016. Ocular findings in infants with microcephaly associated with presumed Zika virus congential infection in Salvador Brazil. *JAMA Ophthalmol.* [Epub ahead of print.] doi:10.1001/jamaophthalmol.

37. **Filipe AR, Martins CM, Rocha H.** 1973. Laboratory infection with Zika virus after vaccination against yellow fever. *Arch Gesamte Virusforsch* 43:315–319.

38. **Dupont-Rouzeyrol M, O'Connor O, Calcez E, John M, Grangeon JP.** 2015. Co-infection with Zika and Dengue viruses in 2 patients, New Caledonia 2014. *Emerg Infect Dis* 21:381–382.

39. **Slenczka W, Piepenburg G, Siegert R.** 1968. "Marburg virus": antigen demonstration in the organs of infected guinea pigs. *Ger Med Mon* XIII:524–529.

40. **Musso D, Nhan T, Robin E, Roche C, Bierlaire D, Zisou K, Shan Yan A, Cao-Lormeau VM, Broult J.** 2014. Potential for Zika virus transmission through blood transfusion demonstrated during an outbreak in French Polynesia, November 2013 to February 2014. *Euro Surveill* 19:20761. http://www.eurosurveillance.org/ViewArticle.aspx?ArticleId=20761.

41. **Oehler E, Watrin L, Larre P, Lepanc-Goffart I, Lastère S, Baudouin L, Mallet HP, Musso D, Ghawche F.** 2014. Zika virus infection complicated by Guillain Barré syndrome: case report, French Polynesia, December 2013. *Euro Surveill* 19:pii:20720. http://www.eurosurveillance.org/ViewArticle.aspx?ArticleId=20720.

42. **Bielefeldt-Ohmann H, Smirnova NP, Tolnay AE, Webb BT, Antoniazzi AQ, van Campen H, Hansen TR.** 2012. Neuro-invasion by a 'Trojan Horse' strategy and vasculopathy during intra-uterine flavivirus infection. *Int J Exp Pathol* 93:24–33.

43. **Bhattacharya A, Hegazy AN, Deigendesch N, Kosack L, Cupovic J, Kandasamy RK, Hildebrandt A, Merkler D, Kühl AA, Vilagos**

B, Schliehe C, Panse I, Khamina K, Baazim H, Arnold I, Flatz L, Xu HC, Lang PA, Aderem A, Takaoka A, Superti-Furga G, Colinge J, Ludewig B, Löhning M, Bergthaler A. 2015. Superoxide dismutase 1 protects hepatocytes from type I interferon driven oxidative damage. *Immunity* **43:**974–986.

44. **Faye O, Faye O, Diallo D, Diallo M, Weidmann M, Sall AA.** 2013. Quantitative real-time PCR detection of Zika virus and evaluation with field-caught mosquitoes. *Virol J* **10:**311.

45. **Staples JE, Dziuban EJ, Fischer M, Cragan JD, Rasmussen SA, Cannon MJ, Frey MT, Renquist CM, Lanciotti RS, Muñoz JL, Powers AM, Honein MA, Moore CA.** 2016. Interim guidelines for the evaluation and testing of infants with possible congenital Zika virus infection: United States 2016. *MMWR Morb Mortal Wkly Rep* **65:**63–67.

46. **World Health Organization.** 2009. *Dengue: Guidelines for Diagnosis, Treatment, Prevention, and Control.* WHO, Geneva, Switzerland. http://www.who.int/csr/resources/publications/dengue_9789241547871/en/.

47. **Petersen EE, Staples JE, Meaney-Delman D, Fischer M, Ellington SR, Callaghan WM, Jamieson DJ.** 2016. Interim guidelines for pregnant women during a Zika virus outbreak: United States 2016. *MMWR Morb Mortal Wkly Rep* **65:**30–33.

48. **Nasci RS, Wirtz RA, Brogdon WG.** 2015. Protection against mosquitoes, ticks, and other arthropods, p 94. *In* Brunette GW (ed), *CDC Health Information for International Travel 2016.* Oxford University Press, New York NY. http://wwwnc.cdc.gov/travel/yellowbook/2016/the-pre-travel-consultation/protection-against-mosquitoes-ticks-other-arthropods.

49. **Ginier M, Neumayr A, Günther S, Schmidt-Chanasit J, Blum J.** 2016. Zika without symptoms in returning travellers: what are the implications? *Travel Med Infect Dis* **14:**16–20.

50. **Baeten JM, Palanee-Phillips T, Brown ER, Schwartz K, Soko-Torres LE, Govender V, Mgodi MM, Matovvu Kiweewa E, Nair G, Mhlanga E, Siva S, Bekker LG, Jeenarain N, Gaffour Z, Martinson F, Makanani B, Pather A, Naidoo L, Husnik M, Richardson BA, Parikh UM, Mellora JW, Marzinke MA, Hendrix CW, van der Straten A, Ramiee G, Chirenie ZM, Nakabiito C, Taha TE, Jones J, Mayo A, Scheckter R, Berthiaume J, Livant E, Jacobson C, Ndase P, White R, Patterson K, Germuga D, Galaska B, Bunge K, Singh D, Szydlo DVV, Montgomery ET, Mensch BS, Toriesen K, Grossman Cl, Chakhtoura N, Nel A, Rosenberg Z, McGowan I, Hiller S, MTN-020-ASPIRE Study Team.** 2016. Use of vaginal ring containing Dapivirine for HIV-1 prevention in women. *N Engl J Med.* [Epub ahead of print.] doi:10.1056/NEJMoa1506110.

51. **Pan American Health Organization.** 2015. Epidemiological alert: neurological syndrome, congenital malformations, and Zika virus infection. *Implications for public health in the Americas.* World Health Organization, Pan American Health Organization, Washington, DC. http://www.paho.org/hq/index.php?option=com_docman&task=doc_download&Itemid=270&gid=32405&lang=en.

West Nile Virus Infection

10

JAMES J. SEJVAR[1]

VIROLOGY

West Nile virus (WNV) (family *Flaviviridae*) is a member of the Japanese encephalitis serologic complex, which includes Japanese encephalitis, St. Louis encephalitis, Murray Valley encephalitis, and Kunjin viruses (1). The virus was first isolated in 1937 from a febrile patient in the West Nile district of Uganda, making it one of the first arthropod-borne viruses (arboviruses) to be identified. Structurally, it is an enveloped, spherical virus of approximately 40 to 50 nm in diameter with a lipid bilayer membrane surrounding a nucleocapsid core (2).

The WNV genome is single-stranded and positive-sense RNA in structure. The genome codes for seven nonstructural proteins and three structural proteins—the envelope, membrane, and capsid proteins (2–4). The envelope protein interacts with cellular receptors and is important in eliciting humoral immunity (3). The nonstructural proteins have varying functions in viral replication and immune response (5–7).

Serologic and molecular studies in the 1960s suggested strain variations among West Nile viruses from differing locations (8–10). More recent genomic sequencing of the envelope protein has demonstrated two main lineages of

[1]Division of High-Consequence Pathogens and Pathology, National Center for Emerging and Zoonotic Infectious Diseases (NCEZID), Centers for Disease Control and Prevention (CDC), Atlanta, GA 30333.
Emerging Infections 10
Edited by W. Michael Scheld, James M. Hughes and Richard J. Whitley
© 2016 American Society for Microbiology, Washington, DC
doi:10.1128/microbiolspec.EI10-0021-2016

WNV (lineage 1 and lineage 2 viruses) (11). Lineage 1 viruses are widespread and have caused recent large epizootics with high equine mortality in Europe (12, 13) and epidemics of human encephalitis in several African countries, the Middle East, eastern Europe, and North America (14–17). Lineage 2 viruses have been found primarily in southern and central Africa, where they are usually associated with systemic febrile illness without involvement of the central nervous system (CNS). Beginning in the 1990s, geographic spread of lineage 2 viruses was observed in the Mediterranean region and Europe, and a more recent outbreak due to a lineage 2 virus resulted in cases of severe human neurologic illness in Greece in 2010 (18–21).

The lineage 1 virus, which began circulating in the United States in 1999, has an over 99.8% nucleotide homology with viruses isolated in Israel in 1998 and 1999 (9, 11). In addition, this North American strain was closely related to WNV isolates from Romania, Italy, and Russia, which had also experienced outbreaks of WNV with substantial neurologic disease (9–11).

Analysis of WNV isolates in the United States has indicated a slowly evolving genetic divergence in different geographic areas; these variations usually represent less than 0.5% of the genomic sequence and result in only a few amino acid changes in any given isolate (22–27). In 2001, a distinct genetic variant emerged (WN02 strain), which displaced the original New York 1999 strain of the virus as the predominant circulating virus by 2004 (28, 29), and nearly all currently circulating viruses in North America are derived from the WN02 strain. The virus subsequently appears to have reached relative genetic stasis within North America (30).

ECOLOGY

WNV is an arthropod-borne virus (arbovirus) that is maintained in an enzootic cycle between mosquitoes and vertebrate hosts, primarily birds (31, 32). In North America, although the WNV genome has been found in more than 58 mosquito species, *Culex pipiens* (the northern house mosquito), *Culex quinquefasciatus* (the southern house mosquito), and *Culex tarsalis* are the most important vectors (33–35) WNV has also been isolated from ticks in the eastern hemisphere (36), but their role in the enzootic cycle is unclear (37).

In temperate regions, the virus is thought to over-winter in adult mosquitoes (36, 38). The enzootic cycle begins when infected mosquitoes feed on nonimmune birds. High-titer viremia develops in some birds, allowing for transmission of the virus to uninfected mosquitoes and continuation of the cycle. While WNV is able to infect over 100 North American bird species, not all develop high-titer viremia. Some avian species develop mild or no illness, but other species, particularly birds of the *Corvidae* family (crows) in North America, often succumb to infection, resulting in large epizootics with high mortality (39, 40). These bird die-offs have served as important sentinel surveillance indicators of subsequent human infections (40).

Once a sufficient proportion of mosquitoes and amplifying vertebrate hosts are infected, "bridging" mosquito species that feed more frequently on mammals and other nonavian vertebrates become infected. Naturally acquired WNV infection has been seen in numerous avian, reptile, and mammalian species (41–45). However, birds and horses are thought to be the only species substantially involved in the enzootic cycle. Humans and horses are most commonly recognized to develop symptomatic infections, but neither species is thought to significantly contribute to the viral amplification cycle because viremia is brief and of low titer (36).

Nonmosquito Transmission Routes

Nearly all human infections of WNV are due to bites from infected mosquitoes; however, other modes of transmission in humans have been noted. Transfusion-associated WNV transmission was first identified in 2002 when 23 people in the United States were infected after receiving platelets, red blood cells, or plasma from 16 viremic blood donors (46, 47). Routine screening of blood donations was initiated in the United States in 2003, and more than 3,000 infected blood products have been removed from the blood supply (48). However, rare cases of transfusion-associated transmission continue to occur due to blood donations that have virus levels below the limit of detection (49–51).

Also in 2002, transmission of WNV via donated organs was first documented when WNV infection was identified in four re-cipients of organs from a common donor (52). A second transmission occurred in 2005 in which WNV infection occurred in three of four organ recipients from a common WNV-infected donor. This donor was seropositive for WNV IgM antibodies but negative for WNV nucleic acid, suggesting that transmission may be possible in the absence of detectable serum viremia. Since that time, several other cases or clusters of WNV infection acquired through solid organ transplants have been reported in the United States and Europe (53–55).

Other rare transmission circumstances have been identified. Intrauterine transmis-sion has been documented in one case of a mother who was infected with WNV at approximately 27 weeks gestation and later delivered an infant with severe chorioretinitis and lissencephaly (56, 57). Umbilical cord and heel-stick blood from the infant was positive for WNV-specific IgM and neutral-izing antibodies. In 2002, possible transmis-sion via human breast milk was identified (58). Human laboratory-acquired WNV in-fections have been acquired by the percutaneous route (59), and transmission through conjunctival exposure in an occupational setting has been suspected (60).

Geographic Distribution

WNV is one of the most widely distributed of all arboviruses, with extensive distribution throughout Africa, the Middle East, parts of Europe and the former Soviet Union, South Asia, Australia (35, 61), and as of 1999, North, Central, and South America and the Caribbean (62–65).

The first recorded instance of severe neurological disease during a WNV outbreak occurred in Israeli nursing homes in 1957 (66). The virus was then isolated from the brains of three children who died of enceph-alitis in India in 1980 and 1981 (67). Never-theless, severe neurological disease during outbreaks remained relatively uncommon until recent outbreaks in Algeria, 1994 (68); Romania, 1996 (17); Tunisia, 1997 (69); Russia, 1999 (70); United States and Canada, 1999–2004 (71); Israel, 2000 (72); and Sudan, 2002 (73).

The most notable epidemiologic develop-ment associated with WNV infection was the unprecedented outbreak in North America. The virus was first identified in the western hemisphere following an outbreak in New York City in the summer of 1999. Subse-quently, the virus spread rapidly across the United States (71); the 2002 and 2003 seasons were the largest outbreaks of WNV neuro-logic illness recorded to date, with the 2003 season representing the largest outbreak of WNV to date. The incidence of reported WNV illnesses in the United States and Canada has subsequently relatively stabilized, and since approximately 2004, the number of reported cases in the United States has remained relatively stable or decreased, sug-gesting a more endemic pattern (Table 1), the exception being 2012, which witnessed the largest outbreak of WNV in the United States since 2003. As of 2014, nearly 50,000 human cases of WNV illness and 1,760 deaths had been reported in the United States (Fig. 1), with the highest incidence of disease in the Western and Mountain regions (Fig. 2) (48, 74, 75). In Canada, WNV was first detected in southern Ontario in 2001 and by 2002, had spread to Manitoba, Quebec, Nova Scotia, and Saskatchewan (76). By 2003, the virus' distribution extended into New Brunswick

TABLE 1 Reported West Nile virus disease cases in humans, United States, 1999–2014

Year	Number of cases				
	Total	WNND	WNF/Other	Deaths	No. of U.S. states
1999–2002	4,305	3,088	1,217	303	39[a]
2003	9,862	2,866	6,996	264	45[a]
2004	2,539	1,148	1,391	100	40[a]
2005	3,000	1,309	1,691	119	43[b]
2006	4,269	1,495	2,774	177	43[a]
2007	3,630	1,227	2,403	124	43
2008	1,356	689	667	44	45[a]
2009	720	386	334	32	37[a]
2010	1,021	629	392	57	40[b]
2011	712	486	226	43	43[a]
2012	5,674	2,873	2,801	286	48[a]
2013	2,469	1,276	1,202	119	47[a]
2014	2,205	1,347	858	97	42[a]

[a]Plus Washington, DC.

and Alberta. Since that time, cases of human illness have continued to be reported from British Columbia, Quebec, Alberta, Manitoba, Saskatchewan, and Ontario (77).

WNV activity in the remainder of the world has been less dramatic. WNV was first detected south of the U.S. border in 2001, when a resident of the Cayman Islands developed WNV encephalitis (78). In 2002, WNV was isolated from a dead common raven in Tabasco State, Mexico (63), and in 2003, WNV RNA was detected in brain tissue of a dead horse from Nuevo Leon State, Mexico (22). Since that time, serologic evidence in birds and horses suggests that WNV is present in multiple Caribbean and Central and South American countries, with evidence of infection as far south as Argentina (79–82). Despite the apparent widespread distribution of WNV in Latin America and the Caribbean,

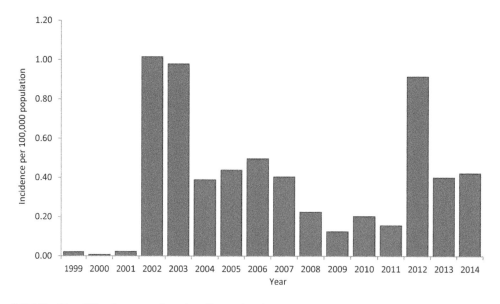

FIGURE 1 West Nile virus neuroinvasive disease incidence reported to the CDC by year, 1999–2014.

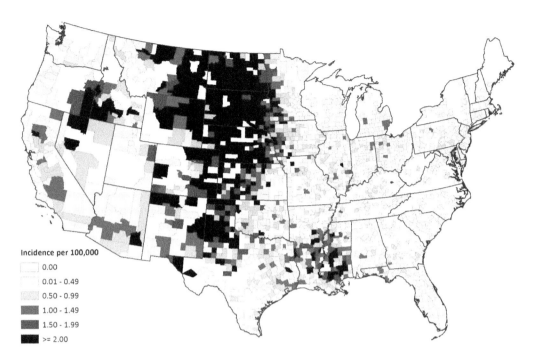

FIGURE 2 **Average annual incidence of West Nile virus neuroinvasive disease reported to the CDC by county, 1999–2014.**

as determined by serological studies of birds and horses, few cases of human illness have been reported. The reason for this is unclear but may be due to the presence of other endemic flaviviruses (such as dengue virus), which may provide some cross-protection against severe WNV disease, a decrease in virulence of the strains in Latin America due to selection of attenuated strains in migrating birds or ecological conditions, less robust surveillance, or other geographic or epidemiologic factors (81).

In the Mediterranean region and Europe, WNV circulation has been recognized since the 1960s. Large outbreaks of human illness occurred in Romania in 1996 and Russia in 1999 caused by a lineage 1 virus and resulting in large numbers of cases of encephalitis. Sporadic human and equine WNV outbreaks have been described in France, Spain, the Czech Republic, and Italy. In 2004, a lineage 2 virus of central African origin was detected in birds in Hungary, the first time a lineage 2

virus was identified in Europe (83); a lineage 2 virus was also responsible for recent outbreaks of human illness in Greece and Italy (18–21, 84).

Several large outbreaks of human encephalitic illness have occurred in Israel since the 1950s, and it is thought that the WNV strain that emerged in North America was derived from a virus causing epizootic illness among farmed geese in Israel in 1998. Serologic evidence of WNV infection in humans has also been identified in a number of other Middle Eastern and South Asian countries.

WNV in sub-Saharan Africa has predominantly been lineage 2 viruses, historically associated with sporadic cases of zoonotic and human illness. However, a large outbreak of human WNV illness was described in South Africa in 1974, with over 18,000 cases of febrile illness reported (85). Lineage 1 viruses have also been identified in several African countries (16). In Australia, Kunjin virus, a lineage 1 variant of WNV, is endemic and has been recognized to cause sporadic cases of human and equine illness. Human illness with Kunjin virus is generally mild and nonencephalitic (86, 87).

PATHOGENESIS OF HUMAN INFECTION

Following natural infection through a mosquito bite, WNV is thought to replicate in regional lymphoid tissue and the spleen, after which a viremia develops. In otherwise healthy people, viremia usually peaks between 2 and 4 days after infection and prior to illness onset (88–90); viremia begins to decline once clinical illness begins. In immunodeficient people, persistence of virus may be more prolonged (52, 89). In less than 1% of infected people, viremia results in dissemination to the CNS. The exact mechanism by which WNV is able to invade the CNS is unknown, but data from animal models suggest that peripheral production of tumor necrosis factor alpha leads to increased blood–brain barrier permeability, perhaps facilitating virus entry (91). Other hypothesized entry routes include infection of cerebral endothelial cells and migration across the cell to brain parenchyma, migration of WNV-infected leukocytes through tight junctions, and direct viral shedding through choroid plexus. Data also suggest that WNV may be transported through peripheral nerve axons in a retrograde fashion, leading to CNS invasion (92). Following neuroinvasion, the virus directly infects neurons, and less frequently, astrocytes, leading to neuronophagia and cell death. Histopathologic changes in human WNV infection are characterized by the presence of microglial nodules composed of lymphocytes and histiocytes; leptomeningeal mononuclear inflammatory infiltrates are present in cases of meningitis. CD8 T-lymphocytes represent the predominant inflammatory cell type in the nodules and infiltrates (93, 94).

While nearly all brain regions may be affected, WNV appears to have a specific neurotropism for neurons in the basal ganglia, thalamus, and brainstem (particularly the medulla and pons). This correlates well with the predominant clinical symptomatology demonstrated by people with WNV encephalitis. Spinal cord pathology is significant for involvement of ventral and dorsal gray and white matter and nerve roots, with a particular predilection for spinal cord anterior horn cells (94, 95). This results in multisegmental, patchy involvement similar to that seen with poliovirus infection (96). This involvement correlates clinically with the multifocal and often segmental distribution of weakness observed in cases of WNV anterior myelitis, or acute flaccid myelitis (AFM). Inflammation of spinal and cranial nerve roots, resulting in radiculitis, may also be seen (97).

EPIDEMIOLOGY OF HUMAN INFECTION AND ILLNESS

Epidemiologic studies of human WNV infection in the United States suggest that the majority of infections are clinically silent (17, 98). Following large epidemics in North America and Europe, an estimated 2 to 3% of the population were infected in a given year (17, 98–100). Serological surveys indicate that even in areas experiencing large outbreaks, less than 5% of the population may have been exposed to the virus (17, 71, 98, 99).

In temperate regions, human WNV infection incidence increases in early summer and peaks in August or early September. In milder climates, transmission may be seen year round. In the United States, within large regional WNV epidemics, the incidence of human disease varies markedly from county to county, suggesting the importance of local ecological conditions (Fig. 2) (74).

Risk Factors for Severe Disease and Death

Of all infected people, fewer than 1% develop West Nile virus neuroinvasive disease

(WNND), which is manifested as aseptic meningitis, encephalitis, or anterior (polio) myelitis (AFM). Although WNND has been reported among all ages, the proportion of those who progress to WNND is greater among older than younger people (101). Serologic surveys in Romania and New York City indicate that WNV infection incidence is relatively consistent across all age groups during outbreaks (17, 98). However, surveillance data from the United States indicate that age is the most important host risk factor for development of neuroinvasive disease after infection. The incidence of neuroinvasive disease increases approximately 1.5-fold for each decade of life, resulting in a risk approximately 30 times greater for people 80 to 90 years old compared to children younger than 10 years old (101). During outbreaks, hospitalized patients older than 70 years of age had case fatality rates of 15% in Romania (17) and 29% in Israel (72). Encephalitis with severe muscle weakness and change in the level of consciousness were also prominent clinical risk factors predicting fatal outcome (72, 102).

Based upon a limited number of cases, patients who acquire WNV from infected donor organs are likely at higher risk for severe neurologic disease and death compared with patients infected through mosquito bites (53, 103). The risk of severe neurologic disease among other organ transplant recipients is not well-defined and may be related to the interval between infection and transplantation or type of posttransplant immunosuppressive therapy. A seroprevalence study carried out in a Canadian outpatient transplant clinic following a WNV epidemic in 2002 indicated that the risk of neuroinvasive disease following infection was 40% (95% confidence interval 16 to 80%) (104). During that epidemic, transplant patients were approximately 40 times more likely than the population at large to develop WNND (105). However, another study assessed seropositivity and incidence of WNND among 194 solid organ transplant recipients and 195 controls, found no significant differ-

ence in seropositivity for WNV IgG between the groups, and determined that the incidence of WNND among the seropositive transplant recipients was relatively low (106).

Aside from age and organ transplantation, other independent risk factors for WNND have been challenging to identify. Hypertension, cerebrovascular disease, renal disease, and diabetes have variably been identified as possible risk factors for WNND in various risk factor studies, and prior immunosuppression has been associated with a fatal outcome (72, 102, 107–111). The incidence of neuroinvasive disease and the probability of death after acquiring neuroinvasive disease seem to be slightly higher in men than women (101).

CLINICAL MANIFESTATIONS OF HUMAN WNV INFECTION

The understanding of the spectrum of illness due to WNV infection in humans has expanded since the establishment of WNV in North America, and a number of previously underrecognized syndromes have been characterized (112–115). It is estimated that more than 80% of infected people remain asymptomatic. Of those who develop symptoms, the vast majority develop an acute, systemic febrile illness ("West Nile fever" [WNF]); less than 1% of infected people develop neuroinvasive disease including aseptic meningitis ("West Nile meningitis" [WNM]), encephalitis ("West Nile encephalitis" [WNE]), or an acute poliomyelitis-like syndrome ("West Nile virus–associated acute flaccid myelitis" [WNV-associated AFM]) (35, 116). WNM makes up the largest percentage of neuroinvasive disease cases in younger age groups, while the proportion of encephalitis increases in older age groups. The clinical picture among people with WNV infection may not always be clear-cut, and sometimes the clinical features of WNF, WNM, and WNE may overlap. For example, patients may develop altered mental status due to severe systemic illness, without true histo-pathologic or radiologic evidence of cerebral inflammation or "encephalitis" in the patho-physiologic sense. Similarly, patients presenting with fever, headache, and "neck stiffness" may not undergo lumbar puncture to demonstrate pleocytosis and, consequently, a diagnosis of West Nile "meningitis" may not be reported. Despite these limitations, the clinical syndrome in most people with WNV illness may generally be discerned on clinical grounds.

WNF

WNF is the predominant clinical syndrome seen in most infected people. All ages may be affected, but data suggest that the incidence of WNF may be higher among younger individuals (101, 114, 117, 118). Following an incubation period of approximately 2 to 14 days, infected people experience the abrupt onset of fever, headache, fatigue, and myalgias. Gastrointestinal complaints, including nausea and vomiting, may be predominant, leading to dehydration.

Occasionally a rash may be noted; this rash tends to be morbilliform, maculopapular, and nonpruritic, and it predominates over the torso and extremities, sparing the palms and soles (119–122). The rash may be transient, lasting less than 24 hours in some people. Rash appears to be more frequently seen in WNF than in more severe illness manifestations (WNM or WNE) (119). In addition, rash is more frequently observed among younger people than among older people (119). Whether the presence of a rash correlates with host immune or cytokine response to infection remains unknown.

Most patients experience complete recovery. Some otherwise healthy people, however, may continue to experience persistent fatigue, headaches, and difficulties concentrating for days or weeks following infection (123). In particular, profound fatigue, sometimes interfering with work or school activities, may last for months among people

recovering from WNF (124). Deaths among those with WNF occur primarily among older people and the immunocompromised population and are frequently attributable to cardiopulmonary complications (125).

Neuroinvasive Disease

WNM

WNM is clinically similar to other viral meningitides, with the abrupt onset of fever and headache, as well as meningeal signs, including nuchal rigidity, Kernig's and/or Brudzinski's signs, and photophobia or phonophobia. The associated headache may be severe, requiring hospitalization for pain control; associated gastrointestinal disturbance may result in dehydration, exacerbating head pain, and systemic symptoms (124). WNM is generally associated with a favorable outcome, though similar to WNF, some patients experience persistent headache, fatigue, and myalgias (112, 124).

Cerebrospinal fluid (CSF) examination is characterized by a modest pleocytosis, generally less than 500 cells/mm^3. While this pleocytosis is usually lymphocytic, CSF obtained soon after the onset of symptoms may show a neutrophilic predominance (126, 127).

WNE

WNE may range in severity from a mild, self-limited confusional state to severe encephalopathy, coma, and death. Several neurological syndromes, primarily extrapyramidal disorders, have been observed in patients with WNE (112, 114, 115, 128). Increased intracranial pressure and cerebral edema are infrequently associated with WNE.

Depending on the study, anywhere between 20 and 70% of patients with WNE have abnormal findings on brain magnetic resonance imaging (MRI). However, even in cases of severe WNE, the MRI may be normal, abnormal findings may not be apparent until several weeks after onset of illness, or such findings may be apparent only on diffusion-weighted imaging (129–131). The most characteristic MRI findings in patients with WNE are bilateral signal abnormalities in the basal ganglia and thalami on T2-, FLAIR, and diffusion-weighted image sequences, indicating the viral neurotropism for these deep gray structures (Fig. 3). These MRI findings, which may be seen in other flaviviral encephalitides, may be indicative but not diagnostic for WNE. Electroencephalographic abnormalities may be present in the form of generalized slowing, frequently anteriorly or temporally predominant, and triphasic sharp waves (132, 133). These electroencephalographic abnormalities, however, are also nonspecific. Overt seizures appear to be relatively uncommon with WNE and are estimated to occur in 3 to 6% of patients (94). CSF abnormalities in patients with WNE are the same as those seen in WNM, characterized by moderate lymphocytic pleocytosis, elevated protein, and normal glucose. One large study suggested that the mean CSF white blood cell count in patients with WNE was 227 cells/mm^3 (median, 90 cells/mm^3) (134).

Patients with WNE frequently develop a coarse tremor, particularly in the upper extremities. The tremor tends to be postural and may have a kinetic component (112, 113, 115, 128). Myoclonus, predominantly of the upper extremities and facial muscles, may occur and may be present during sleep. Features of parkinsonism, including hypomimia, bradykinesia, and postural instability, may be seen and can be associated with falls and functional difficulties (112, 135). Cerebellar ataxia, with associated truncal instability and gait disturbance leading to falls, has been described (115, 128, 136). These abnormal movements usually follow the onset of mental status changes and typically resolve over time; however, tremor and parkinsonism may persist in patients recovering from severe encephalitis (112, 114).

The development of these movement disorders in WNE is due to specific neurotropism of WNV for extrapyramidal structures; there is frequent involvement of the brainstem (particularly the medulla and pons), the deep gray matter nuclei,

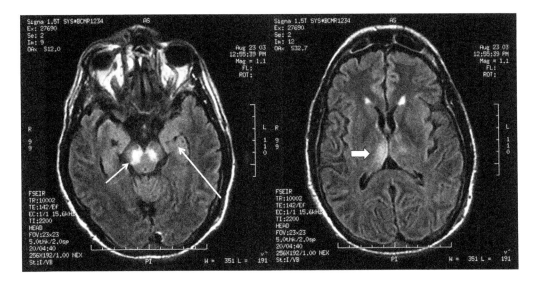

FIGURE 3 Fluid-attenuated inversion recovery magnetic resonance imaging sequence of the brain of a patient with West Nile virus encephalitis with associated parkinsonism and tremor, displaying signal abnormality in the substantia nigra (short arrow), the mesial temporal lobe (long arrow), and right posterior thalamus (thick arrow).

particularly the substantia nigra of the basal ganglia and the thalami, and the cerebellum (137–139). This clinico-pathologic correlation may be extended to the neuroimaging findings in WNE, as noted above.

Weakness and paralysis

Acute weakness is associated with WNV infection; most cases of paralysis are due to viral involvement of the lower motor neurons of the spinal cord (anterior horn cells), resulting in a condition identical to that caused by polio virus and referred to as acute flaccid myelitis (AFM) (127, 140–144). The clinical features of WNV-associated AFM are characteristic and dramatic and should be easily differentiated from the characteristic diffuse "muscle weakness" described by many people with severe fatigue associated with WNV infection (Table 2). WNV-associated AFM generally develops soon after illness onset, usually within the first 24 to 48 hours. Limb paralysis generally develops rapidly and may be abrupt, occasionally raising clinical concern about stroke (145, 146). The weakness is usually asymmetric and often results in monoplegia. Patients with severe and extensive spinal cord involvement develop a more symmetric dense quadriplegia. Central facial weakness, frequently bilateral, can also be seen (140). Sensory loss or numbness is generally absent, though some patients experience intense pain in the affected limbs just before or during the onset of weakness, and this limb pain may be persistent (127).

In some people, involvement of respiratory muscle innervation leading to diaphragmatic and intercostal muscle paralysis may result in respiratory failure requiring emergent endotracheal intubation (127, 147). Involvement of the lower brainstem, including the motor nuclei of the vagus and glossopharyngeal nerves, is similar to that seen in poliovirus infection and appears to be the genesis of this syndrome (94, 95). Respiratory involvement in WNV-associated AFM is associated with high morbidity and mortality, and among survivors, prolonged ventilatory support lasting months may be required (127). Patients who develop bulbar findings, such as dysarthria, dysphagia, or loss of gag reflex, are at greater risk for respiratory failure and should be monitored closely.

Electrodiagnostic studies (electromyography/nerve conduction studies) display findings consistent with a motor axonopathy with little or no demyelinating changes and preservation of sensory nerve potentials (148, 149). Spinal MRI may show signal

TABLE 2 Clinical and electrodiagnostic features of West Nile virus–associated acute flaccid paralysis

Characteristic	West Nile poliomyelitis	Guillain-Barré syndromes	Fatigue
Timing of onset	Acute phase of infection	1–8 weeks following acute infection	Acute infection
Fever and leukocytosis	Present	Absent	Present
Weakness distribution	Asymmetric; occasional monoplegia	Generally symmetric; proximal and distal muscles	Generalized, subjective, but neurologic examination normal
Sensory symptoms	Absence of numbness, paresthesias, or sensory loss; pain often present	Painful distal paresthesias and sensory loss	Generally absent
Bowel/bladder involvement	Often present	Rare	Not present
Concurrent encephalopathy	Often present	Generally absent	May be seen with fever, meningitis, or encephalitis
CSF profile	Pleocytosis and elevated protein	No pleocytosis; elevated protein (albuminocytologic dissociation)	Pleocytosis and elevated protein in the setting of meningitis/encephalitis

abnormalities in the anterior spinal cord, consistent with anterior horn cell damage; ventral nerve root enhancement may be seen as well (Fig. 4).

Other forms of acute flaccid paralysis, including radiculopathy and the acute demyelinating polyradiculoneuropathy form of Guillain-Barré syndrome, have also been associated with WNV infection (97, 150). However, these syndromes appear to be far less common than WNV-associated AFM and may be differentiated on the basis of clinical and electrophysiologic features (Table 2). The weakness associated with the Guillain-Barré syndrome is usually symmetric and ascending and is associated with sensory and autonomic dysfunction. Additionally, CSF examination generally shows elevated protein in the absence of pleocytosis ("cytoalbuminologic dissociation"), and electrodiagnostic studies are consistent with a predominantly demyelinating polyneuropathy.

Recovery of limb strength in people with WNV-associated AFM is variable (127, 151).

However, persistent weakness and associated functional disability appears to be the rule, at least in the short term, and prolonged physical and occupational therapy may be required. Most limb strength recovery occurs within the first 6 to 8 months after acute illness, following which improvement appears to plateau (151, 152). In particular, quadriplegia and respiratory failure are associated with high morbidity and mortality, and recovery is slow and incomplete (127). More than 50% of the mortality associated with WNV-associated AFM occurs in patients with acute neuromuscular respiratory failure; of patients who survive respiratory failure due to WNV-associated AFM, a substantial number require prolonged tracheostomy or long-term supplemental oxygen (127, 152). In general, less profound initial weakness may be associated with more rapid and more complete strength recovery (127). However, even patients with initially severe and profound paralysis may experience substantial recovery (127, 151); thus, the initial severity of

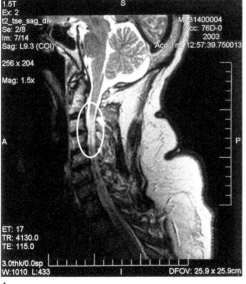
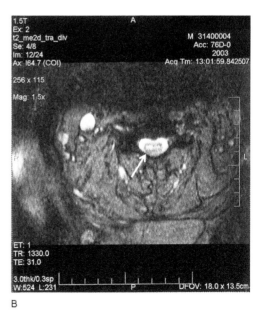

FIGURE 4 Sagittal (A) and axial (B) T2-weighted magnetic resonance imaging of the cervical spinal cord of a patient with bilateral upper extremity paralysis and respiratory failure from West Nile poliomyelitis, displaying increased signal in the anterior spinal cord (circle and arrow).

paralysis should not be used as a prognosticator of eventual outcome. This recovery phenomenon is thought to be due to the involvement of a large number of motor neurons which may initially be reversibly damaged but are able to recover (144). Electrodiagnostic studies may be useful in predicting recovery of muscle strength, with subsequent improvement correlating with motor unit number estimate values (97, 144). Although case reports have suggested the occurrence of relapsing or delayed-onset cases of WNV-associated AFM (153), the long-term clinical and functional outcomes in patients with WNV-associated AFM is still evolving, and whether there may be the subsequent development of a delayed, "postpolio"-like syndrome years after acute illness is unknown.

Other Clinical Manifestations

Ocular manifestations, including chorioretinitis and vitritis, are perhaps the most commonly reported sequelae of WNV infection following WNND (154–159). The chorioretinal lesions have been described as multifocal and with a "target-like" appearance (155); retinal hemorrhages have also been noted. Lesions tend to be clustered primarily in the temporal and nasal regions of the periphery of the fundus. The distribution and appearance of the chorioretinal lesions have been suggested to be distinctive for WNV infection (154). One study in Tunisia identified chorioretinitis in 20 (69%) of 29 patients with laboratory-confirmed, symptomatic WNV infection (160); the authors concluded that ophthalmoscopic examination should be performed on all patients with suspected WNV disease.

An inflammatory vitritis has occurred concomitantly with the chorioretinitis and may be significant enough to obscure the optic disc. Symptomatic people describe gradual visual blurring and loss of vision, floaters, and flashes. Although experience with management is limited, improvement both in symptoms and in underlying chorio-retinal lesions has been observed following treatment with intraocular corticosteroids (155). To date, WNV has not been isolated intraorbitally.

Several other clinical manifestations have been described in association with WNV infection but have been described mostly in case reports or small case series, and a definitive causal association with WNV infection is less substantiated. Rhabdomyolysis has been reported in the temporal setting of WNV infection (140, 145), suggesting a viral myositis, but the presence of virus in muscle tissue has not been observed. Hepatitis and pancreatitis have been reported in cases of severe WNV infection (93, 161), and WNV has been identified in hepatic and pancreatic specimens at autopsy, suggesting that viscerotropic WNV disease may be an infrequent manifestation of infection. Myocarditis has been seen pathologically in WNV infection, and cardiac arrhythmias have occurred in people with WNP, suspected to be due to autonomic dysfunction (96)

A study published in 2010 identified WNV RNA in the urine of 5 (20%) of 25 patients at up to 7 years following acute WNV illness (162). Four of the patients with WNV RNA in their urine reported persistent subjective symptoms, and one patient had developed renal failure after acute illness. However, one subsequent study found no WNV RNA in urine samples collected from 40 patients at 6.5 years after acute WNV disease, and another study detected WNV RNA in the urine of only 1 (1.6%) of 63 persons tested <5 months after initial acute WNV infection (163, 164). The frequency and clinical implications of persistent WNV RNA in urine are unknown, and additional data are needed.

PEDIATRIC WNV INFECTION

Most children with symptomatic WNV infection present with WNF; neuroinvasive disease, when it occurs, is frequently meningitis (88, 165, 166). However, poliomyelitis

(167, 168), fatal encephalitis (169), rhombo-encephalitis (170), and hepatitis (171) have been described in children with WNV infection. Similar to adults, immunocompromised children may be more susceptible to more severe illness (172).

WNV LONG-TERM OUTCOMES

There is a growing body of literature defining the long-term neurologic and functional outcomes of WNV encephalitis. As with many other viral encephalitides, initial severe neurologic illness does not necessarily correlate with eventual outcome, and some patients with initial severe encephalopathy with associated coma may experience dramatic recovery and minimal sequelae (112). However, others experience persistent neurologic dysfunction, including movement disorders, headaches, fatigue, and cognitive complaints. Large hospital-based series suggest that patients with severe WNV encephalitis frequently require assistance with daily activities following acute care discharge (113, 114). Patients often report substantial functional and cognitive difficulties for up to a year following acute infection, and only 37% of patients in the 1999 New York City outbreak achieved full recovery at 1 year (173). Of 265 people who developed symptomatic WNV infection in Idaho between 2006 and 2008, 53% reported one or more persistent symptoms 6 months or more following acute illness; the most frequent complaints were fatigue, muscle aches, and difficulties with memory and concentration (174). Cognitive complaints including difficulties with attention and concentration have been described among patients recovering from WNE and suggest a predominantly subcortical type of cognitive dysfunction based on prominent thalamic and basal ganglia involvement (112). However, limited formal neuropsychometric assessments have been performed. A few studies have shown that patients recovering from WNV illness demonstrate measurable neurocognitive deficits on standardized testing as long as 1 year after acute illness (175, 176). Other studies have shown that people recovering from WNV illness do not perform significantly differently on standardized neurocognitive assessments based upon nature of clinical illness compared to unaffected people (124). However, self-reported fatigue and somatic and cognitive complaints are common among people recovering from WNV illness, and subjective complaints and poorer performance on self-reported functionality indices as compared to normative data have been seen in patients months or years following acute illness (173, 177). One study has suggested normalization of self-reported symptoms within 1 year of acute illness (178). Neuropsychiatric symptoms, including depression, anxiety, and apathy, have been reported by patients recovering from WNE (112, 179, 180).

Fatality rates range from 10 to 20% among patients with severe neuroinvasive disease (101, 114).

DIAGNOSIS

The diagnosis of WNV infection may be suspected clinically by the onset of fever, aseptic meningitis, encephalitis, or paralysis in the setting of known WNV transmission or mosquito activity. The clinical features of tremor, myoclonus, and parkinsonism may be helpful in diagnosing WNE in the setting of a WNV epidemic. WNV-associated AFM often has a dramatic clinical presentation and should be suspected in any person who develops acute flaccid paralysis during periods of WNV transmission. Other etiologies of flaccid paralysis, most importantly Guillain-Barré syndrome, must also be considered, however, and can be distinguished from WNV-associated AFM on the basis of clinical and laboratory findings (Table 2). In general, routine laboratory, radiologic, and neuroimaging testing are unhelpful in the confirmation of WNV infection but are useful in excluding other etiologies of meningitis, encephalitis, and flaccid paralysis.

The diagnosis of WNV infection is typically made by demonstrating WNV-specific IgM antibodies in serum or CSF. The presence of WNV-specific IgM is usually good evidence of recent WNV infection but, due to serologic cross-reactivity among the flaviviruses, may indicate infection with another closely related flavivirus (e.g., St. Louis encephalitis or dengue virus) (181). Because WNV-specific IgM antibodies can persist in serum in some patients for over a year, with some data suggesting IgM persistence up to 3 years after acute infection (182), a positive test result occasionally may reflect past infection (183). The detection of WNV-specific IgM in the CSF of a patient with a clinically compatible illness is generally considered evidence of recent infection, although IgM antibodies have been found in three patients at 3 to 6 months after their acute illness (184). Serum collected within 8 days of illness onset may lack detectable IgM, and the test may need to be repeated on a convalescent-phase sample. IgG antibody generally is detectable shortly after IgM and persists for years. Plaque-reduction neutralization tests can be performed to measure virus-specific neutralizing antibodies (181, 185). A 4-fold or greater rise in virus-specific neutralizing antibodies between acute- and convalescent-phase serum specimens collected 2 to 3 weeks apart may be used to confirm recent WNV infection and to discriminate between cross-reacting antibodies from closely related flaviviruses. While commercial assays for detection of WNV-specific antibodies are widely available, their sensitivities and specificities may vary. In the United States, confirmatory testing is available at the Centers for Disease Control and Prevention Division of Vector-Borne Diseases and many local and state health department laboratories.

Although the "gold standard" for diagnosis of WNV infection is isolation of virus from biological specimens (e.g., blood, serum, CSF, or tissues, particularly CNS), this is infrequently achieved because the virus is often cleared from the blood by the time of illness onset. Virus isolation by culture is difficult to perform, is of low yield, and can be performed only in laboratories with proper biosafety containment facilities. Nucleic acid amplification tests (PCR techniques) are available for detection of WNV RNA in clinical samples but are of limited sensitivity for many of the same reasons that isolation is not ideal for diagnosis. Results of viral culture and nucleic acid amplification tests are more likely to be positive with samples from elderly or immunocompromised hosts (186, 187). Immunohistochemical staining can detect WNV antigen in formalin-fixed tissue (138). Negative results of these tests do not exclude WNV infection.

MANAGEMENT

There is currently no definitive treatment for WNV infection. Prevention of infection through protection from mosquito bites is therefore critical and is an important public health measure. In the absence of definitive antiviral treatment, management of illness due to WNV infection remains supportive. Patients with otherwise uncomplicated WNF generally do not require specific intervention, though control of headache and rehydration may sometimes be needed. However, people with documented WN viremia and patients with WNF in which other risk factors, including older age and underlying immunosuppression, are present should be observed for progression to more severe neuroinvasive disease. Patients with severe WNM may also require pain control for severe headache, and dehydration due to associated nausea and vomiting may require hospitalization for rehydration. In patients with WNE, attention to level of alertness and airway protection is important. While seizures and increased intracranial pressure have been infrequently reported with WNE, if present, they should be managed appropriately.

Patients with WNV-associated AFM may not have concurrent meningitis or encephalitis, and thus WNV infection may not initially be suspected. This may result in the implementation of inappropriate diagnostic procedures or treatment modalities, including anticoagulation for suspected acute stroke or muscle biopsy for suspected myopathy. WNV infection should be suspected in people developing acute asymmetric paralysis, particularly if accompanied by other signs of infection. Patients developing early dysarthria and dysphagia are at higher risk for subsequent acute respiratory failure (127); for this reason, hospitalization and observation of patients with AFM is advised, and the development of dysarthria and dysphagia should be viewed with concern. Management of poliomyelitis due to poliovirus suggests that initiation of aggressive physical activity during the acute febrile period of illness is associated with more profound and persistent weakness (188); in the absence of additional data, avoidance of aggressive physical activity during the acute febrile illness or during the initial 48 to 72 hours of weakness in WNV-associated AFM would be reasonable.

The fact that WN viremia in humans is short-lived and is usually cleared by the time of clinical presentation presents a substantial theoretical obstacle for specific antiviral therapies. Any therapeutic agent would have to reduce intracellular virus load and/or prevent viral spread in the CNS and possibly reduce the inflammatory response to infection to be effective. The recent use of several therapeutic modalities, including antiviral agents, nucleic acid analogues and missense sequences, immunomodulating agents, and angiotensin-receptor blockers, has been outside the setting of carefully controlled, randomized, blinded, placebo-controlled trials; thus, anecdotal reports of the effectiveness of these agents are unsubstantiated. However, such anecdotal reports of effectiveness and the clinical desire to provide an intervention have led to empiric use.

The antiviral agent ribavirin has demonstrated *in vitro* activity against WNV infection, but efficacy has not yet been demonstrated in animal models or humans (189, 190). The agent was used in an uncontrolled, nonblinded fashion in a group of patients with WNV neuroinvasive disease in Israel in 2000 and was found to be ineffective and potentially harmful (72). The immunomodulating agent interferon-α, while again showing *in vitro* inhibition of cytotoxicity due to WNV (191), has not been fully evaluated in animal models, and data from an open-label, nonblinded trial in the United States have not suggested clear benefit. The use of interferon-α in the treatment of the closely related Japanese encephalitis virus suggested no benefit (192).

Animal models and anecdotal reports have suggested the efficacy of high-titer WNV-specific intravenous immune globulin from pooled donors (Omr-IgG-am) (193–195) and humanized monoclonal WNV antibodies targeting the envelope protein of the virus (MGAWN1) (196–199). However, animal models suggest that efficacy is greatest if these therapeutics are given prior to or very shortly after onset of clinical illness, and attempts at human randomized clinical trials to assess the efficacy of these therapeutic agents have been unsuccessful, largely due to the challenge of enrolling a sufficient number of subjects within a likely therapeutic window. Neither of these products is licensed or available for use in the United States.

PREVENTION

Given the absence of definitive treatment for WNV infection, prevention remains the cornerstone of management of human WNV from a public health standpoint. Prevention may take the form of community-based programs and personal protection. Public mosquito control programs to reduce vector populations are employed to different degrees in various communities in North America and may involve removal of mosquito breeding sites, employing larvicide, and spraying for adult mosquitoes. Personal protective measures include limiting outdoor activities at dawn and dusk when mosquito activity is high, covering exposed skin with long sleeves and pants, and using insect repellent. The most effective repellents for use on skin are products that contain either diethyltoluamide (DEET), picaridin (KBR 3023), IR3535, or oil of lemon eucalyptus (200–204). In general, higher concentrations of active ingredient provide longer durations of protection, regardless of the active ingredient. Permethrin is an effective insecticide and repellent approved for use on clothing or fabrics but not on skin.

Although several candidate WNV vaccines are being evaluated, none are licensed or available for use in humans (205–208). Four WNV vaccines are licensed in the United States for use in horses (206, 209, 210). It is unclear if vaccination with related flavivirus vaccines (e.g., Japanese encephalitis or yellow fever) provides significant protection against WNV disease (211–217). Though it is likely that an effective WNV vaccine for humans can be developed, the cost-effectiveness and commercial viability of such a vaccine remains uncertain.

CONCLUSIONS

The arrival and subsequent spread of WNV infection throughout North America has served as a reminder of the capacity for emerging and re-emerging pathogens to move into and thrive in new settings. The future epidemiologic pattern of WNV infection in North America, and indeed worldwide, remains unclear. Whereas WNV infection in the United States appears to have reached an endemic pattern, the possibility of large future outbreaks remains, and re-emergence of WNV in European countries raises the possibility of significant WNV activity globally. The long-term functional and cognitive outcomes of people with WNV illness continue to be elucidated and will have significant implications on the assessment of overall disease burden. The challenges of definitive treatment and prevention of WNV infection will require further research.

ACKNOWLEDGMENTS

The author has no financial relationships relevant to this article to disclose. The findings and conclusions in this report are those of the author and do not necessarily represent the official position of the Centers for Disease Control and Prevention.

CITATION

Sejvar JJ. 2016. West Nile virus infection. Microbiol Spectrum 4(3):EI10-0021-2016.

REFERENCES

1. **Mackenzie JS, Barrett AD, Deubel V.** 2002. The Japanese encephalitis serological group of flaviviruses: a brief introduction to the group. *Curr Top Microbiol Immunol* **267:**1–10.
2. **Chambers TJ, Halevy M, Nestorowicz A, Rice CM, Lustig S.** 1998. West Nile virus envelope proteins: nucleotide sequence analysis of strains differing in mouse neuroinvasiveness. *J Gen Virol* **79:**2375–2380.
3. **Monath T, Heinz F.** 1996. Flaviviruses, p 961–1034. *In* Fields B, Knipe D, Howley P (ed), *Fields Virology*, 3rd ed, vol I. Lippincott-Raven, Philadelphia, PA.
4. **Lanciotti RS, Roehrig JT, Deubel V, Smith J, Parker M, Steele K, Crise B, Volpe KE, Crabtree MB, Scherret JH, Hall RA, MacKenzie JS, Cropp CB, Panigrahy B, Ostlund E, Schmitt B, Malkinson M, Banet C, Weissman J, Komar N, Savage HM, Stone W, McNamara T, Gubler DJ.** 1999. Origin of the West Nile virus responsible for an outbreak of encephalitis in the northeastern United States. *Science* **286:**2333–2337.
5. **Falkler WA, Jr, Diwan AR, Halstead SB.** 1973. Human antibody to dengue soluble complement-fixing (SCF) antigens. *J Immunol* **111:**1804–1809.
6. **Murthy HM, Clum S, Padmanabhan R.** 1999. Dengue virus NS3 serine protease. Crystal

structure and insights into interaction of the active site with substrates by molecular modeling and structural analysis of mutational effects. *J Biol Chem* **274**:5573–5580.

7. **Clum S, Ebner KE, Padmanabhan R.** 1997. Cotranslational membrane insertion of the serine proteinase precursor NS2B-NS3(Pro) of dengue virus type 2 is required for efficient *in vitro* processing and is mediated through the hydrophobic regions of NS2B. *J Biol Chem* **272**:30715–30723.

8. **Parks JJ, Ganaway JR, Price WH.** 1958. Studies on immunologic overlap among certain arthropod-borne viruses. III. A laboratory analysis of three strains of West Nile virus which have been studied in human cancer patients. *Am J Hyg* **68**:106–119.

9. **Nir Y, Goldwasser R, Lasowski Y, Margalit J.** 1968. Isolation of West Nile virus strains from mosquitoes in Israel. *Am J Epidemiol* **87**:496–501.

10. **Savage HM, Ceianu C, Nicolescu G, Karabatsos N, Lanciotti R, Vladimirescu A, Laiv L, Ungureanu A, Romanca C, Tsai TF.** 1999. Entomologic and avian investigations of an epidemic of West Nile fever in Romania in 1996, with serologic and molecular characterization of a virus isolate from mosquitoes. *Am J Trop Med Hyg* **61**:600–611.

11. **Lanciotti RS, Ebel GD, Deubel V, Kerst AJ, Murri S, Meyer R, Bowen M, McKinney N, Morrill WE, Crabtree MB, Kramer LD, Roehrig JT.** 2002. Complete genome sequences and phylogenetic analysis of West Nile virus strains isolated from the United States, Europe, and the Middle East. *Virology* **298**:96–105.

12. **Castillo-Olivares J, Wood J.** 2004. West Nile virus infection of horses. *Vet Res* **35**:467–483.

13. **Murgue B, Murri S, Zientara S, Durand B, Durand JP, Zeller H.** 2001. West Nile outbreak in horses in southern France, 2000: the return after 35 years. *Emerg Infect Dis* **7**:692–696.

14. **L'Vov DK, Kovtunov AI, Iashkulov KB, Gromashevskii VL, Dzharkenov AF, Shchelkanov M, Kulikova LN, Savage HM, Chimidova NM, Mikhaliaeva LB, Vasil'ev AV, Galkina IV, Prilipov AG, Kinney RM, Samokhvalov EI, Bushkieva B, Gubler DJ, Al'khovskii SK, Aristova VA, Deriabin PG, Butenko AM, Moskvina TM, L'Vov DN, Zlobina LV, Liapina OV, Sadykova GK, Shatalov AG, Usachev VE, Voronina AG, Luneva LI.** 2004. Circulation of West Nile virus (*Flaviviridae, Flavivirus*) and some other arboviruses in the ecosystems of Volga delta, Volga-Akhtuba floodlands and adjoining arid regions (2000-2002). *Vopr Virusol* **49**:45–51. (InRussian).

15. **Zeller HG, Schuffenecker I.** 2004. West Nile virus: an overview of its spread in Europe and the Mediterranean basin in contrast to its spread in the Americas. *Eur J Clin Microbiol Infect Dis* **23**:147–156.

16. **Weinberger M, Pitlik SD, Gandacu D, Lang R, Nassar F, Ben David D, Rubinstein E, Izthaki A, Mishal J, Kitzes R, Siegman-Igra Y, Giladi M, Pick N, Mendelson E, Bin H, Shohat T.** 2001. West Nile fever outbreak, Israel, 2000: epidemiologic aspects. *Emerg Infect Dis* **7**:686–691.

17. **Tsai TF, Popovici F, Cernescu C, Campbell GL, Nedelcu NI.** 1998. West Nile encephalitis epidemic in southeastern Romania. *Lancet* **352**:767–771.

18. **Anastasiadou A, Economopoulou A, Kakoulidis I, Zilidou R, Butel D, Zorpidou D, Ferentinos G, Markou P, Kougas E, Papa A.** 2011. Non-neuroinvasive West Nile virus infections during the outbreak in Greece. *Clin Microbiol Infect* **17**:1681–1683.

19. **Danis K, Papa A, Papanikolaou E, Dougas G, Terzaki I, Baka A, Vrioni G, Kapsimali V, Tsakris A, Kansouzidou A, Tsiodras S, Vakalis N, Bonovas S, Kremastinou J.** 2011. Ongoing outbreak of West Nile virus infection in humans, Greece, July to August 2011. *Euro Surveill* **16**:19951. http://www.eurosurveillance.org/ViewArticle.aspx?ArticleId=19951.

20. **Danis K, Papa A, Theocharopoulos G, Dougas G, Athanasiou M, Detsis M, Baka A, Lytras T, Mellou K, Bonovas S, Panagiotopoulos T.** 2011. Outbreak of West Nile virus infection in Greece, 2010. *Emerg Infect Dis* **17**:1868–1872.

21. **Papa A, Xanthopoulou K, Gewehr S, Mourelatos S.** 2011. Detection of West Nile virus lineage 2 in mosquitoes during a human outbreak in Greece. *Clin Microbiol Infect* **17**:1176–1180.

22. **Blitvich BJ, Fernandez-Salas I, Contreras-Cordero JF, Lorono-Pino MA, Marlenee NL, Diaz FJ, Gonzalez-Rojas JI, Obregon-Martinez N, Chiu-Garcia JA, Black WC, 4th, Beaty BJ.** 2004. Phylogenetic analysis of West Nile virus, Nuevo Leon State, Mexico. *Emerg Infect Dis* **10**:1314–1317.

23. **Beasley DW, Davis CT, Guzman H, Vanlandingham DL, Travassos da Rosa AP, Parsons RE, Higgs S, Tesh RB, Barrett AD.** 2003. Limited evolution of West Nile virus has occurred during its southwesterly spread in the United States. *Virology* **309**:190–195.

24. **Davis CT, Beasley DW, Guzman H, Raj R, D'Anton M, Novak RJ, Unnasch TR, Tesh RB, Barrett AD.** 2003. Genetic variation among temporally and geographically distinct West

Nile virus isolates, United States, 2001, 2002. *Emerg Infect Dis* **9:**1423–1429.

25. **Davis CT, Beasley DW, Guzman H, Siirin M, Parsons RE, Tesh RB, Barrett AD.** 2004. Emergence of attenuated West Nile virus variants in Texas, 2003. *Virology* **330:**342–350.

26. **Ebel GD, Carricaburu J, Young D, Bernard KA, Kramer LD.** 2004. Genetic and phenotypic variation of West Nile virus in New York, 2000-2003. *Am J Trop Med Hyg* **71:**493–500.

27. **Granwehr BP, Li L, Davis CT, Beasley DW, Barrett AD.** 2004. Characterization of a West Nile virus isolate from a human on the Gulf Coast of Texas. *J Clin Microbiol* **42:**5375–5377.

28. **Herring BL, Bernardin F, Caglioti S, Stramer S, Tobler L, Andrews W, Cheng L, Rampersad S, Cameron C, Saldanha J, Busch MP, Delwart E.** 2007. Phylogenetic analysis of WNV in North American blood donors during the 2003-2004 epidemic seasons. *Virology* **363:**220–228.

29. **Grinev A, Daniel S, Stramer S, Rossmann S, Caglioti S, Rios M.** 2008. Genetic variability of West Nile virus in US blood donors, 2002-2005. *Emerg Infect Dis* **14:**436–444.

30. **Davis CT, Li L, May FJ, Bueno R Jr, Dennett JA, Bala AA, Guzman H, Quiroga-Elizondo D, Tesh RB, Barrett AD.** 2007. Genetic stasis of dominant West Nile virus genotype, Houston, Texas. *Emerg Infect Dis* **13:**601–604.

31. **Hubalek Z, Halouzka J.** 1999. West Nile fever: a reemerging mosquito-borne viral disease in Europe. *Emerg Infect Dis* **5:**643–650.

32. **Hayes CG.** 2001. West Nile virus: Uganda, 1937, to New York City, 1999. *Ann N Y Acad Sci* **951:**25–37.

33. **Centers for Disease Control and Prevention.** 2002. Provisional surveillance summary of the West Nile virus epidemic: United States, January-November 2002. *MMWR Morb Mortal Wkly Rep* **51:**1129–1133.

34. **Brault AC.** 2009. Changing patterns of West Nile virus transmission: altered vector competence and host susceptibility. *Vet Res* **40:**43.

35. **Campbell GL, Marfin AA, Lanciotti RS, Gubler DJ.** 2002. West Nile virus. *Lancet Infect Dis* **2:**519–529.

36. **Hayes C.** 1989. West Nile fever, p 59–88. *In* Monath T (ed), *The Arboviruses: Epidemiology and Ecology*, vol V. CRC Press, Boca Raton, FL.

37. **Lawrie CH, Uzcategui NY, Gould EA, Nuttall PA.** 2004. Ixodid and argasid tick species and West Nile virus. *Emerg Infect Dis* **10:**653–657.

38. **Nasci RS, Savage HM, White DJ, Miller JR, Cropp BC, Godsey MS, Kerst AJ, Bennett P, Gottfried K, Lanciotti RS.** 2001. West Nile virus in overwintering *Culex* mosquitoes, New York City, 2000. *Emerg Infect Dis* **7:**742–744.

39. **Komar N, Panella NA, Burns JE, Dusza SW, Mascarenhas TM, Talbot TO.** 2001. Serologic evidence for West Nile virus infection in birds in the New York City vicinity during an outbreak in 1999. *Emerg Infect Dis* **7:**621–625.

40. **Eidson M, Komar N, Sorhage F, Nelson R, Talbot T, Mostashari F, McLean R.** 2001. Crow deaths as a sentinel surveillance system for West Nile virus in the northeastern United States, 1999. *Emerg Infect Dis* **7:**615–620.

41. **Marfin AA, Petersen LR, Eidson M, Miller J, Hadler J, Farello C, Werner B, Campbell GL, Layton M, Smith P, Bresnitz E, Cartter M, Scaletta J, Obiri G, Bunning M, Craven RC, Roehrig JT, Julian KG, Hinten SR, Gubler DJ.** 2001. Widespread West Nile virus activity, eastern United States, 2000. *Emerg Infect Dis* **7:**730–735.

42. **Komar N.** 2000. West Nile viral encephalitis. *Rev Sci Tech* **19:**166–176.

43. **Heinz-Taheny KM, Andrews JJ, Kinsel MJ, Pessier AP, Pinkerton ME, Lemberger KY, Novak RJ, Dizikes GJ, Edwards E, Komar N.** 2004. West Nile virus infection in free-ranging squirrels in Illinois. *J Vet Diagn Invest* **16:**186–190.

44. **Miller DL, Mauel MJ, Baldwin C, Burtle G, Ingram D, Hines ME 2nd, Frazier KS.** 2003. West Nile virus in farmed alligators. *Emerg Infect Dis* **9:**794–799.

45. **Bunning ML, Bowen RA, Cropp CB, Sullivan KG, Davis BS, Komar N, Godsey MS, Baker D, Hettler DL, Holmes DA, Biggerstaff BJ, Mitchell CJ.** 2002. Experimental infection of horses with West Nile virus. *Emerg Infect Dis* **8:**380–386.

46. **Pealer LN, Marfin AA, Petersen LR, Lanciotti RS, Page PL, Stramer SL, Stobierski MG, Signs K, Newman B, Kapoor H, Goodman JL, Chamberland ME.** 2003. Transmission of West Nile virus through blood transfusion in the United States in 2002. *N Engl J Med* **349:**1236–1245.

47. **Harrington T, Kuehnert MJ, Kamel H, Lanciotti RS, Hand S, Currier M, Chamberland ME, Petersen LR, Marfin AA.** 2003. West Nile virus infection transmitted by blood transfusion. *Transfusion* **43:**1018–1022.

48. **Centers for Disease Control and Prevention.** 2011. West Nile virus disease and other arboviral diseases: United States, 2010. *MMWR Morb Mortal Wkly Rep* **60:**1009–1013.

49. **Petersen LR, Epstein JS.** 2005. Problem solved? West Nile virus and transfusion safety. *N Engl J Med* **353:**516–517.

50. **Centers for Disease Control and Prevention.** 2009. West Nile virus transmission via organ

transplantation and blood transfusion: Louisiana, 2008. *MMWR Morb Mortal Wkly Rep* **58:**1263–1267.

51. **Centers for Disease Control and Prevention.** 2007. West Nile virus transmission through blood transfusion: South Dakota, 2006. *MMWR Morb Mortal Wkly Rep* **56:**76–79.

52. **Iwamoto M, Jernigan DB, Guasch A, Trepka MJ, Blackmore CG, Hellinger WC, Pham SM, Zaki S, Lanciotti RS, Lance-Parker SE, DiazGranados CA, Winquist AG, Perlino CA, Wiersma S, Hillyer KL, Goodman JL, Marfin AA, Chamberland ME, Petersen LR.** 2003. Transmission of West Nile virus from an organ donor to four transplant recipients. *N Engl J Med* **348:**2196–2203.

53. **Rhee C, Eaton EF, Concepcion W, Blackburn BG.** 2011. West Nile virus encephalitis acquired via liver transplantation and clinical response to intravenous immunoglobulin: case report and review of the literature. *Transpl Infect Dis* **13:**312–317.

54. **Nett RJ, Kuehnert MJ, Ison MG, Orlowski JP, Fischer M, Staples JE.** 2012. Current practices and evaluation of screening solid organ donors for West Nile virus. *Transpl Infect Dis* **14:**268–277.

55. **Costa AN, Capobianchi MR, Ippolito G, Palu G, Barzon L, Piccolo G, Andreetta B, Filippetti M, Fehily D, Lombardini L, Grossi P.** 2011. West Nile virus: the Italian national transplant network reaction to an alert in the north-eastern region, Italy 2011. *Euro Surveill* **16:**19991. http://www.eurosurveillance.org/ViewArticle.aspx?ArticleId=19991.

56. **Alpert SG, Fergerson J, Noel LP.** 2003. Intrauterine West Nile virus: ocular and systemic findings. *Am J Ophthalmol* **136:**733–735.

57. **Centers for Disease Control and Prevention.** 2002. Intrauterine West Nile virus infection: New York, 2002. *MMWR Morb Mortal Wkly Rep* **51:**1135–1136.

58. **Centers for Disease Control and Prevention.** 2002. Possible West Nile virus transmission to an infant through breast-feeding: Michigan, 2002. *MMWR Morb Mortal Wkly Rep* **51:**877–878.

59. **Centers for Disease Control and Prevention.** 2002. Laboratory-acquired West Nile virus infections: United States, 2002. *MMWR Morb Mortal Wkly Rep* **51:**1133–1135.

60. **Fonseca K, Prince GD, Bratvold J, Fox JD, Pybus M, Preksaitis JK, Tilley P.** 2005. West Nile virus infection and conjunctival exposure. *Emerg Infect Dis* **11:**1648–1649.

61. **Petersen LR, Roehrig JT.** 2001. West Nile virus: a reemerging global pathogen. *Emerg Infect Dis* **7:**611–614.

62. **Gubler DJ.** 2001. Human arbovirus infections worldwide. *Ann N Y Acad Sci* **951:**13–24.

63. **Estrada-Franco JG, Navarro-Lopez R, Beasley DW, Coffey L, Carrara AS, Travassos da Rosa A, Clements T, Wang E, Ludwig GV, Cortes AC, Ramirez PP, Tesh RB, Barrett AD, Weaver SC.** 2003. West Nile virus in Mexico: evidence of widespread circulation since July 2002. *Emerg Infect Dis* **9:**1604–1607.

64. **Cruz L, Cardenas VM, Abarca M, Rodriguez T, Reyna RF, Serpas MV, Fontaine RE, Beasley DW, Da Rosa AP, Weaver SC, Tesh RB, Powers AM, Suarez-Rangel G.** 2005. Short report: serological evidence of West Nile virus activity in El Salvador. *Am J Trop Med Hyg* **72:**612–615.

65. **Health Canada.** 2005. West Nile virus weekly surveillance report, on Centre for Infectious Disease Prevention & Control, and the National Microbiology Laboratory of the Public Health Agency of Canada. http://www.phac-aspc.gc.ca/wnv-vwn/mon-hmnsurv-2005-eng.php.

66. **Spigland I, Jasinska-Klingberg W, Hofshi E, Goldblum N.** 1958. Clinical and laboratory observations in an outbreak of West Nile fever in Israel in 1957. *Harefuah* **54:**275–280. (English and French abstracts 280–281) (In French).

67. **George S, Gourie-Devi M, Rao JA, Prasad SR, Pavri KM.** 1984. Isolation of West Nile virus from the brains of children who had died of encephalitis. *Bull World Health Organ* **62:**879–882.

68. **Le Guenno B, Bougermouh A, Azzam T, Bouakaz R.** 1996. West Nile: a deadly virus? *Lancet* **348:**1315.

69. **Murgue B, Murri S, Triki H, Deubel V, Zeller HG.** 2001. West Nile in the Mediterranean basin: 1950-2000. *Ann N Y Acad Sci* **951:**117–126.

70. **Platonov AE.** 2001. West Nile encephalitis in Russia 1999-2001: were we ready? Are we ready? *Ann N Y Acad Sci* **951:**102–116.

71. **Petersen LR, Hayes EB.** 2004. Westward ho? The spread of West Nile virus. *N Engl J Med* **351:**2257–2259.

72. **Chowers MY, Lang R, Nassar F, Ben-David D, Giladi M, Rubinshtein E, Itzhaki A, Mishal J, Siegman-Igra Y, Kitzes R, Pick N, Landau Z, Wolf D, Bin H, Mendelson E, Pitlik SD, Weinberger M.** 2001. Clinical characteristics of the West Nile fever outbreak, Israel, 2000. *Emerg Infect Dis* **7:**675–678.

73. **Depoortere E, Kavle J, Keus K, Zeller H, Murri S, Legros D.** 2004. Outbreak of West Nile virus causing severe neurological involvement in children, Nuba Mountains, Sudan, 2002. *Trop Med Int Health* **9:**730–736.

74. **Lindsey NP, Staples JE, Lehman JA, Fischer M, Centers for Disease Control and Prevention.**

2010. Surveillance for human West Nile virus disease: United States, 1999-2008. *MMWR Surveill Summ* **59:**1–17.

75. **Lindsey NP, Lehman JA, Staples JE, Fischer M.** 2015. West Nile virus and other nationally notifiable arboviral diseases: United States, 2014. *MMWR Morb Mortal Wkly Rep* **64:** 929–934.

76. **Drebot MA, Lindsay R, Barker IK, Buck PA, Fearon M, Hunter F, Sockett P, Artsob H.** 2003. West Nile virus surveillance and diagnostics: a Canadian perspective. *Can J Infect Dis* **14:**105–114.

77. **Public Health Agency of Canada.** 2011. Surveillance of West Nile virus. http://www.phac-aspc.gc.ca/wnv-vwn/index-eng.php.

78. **Centers for Disease Control and Prevention.** 2002. West Nile Virus activity: United States, 2001. *MMWR Morb Mortal Wkly Rep* **51:**497–501.

79. **Adrian Diaz L, Komar N, Visintin A, Dantur Juri MJ, Stein M, Lobo Allende R, Spinsanti L, Konigheim B, Aguilar J, Laurito M, Almiron W, Contigiani M.** 2008. West Nile virus in birds, Argentina. *Emerg Infect Dis* **14:**689–691.

80. **Morales MA, Barrandeguy M, Fabbri C, Garcia JB, Vissani A, Trono K, Gutierrez G, Pigretti S, Menchaca H, Garrido N, Taylor N, Fernandez F, Levis S, Enria D.** 2006. West Nile virus isolation from equines in Argentina, 2006. *Emerg Infect Dis* **12:**1559–1561.

81. **Petersen LR, Hayes EB.** 2008. West Nile virus in the Americas. *Med Clin North Am* **92:**1307–1322,ix.

82. **Pauvolid-Correa A, Morales MA, Levis S, Figueiredo LT, Couto-Lima D, Campos Z, Nogueira MF, da Silva EE, Nogueira RM, Schatzmayr HG.** 2011. Neutralising antibodies for West Nile virus in horses from Brazilian Pantanal. *Mem Inst Oswaldo Cruz* **106:**467–474.

83. **Calistri P, Giovannini A, Hubalek Z, Ionescu A, Monaco F, Savini G, Lelli R.** 2010. Epidemiology of West Nile in Europe and in the Mediterranean basin. *Open Virol J* **4:**29–37.

84. **Barzon L, Pacenti M, Cusinato R, Cattai M, Franchin E, Pagni S, Martello T, Bressan S, Squarzon L, Cattelan A, Pellizzer G, Scotton P, Beltrame A, Gobbi F, Bisoffi Z, Russo F, Palu G.** 2011. Human cases of West Nile Virus infection in north-eastern Italy, 15 June to 15 November 2010. *Euro Surveill* **16:**19949. http://www.eurosurveillance.org/ViewArticle.aspx?ArticleId=19949.

85. **McIntosh BM, Jupp PG, dos Santos I, Meenehan GM.** 1976. Epidemics of West Nile and Sindbis viruses in South Africa with *Culex* (*Culex*) *univittatus* Theobald as vector. *S Afr J Sci* **72:**295–300.

86. **Hall RA, Scherret JH, Mackenzie JS.** 2001. Kunjin virus: an Australian variant of West Nile? *Ann N Y Acad Sci* **951:**153–160.

87. **Gray TJ, Burrow JN, Markey PG, Whelan PI, Jackson J, Smith DW, Currie BJ.** 2011. West Nile virus (Kunjin subtype) disease in the northern territory of Australia: a case of encephalitis and review of all reported cases. *Am J Trop Med Hyg* **85:**952–956.

88. **Hayes EB, O'Leary DR.** 2004. West Nile virus infection: a pediatric perspective. *Pediatrics* **113:**1375–1381.

89. **Southam CM, Moore AE.** 1952. Clinical studies of viruses as antineoplastic agents with particular reference to Egypt 101 virus. *Cancer* **5:**1025–1034.

90. **Southam CM, Moore AE.** 1954. Induced virus infections in man by the Egypt isolates of West Nile virus. *Am J Trop Med Hyg* **3:**19–50.

91. **Diamond MS, Klein RS.** 2004. West Nile virus: crossing the blood-brain barrier. *Nat Med* **10:**1294–1295.

92. **Samuel MA, Wang H, Siddharthan V, Morrey JD, Diamond MS.** 2007. Axonal transport mediates West Nile virus entry into the central nervous system and induces acute flaccid paralysis. *Proc Natl Acad Sci USA* **104:**17140–17145.

93. **Sampson BA, Ambrosi C, Charlot A, Reiber K, Veress JF, Armbrustmacher V.** 2000. The pathology of human West Nile virus infection. *Hum Pathol* **31:**527–531.

94. **Doron SI, Dashe JF, Adelman LS, Brown WF, Werner BG, Hadley S.** 2003. Histopathologically proven poliomyelitis with quadriplegia and loss of brainstem function due to West Nile virus infection. *Clin Infect Dis* **37:** e74–e77.

95. **Agamanolis DP, Leslie MJ, Caveny EA, Guarner J, Shieh WJ, Zaki SR.** 2003. Neuropathological findings in West Nile virus encephalitis: a case report. *Ann Neurol* **54:**547–551.

96. **Fratkin JD, Leis AA, Stokic DS, Slavinski SA, Geiss RW.** 2004. Spinal cord neuropathology in human West Nile virus infection. *Arch Pathol Lab Med* **128:**533–537.

97. **Park M, Hui JS, Bartt RE.** 2003. Acute anterior radiculitis associated with West Nile virus infection. *J Neurol Neurosurg Psychiatry* **74:**823–825.

98. **Mostashari F, Bunning ML, Kitsutani PT, Singer DA, Nash D, Cooper MJ, Katz N, Liljebjelke KA, Biggerstaff BJ, Fine AD, Layton MC, Mullin SM, Johnson AJ, Martin DA, Hayes EB, Campbell GL.** 2001. Epidemic West Nile encephalitis, New York, 1999: results of a household-based seroepidemiological survey. *Lancet* **358:**261–264.

99. **Centers for Disease Control and Prevention.** 2001. Serosurveys for West Nile virus infection: New York and Connecticut counties, 2000. *MMWR Morb Mortal Wkly Rep* **50:**37–39.

100. **McCarthy TA, Hadler JL, Julian K, Walsh SJ, Biggerstaff BJ, Hinten SR, Baisley C, Iton A, Brennan T, Nelson RS, Achambault G, Marfin AA, Petersen LR.** 2001. West Nile virus serosurvey and assessment of personal prevention efforts in an area with intense epizootic activity: Connecticut, 2000. *Ann N Y Acad Sci* **951:**307–316.

101. **O'Leary DR, Marfin AA, Montgomery SP, Kipp AM, Lehman JA, Biggerstaff BJ, Elko VL, Collins PD, Jones JE, Campbell GL.** 2004. The epidemic of West Nile virus in the United States, 2002. *Vector Borne Zoonotic Dis* **4:**61–70.

102. **Nash D, Mostashari F, Fine A, Miller J, O'Leary D, Murray K, Huang A, Rosenberg A, Greenberg A, Sherman M, Wong S, Layton M.** 2001. The outbreak of West Nile virus infection in the New York City area in 1999. *N Engl J Med* **344:**1807–1814.

103. **Nett RJ, Kuehnert MJ, Ison MG, Orlowski JP, Fischer M, Staples JE.** 2012. Current practices and evaluation of screening solid organ donors for West Nile virus. *Transpl Infect Dis* **14:**268–277.

104. **Kumar D, Drebot MA, Wong SJ, Lim G, Artsob H, Buck P, Humar A.** 2004. A seroprevalence study of West Nile virus infection in solid organ transplant recipients. *Am J Transplant* **4:**1883–1888.

105. **Kumar D, Prasad GV, Zaltzman J, Levy GA, Humar A.** 2004. Community-acquired West Nile virus infection in solid-organ transplant recipients. *Transplantation* **77:**399–402.

106. **Freifeld AG, Meza J, Schweitzer B, Shafer L, Kalil AC, Sambol AR.** 2010. Seroprevalence of West Nile virus infection in solid organ transplant recipients. *Transpl Infect Dis* **12:**120–126.

107. **Murray KO, Koers E, Baraniuk S, Herrington E, Carter H, Sierra M, Kilborn C, Arafat R.** 2009. Risk factors for encephalitis from West Nile virus: a matched case-control study using hospitalized controls. *Zoonoses Public Health* **56:**370–375.

108. **Patnaik JL, Harmon H, Vogt RL.** 2006. Follow-up of 2003 human West Nile virus infections, Denver, Colorado. *Emerg Infect Dis* **12:**1129–1131.

109. **Jean CM, Honarmand S, Louie JK, Glaser CA.** 2007. Risk factors for West Nile virus neuroinvasive disease, California, 2005. *Emerg Infect Dis* **13:**1918–1920.

110. **Murray K, Baraniuk S, Resnick M, Arafat R, Kilborn C, Cain K, Shallenberger R, York TL,** Martinez D, Hellums JS, Hellums D, Malkoff M, Elgawley N, McNeely W, Khuwaja SA, Tesh RB. 2006. Risk factors for encephalitis and death from West Nile virus infection. *Epidemiol Infect* **134:**1325–1332.

111. **Bode AV, Sejvar JJ, Pape WJ, Campbell GL, Marfin AA.** 2006. West Nile virus disease: a descriptive study of 228 patients hospitalized in a 4-county region of Colorado in 2003. *Clin Infect Dis* **42:**1234–1240.

112. **Sejvar JJ, Haddad MB, Tierney BC, Campbell GL, Marfin AA, Van Gerpen JA, Fleischauer A, Leis AA, Stokic DS, Petersen LR.** 2003. Neurologic manifestations and outcome of West Nile virus infection. *JAMA* **290:**511–515.

113. **Emig M, Apple DJ.** 2004. Severe West Nile virus disease in healthy adults. *Clin Infect Dis* **38:**289–292.

114. **Pepperell C, Rau N, Krajden S, Kern R, Humar A, Mederski B, Simor A, Low DE, McGeer A, Mazzulli T, Burton J, Jaigobin C, Fearon M, Artsob H, Drebot MA, Halliday W, Brunton J.** 2003. West Nile virus infection in 2002: morbidity and mortality among patients admitted to hospital in southcentral Ontario. *CMAJ* **168:**1399–1405.

115. **Sayao AL, Suchowersky O, Al-Khathaami A, Klassen B, Katz NR, Sevick R, Tilley P, Fox J, Patry D.** 2004. Calgary experience with West Nile virus neurological syndrome during the late summer of 2003. *Can J Neurol Sci* **31:**194–203.

116. **Granwehr BP, Lillibridge KM, Higgs S, Mason PW, Aronson JF, Campbell GA, Barrett AD.** 2004. West Nile virus: where are we now? *Lancet Infect Dis* **4:**547–556.

117. **Brown JA, Factor DL, Tkachencko N, Templeton SM, Crall ND, Pape WJ, Bauer MJ, Ambruso DR, Dickey WC, Marfin AA.** 2007. West Nile viremic blood donors and risk factors for subsequent West Nile fever. *Vector Borne Zoonotic Dis* **7:**479–488.

118. **Hayes EB, Gubler DJ.** 2006. West Nile virus: epidemiology and clinical features of an emerging epidemic in the United States. *Annu Rev Med* **57:**181–194.

119. **Ferguson DD, Gershman K, LeBailly A, Petersen LR.** 2005. Characteristics of the rash associated with West Nile virus fever. *Clin Infect Dis* **41:**1204–1207.

120. **Del Giudice P, Schuffenecker I, Zeller H, Grelier M, Vandenbos F, Dellamonica P, Counillon E.** 2005. Skin manifestations of West Nile virus infection. *Dermatology* **211:**348–350.

121. **Gorsche R, Tilley P.** 2005. The rash of West Nile virus infection. *CMAJ* **172:**1440.

122. **Anderson RC, Horn KB, Hoang MP, Gottlieb E, Bennin B.** 2004. Punctate exanthem of

West Nile virus infection: report of 3 cases. *J Am Acad Dermatol* 51:820–823.

123. **Watson JT, Pertel PE, Jones RC, Siston AM, Paul WS, Austin CC, Gerber SI.** 2004. Clinical characteristics and functional outcomes of West Nile fever. *Ann Intern Med* 141:360–365.

124. **Sejvar JJ, Curns AT, Welburg L, Jones JF, Lundgren LM, Capuron L, Pape J, Reeves WC, Campbel GL.** 2008. Neurocognitive and functional outcomes in persons recovering from West Nile virus illness. *J Neuropsychol* 2:477–499.

125. **Sejvar JJ, Lindsey NP, Campbell GL.** 2011. Primary causes of death in reported cases of fatal West Nile fever, United States, 2002-2006. *Vector Borne Zoonotic Dis* 11:161–164.

126. **Crichlow R, Bailey J, Gardner C.** 2004. Cerebrospinal fluid neutrophilic pleocytosis in hospitalized West Nile virus patients. *J Am Board Fam Pract* 17:470–472.

127. **Sejvar JJ, Bode AV, Marfin AA, Campbell GL, Ewing D, Mazowiecki M, Pavot PV, Schmitt J, Pape J, Biggerstaff BJ, Petersen LR.** 2005. West Nile virus-associated flaccid paralysis. *Emerg Infect Dis* 11:1021–1027.

128. **Burton JM, Kern RZ, Halliday W, Mikulis D, Brunton J, Fearon M, Pepperell C, Jaigobin C.** 2004. Neurological manifestations of West Nile virus infection. *Can J Neurol Sci* 31:185–193.

129. **Brilla R, Block M, Geremia G, Wichter M.** 2004. Clinical and neuroradiologic features of 39 consecutive cases of West Nile virus meningoencephalitis. *J Neurol Sci* 220:37–40.

130. **Ali M, Safriel Y, Sohi J, Llave A, Weathers S.** 2005. West Nile virus infection: MR imaging findings in the nervous system. *AJNR Am J Neuroradiol* 26:289–297.

131. **Petropoulou KA, Gordon SM, Prayson RA, Ruggierri PM.** 2005. West Nile virus meningoencephalitis: MR imaging findings. *AJNR Am J Neuroradiol* 26:1986–1995.

132. **Rodriguez AJ, Westmoreland BF.** 2007. Electroencephalographic characteristics of patients infected with West Nile virus. *J Clin Neurophysiol* 24:386–389.

133. **Gandelman-Marton R, Kimiagar I, Itzhaki A, Klein C, Theitler J, Rabey JM.** 2003. Electroencephalography findings in adult patients with West Nile virus-associated meningitis and meningoencephalitis. *Clin Infect Dis* 37:1573–1578.

134. **Tyler KL, Pape J, Goody RJ, Corkill M, Kleinschmidt-DeMasters BK.** 2006. CSF findings in 250 patients with serologically confirmed West Nile virus meningitis and encephalitis. *Neurology* 66:361–365.

135. **Robinson RL, Shahida S, Madan N, Rao S, Khardori N.** 2003. Transient parkinsonism in West Nile virus encephalitis. *Am J Med* 115:252–253.

136. **Kanagarajan K, Ganesh S, Alakhras M, Go ES, Recco RA, Zaman MM.** 2003. West Nile virus infection presenting as cerebellar ataxia and fever: case report. *South Med J* 96:600–601.

137. **Kelley TW, Prayson RA, Ruiz AI, Isada CM, Gordon SM.** 2003. The neuropathology of West Nile virus meningoencephalitis. A report of two cases and review of the literature. *Am J Clin Pathol* 119:749–753.

138. **Guarner J, Shieh WJ, Hunter S, Paddock CD, Morken T, Campbell GL, Marfin AA, Zaki SR.** 2004. Clinicopathologic study and laboratory diagnosis of 23 cases with West Nile virus encephalomyelitis. *Hum Pathol* 35:983–990.

139. **Bosanko CM, Gilroy J, Wang AM, Sanders W, Dulai M, Wilson J, Blum K.** 2003. West nile virus encephalitis involving the substantia nigra: neuroimaging and pathologic findings with literature review. *Arch Neurol* 60:1448–1452.

140. **Jeha LE, Sila CA, Lederman RJ, Prayson RA, Isada CM, Gordon SM.** 2003. West Nile virus infection: a new acute paralytic illness. *Neurology* 61:55–59.

141. **Leis AA, Stokic DS, Polk JL, Dostrow V, Winkelmann M.** 2002. A poliomyelitis-like syndrome from West Nile virus infection. *N Engl J Med* 347:1279–1280.

142. **Glass JD, Samuels O, Rich MM.** 2002. Poliomyelitis due to West Nile virus. *N Engl J Med* 347:1280–1281.

143. **Sejvar JJ, Leis AA, Stokic DS, Van Gerpen JA, Marfin AA, Webb R, Haddad MB, Tierney BC, Slavinski SA, Polk JL, Dostrow V, Winkelmann M, Petersen LR.** 2003. Acute flaccid paralysis and West Nile virus infection. *Emerg Infect Dis* 9:788–793.

144. **Li J, Loeb JA, Shy ME, Shah AK, Tselis AC, Kupski WJ, Lewis RA.** 2003. Asymmetric flaccid paralysis: a neuromuscular presentation of West Nile virus infection. *Ann Neurol* 53:703–710.

145. **Kulstad EB, Wichter MD.** 2003. West Nile encephalitis presenting as a stroke. *Ann Emerg Med* 41:283.

146. **Berner YN, Lang R, Chowers MY.** 2002. Outcome of West Nile fever in older adults. *J Am Geriatr Soc* 50:1844–1846.

147. **Fan E, Needham DM, Brunton J, Kern RZ, Stewart TE.** 2004. West Nile virus infection in the intensive care unit: a case series and literature review. *Can Respir J* 11:354–358.

148. **Leis AA, Stokic DS, Webb RM, Slavinski SA, Fratkin J.** 2003. Clinical spectrum of muscle

weakness in human West Nile virus infection. *Muscle Nerve* **28**:302–308.

149. **Al-Shekhlee A, Katirji B.** 2004. Electrodiagnostic features of acute paralytic poliomyelitis associated with West Nile virus infection. *Muscle Nerve* **29**:376–380.

150. **Ahmed S, Libman R, Wesson K, Ahmed F, Einberg K.** 2000. Guillain-Barre syndrome: an unusual presentation of West Nile virus infection. *Neurology* **55**:144–146.

151. **Cao NJ, Ranganathan C, Kupsky WJ, Li J.** 2005. Recovery and prognosticators of paralysis in West Nile virus infection. *J Neurol Sci* **236**:73–80.

152. **Sejvar JJ, Bode AV, Marfin AA, Campbell GL, Pape J, Biggerstaff BJ, Petersen LR.** 2006. West Nile virus-associated flaccid paralysis outcome. *Emerg Infect Dis* **12**:514–516.

153. **Sejvar JJ, Davis LE, Szabados E, Jackson AC.** 2010. Delayed-onset and recurrent limb weakness associated with West Nile virus infection. *J Neurovirol* **16**:93–100.

154. **Hershberger VS, Augsburger JJ, Hutchins RK, Miller SA, Horwitz JA, Bergmann M.** 2003. Chorioretinal lesions in nonfatal cases of West Nile virus infection. *Ophthalmology* **110**:1732–1736.

155. **Adelman RA, Membreno JH, Afshari NA, Stoessel KM.** 2003. West Nile virus chorioretinitis. *Retina* **23**:100–101.

156. **Bains HS, Jampol LM, Caughron MC, Parnell JR.** 2003. Vitritis and chorioretinitis in a patient with West Nile virus infection. *Arch Ophthalmol* **121**:205–207.

157. **Kuchtey RW, Kosmorsky GS, Martin D, Lee MS.** 2003. Uveitis associated with West Nile virus infection. *Arch Ophthalmol* **121**:1648–1649.

158. **Shaikh S, Trese MT.** 2004. West Nile virus chorioretinitis. *Br J Ophthalmol* **88**:1599–1560.

159. **Vandenbelt S, Shaikh S, Capone A, Jr, Williams GA.** 2003. Multifocal choroiditis associated with West Nile virus encephalitis. *Retina* **23**:97–99.

160. **Khairallah M, Ben Yahia S, Ladjimi A, Zeghidi H, Ben Romdhane F, Besbes L, Zaouali S, Messaoud R.** 2004. Chorioretinal involvement in patients with West Nile virus infection. *Ophthalmology* **111**:2065–2070.

161. **Perelman A, Stern J.** 1974. Acute pancreatitis in West Nile fever. *Am J Trop Med Hyg* **23**:1150–1152.

162. **Murray K, Walker C, Herrington E, Lewis JA, McCormick J, Beasley DW, Tesh RB, Fisher-Hoch S.** 2010. Persistent infection with West Nile virus years after initial infection. *J Infect Dis* **201**:2–4.

163. **Gibney KB, Lanciotti RS, Sejvar JJ, Nugent CT, Linnen JM, Delorey MJ, Lehman JA,** Boswell EN, Staples JE, Fischer M. 2011. West Nile virus RNA not detected in urine of 40 people tested 6 years after acute West Nile virus disease. *J Infect Dis* **203**:344–347.

164. **Baty SA, Gibney KB, Staples JE, Patterson AB, Levy C, Lehman J, Wadleigh T, Feld J, Lanciotti R, Nugent CT, Fischer M.** 2012. Evaluation for West Nile Virus (WNV) RNA in Urine of Patients Within 5 Months of WNV Infection. *J Infect Dis* **205**:1476–1477.

165. **Lindsey NP, Hayes EB, Staples JE, Fischer M.** 2009. West Nile virus disease in children, United States, 1999-2007. *Pediatrics* **123**:e1084–e1089.

166. **Civen R, Villacorte F, Robles DT, Dassey DE, Croker C, Borenstein L, Harvey SM, Mascola L.** 2006. West Nile virus infection in the pediatric population. *Pediatr Infect Dis J* **25**:75–78.

167. **Heresi GP, Mancias P, Mazur LJ, Butler IJ, Murphy JR, Cleary TG.** 2004. Poliomyelitis-like syndrome in a child with West Nile virus infection. *Pediatr Infect Dis J* **23**:788–789.

168. **Vidwan G, Bryant KK, Puri V, Stover BH, Rabalais GP.** 2003. West Nile virus encephalitis in a child with left-side weakness. *Clin Infect Dis* **37**:e91–e94.

169. **Carey DE, Rodrigues FM, Myers RM, Webb JK.** 1968. Arthropod-borne viral infections in children in Vellore, South India, with particular reference to dengue and West Nile viruses. *Indian Pediatr* **5**:285–296.

170. **Nichter CA, Pavlakis SG, Shaikh U, Cherian KA, Dobrosyzcki J, Porricolo ME, Chatturvedi I.** 2000. Rhombencephalitis caused by West Nile fever virus. *Neurology* **55**:153.

171. **Yim R, Posfay-Barbe KM, Nolt D, Fatula G, Wald ER.** 2004. Spectrum of clinical manifestations of West Nile virus infection in children. *Pediatrics* **114**:1673–1675.

172. **Ravindra KV, Freifeld AG, Kalil AC, Mercer DF, Grant WJ, Botha JF, Wrenshall LE, Stevens RB.** 2004. West Nile virus-associated encephalitis in recipients of renal and pancreas transplants: case series and literature review. *Clin Infect Dis* **38**:1257–1260.

173. **Klee AL, Maidin B, Edwin B, Poshni I, Mostashari F, Fine A, Layton M, Nash D.** 2004. Long-term prognosis for clinical West Nile virus infection. *Emerg Infect Dis* **10**:1405–1411.

174. **Cook RL, Xu X, Yablonsky EJ, Sakata N, Tripp JH, Hess R, Piazza P, Rinaldo CR.** 2010. Demographic and clinical factors associated with persistent symptoms after West Nile virus infection. *Am J Trop Med Hyg* **83**:1133–1136.

175. Haaland KY SJ, Pergam S, Echevarria LA, Davis LE, Goade D, Harnar J, Nfchissey RA, Sewel CM, Ettestad P. 2006. Mental status after West Nile virus infection. *Emerg Infect Dis* **12:**1260–1262.

176. Sadek JR, Pergam SA, Harrington JA, Echevarria LA, Davis LE, Goade D, Harnar J, Nofchissey RA, Sewell CM, Ettestad P, Haaland KY. 2010. Persistent neuropsychological impairment associated with West Nile virus infection. *J Clin Exp Neuropsychol* **32:**81–87.

177. Carson PJ, Konewko P, Wold KS, Mariani P, Goli S, Bergloff P, Crosby RD. 2006. Long-term clinical and neuropsychological outcomes of West Nile virus infection. *Clin Infect Dis* **43:**723–730.

178. Loeb M, Hanna S, Nicolle L, Eyles J, Elliott S, Rathbone M, Drebot M, Neupane B, Fearon M, Mahony J. 2008. Prognosis after West Nile virus infection. *Ann Intern Med* **149:**232–241.

179. Berg PJ, Smallfield S, Svien L. 2010. An investigation of depression and fatigue post West Nile virus infection. *S D Med* **63:**127–129,131–133.

180. Murray KO, Resnick M, Miller V. 2007. Depression after infection with West Nile virus. *Emerg Infect Dis* **13:**479–481.

181. Martin DA, Biggerstaff BJ, Allen B, Johnson AJ, Lanciotti RS, Roehrig JT. 2002. Use of immunoglobulin M cross-reactions in differential diagnosis of human flaviviral encephalitis infections in the United States. *Clin Diagn Lab Immunol* **9:**544–549.

182. Papa A, Anastasiadou A, Delianidou M. 2015. West Nile virus IgM and IgG antibodies three years post-infection. *Hippokratia* **19:**34–36.

183. Roehrig JT, Nash D, Maldin B, Labowitz A, Martin DA, Lanciotti RS, Campbell GL. 2003. Persistence of virus-reactive serum immunoglobulin M antibody in confirmed West Nile virus encephalitis cases. *Emerg Infect Dis* **9:**376–379.

184. Kapoor H, Signs K, Somsel P, Downes FP, Clark PA, Massey JP. 2004. Persistence of West Nile virus (WNV) IgM antibodies in cerebrospinal fluid from patients with CNS disease. *J Clin Virol* **31:**289–291.

185. Martin DA, Muth DA, Brown T, Johnson AJ, Karabatsos N, Roehrig JT. 2000. Standardization of immunoglobulin M capture enzyme-linked immunosorbent assays for routine diagnosis of arboviral infections. *J Clin Microbiol* **38:**1823–1826.

186. Koepsell SA, Freifeld AG, Sambol AR, McComb RD, Kazmi SA. 2010. Seronegative naturally acquired West Nile virus encephalitis in a renal and pancreas transplant recipient. *Transpl Infect Dis* **12:**459–464.

187. Penn RG, Guarner J, Sejvar JJ, Hartman H, McComb RD, Nevins DL, Bhatnagar J, Zaki SR. 2006. Persistent neuroinvasive West Nile virus infection in an immunocompromised patient. *Clin Infect Dis* **42:**680–683.

188. Guyton A. 1949. Reaction of the body to poliomyelitis and the recovery process. *Arch Int Med* **83:**27.

189. Jordan I, Briese T, Fischer N, Lau JY, Lipkin WI. 2000. Ribavirin inhibits West Nile virus replication and cytopathic effect in neural cells. *J Infect Dis* **182:**1214–1217.

190. Ferrara EA, Oishi JS, Wannemacher RW, Jr, Stephen EL. 1981. Plasma disappearance, urine excretion, and tissue distribution of ribavirin in rats and rhesus monkeys. *Antimicrob Agents Chemother* **19:**1042–1049.

191. Morrey JD, Day CW, Julander JG, Blatt LM, Smee DF, Sidwell RW. 2004. Effect of interferon-alpha and interferon-inducers on West Nile virus in mouse and hamster animal models. *Antivir Chem Chemother* **15:**101–109.

192. Solomon T, Dung NM, Wills B, Kneen R, Gainsborough M, Diet TV, Thuy TT, Loan HT, Khanh VC, Vaughn DW, White NJ, Farrar JJ. 2003. Interferon alfa-2a in Japanese encephalitis: a randomised double-blind placebo-controlled trial. *Lancet* **361:**821–826.

193. Diamond MS, Shrestha B, Marri A, Mahan D, Engle M. 2003. B cells and antibody play critical roles in the immediate defense of disseminated infection by West Nile encephalitis virus. *J Virol* **77:**2578–2586.

194. Shimoni Z, Niven MJ, Pitlick S, Bulvik S. 2001. Treatment of West Nile virus encephalitis with intravenous immunoglobulin. *Emerg Infect Dis* **7:**759.

195. Agrawal AG, Petersen LR. 2003. Human immunoglobulin as a treatment for West Nile virus infection. *J Infect Dis* **188:**1–4.

196. Oliphant T, Engle M, Nybakken GE, Doane C, Johnson S, Huang L, Gorlatov S, Mehlhop E, Marri A, Chung KM, Ebel GD, Kramer LD, Fremont DH, Diamond MS. 2005. Development of a humanized monoclonal antibody with therapeutic potential against West Nile virus. *Nat Med* **11:**522–530.

197. Beigel JH, Nordstrom JL, Pillemer SR, Roncal C, Goldwater DR, Li H, Holland PC, Johnson S, Stein K, Koenig S. 2010. Safety and pharmacokinetics of single intravenous dose of MGAWN1, a novel monoclonal antibody to West Nile virus. *Antimicrob Agents Chemother* **54:**2431–2436.

198. Morrey JD, Siddharthan V, Olsen AL, Roper GY, Wang H, Baldwin TJ, Koenig S, Johnson

S, Nordstrom JL, Diamond MS. 2006. Humanized monoclonal antibody against West Nile virus envelope protein administered after neuronal infection protects against lethal encephalitis in hamsters. *J Infect Dis* **194**: 1300–1308.

199. **Smeraski CA, Siddharthan V, Morrey JD.** 2011. Treatment of spatial memory impairment in hamsters infected with West Nile virus using a humanized monoclonal antibody MGAWN1. *Antiviral Res* **91**:43–49.

200. **Barnard DR, Xue RD.** 2004. Laboratory evaluation of mosquito repellents against *Aedes albopictus*, *Culex nigripalpus*, and *Ochlerotatus triseriatus* (*Diptera*: *Culicidae*). *J Med Entomol* **41**:726–730.

201. **Frances SP, Van Dung N, Beebe NW, Debboun M.** 2002. Field evaluation of repellent formulations against daytime and nighttime biting mosquitoes in a tropical rainforest in northern Australia. *J Med Entomol* **39**:541–544.

202. **Frances SP, Waterson DG, Beebe NW, Cooper RD.** 2004. Field evaluation of repellent formulations containing deet and picaridin against mosquitoes in Northern Territory, Australia. *J Med Entomol* **41**:414–417.

203. **Costantini C, Badolo A, Ilboudo-Sanogo E.** 2004. Field evaluation of the efficacy and persistence of insect repellents DEET, IR3535, and KBR 3023 against *Anopheles gambiae* complex and other Afrotropical vector mosquitoes. *Trans R Soc Trop Med Hyg* **98**:644–652.

204. **Zielinski-Gutierrez E, Wirtz RA, Nasci RS, Brogdon WG.** 2012. Chapter 2: The pre-travel consultation counseling & advice for travelers; protection against mosquitoes, ticks, & other insects & arthropods. http://wwwnc.cdc.gov/travel/page/yellowbook-2012-home.htm.

205. **Hall RA, Khromykh AA.** 2004. West Nile virus vaccines. *Expert Opin Biol Ther* **4**:1295–1305.

206. **Chang GJ, Kuno G, Purdy DE, Davis BS.** 2004. Recent advancement in flavivirus vaccine development. *Expert Rev Vaccines* **3**:199–220.

207. **Monath TP, Liu J, Kanesa-Thasan N, Myers GA, Nichols R, Deary A, McCarthy K, Johnson C, Ermak T, Shin S, Arroyo J, Guirakhoo F, Kennedy JS, Ennis FA, Green S, Bedford P.** 2006. A live, attenuated recombinant West Nile virus vaccine. *Proc Natl Acad Sci USA* **103**:6694–6699.

208. **Pletnev AG, Claire MS, Elkins R, Speicher J, Murphy BR, Chanock RM.** 2003. Molecularly engineered live-attenuated chimeric West Nile/dengue virus vaccines protect rhesus monkeys from West Nile virus. *Virology* **314**:190–195.

209. **Siger L, Bowen R, Karaca K, Murray M, Jagannatha S, Echols B, Nordgren R, Minke JM.** 2006. Evaluation of the efficacy provided by a recombinant canarypox-vectored equine West Nile virus vaccine against an experimental West Nile virus intrathecal challenge in horses. *Vet Ther* **7**:249–256.

210. **Ng T, Hathaway D, Jennings N, Champ D, Chiang YW, Chu HJ.** 2003. Equine vaccine for West Nile virus. *Dev Biol (Basel)* **114**:221–227.

211. **Monath TP.** 2002. Editorial: jennerian vaccination against West Nile virus. *Am J Trop Med Hyg* **66**:113–114.

212. **Mansfield KL, Horton DL, Johnson N, Li L, Barrett AD, Smith DJ, Galbraith SE, Solomon T, Fooks AR.** 2011. Flavivirus-induced antibody cross-reactivity. *J Gen Virol* **92**:2821–2829.

213. **Johnson BW, Kosoy O, Martin DA, Noga AJ, Russell BJ, Johnson AA, Petersen LR.** 2005. West Nile virus infection and serologic response among persons previously vaccinated against yellow fever and Japanese encephalitis viruses. *Vector Borne Zoonotic Dis* **5**:137–145.

214. **Tang F, Zhang JS, Liu W, Zhao QM, Zhang F, Wu XM, Yang H, Ly H, Cao WC.** 2008. Failure of Japanese encephalitis vaccine and infection in inducing neutralizing antibodies against West Nile virus, People's Republic of China. *Am J Trop Med Hyg* **78**:999–1001.

215. **Yamshchikov G, Borisevich V, Kwok CW, Nistler R, Kohlmeier J, Seregin A, Chaporgina E, Benedict S, Yamshchikov V.** 2005. The suitability of yellow fever and Japanese encephalitis vaccines for immunization against West Nile virus. *Vaccine* **23**:4785–4792.

216. **Kanesa-Thasan N, Putnak JR, Mangiafico JA, Saluzzo JE, Ludwig GV.** 2002. Short report: absence of protective neutralizng antibodies to West Nile virus in subjects following vaccination with Japanese encephalitis or dengue vaccines. *Am J Trop Med Hyg* **66**:115–116.

217. **Lobigs M, Diamond MS.** 2012. Feasibility of cross-protective vaccination against flaviviruses of the Japanese encephalitis serocomplex. *Expert Rev Vaccines* **11**:177–187.

Mobilization of Carbapenemase-Mediated Resistance in Enterobacteriaceae

11

AMY MATHERS[1,2]

INTRODUCTION

After decades of worry, extreme drug resistance has become an unfortunate reality in many hospitals around the world. Rather than arriving in the form of vancomycin-resistant *Staphylococcus aureus* or pan-drug-resistant tuberculosis, extreme drug resistance has emerged in enteric Gram-negative bacilli. Essentially unheard of prior to 2003, in 2011 11% of *Klebsiella pneumoniae* isolates from intensive care units in the United States were resistant to carbapenems, with an attributable mortality rate of 40% from associated invasive infections (1–3). From a recent World Health Organization report, carbapenem resistance in *Klebsiella pneumoniae* had been seen in almost all countries that had data, and some countries reported carbapenem resistance rates of more than 50% (4). The Centers for Disease Control and Prevention (CDC) listed carbapenem-resistant *Enterobacteriaceae* as one of the three most urgent groups of drug-resistant microbes threatening human health in the United States (5).

The epidemiology of carbapenem resistance in *Enterobacteriaceae* around the globe has been dominated by the dissemination of three distinct Ambler classes of β-lactamases with carbapenem-hydrolyzing activity, the carbapenemases.

[1]Division of Infectious Diseases and International Health, Department of Medicine; [2]Clinical Microbiology, Department of Pathology, University of Virginia Health System, Charlottesville, VA 22911
Emerging Infections 10
Edited by W. Michael Scheld, James M. Hughes and Richard J. Whitley
© 2016 American Society for Microbiology, Washington, DC
doi:10.1128/microbiolspec.EI10-0010-2015

In almost all cases, the genes for carbapenem resistance are carried not on the chromosome of a successful lineage of bacteria but rather on mobile elements of DNA which can be shared and spread between bacteria (6). This means that a previously susceptible member of the *Enterobacteriaceae* can acquire a single gene and become resistant to the majority of β-lactam antibiotics, including carbapenems.

Interestingly, the epidemiology around the globe has been slightly different, with unique carbapenemases having a different pattern of dissemination. This may be driven largely by the distinct mobile genetic location of the carbapenemase gene. The unique mobile elements surrounding the different carbapenemase genes may be best suited for specific bacterial host ranges and environments. The concept of tracking a gene of resistance rather than a strain or species of bacteria may be central to slowing the spread of resistance. In this chapter, I explore carbapenemase-mediated resistance in *Enterobacteriaceae*, including clinical context, epidemiology, and detection. I also examine the potential impact mobile elements have on the epidemiology of the extreme drug resistance and why understanding modes of genetic mobility may need to be considered in understanding the spread of these extremely antibiotic-resistant organisms.

CLINICAL CONTEXT OF CARBAPENEMASES

Enterobacteriaceae (e.g., *Escherichia coli*, *Klebsiella*, *Enterobacter*, *Citrobacter*, *Serratia*, and *Proteus*) are among the most frequently identified agents for a variety of serious bacterial infections. They account for 21% of all nosocomial infections (e.g., sepsis, ∼30%; pneumonia, 15 to 20%; urinary tract infections, ∼90%; and intra-abdominal infections, ∼90%) (7–12). Carbapenems had long been held as the last-line agents against extended-spectrum-β-lactamase (ESBL)-producing *Enterobacteriaceae*. In general, carbapenem resistance negatively impacts patient outcomes (1, 13–15). In a large case-control study, carbapenem resistance increased overall mortality (48% versus 20%; $P < 0.001$) and attributable mortality (38% versus 12%; $P < 0.001$) for invasive *K. pneumoniae* infections matched with carbapenem-susceptible isolates (1).

Dissemination of carbapenemase genes is the primary cause of carbapenem resistance around the globe. A carbapenemase is a β-lactamase which has high affinity for carbapenem hydrolysis. Acquisition of a carbapenemase gene by *Enterobacteriaceae* may then result in the destruction and often clinical failure of this previously effective agent. Often these *Enterobacteriaceae* are multidrug resistant and other classes of antimicrobials are also ineffective, leaving the patient with few treatment options.

Carbapenemases can be placed into different classes depending on their biochemical and molecular characteristics, including metallocarbapenemase (e.g., New Delhi metallo-β-lactamase [NDM-1]), serine carbapenemase (e.g., *K. pneumoniae* carbapenemase [KPC]), and a group of penicillinases typically associated with carbapenem resistance in *Acinetobacter baumannii* (oxacillinase [OXA]) (16–18). In *Enterobacteriaceae*, the genetic elements encoding carbapenemases are typically contained within replicative transposons carried by plasmids that frequently harbor additional drug resistance determinants, thus enabling rapid horizontal transmissibility of multidrug resistance (19–24). Understanding the differences between the primary enzymes can be challenging but important in determining the antibiotic agents which may be effective. This will likely become more relevant as an increasing number of therapeutics which target specific carbapenemases become clinically available. For example, the traditional β-lactamase inhibitors, clavulanic acid, tazobactam, and sulbactam, do not have clinically relevant activity for metallo-β-lactamases, oxacillinases, or KPC, whereas the newly approved drug avibactam has strong affinity to inhibit KPC and therefore could be an effective therapeutic (25). The general classification of carbapenemases is shown in Table 1.

DISTINCT EPIDEMIOLOGIES OF THE MAJOR CARBAPENEMASES

The focus of this chapter is on the three most widely seen and rapidly emergent carbapenemases: NDM, KPC, and oxacillinase-48-like (OXA-48-like). The genes (*bla*) that encode these three carbapenemases all demonstrate unique epidemiological stories.

KPC has been the most frequently reported carbapenemase, with the highest number of clinical cases around the globe. KPC was first described in North Carolina in a case in 1996 (26). There were no further reports or identified isolates until 2001, when a few carbapenem-resistant *K. pneumoniae* isolates were seen in New York City. By 2005, KPC was carried by half of the *K. pneumoniae* organisms in some intensive care units in multiple New York City hospitals (27). Around the same time, KPC-producing *Enterobacteriaceae* were described in the Caribbean, South America, China, and Israel (28–30). Initial outbreak descriptions were dominated by a highly related strain of *K. pneumoniae*. This high-risk clone, multilocus sequence type 258 (ST258), has been successfully transmitted around the globe and has dominated almost all locations where KPC has been described. The majority of clinical cases are still confined to patients who have hos-

pital exposure, complex medical histories, and receipt of antibiotics (31, 32). The regions of endemicity have increased in number and now include Italy and Greece (Fig. 1A). Israel, which undertook a national effort to eliminate the spread, has been the only country with a decrease in the number of infected patients. However, KPC-producing ST258 *K. pneumoniae* still persists (33).

The OXA-48-like enzymes present a different challenge for understanding transmission and gene movement as several of the alleles likely arose independently and should likely be considered several different outbreaks with unique epidemiology. The focus here is on bla_{OXA-48} and $bla_{OXA-181}$. The first case of a bla_{OXA-48}-positive *K. pneumoniae* isolate was seen in Turkey in 2001 (34). It then spread to Western Europe and escaped detection for a period of time, as the enzyme does not always confer full carbapenem resistance or cephalosporin resistance, and was found in multiple species (35). This enzyme has now been described as the dominant carbapenemase in *Enterobacteriaceae* in Northern Africa, the Gulf States of the Persian Gulf, and some countries in Western Europe (35, 36) (Fig. 1B). It does appear that in most described outbreaks, patients have had health care exposure (37). The other major class D carbapenemase in *Enterobacteriaceae* is $bla_{OXA-181}$. This gene has been described for several isolates from India and is often coproduced with another carbapenemase, such as NDM (38, 39). Less is known about the full epidemiology of this enzyme, but it has

TABLE 1 Ambler class β-lactamases with efficient carbapenem hydrolysis found in *Enterobacteriaceae*[a]

Class[b]	β-Lactamase type	Frequent enzyme(s)	Obscure enzyme(s)	Spectrum
A	Penicillinases	KPC	IMI, SME, GES	PCNs, cephalosporins, aztreonam, carbapenems
B	Metallo-β-lactamases	NDM, IMP, VIM	SIM, AIM, GIM	Same as above except aztreonam
D	Oxacillinases	OXA-48, -181	OXA-163	±aztreonam, ±cephalosporin

[a]Abbreviations: KPC, *Klebsiella pneumoniae* carbapenemase; IMI, imipenemase; SME, *Serratia marcescens* enzyme; GES, Guiana extended spectrum; PCN, penicillin; NDM, New Delhi metallo-β-lactamase; IMP, active on imipenem; VIM, Verona integron-encoded metallo-β-lactamase; SIM, Seoul imipenemase; AIM, Adelaide imipenemase; GIM, German imipenemase; OXA, oxacillinase.
[b]Ambler class C cephalosporinases do not demonstrate efficient carbapenem hydrolysis and therefore are not listed.

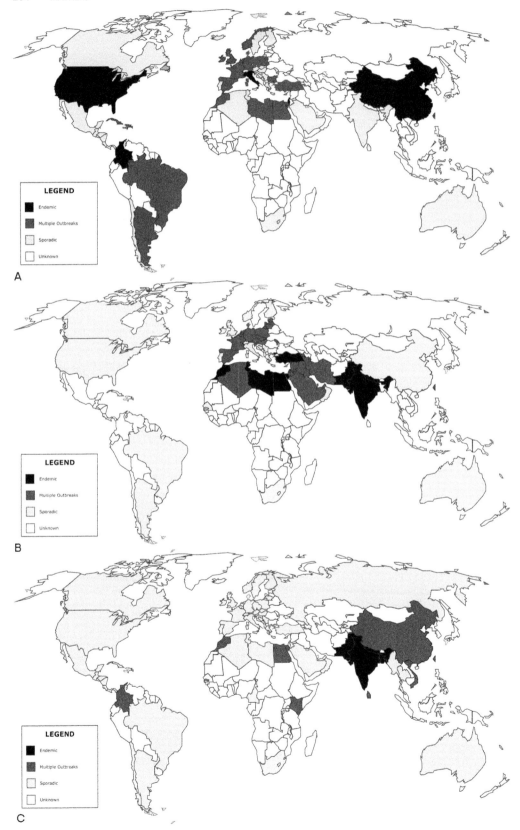

been described in multiple genetic contexts and likely arose relatively independently of bla_{OXA-48} (40).

NDM is the most recent carbapenemase to be identified after a description of isolates in India, Pakistan, and the United Kingdom in 2008 (22). The epidemiology of NDM differs from that of the non-metallo-β-lactamases, as it has been seen in multiple species and epidemiologic locations. This enzyme has been found in drinking water in India, and although most clinical descriptions of infection involve nosocomial transmission, it appears that the barrier for community acquisition is likely lower and the enzyme does not remain confined to health care-exposed patients only (41). Microbiologically, NDM has also been seen in multiple *Enterobacteriaceae* species and even within the same host has a high degree of species and strain variability (42). The global epidemiology of this enzyme has largely dominated India, Pakistan, and Southeast Asia, but the enzyme has also been frequently imported, with resultant outbreaks (43) (Fig. 1C). It appears too early in the outbreak to understand completely if this enzyme will have global dominance similar to that of KPC; however, there is no barrier to this occurring.

CHALLENGES OF DETECTION OF A CARBAPENEMASE IN A CLINICAL MICROBIOLOGY LABORATORY

Determination of antibiotic sensitivities in a clinical microbiology laboratory is most often done by assessing the MIC against the antibiotic tested. The MIC at which an organism is considered susceptible in the United States is governed by the Clinical Laboratory and Standards Institute (CLSI) and Food and Drug Administration (FDA). The MIC cutoff for susceptibly is based largely on drug levels achievable in serum and, when possible, animal model and/or clinical outcome data (44). When PCR-confirmed KPC-producing bacteria began to spread, it was soon recognized that many isolates were in the range of susceptible (45–47). Reports of clinical failures soon followed, describing infections with KPC-producing *Enterobacteriaceae* treated with a carbapenem alone despite a MIC within the range achievable in serum (48–51). The inability of a MIC alone to predict clinical success in the setting of carbapenemases compelled the CLSI to generate an alternate approach (52).

In 2009, the CLSI recommended that clinical laboratories perform a phenotypic carbapenemase test for *Enterobacteriaceae* suspicious for carbapenemase production but falling within a range of previously determined susceptibility (53). However, phenotypic tests can give false-positive and false-negative results as to the presence of a carbapenemase, and results vary depending on the experience of the laboratory technician. In June 2010, the CLSI amended their former recommendations and effectively replaced phenotypic testing for carbapenemase production with lower breakpoints (54). The lower breakpoints have better sensitivity for carbapenemase detection in clinical isolates and also make it possible for testing to be done in all clinical laboratories. However, this creates a problem of understanding the dissemination of carbapenemases within a hospital and/or within a region. Another issue which arises occurs because not all carbapenem resistance in *Enterobacteriaceae* is due to acquisition of a carbapenemase gene. The other major mechanism of carbapenem resistance in *Enterobacteriaceae* is through a combination of decreased outer membrane permeability and increased nonspecific β-lactamase activity (55–58). However,

FIGURE 1 Global epidemiology of three major carbapenemase enzymes in *Enterobacteriaceae*. (A) Distribution of KPC; (B) distribution of OXA-48; (C) distribution of NDM. Legend colors (darkest to lightest): endemic, multiple outbreaks, sporadic, unknown.

carbapenemase-producing *Enterobacteriaceae* are thought to be at higher risk for nosocomial dissemination, as maintaining porin loss confers fitness cost to the bacteria, making this mechanism a lower risk for causing a sustained outbreak (56). Therefore, it is ideal to understand when a carbapenemase is present and apply strict epidemiologic interventions to prevent nosocomial spread (59, 60). If continued carbapenemase inhibitors with a specific spectrum become therapeutics (e.g., avibactam), understanding the enzyme present may be relevant in clinical decision making.

Other challenges with detection arise due to the bacterial species variability of isolates which carry a carbapenemase. For example, in my institution, investigators have seen multiple strains and species with various degrees of phenotypic resistance from multiple mechanisms, and therefore, the task of identification for a clinical laboratory is often overwhelming (61, 62). Guidance from the CDC on clinical microbiology screening has recommended that laboratories focus on *K. pneumoniae* and *E. coli*; however, depending on the outbreak, a carbapenemase gene can move among different species and strains, and this could miss many isolates depending on the outbreak (63). This is in direct contrast to resistance in some Gram-positive organisms, such as *Staphylococcus aureus*, in which the presence of *mecA* is responsible for almost all methicillin resistance seen globally. Also, even with the lowered breakpoints, not all of the isolates that carry a carbapenemase will demonstrate full phenotypic resistance to all carbapenems by susceptibility testing (62). It is very difficult for laboratory technicians to notice all variability across species with carbapenem resistance and know when an isolate needs further investigation, especially at small community hospital laboratories.

Screening with a molecular diagnostic could address many of these issues, but to run a PCR on all isolates would be extremely costly for laboratories where there are finite resources (64). This therefore would lead back to labs having the ability to identify high-risk isolates to target expensive molecular diagnostics. Reporting the molecular information also implies the presence of clinicians and infection control practitioners who can then interpret the data and this expertise may not be present in all hospitals around the world.

The final issue which is related to detection of carbapenemase-producing *Enterobacteriaceae* arises from our current approaches to molecular epidemiology of outbreaks and transmission. Most of the tools of molecular epidemiology relate to tracking a group of highly related bacteria based on chromosomal DNA. However, the carbapenemase gene rarely associates with the chromosomal DNA and can mobilize to different strains even during an outbreak (24). Even with the high resolution of whole-genome sequencing, tracking mobile elements through a bacterial population takes a great effort and requires costly long-read sequencing to fully resolve structures. Even when the mobile elements from outbreak strains can be fully analyzed, if there are gaps in the strains collected, it can be difficult to apply molecular epidemiology to string together relatedness and evolution to understand routes of transmission.

THE IMPACT OF THE GENETIC CONTEXT ON MOBILITY OF DIFFERENT CARBAPENEMASE GENES

As described above, the three most globally relevant carbapenemase genes have very different epidemiologies. This may be driven largely by the genetic environment surrounding the gene rather than the carbapenemase gene or enzyme it produces. *Enterobacteriaceae* have an incredible ability to evolve through horizontal gene transfer (Fig 2). With antibiotics widely used in health care and agriculture, acquisition of a plasmid which encodes antibiotic resistance can provide a selective advantage, but there may be other, unknown selective advantages for particular

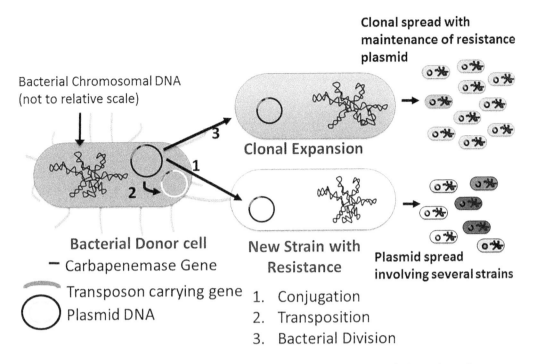

FIGURE 2 **Schematic of mechanisms of mobility of carbapenemase genes in *Enterobacteriaceae*.**

environments which are not as readily apparent. KPC, NDM, and OXA-48 are most frequently described to occur on plasmids which can mobilize between bacteria via conjugation. The range of species that will maintain any given plasmid is thought to be dependent on interplay between the host range of the plasmid and the bacterial host species. In addition, all three carbapenemase genes discussed at length in this chapter are located within a mobile transposon within a plasmid. A transposon can also mobilize to new genetic locations within a bacterial cell and integrate into DNA, which can provide the potential for further benefit to the bacterial host.

As described above, the majority of KPC outbreak descriptions detail a highly successful strain of *K. pneumoniae* as being introduced and disseminating among patients in a health care setting. This occurs even though the KPC gene is carried on a mobile plasmid which could disseminate among other species. Plasmid transfer via conjugation occurs at a surprisingly low rate clinically. It appears that the most common bla_{KPC} plasmid, pKpQiL, may provide additional benefit to the *K. pneumoniae* strain (65). When the bla_{KPC} plasmid is lost, the ST258 strains do not appear as well suited for success in a health care environment (66). The plasmids that carry bla_{KPC} in the ST258 *K. pneumoniae* are all also narrow-host-range type plasmids, which may also provide insight into why bla_{KPC} plasmids do not frequently mobilize to other species from ST258 *K. pneumoniae* (65).

The epidemiology of OXA-48 has also been potentially driven by the genetic environment rather than the gene itself. Original descriptions of bla_{OXA-48} were in differing strains of *E. coli* and *K. pneumoniae* with a conserved broad-host-range IncL/M, 62.5-kb plasmid (67). In contrast to the initial KPC descriptions, there were multiple strains and species involved as the outbreak evolved, while the plasmid remained relatively conserved, indicating likely plasmid mobilization and maintenance in multiple bacterial backgrounds. The OXA-48 gene is also located within a mobile composite transposon, Tn*1999*. Interestingly, in the widely spread bla_{OXA-48} IncL/M plasmid, Tn*1999* is inserted into a transfer inhibition (*tir*) gene which, when functional, decreases conjugation rates (68, 69). This *tir* gene disruption likely also contributes to the high rate of plasmid mobility which has promoted the multispecies epidemiology of the bla_{OXA-48} outbreak seen in Europe and Northern Africa.

Finally, bla_{NDM} has been identified in the largest number of different bacterial contexts and on multiple different plasmids, indicating that the mobility of the transposon associated with bla_{NDM} has been the most promiscuous from the outset. For example, one review found at least eight different incompatibility plasmid types and 22 different bla_{NDM} plasmid sizes in *E. coli* and *K. pneumoniae* from around the world (70). The immediate genetic environment adjacent to bla_{NDM} consists of an insertion sequence (IS*Aba125*) and a bleomycin resistance gene. The origin of bla_{NDM} mobility may have developed in *Acinetobacter baumannii* with a composite transposon, Tn*125*, where bla_{NDM} is located between two copies of IS*Aba125*. Several truncated versions of the Tn*125* have been described in almost all worldwide descriptions of bla_{NDM} (71), indicating that it was likely truncated over time after originating in *A. baumannii*. NDM has been identified with a much higher degree of epidemiologic and genetic diversity than in the majority of descriptions of OXA-48 and KPC. A recent account described NDM in *Pseudomonas aeruginosa*, *Acinetobacter* spp., and *Aeromonas* spp. as well as *Enterobacteriaceae* in multiple locations in the environment in Dhaka (72). Some of the environmental success has been attributed to the bleomycin gene, which may be advantageous for an environmental organism, as there could be low-level bleomycin-like compounds which result in bacterial toxicity (70). The high degree of horizontal gene transfer associated with bla_{NDM} is not confined to the environment, as this diversity has also been described clinically with a recent report of 11 different bacterial strains with multiple different plasmid types all carrying bla_{NDM} isolated from just four patients in Pakistan (42).

CONCLUSIONS

A recent World Health Organization report states that antimicrobial resistance is "a problem so serious that it threatens the achievements of modern medicine" (4). Ultimately, the medical community faces many new challenges posed by the wide dissemination of very successful genes of drug resistance between bacteria. Approaching this new type of clinically relevant resistance as gene-based outbreaks will challenge our current models of surveillance, molecular tracking, and detection. We will be required to realize the factors which contribute to horizontal gene transfer to understand the epidemiology and therefore the approach to slow the spread of these genes. The spread of organisms that carry multiple antimicrobial resistance mechanisms is anticipated to be more widely seen around the globe in the coming years, likely with significant clinical consequences. Carbapenemase-producing *Enterobacteriaceae* have all the qualities of an emerging infectious pathogen, with the ability to evolve and adapt central to their global success. Our ability to control the threat of continued spread will present new frontiers for the microbiology community and require that we adapt our methods of detection, molecular epidemiology, and infection control in ways that we have not yet fully realized but will likely bring new challenges.

CITATION

Mathers A. 2016. Mobilization of carbapenemase-mediated resistance in *Enterobacteriaceae*. Microbiol Spectrum 4(3):EI10-0010-2015.

REFERENCES

1. **Patel G, Huprikar S, Factor SH, Jenkins SG, Calfee DP.** 2008. Outcomes of carbapenem-resistant *Klebsiella pneumoniae* infection and the impact of antimicrobial and adjunctive therapies. *Infect Control Hosp Epidemiol* **29:**1099–1106.

2. **Centers for Disease Control and Prevention.** 2013. Vital signs: carbapenem-resistant *Enterobacteriaceae*. *MMWR Morb Mortal Wkly Rep* **62:**165–170.

3. **Falagas ME, Tansarli GS, Karageorgopoulos DE, Vardakas KZ.** 2014. Deaths attributable to carbapenem-resistant *Enterobacteriaceae* infections. *Emerg Infect Dis* **20:**1170–1175.

4. **World Health Organization.** 2014. *Antimicrobial Resistance: A Global Report on Surviellence.* World Health Organization, Geneva, Switzerland.

5. **Centers for Disease Control and Prevention.** 2013. *Antibiotic Resistance Threats in the United States.* Centers for Disease Control and Prevention, Atlanta, GA.

6. **Munoz-Price LS, Poirel L, Bonomo RA, Schwaber MJ, Daikos GL, Cormican M, Cornaglia G, Garau J, Gniadkowski M, Hayden MK, Kumarasamy K, Livermore DM, Maya JJ, Nordmann P, Patel JB, Paterson DL, Pitout J, Villegas MV, Wang H, Woodford N, Quinn JP.** 2013. Clinical epidemiology of the global expansion of *Klebsiella pneumoniae* carbapenemases. *Lancet Infect Dis* **13:**785–796.

7. **Hidron AI, Edwards JR, Patel J, Horan TC, Sievert DM, Pollock DA, Fridkin SK.** 2008. NHSN annual update: antimicrobial-resistant pathogens associated with healthcare-associated infections: annual summary of data reported to the National Healthcare Safety Network at the Centers for Disease Control and Prevention, 2006–2007. *Infect Control Hosp Epidemiol* **29:** 996–1011.

8. **Solomkin JS, Yellin AE, Rotstein OD, Christou NV, Dellinger EP, Tellado JM, Malafaia O, Fernandez A, Choe KA, Carides A, Satishchandran V, Teppler H.** 2003. Ertapenem versus piperacillin/tazobactam in the treatment of complicated intraabdominal infections: results of a double-blind, randomized comparative phase III trial. *Ann Surg* **237:**235–245.

9. **Biedenbach DJ, Moet GJ, Jones RN.** 2004. Occurrence and antimicrobial resistance pattern comparisons among bloodstream infection isolates from the SENTRY Antimicrobial Surveillance Program (1997–2002). *Diagn Microbiol Infect Dis* **50:**59–69.

10. **Martin GS, Mannino DM, Eaton S, Moss M.** 2003. The epidemiology of sepsis in the United States from 1979 through 2000. *N Engl J Med* **348:**1546–1554.

11. **Kollef MH, Shorr A, Tabak YP, Gupta V, Liu LZ, Johannes RS.** 2005. Epidemiology and outcomes of health-care-associated pneumonia: results from a large US database of culture-positive pneumonia. *Chest* **128:**3854–3862.

12. **Gaynes R, Edwards JR.** 2005. Overview of nosocomial infections caused by gram-negative bacilli. *Clin Infect Dis* **41:**848–854.

13. **Marchaim D, Navon-Venezia S, Schwaber MJ, Carmeli Y.** 2008. Isolation of imipenem-resistant *Enterobacter* species: emergence of KPC-2 carbapenemase, molecular characterization, epidemiology, and outcomes. *Antimicrob Agents Chemother* **52:**1413–1418.

14. **Borer A, Saidel-Odes L, Riesenberg K, Eskira S, Peled N, Nativ R, Schlaeffer F, Sherf M.** 2009. Attributable mortality rate for carbapenem-resistant *Klebsiella pneumoniae* bacteremia. *Infect Control Hosp Epidemiol* **30:**972–976.

15. **Neonakis IK, Samonis G, Messaritakis H, Baritaki S, Georgiladakis A, Maraki S, Spandidos DA.** 2010. Resistance status and evolution trends of *Klebsiella pneumoniae* isolates in a university hospital in Greece: ineffectiveness of carbapenems and increasing resistance to colistin. *Chemotherapy* **56:**448–452.

16. **Poirel L, Pitout JD, Nordmann P.** 2007. Carbapenemases: molecular diversity and clinical consequences. *Future Microbiol* **2:**501–512.

17. **Thomson KS.** 2010. Extended-spectrum-beta-lactamase, AmpC, and carbapenemase issues. *J Clin Microbiol* **48:**1019–1025.

18. **Bush K.** 2010. Alarming beta-lactamase-mediated resistance in multidrug-resistant *Enterobacteriaceae*. *Curr Opin Microbiol* **13:** 558–564.

19. **Tato M, Coque TM, Ruiz-Garbajosa P, Pintado V, Cobo J, Sader HS, Jones RN, Baquero F, Canton R.** 2007. Complex clonal and plasmid epidemiology in the first outbreak of *Enterobacteriaceae* infection involving VIM-1 metallo-beta-lactamase in Spain: toward endemicity? *Clin Infect Dis* **45:**1171–1178.

20. **Mathers AJ, Cox HL, Bonatti H, Kitchel B, Brassinga AK, Wispelwey B, Sawyer RG, Pruett TL, Hazen KC, Patel JB, Sifri CD.** 2009. Fatal cross infection by carbapenem-resistant *Klebsiella* in two liver transplant recipients. *Transpl Infect Dis* **11:**257–265.

21. **Carattoli A, Aschbacher R, March A, Larcher C, Livermore DM, Woodford N.** 2010. Complete nucleotide sequence of the IncN plasmid pKOX105 encoding VIM-1, QnrS1 and SHV-12 proteins in *Enterobacteriaceae* from Bolzano, Italy compared with IncN plasmids encoding

KPC enzymes in the USA. *J Antimicrob Chemother* **65:**2070–2075.

22. **Kumarasamy KK, Toleman MA, Walsh TR, Bagaria J, Butt F, Balakrishnan R, Chaudhary U, Doumith M, Giske CG, Irfan S, Krishnan P, Kumar AV, Maharjan S, Mushtaq S, Noorie T, Paterson DL, Pearson A, Perry C, Pike R, Rao B, Ray U, Sarma JB, Sharma M, Sheridan E, Thirunarayan MA, Turton J, Upadhyay S, Warner M, Welfare W, Livermore DM, Woodford N.** 2010. Emergence of a new antibiotic resistance mechanism in India, Pakistan, and the UK: a molecular, biological, and epidemiological study. *Lancet Infect Dis* **10:**597–602.

23. **Moellering RC Jr.** 2010. NDM-1—a cause for worldwide concern. *N Engl J Med* **363:**2377–2379.

24. **Mathers AJ, Cox HL, Kitchel B, Bonatti H, Brassinga AK, Carroll J, Scheld WM, Hazen KC, Sifri CD.** 2011. Molecular dissection of an outbreak of carbapenem-resistant Enterobacteriaceae reveals intergenus KPC carbapenemase transmission through a promiscuous plasmid. *mBio* **2:**e00204-11.

25. **Dupont H, Gaillot O, Goetgheluck AS, Plassart C, Emond JP, Lecuru M, Gaillard N, Derdouri S, Lemaire B, Girard de Courtilles M, Cattoir V, Mammeri H.** 2016. Molecular characterization of carbapenem-non-susceptible enterobacterial isolates collected during a prospective interregional survey in France and susceptibility to the novel ceftazidime-avibactam and aztreonam-avibactam combinations. *Antimicrob Agents Chemother* **60:**215–221.

26. **Yigit H, Queenan AM, Anderson GJ, Domenech-Sanchez A, Biddle JW, Steward CD, Alberti S, Bush K, Tenover FC.** 2001. Novel carbapenem-hydrolyzing beta-lactamase, KPC-1, from a carbapenem-resistant strain of *Klebsiella pneumoniae. Antimicrob Agents Chemother* **45:**1151–1161.

27. **Bratu S, Landman D, Haag R, Recco R, Eramo A, Alam M, Quale J.** 2005. Rapid spread of carbapenem-resistant *Klebsiella pneumoniae* in New York City: a new threat to our antibiotic armamentarium. *Arch Intern Med* **165:**1430–1435.

28. **Navon-Venezia S, Leavitt A, Schwaber MJ, Rasheed JK, Srinivasan A, Patel JB, Carmeli Y.** 2009. First report on a hyperepidemic clone of KPC-3-producing *Klebsiella pneumoniae* in Israel genetically related to a strain causing outbreaks in the United States. *Antimicrob Agents Chemother* **53:**818–820.

29. **Shen P, Wei Z, Jiang Y, Du X, Ji S, Yu Y, Li L.** 2009. Novel genetic environment of the carbapenem-hydrolyzing beta-lactamase KPC-2 among *Enterobacteriaceae* in China. *Antimicrob Agents Chemother* **53:**4333–4338.

30. **Villegas MV, Lolans K, Correa A, Kattan JN, Lopez JA, Quinn JP, Colombian Nosocomial Resistance Study Group.** 2007. First identification of *Pseudomonas aeruginosa* isolates producing a KPC-type carbapenem-hydrolyzing beta-lactamase. *Antimicrob Agents Chemother* **51:**1553–1555.

31. **da Silva RM, Traebert J, Galato D.** 2012. *Klebsiella pneumoniae* carbapenemase (KPC)-producing *Klebsiella pneumoniae*: a review of epidemiological and clinical aspects. *Expert Opin Biol Ther* **12:**663–671.

32. **Papadimitriou-Olivgeris M, Marangos M, Fligou F, Christofidou M, Bartzavali C, Anastassiou ED, Filos KS.** 2012. Risk factors for KPC-producing *Klebsiella pneumoniae* enteric colonization upon ICU admission. *J Antimicrob Chemother* **67:**2976–2981.

33. **Adler A, Hussein O, Ben-David D, Masarwa S, Navon-Venezia S, Schwaber MJ, Carmeli Y, Post-Acute-Care Hospital Carbapenem-Resistant Enterobacteriaceae Working Group.** 2015. Persistence of *Klebsiella pneumoniae* ST258 as the predominant clone of carbapenemase-producing *Enterobacteriaceae* in post-acute-care hospitals in Israel, 2008–13. *J Antimicrob Chemother* **70:**89–92.

34. **Poirel L, Heritier C, Tolun V, Nordmann P.** 2004. Emergence of oxacillinase-mediated resistance to imipenem in *Klebsiella pneumoniae. Antimicrob Agents Chemother* **48:**15–22.

35. **Glupczynski Y, Huang TD, Bouchahrouf W, Rezende de Castro R, Bauraing C, Gerard M, Verbruggen AM, Deplano A, Denis O, Bogaerts P.** 2012. Rapid emergence and spread of OXA-48-producing carbapenem-resistant *Enterobacteriaceae* isolates in Belgian hospitals. *Int J Antimicrob Agents* **39:**168–172.

36. **Zowawi HM, Sartor AL, Balkhy HH, Walsh TR, Al Johani SM, AlJindan RY, Alfaresi M, Ibrahim E, Al-Jardani A, Al-Abri S, Al Salman J, Dashti AA, Kutbi AH, Schlebusch S, Sidjabat HE, Paterson DL.** 2014. Molecular characterization of carbapenemase-producing *Escherichia coli* and *Klebsiella pneumoniae* in the countries of the Gulf Cooperation Council: dominance of OXA-48 and NDM producers. *Antimicrob Agents Chemother* **58:**3085–3090.

37. **Palacios-Baena ZR, Oteo J, Conejo C, Larrosa MN, Bou G, Fernández-Martínez M, González-López JJ, Pintado V, Martínez-Martínez L, Merino M, Pomar V, Mora-Rillo M, Rivera MA, Oliver A, Ruiz-Carrascoso G, Ruiz-Garbajosa P, Zamorano L, Bautista V, Ortega A, Morales I, Pascual Á, Campos J, Rodríguez-**

Baño J, GEIH-GEMARA (SEIMC) and REIPI Group for CPE. 2016. Comprehensive clinical and epidemiological assessment of colonisation and infection due to carbapenemase-producing *Enterobacteriaceae* in Spain. *J Infect* **72:**152–160.

38. **Cho SY, Huh HJ, Baek JY, Chung NY, Ryu JG, Ki CS, Chung DR, Lee NY, Song JH.** 2015. *Klebsiella pneumoniae* co-producing NDM-5 and OXA-181 carbapenemases, South Korea. *Emerg Infect Dis* **21:**1088–1089.

39. **Castanheira M, Deshpande LM, Mathai D, Bell JM, Jones RN, Mendes RE.** 2011. Early dissemination of NDM-1- and OXA-181-producing *Enterobacteriaceae* in Indian hospitals: report from the SENTRY Antimicrobial Surveillance Program, 2006–2007. *Antimicrob Agents Chemother* **55:**1274–1278.

40. **Kayama S, Koba Y, Shigemoto N, Kuwahara R, Kakuhama T, Kimura K, Hisatsune J, Onodera M, Yokozaki M, Ohge H, Sugai M.** 2015. Imipenem-susceptible, meropenem-resistant *Klebsiella pneumoniae* producing OXA-181 in Japan. *Antimicrob Agents Chemother* **59:**1379–1380.

41. **Walsh TR, Weeks J, Livermore DM, Toleman MA.** 2011. Dissemination of NDM-1 positive bacteria in the New Delhi environment and its implications for human health: an environmental point prevalence study. *Lancet Infect Dis* **11:**355–362.

42. **Wailan AM, Sartor AL, Zowawi HM, Perry JD, Paterson DL, Sidjabat HE.** 2015. Genetic contexts of blaNDM-1 in patients carrying multiple NDM-producing strains. *Antimicrob Agents Chemother* **59:**7405–7410.

43. **Epson EE, Pisney LM, Wendt JM, MacCannell DR, Janelle SJ, Kitchel B, Rasheed JK, Limbago BM, Gould CV, Kallen AJ, Barron MA, Bamberg WM.** 2014. Carbapenem-resistant *Klebsiella pneumoniae* producing New Delhi metallo-β-lactamase at an acute care hospital, Colorado, 2012. *Infect Control Hosp Epidemiol* **35:**390–397.

44. **Clinical Laboratory and Standards Institute.** 2012. *Performance Standards for Antimicrobial Susceptibility Testing. M100-S22.* Clinical and Laboratory Standards Institute, Wayne, PA.

45. **McGettigan SE, Andreacchio K, Edelstein PH.** 2009. Specificity of ertapenem susceptibility screening for detection of *Klebsiella pneumoniae* carbapenemases. *J Clin Microbiol* **47:**785–786.

46. **Tenover FC, Kalsi RK, Williams PP, Carey RB, Stocker S, Lonsway D, Rasheed JK, Biddle JW, McGowan JE Jr, Hanna B.** 2006. Carbapenem resistance in *Klebsiella pneumoniae* not detected by automated susceptibility testing. *Emerg Infect Dis* **12:**1209–1213.

47. **Anderson KF, Lonsway DR, Rasheed JK, Biddle J, Jensen B, McDougal LK, Carey RB, Thompson A, Stocker S, Limbago B, Patel JB.** 2007. Evaluation of methods to identify the *Klebsiella pneumoniae* carbapenemase in *Enterobacteriaceae. J Clin Microbiol* **45:**2723–2725.

48. **Daikos GL, Petrikkos P, Psichogiou M, Kosmidis C, Vryonis E, Skoutelis A, Georgousi K, Tzouvelekis LS, Tassios PT, Bamia C, Petrikkos G.** 2009. Prospective observational study of the impact of VIM-1 metallo-beta-lactamase on the outcome of patients with *Klebsiella pneumoniae* bloodstream infections. *Antimicrob Agents Chemother* **53:**1868–1873.

49. **Weisenberg SA, Morgan DJ, Espinal-Witter R, Larone DH.** 2009. Clinical outcomes of patients with *Klebsiella pneumoniae* carbapenemase-producing *K. pneumoniae* after treatment with imipenem or meropenem. *Diagn Microbiol Infect Dis* **64:**233–235.

50. **Falcone M, Mezzatesta ML, Perilli M, Forcella C, Giordano A, Cafiso V, Amicosante G, Stefani S, Venditti M.** 2009. Infections with VIM-1 metallo-β-lactamase-producing *Enterobacter cloacae* and their correlation with clinical outcome. *J Clin Microbiol* **47:**3514–3519.

51. **Daikos GL, Markogiannakis A.** 2011. Carbapenemase-producing *Klebsiella pneumoniae*: (when) might we still consider treating with carbapenems? *Clin Microbiol Infect* **17:**1135–1141.

52. **Clinical Laboratory and Standards Institute.** 2010. *Performance Standards for Antimicrobial Susceptibility Testing. M100-S20 U.* Clinical and Laboratory Standards Institute, Wayne, PA.

53. **Clinical Laboratory and Standards Institute.** 2009. *Performance Standards for Antimicrobial Susceptibility Testing. M100-S19.* Clinical and Laboratory Standards Institute, Wayne, PA.

54. **Clinical Laboratory and Standards Institute.** 2010. *Performance Standards for Antimicrobial Susceptibility Testing. M100-S20,* 20th ed. Clinical and Laboratory Standards Institute, Wayne, PA.

55. **Ruiz E, Ocampo-Sosa AA, Rezusta A, Revillo MJ, Roman E, Torres C, Martinez-Martinez L.** 2012. Acquisition of carbapenem resistance in multiresistant *Klebsiella pneumoniae* strains harbouring bla$_{CTX-M-15}$, qnrS1 and aac (6')-Ib-cr genes. *J Med Microbiol* **61**(Part 5)**:**672–677.

56. **Doumith M, Ellington MJ, Livermore DM, Woodford N.** 2009. Molecular mechanisms disrupting porin expression in ertapenem-resistant *Klebsiella* and *Enterobacter* spp. clinical isolates from the UK. *J Antimicrob Chemother* **63:**659–667.

57. **Bennett JW, Mende K, Herrera ML, Yu X, Lewis JS 2nd, Wickes BL, Jorgensen JH, Murray CK.** 2010. Mechanisms of carbapenem resistance among a collection of *Enterobacteriaceae* clinical isolates in a Texas city. *Diagn Microbiol Infect Dis* **66**:445–448.

58. **Davies TA, Marie Queenan A, Morrow BJ, Shang W, Amsler K, He W, Lynch AS, Pillar C, Flamm RK.** 2011. Longitudinal survey of carbapenem resistance and resistance mechanisms in *Enterobacteriaceae* and non-fermenters from the USA in 2007–09. *J Antimicrob Chemother* **66**:2298–2307.

59. **Garcia-Sureda L, Domenech-Sanchez A, Barbier M, Juan C, Gasco J, Alberti S.** 2011. OmpK26, a novel porin associated with carbapenem resistance in *Klebsiella pneumoniae*. *Antimicrob Agents Chemother* **55**:4742–4747.

60. **García-Fernández A, Miriagou V, Papagiannitsis CC, Giordano A, Venditti M, Mancini C, Carattoli A.** 2010. An ertapenem-resistant extended-spectrum-beta-lactamase-producing *Klebsiella pneumoniae* clone carries a novel OmpK36 porin variant. *Antimicrob Agents Chemother* **54**:4178–4184.

61. **Mathers AJ, Hazen KC, Carroll J, Yeh AJ, Cox HL, Bonomo RA, Sifri CD.** 2013. First clinical cases of OXA-48-producing carbapenem-resistant *Klebsiella pneumoniae* in the United States: the "menace" arrives in the New World. *J Clin Microbiol* **51**:680–683.

62. **Mathers AJ, Carroll J, Sifri CD, Hazen KC.** 2013. Modified Hodge test versus indirect carbapenemase test: prospective evaluation of a phenotypic assay for detection of *Klebsiella pneumoniae* carbapenemase (KPC) in *Enterobacteriaceae*. *J Clin Microbiol* **51**:1291–1293.

63. **Centers for Disease Control and Prevention.** 2009. Guidance for control of infections with carbapenem-resistant or carbapenemase-producing *Enterobacteriaceae* in acute care facilities. *MMWR Morb Mortal Wkly Rep* **58**:256–260.

64. **Mathers AJ, Poulter M, Dirks D, Carroll J, Sifri CD, Hazen KC.** 2014. Clinical microbiology costs for methods of active surveillance for *Klebsiella pneumoniae* carbapenemase-producing *Enterobacteriaceae*. *Infect Control Hosp Epidemiol* **35**:350–355.

65. **Mathers AJ, Peirano G, Pitout JD.** 2015. The role of epidemic resistance plasmids and international high-risk clones in the spread of multidrug-resistant *Enterobacteriaceae*. *Clin Microbiol Rev* **28**:565–591.

66. **Adler A, Paikin S, Sterlin Y, Glick J, Edgar R, Aronov R, Schwaber MJ, Carmeli Y.** 2012. A swordless knight: epidemiology and molecular characteristics of the blaKPC-negative sequence type 258 *Klebsiella pneumoniae* clone. *J Clin Microbiol* **50**:3180–3185.

67. **Poirel L, Potron A, Nordmann P.** 2012. OXA-48-like carbapenemases: the phantom menace. *J Antimicrob Chemother* **67**:1597–1606.

68. **Poirel L, Bonnin RA, Nordmann P.** 2012. Genetic features of the widespread plasmid coding for the carbapenemase OXA-48. *Antimicrob Agents Chemother* **56**:559–562.

69. **Potron A, Poirel L, Nordmann P.** 2014. Derepressed transfer properties leading to the efficient spread of the plasmid encoding carbapenemase OXA-48. *Antimicrob Agents Chemother* **58**:467–471.

70. **Johnson AP, Woodford N.** 2013. Global spread of antibiotic resistance: the example of New Delhi metallo-β-lactamase (NDM)-mediated carbapenem resistance. *J Med Microbiol* **62**:499–513.

71. **Dortet L, Poirel L, Nordmann P.** 2014. Worldwide dissemination of the NDM-type carbapenemases in Gram-negative bacteria. *Biomed Res Int* **2014**:249856.

72. **Toleman MA, Bugert JJ, Nizam SA.** 2015. Extensively drug-resistant New Delhi metallo-β-lactamase-encoding bacteria in the environment, Dhaka, Bangladesh, 2012. *Emerg Infect Dis* **21**:1027–1030.

Antimicrobial Resistance Expressed by *Neisseria gonorrhoeae*: A Major Global Public Health Problem in the 21st Century

12

MAGNUS UNEMO,[1] CARLOS DEL RIO,[2] and WILLIAM M. SHAFER[3,4]

GONORRHEA AND *NEISSERIA GONORRHOEAE*

The sexually transmitted infection gonorrhea is a very old malady that can be traced to ancient Chinese, Egyptian, Roman, and Greek literature as well as in the Old Testament of the Bible (Leviticus 15:1–3). *Neisseria gonorrhoeae* (gonococcus), the obligate human pathogen and etiological agent of gonorrhea, is primarily transmitted from an infected individual by direct human-to-human contact between the mucosal membranes of the urogenital tract, anal canal, and the oropharynx, usually during sexual activities. Neonates can be infected during passage through the birth canal if the mother has urogenital gonorrhea. After transmission, *N. gonorrhoeae* causes urethritis in males and cervicitis in females. Relatively few males (≤10%) but a large proportion of females (≥50%) can have an asymptomatic urogenital infection. Rectal and pharyngeal gonorrhea is commonly asymptomatic in both genders. These infections are most frequently identified in men who have sex with men (MSM), but dependent on sexual practice, they can be encountered in both

[1]WHO Collaborating Centre for Gonorrhoea and Other STIs, Department of Laboratory Medicine, Microbiology, Örebro University Hospital, SE-701 85 Örebro, Sweden; [2]Hubert Department of Global Health, Rollins School of Public Health of Emory University and Department of Medicine, Division of Infectious Diseases; [3]Department of Microbiology and Immunology, Emory University School of Medicine, Atlanta, GA 30322; [4]Veterans Affairs Medical Center (Atlanta), Decatur, GA 30033.

Emerging Infections 10
Edited by W. Michael Scheld, James M. Hughes and Richard J. Whitley
© 2016 American Society for Microbiology, Washington, DC
doi:10.1128/microbiolspec.EI10-0009-2015

genders in many settings. Urogenital infections, if untreated, might ascend to the upper genital tract and result in severe reproductive complications (mostly, but not only, in females), such as pelvic inflammatory disease in women and epididymitis (rare) in men, that can result in infertility or, for women, even loss of life through ectopic pregnancy. Gonococcal infections also facilitate the transmission and acquisition of HIV (1–4). *N. gonorrhoeae* may also cause conjunctivitis, mostly in neonates (ophthalmia neonatorum) infected by their mothers during delivery but also in adults. Conjunctivitis may, if untreated, result in blindness. Disseminated gonococcal infection is an uncommon complication of gonococcal infection; although it is rare, this can lead to, for example, arthritis, meningitis, and endocarditis (1, 2, 5, 6).

Gonorrhea has remained a major global public health concern, and in 2012, the World Health Organization (WHO) estimated 78.3 million cases among adults (15 to 49 years of age) worldwide. The largest burdens were in the WHO Western Pacific region (35.2 million cases), WHO South-East Asia region (11.4 million cases), and WHO Africa region (11.4 million cases) (7). Nevertheless, the number of reported cases is much lower, particularly from resource-poor settings, than the true number of cases due to poor diagnostics, lack of laboratory testing, and incomplete case reporting. In the United States, gonorrhea is the second most commonly reported notifiable disease. In 2013, a total of 333,004 cases of gonorrhea were reported, and the national gonorrhea rate was 106.1 cases per 100,000 population (http://www.cdc.gov/std/stats13/gonorrhea.htm). As in previous years, the South had the highest rate of reported gonorrhea cases (128.6 cases per 100,000 population), followed by the Midwest (108.6 cases per 100,000 population), Northeast (85.5 cases per 100,000 population), and West (83.5 cases per 100,000 population).

In the absence of a gonococcal vaccine, public health control of gonorrhea relies entirely on appropriate generalized and targeted prevention efforts, sexual contact notification, epidemiological surveillance, diagnosis, and particularly the availability of effective antimicrobial treatment. *N. gonorrhoeae* was initially highly susceptible to many antimicrobials. However, since the introduction of sulfonamides for treatment of gonorrhea in the 1930s *N. gonorrhoeae* has repeatedly shown an extraordinary capacity to develop resistance to all antimicrobials introduced for treatment during the past 70 to 80 years. Currently, the prevalence of gonococcal strains with resistance to most antimicrobials previously recommended for treatment (e.g., sulfonamides, penicillins, early-generation cephalosporins, tetracyclines, macrolides, and fluoroquinolones) is high in many settings. The recent emergence of resistance to the extended-spectrum cephalosporins (ESCs) cefixime and ceftriaxone, and emergence of *N. gonorrhoeae* strains exhibiting high-level clinical resistance to all ESCs (8–12), combined with resistance to nearly all other available gonorrhea antimicrobials (including azithromycin, which is now recommended with ceftriaxone in dual therapy of gonorrhea), is of grave concern (1, 11–20). The ESCs are at the front line of antimicrobial therapy, and treatment failures particularly with cefixime, but also sporadically with ceftriaxone (mainly pharyngeal gonorrhea), have been verified in Japan, Australia, several European countries, Canada, and South Africa (11, 12, 21). This developing situation requires immediate international attention and resources internationally. The emergence of resistance to ESCs is a public health concern also in the United States, and in 2013, the U.S. Centers for Disease Control and Prevention (CDC) included *N. gonorrhoeae* on the list of organisms for which drug resistance is an urgent public health threat (http://www.cdc.gov/drugresistance/pdf/ar-threats-2013-508.pdf). *N. gonorrhoeae* has additionally been classified by the CDC as a "superbug" and the prospect of untreatable gonorrhea was voiced in 2012 by both the CDC (18) and WHO (1). Clearly, we are now facing a threatening major public health crisis that could result in significant reproductive morbidity (including infertility) and socioeconomic cost worldwide.

ANTIMICROBIAL RESISTANCE IN *NEISSERIA GONORRHOEAE*

Mechanisms of Antimicrobial Resistance

For rapid adaptation and survival in hostile environments, *N. gonorrhoeae* has an extraordinary capacity to alter its DNA because it is naturally competent for transformation during its entire life cycle and it can also, particularly when exposed to selective pressure, effectively change its genome through all types of mutations. In this way, *N. gonorrhoeae* has evolved and acquired or developed all known mechanisms of physiological resistance to all antimicrobials used for treatment, e.g., (i) antimicrobial destruction or modification by enzymes (e.g., the action of β-lactamases; see below), (ii) target modification or protection-reducing affinity for the antimicrobials, (iii) decreased influx of antimicrobials, and (iv) increased efflux of antimicrobials (12). Most gonococcal antimicrobial resistance (AMR) determinants are located chromosomally, and only the *bla*$_{TEM}$ gene (22, 23) and the *tetM* gene (24), which result in high-level resistance to penicillin and tetracycline, respectively, are known to be plasmid borne; these determinants can be transferred between gonococcal strains by transformation or conjugation. For many antimicrobials and AMR determinants, acquisition of a single AMR determinant confers only an incremental MIC increase without clinical importance (i.e., the MIC remains below the so-called resistance breakpoint). Importantly, however, the cumulative effects of several AMR determinants and their interactions can ultimately result in AMR of clinical importance that would result

in clinical treatment failure if the particular antibiotic was used in monotherapy. The known gonococcal AMR determinants and mechanisms of action are summarized in Table 1 (12).

In general, AMR strains of different bacterial species have advantages both *in vitro* and *in vivo* over antimicrobial-susceptible strains in the presence of the specific antimicrobial; however, the AMR strains also frequently have lower fitness in the absence of the antimicrobial (25–27). This decreased fitness of the AMR strains can, however, be restored through compensatory mutations, which frequently occur *in vitro* and most likely also *in vivo*. In *N. gonorrhoeae*, most of the AMR mechanisms do not appear to cause significantly lower biological fitness (with or without compensatory mutations), which results in the persistence of AMR strains also in the absence of obvious antimicrobial selection from the gonorrhea treatment (12). Nevertheless, a general antimicrobial pressure in the community due to the use of antimicrobials for other infectious diseases remains. Some AMR determinants (e.g., *mtrR* and *gyrA* mutations) might even enhance the fitness of at least some *N. gonorrhoeae* strains (28, 29). Unfortunately, this shows that the prospect of being able to use earlier abandoned antimicrobials, such as penicillin, tetracycline, or fluoroquinolones, for gonorrhea treatment is extremely unlikely (11, 12, 15).

Below, we describe AMR systems identified in gonococci from a historical perspective based on the timeline of introduction of a particular antimicrobial for treatment of gonorrhea.

Sulfonamide Resistance

Sulfonamides target the bacterial dihydropteroate synthase enzymes to inhibit folic acid synthesis in the gonococci. Since sulfonamides were introduced as the first antimicrobials for treatment of gonorrhea in the mid-1930s, *N. gonorrhoeae* has repeatedly shown an extraordinary capacity to develop

TABLE 1 Main antimicrobial resistance determinants in *Neisseria gonorrhoeae* for previously and currently recommended antimicrobials for treatment of gonorrhea (adapted from reference 12)

Antimicrobial(s)	Resistance determinants/mechanism
Sulfonamides	Dilution of antimicrobial by oversynthesis of *p*-aminobenzoic acid
	folP mutations: SNPs or mosaic *folP* gene, including commensal *Neisseria* sequences
Penicillins	*penA* mutations: D345 amino acid insertion in PBP2 plus 4–8 associated amino acid alterations in the PBP2 carboxyl-terminal region or mosaic *penA* alleles, encoding up to 70 PBP2 amino acid alterations, including sequences from nongonococcal *Neisseria* species
	mtrR mutations: in promoter (frequently a single A deletion in the 13-bp inverted repeat sequence) or coding sequence (usually a G45D amino acid alteration)
	porB1b (*penB*) SNPs: alterations in amino acid codons G120 and A121D of PorB1b
	pilQ SNP: E666K alteration (found only in laboratory strains)
	ponA SNP: "*ponA1* determinant" (L421P alteration)
	"Factor X": unknown nontransformable determinant
	Penicillinase (TEM-1 or TEM-135)-encoding plasmids
Tetracyclines	*rpsJ* SNP: V57M alteration
	mtrR mutations; see above
	penB mutations; see above
	pilQ mutation; see above
	TetM-encoding plasmids
Spectinomycin	16S rRNA SNP: C1192U substitution
	rpsE mutations: T24P alteration, V25 deletion, and K26E alteration
Fluoroquinolones	*gyrA* SNPs: frequently S91F, D95N, and D95G alterations
	parC SNPs: frequently D86N, S88P, and E91K alterations
Macrolides	*23S rRNA* SNPs: C2611T and A2059G, resulting in low-level and high-level resistances, respectively
	mtrR mutations; see above. Additional more rare macrolide resistance determinants exist (12).
Extended-spectrum cephalosporins	Mosaic *penA* alleles: mosaic *penA* alleles, encoding up to 70 PBP2 amino acid alterations, including sequences from nongonococcal *Neisseria* species. Amino acid alterations confirmed to contribute to resistance include A311V, I312M, V316T, V316P, T483S, A501P, A501V, N512Y, and G545S.
	penA SNPs: A501V and A501T alterations in nonmosaic alleles
	mtrR mutations; see above
	penB mutations; see above
	"Factor X": unknown nontransformable determinant

resistance to all antimicrobials introduced for treatment during the past 70 to 80 years. Already by the late 1940s, >90% of *N. gonorrhoeae* isolates were resistant *in vitro* to sulfonamides (30, 31), and their use was halted in the United States due to the high prevalence of strains exhibiting resistance. Sulfonamide resistance can be due to oversynthesis of *p*-aminobenzoic acid or alterations in the *folP* gene encoding the drug target dihydropteroate synthase (32–34).

Penicillin Resistance

β-Lactam antimicrobials, such as penicillins and cephalosporins, inhibit the peptidogly-can cross-links in the bacterial cell wall through binding of the β-lactam ring to transpeptidase enzymes (penicillin-binding proteins [PBPs]). Penicillin was discovered accidently by Alexander Fleming in 1928, but it took until 1943 before penicillin was adequately validated to be highly effective for gonococcal urethritis. Penicillin rapidly became the recommended first-line treatment for gonorrhea (35, 36). However, during the following decades the penicillin MICs in gonococcal strains increased, due to emergence of chromosomal AMR determinants, and the recommended doses had to be progressively increased for cure (12, 15, 37–43). The emergence and subsequent international spread of two types of β-lactamase-encoding plasmids, originating in Southeast Asia and sub-Saharan West Africa, in certain gonococcal strains from the United States and United Kingdom in 1976, which caused high-level resistance to penicillin (22, 23), reinforced the fear that the effectiveness of penicillin might soon end. Nevertheless, the main reason to abandon penicillin as a first-line treatment in the United States and many other countries about a decade later was the emergence of chromosomally mediated clinical resistance to penicillin (44, 45). Currently, gonococcal strains with plasmid-mediated and/or chromosomally mediated resistance to penicillin are common globally (4, 11, 12, 15, 46–54). Gonococcal strains with plasmid-mediated resistance to penicillin usually contain plasmids with a bla_{TEM-1} or $bla_{TEM-135}$ gene encoding a TEM-1 or TEM-135 type of β-lactamase. This enzyme hydrolyzes the cyclic amide bond of β-lactamase-susceptible penicillins, opening the β-lactam ring and rendering the penicillin inactive. Chromosomally mediated penicillin resistance in gonococci is due to specific mutations that modify the target proteins (primary target PBP2 encoded by the *penA* gene and PBP1 encoded by the *ponA* gene), increased efflux of penicillin through the efflux pump MtrCDE due to mutations that increase expression of the *mtrCDE* operon, and decreased influx of penicillin through the porin PorB (interestingly, this phenotype is apparent only in strains with the *mtrR* resistance determinant) and, at least in laboratory isolates, through the pore-forming secretin PilQ (see the work of Unemo and Shafer [12] for an extensive review of these AMR systems). Nevertheless, the described *pilQ* mutations will most likely not be found in any clinical *N. gonorrhoeae* isolates because they destroy the proper formation of the type IV pili, which are essential for gonococcal pathogenesis (55). Finally, at least one nontransformable unknown resistance determinant, the so-called "factor X," exists (11, 12).

Tetracycline Resistance

Tetracyclines inhibit the binding of aminoacyl-tRNA to the mRNA-ribosome complex by binding to the 30S ribosomal subunit, resulting in an inhibition of protein synthesis. Tetracyclines were used early in clinical medicine to treat gonorrhea, particularly in patients with penicillin allergy. Nevertheless, the tetracycline MICs in *N. gonorrhoeae* strains increased over time, due to an accumulation of chromosomal resistance determinants (40). In the mid-1980s, the emergence of *tetM*-possessing conjugative plasmids (24) causing high-level tetracycline resistance resulted in the exclusion of tetracycline from treatment guidelines in the United States and in many other countries worldwide. These gonococcal strains with plasmid-mediated resistance to tetracyclines are now widespread internationally (4, 11, 12, 15, 46–52). TetM confers resistance to tetracycline by binding to the ribosomes and causing the release of tetracycline, thereby permitting protein synthesis to proceed. Chromosomally mediated tetracycline resistance in *N. gonorrhoeae* is due to mutations that modify the target (ribosomal protein S10 encoded by the *rpsJ* gene), increased efflux through the MtrCDE efflux pump, and decreased influx through the PorB porin (12).

Spectinomycin Resistance

Spectinomycin binds to the 30S ribosomal subunit of the bacterium and inhibits protein translation. In detail, spectinomycin interacts with 16S rRNA and during polypeptide elongation blocks the elongation factor G-catalyzed translocation of the peptidyl-tRNA from the A site to the P site. After the emergence of plasmid-mediated high-level resistance to penicillin, the aminocyclitol spectinomycin, synthesized in the early 1960s, was frequently used for treatment of these cases (56, 57). Nevertheless, by 1967, the first spectinomycin-resistant gonococcal strain was reported in the Netherlands

(58). In 1981 in Korea, spectinomycin was introduced as first-line gonorrhea treatment in U.S. military personnel. Only 4 years later, 8.2% of the gonorrhea cases showed clinical resistance to spectinomycin (59). Subsequently, spectinomycin was abandoned as a first-line monotherapy for gonorrhea internationally. In addition, spectinomycin was never a good drug to treat pharyngeal gonococcal infection. Currently, particularly high-level spectinomycin resistance in *N. gonorrhoeae* strains is exceedingly rare globally, including in South Korea, where no spectinomycin-resistant gonococcal strain has been identified since 1993, despite spectinomycin being frequently used in the treatment of gonorrhea (60). However, spectinomycin is currently not frequently used in most countries (and is often not available), and resistance might be rapidly selected if spectinomycin is introduced as a first-line treatment (61–63). Spectinomycin is not available in the United States. High-level resistance to spectinomycin (MIC > 1,024 µg/ml) in *N. gonorrhoeae* was early shown to be caused by a C1192U single nucleotide polymorphism (SNP) in the spectinomycin-binding region of helix 34 in 16S rRNA (64, 65). Recently, specific alterations in the *rpsE*-encoded 30S ribosomal protein S5 were also confirmed to result in high-level or low-level spectinomycin resistance (128 µg/ml) (12, 66, 67).

Fluoroquinolone Resistance

Fluoroquinolones act by inhibition of DNA gyrase and topoisomerase IV. Bacterial DNA gyrase and topoisomerase IV belong to the type II topoisomerases, are highly conserved, and are essential for the metabolism of DNA in the bacterial cell. Their actions include breaking and rejoining the double-stranded DNA in a reaction that is coupled with ATP hydrolysis in the bacterial cell. Fluoroquinolones, particularly ciprofloxacin but also ofloxacin, were first-line recommendations and widely used for empirical gonorrhea

treatment worldwide from the middle or late 1980s onward. However, resistance emerged and spread quickly, initially in the Asian Western Pacific region (68, 69). In some of these countries, ciprofloxacin was abandoned as a first-line treatment by the middle to late 1990s (12, 15). Ciprofloxacin-resistant gonococcal strains were then quickly exported internationally or emerged independently (70–72). In the United States, ciprofloxacin-resistant strains, initially imported from Asia, were prevalent in Hawaii in the year 2000 (73), and these strains were then disseminated first to the West Coast and then to the rest of the United States, predominantly among MSM (74). In 2007, all fluoroquinolones were excluded from the CDC-recommended treatment regimens for gonorrhea (75); it was this exclusion and the discontinuation of penicillin and tetracycline for gonorrhea treatment that elevated *N. gonorrhoeae* to the infamous "superbug" status. Many Asian and European countries had abandoned ciprofloxacin as a first-line option for empirical treatment already in the early to middle 2000s (12, 15). The prevalence of ciprofloxacin-resistant gonococcal strains has remained high globally (4, 11, 12, 15, 46–54). Gonococci develop ciprofloxacin resistance through mutations that reduce the ciprofloxacin binding affinity of DNA gyrase (encoded by the *gyrA* and *gyrB* genes) and topoisomerase IV (encoded by the *parC* and *parE* genes). The primary target gene is *gyrA*; however, isolates with higher levels of resistance additionally have specific SNPs in *parC* (12).

Macrolide Resistance

Macrolides block protein synthesis by binding to the 50S ribosomal subunit, preventing translocation of the peptidyl-tRNA, blocking the peptide exit channel in 50S subunits by interacting with 23S rRNA, and causing ribosomes to release incomplete polypeptides (76). Azithromycin was developed as a synthetic derivative of erythromycin in 1980.

Azithromycin had a significantly higher activity than erythromycin against *N. gonorrhoeae*. Nevertheless, by the middle to late 1990s, resistance to azithromycin was reported from Latin America (77, 78). Resistance to azithromycin subsequently emerged in many countries (47–50, 79). At present, rare *N. gonorrhoeae* strains with high-level azithromycin resistance (MIC ≥ 256 µg/ml) have also been identified in Scotland (80), England (80), Ireland (81), Italy (82), Sweden (83), Australia (84), China (85), Argentina (86), the United States (87), and Canada (88). Currently, azithromycin is not recommended for empirical monotherapy of gonorrhea (2, 12, 21, 80, 89, 90); however, this drug is administered together with ceftriaxone in the dual antimicrobial gonorrhea therapy (2, 91, 92). Gonococcal resistance to azithromycin can result from alterations of the ribosomal target (blocking or reducing the target affinity for the drug), e.g., by rRNA methylase-associated modification or specific SNPs in the peptidyl transferase domain V of 23S rRNA and/or an overexpressed efflux pump system, particularly the MtrCDE efflux pump but also *mef*-encoded and the MacAB efflux pumps (12).

Cephalosporin Resistance

Cephalosporins, like penicillins, inhibit the peptidoglycan cross-links in the bacterial cell wall through binding of the β-lactam ring to transpeptidase enzymes (PBPs). The most frequently used cephalosporins for treatment of gonorrhea have been the ESCs, the injectable ceftriaxone and the orally administered cefixime. No other ESCs have any evident advantages over these (2, 37, 93). However, other oral cephalosporins have been used in different countries (e.g., cefuroxime, cefpodoxime, ceftibuten, cefditoren, and cefdinir [12, 15, 37, 93–95]). During the last two decades, resistance to ESCs in *N. gonorrhoeae* strains appears to have initially emerged in Japan and subsequently spread worldwide. In Japan, many oral ESCs in

different dose regimens, including some with likely subinhibitory ESC concentrations and accordingly suboptimal efficacy, were used for monotherapy that can have selected for ESC resistance (11, 12, 96–100). In 1995, the first cefixime-resistant gonococcal strain was isolated in Kanagawa, Japan. After 1996, the prevalence of isolates with decreased susceptibility or resistance to cefixime significantly increased in Kanagawa, with a peak resistance level of 57.1% in 2002 (101). Also in other regions of Japan, such as Fukuoka and central Japan, the ESC *in vitro* resistance levels increased significantly during this time (97, 100). Clinical resistance to cefixime in regard to treatment failures was also observed early. From 1999 to 2001, eight treatment failures with cefixime (two doses of 200 mg orally, 6 h apart) were reported (99), and four treatment failures with an extended cefixime regimen (200 mg orally twice a day for 3 days) were documented in 2002 and 2003 (102). All oral ESCs were subsequently excluded in 2006 from the Japanese treatment guidelines, and ceftriaxone (1 g intravenously), which is mostly used, cefodizime (1 g intravenously), and spectinomycin (2 g intramuscularly [i.m.]) have been recommended since then for uncomplicated gonorrhea (103). During the last decade, *N. gonorrhoeae* strains with decreased susceptibility and resistance to ESCs have been disseminated mainly globally (11, 12, 15, 46–48, 50, 52–54, 79, 104–108). Treatment failures with cefixime have now been confirmed in Japan, several European countries, Canada, and South Africa, and rare treatment failures with ceftriaxone (only pharyngeal gonorrhea) have been identified in Japan, some European countries, and Australia (21).

The first *N. gonorrhoeae* extensively drug-resistant (XDR) strains showing high-level resistance to all ESCs, as well as resistance to mainly all other therapeutic gonorrhea antimicrobials, have also been identified in Kyoto, Japan (9), Quimper, France (10), and Catalonia, Spain (8). Worryingly, these XDR strains were all identified in high-frequency transmitting populations, i.e., female commercial sex workers or MSM. Nevertheless, based on the intensified surveillance undertaken in Kyoto and Osaka from 2010 and onwards after identification of the first XDR strain (H041), no similar strain with high-level ESC resistance has been identified in that local community (109) or elsewhere. No additional isolates of the XDR strains initially identified in France and Spain have been found. Consequently, this might indicate that these XDR strains suffer from a decreased biological fitness, which is currently under detailed investigation (11, 12, 109). ESC resistance in gonococci is due primarily to mutations that modify the target proteins (PBP2 encoded by the *penA* gene) but also to an increased efflux of ESC through the MtrCDE efflux pump and decreased influx of ESC through the porin PorB (12). The stepwise acquisition and interactions between these AMR determinants have been described for both penicillin (110) and ESCs (111). Mutations in the genes encoding PBP1 or PilQ have not been shown to contribute to ESC resistance yet; however, their contributions to resistance in future ESC-resistant strains cannot be excluded. Finally, as with penicillin resistance, at least one nontransformable unknown resistance determinant ("factor X") also increases the ESC MICs (9–12, 111).

INTERNATIONAL RESPONSES TO THE EMERGENCE OF EXCEEDINGLY DIFFICULT-TO-TREAT OR POSSIBLE UNTREATABLE GONORRHEA

The evolution of AMR, particularly the emergence of ceftriaxone resistance in gonococci, with retained resistance to all previously used therapeutic antimicrobials, and fear of exceedingly difficult-to-treat and even untreatable gonorrhea have resulted in great concern and attention internationally, that is, in lay media, the public health community, and scientific societies (12). Consequently, dual antimicrobial treatment regimens were

introduced as a first-line treatment for uncomplicated anogenital and pharyngeal gonorrhea in United States (91), Canada (112), Australia (113), and Europe (2). These treatment regimens are summarized in Table 2 and mainly include i.m. ceftriaxone (250 mg [91, 112] or 500 mg [2, 113], single dose) together with an oral single dose of azithromycin (1 g [91, 112, 113] or 2 g [2]). Furthermore, in 2012, to control and decrease the spread of multidrug-resistant gonococcal strains, the WHO, CDC, and European Centre for Disease Prevention and Control (ECDPC) published a global action plan and regional response plans, respectively (1, 18–20).

The AMR gonococcal strains do not recognize any borders, and accordingly, international actions, collaborations, and political will, advocacy, research, and funding are essential. Some key components of the WHO global action plan are summarized in Table 3. Briefly, these plans emphasize the need for a substantially increased awareness among clinical microbiologists, scientists, epidemiologists, and clinicians and on political levels, as well as more holistic actions. For example, these plans call for significant improvements in the prevention, diagnosis, contact tracing, treatment, and surveillance of gonorrhea, in order to reduce the global burden of infection, as essential to control the AMR emergence and spread internationally. Linked to this, it is essential to establish and/or strengthen existing strategies for general antimicrobial control (updated and implemented guidelines for appropriate use, selection, supplies, quality, etc.). There is also an urgent need for an enhanced focus on reducing the incidence of gonorrhea in high-risk frequently transmitting populations (such as commercial sex workers and particularly MSM) and effective prevention (e.g., condom use when practicing oral sex), diagnosis, and treatment of pharyngeal gonorrhea, which is significantly more difficult to eradicate and represents an asymptomatic reservoir for gonorrhea and emergence of

TABLE 2 Recommended treatments for uncomplicated *Neisseria gonorrhoeae* infections of the urethra, cervix, rectum, and pharynx in adults and youth in the United States, Canada, Australia, and Europe

Treatment	Recommendation by country			
	USA (91)	Canada (112)	Australia (113)	Europe (2)
First-line treatment for anogenital infections[a]	Ceftriaxone, one dose of 250 mg i.m., plus azithromycin, one dose of 1 g orally	Ceftriaxone, one dose of 250 mg i.m., plus azithromycin, one dose of 1 g orally, or cefixime, one dose of 800 mg orally, plus azithromycin, one dose of 1 g orally	Ceftriaxone, one dose of 500 mg i.m., plus azithromycin, one dose of 1 g orally	Ceftriaxone, one dose of 500 mg i.m., plus azithromycin, one dose of 2 g orally[b]
First-line treatment for pharyngeal infections	Same regimen as for anogenital gonorrhea	Ceftriaxone, one dose of 250 mg i.m., plus azithromycin, one dose of 1 g orally Alternative: cefixime, one dose of 800 mg orally, plus azithromycin, one dose of 1 g orally, or azithromycin, one dose of 2 g orally	Same regimen as for anogenital gonorrhea	Same regimen as for anogenital gonorrhea

[a]Uncomplicated gonococcal infections of the cervix, urethra, and rectum.
[b]Azithromycin tablets may be taken with or without food, but gastrointestinal side effects can be less pronounced if the drug is taken after food.

antimicrobial resistance. Implementation of test of cure is also crucial, particularly for pharyngeal gonorrhea, to identify treatment failures as well as reinfections. It is also evident that the global burden of gonococcal AMR is largely unknown, and accordingly, it is imperative to significantly enhance the quality-assured surveillance of *N. gonorrhoeae* AMR and verified gonorrhea treatment failures (using recommended treatment) locally, nationally, and internationally.

In the age of easy and rapid travelling, a global approach is certainly demanded. Accordingly, the WHO Global Gonococcal Antimicrobial Surveillance Programme (WHO Global GASP) was initiated in the early 1990s but was revisited and relaunched in 2009 (20). The WHO Global GASP network aims

TABLE 3 Key components of the WHO global action plan to control the spread and impact of antimicrobial resistance in *Neisseria gonorrhoeae*

Increase the awareness of appropriate use of antimicrobials among health care providers and consumers, particularly in high-risk frequently transmitting populations, including sex workers and MSM
Improve prevention, diagnosis, treatment, and control of gonorrhea, using prevention messages, interventions, effective and recommended diagnosis and antimicrobial treatment regimens
Systematic monitoring, early detection, and follow-up of clinical treatment failures with recommended treatment using a standard case definition of treatment failure and protocols for confirmation, reporting, and management of failure
Effective drug regulations and prescription policies
Strengthened and quality-assured antimicrobial susceptibility surveillance, particularly in settings with a high gonorrhea burden (and/or *N. gonorrhoeae* antimicrobial resistance), other sexually transmitted infections, and HIV
Build capacity to establish regional networks of laboratories to perform quality-assured gonococcal culture and antimicrobial susceptibility testing
Research to identify novel molecular methods to detect and monitor antimicrobial resistance
Research to identify and/or develop alternative strategies and/or novel antimicrobials (or other therapeutic compounds) for effective gonorrhea treatment (and, ideally, a vaccine)

to recruit laboratories worldwide to monitor gonococcal AMR data using quality-assured methods (with the main focus on ESCs), provide support to establish gonococcal culture and AMR testing, inform public health authorities and revisions of treatment guidelines on trends in gonococcal AMR, optimize early detection of emerging resistance, and identify and confirm treatment failures with ESCs (1, 20). In this work, the WHO Global GASP works collaboratively with other GASPs. For example, in the European Union/European Economic Area, the ECDC is funding the regional Euro-GASP (53, 54, 104, 114–116), and national GASPs have been running for several years in the United Kingdom (117; http://www.hpa.org.uk/Publications/InfectiousDiseases/HIVAndSTIs/GRASPReports/), United States (48, 74, 118, 119; http://www.cdc.gov/std/gisp), and several additional countries. The objectives with these GASPs are to timely monitor trends in resistance (including regional differences), provide high-quality susceptibility data that inform timely revisions of evidence-based empirical management guidelines, and, ideally, identify newly emerging AMR. Disquietingly, longitudinal quality-assured GASPs have been insufficient in some geographic regions (e.g., Latin America and the Caribbean [47, 78]) or have been sporadic or entirely lacking in large geographic regions, such as the WHO Eastern Mediterranean region, Eastern Europe, Central Asia, and Africa (52, 54, 120). It is essential to establish and maintain *N. gonorrhoeae* culture and AMR surveillance in these geographic regions and additional regions globally. This surveillance should ideally be integrated in the diagnostics and/or surveillance of sexually transmitted infections. Furthermore, for international comparison of quality-assured AMR data, ideally MIC-based and, whenever feasible, standardized methods, resistance breakpoints, and internal and external quality assurance should be used. It is also crucial that rapid and effective mechanisms exist to use the valid AMR data to update and implement the empirical management guidelines. Finally, significantly intensified research efforts to develop rapid molecular methods for AMR testing, novel therapeutic strategies, and especially compounds for treatment of gonorrhea need to be a very high priority (1, 12, 121).

GONOCOCCAL ISOLATE SURVEILLANCE PROJECT: AN EXAMPLE OF AN ESSENTIAL RESISTANCE SURVEILLANCE PROGRAM

In the United States, the antimicrobial susceptibility patterns of *N. gonorrhoeae* have been monitored since 1986 through the Gonococcal Isolate Surveillance Project (GISP), a national sentinel surveillance program and the oldest continuously running antimicrobial susceptibility surveillance program in the world (122). Since its inception, the GISP has provided valuable information that has been used to update the CDC's Sexually Transmitted Diseases (STD) Treatment Guidelines as well as provided data used by CDC to modify the treatment recommendations for gonorrhea in real time. For example, data from GISP were pivotal in alerting public health officials about the increasing prevalence of gonorrhea among MSM in the late 1990s (123), the recommendation to avoid the use of fluoroquinolones among MSM with gonorrhea in 2004 (74), and, in 2007, the recommendation that fluoroquinolones not be used for any patient that presents with gonorrhea, leaving ESCs as the only remaining class of antimicrobials recommended for treatment of gonorrhea (124). Furthermore, in 2010, due to concerns regarding emergence of ESC resistance, the CDC introduced recommendations for dual antimicrobial therapy. The CDC's 2010 STD Treatment Guidelines recommended an ESC (ceftriaxone at 250 mg i.m. or cefixime at 400 mg orally) plus azithromycin at 1 g orally or doxycycline at 100 mg orally twice daily for

7 days (125). In 2012, data from the GISP led the CDC to no longer recommend oral cephalosporin for the treatment of gonorrhea. Accordingly, cefixime was excluded from the recommended regimens in the CDC's STD Treatment Guidelines and cefixime was an alternative regimen (together with azithromycin at 1 g orally) only when ceftriaxone was not available (126). In 2015, due to the high prevalence of tetracycline resistance among GISP isolates, particularly those with elevated cefixime MICs, doxycycline was excluded from the recommended regimen. Consequently, the CDC's 2015 STD Treatment Guidelines recommend for the treatment of uncomplicated urogenital, anogenital, and pharyngeal gonorrhea only dual therapy with a single i.m. injection of ceftriaxone (250 mg) plus azithromycin at 1 g orally (91). Clearly the emergence and spread of ESC-resistant *N. gonorrhoeae* would severely limit the treatment options for gonorrhea in the United States and globally. As mentioned above, in response to the threat of ESC-resistant *N. gonorrhoeae*, the Division of STD Prevention at the CDC has developed a response plan (18) that includes the GISP as a critical component of the surveillance for ESC-resistant *N. gonorrhoeae*.

GISP is a collaborative project among selected STD clinics, five regional laboratories, and the CDC (Fig. 1). In GISP, *N. gonorrhoeae* specimens and demographic and clinical data of corresponding patients are collected each month from the first 25 men who attend the participating STD clinics in 26 selected U.S. cities and who have also been diagnosed with urethral gonorrhea (presumptive or confirmed diagnosis). These isolates are then shipped to one of five regional laboratories (Atlanta, GA; Baltimore, MD; Birmingham, AL; Seattle, WA; and Austin, TX), where they are confirmed as *N. gonorrhoeae*, tested for β-lactamase production using the nitrocefin test, and analyzed for antimicrobial susceptibility by agar dilution. The antimicrobials tested are ceftriaxone, cefixime, azithromycin, ciprofloxacin, gentamicin, penicillin G, and tetracycline. More information can be found in the GISP protocol available at http://www.cdc.gov/std/gisp/gisp-protocol-feb-2015_v3.pdf. Results are interpreted according to criteria recommended by the Clinical and

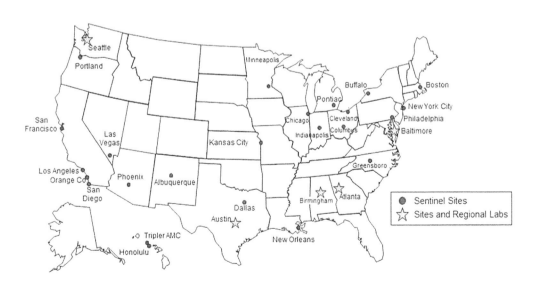

FIGURE 1 Gonococcal Isolate Surveillance Project (GISP) sentinel sites and regional laboratories in 2015. Courtesy of Centers for Diseases Control and Prevention (http://www.cdc.gov/std/gisp/gisp-map.htm).

Laboratory Standards Institute (CLSI) or, when CLSI criteria do not exist, according to expert opinion of what constitutes decreased susceptibility or resistance. The results of these tests are then transmitted to the CDC, where they are collated and analyzed together with the demographic and clinical data (see below). If isolates meet the predefined "alert value" MIC, the isolates are retested to confirm the result and CDC and the sentinel sites are notified. The demographic and clinical data submitted for each GISP patient include date and place of specimen collection, age, age and sex of sex partner, ethnicity, race (census categories), presence of symptoms, treatment for gonorrhea, HIV status, and history of previous gonorrhea, travel outside the United States during the previous 60 days, giving or receiving drugs or money for sex in the previous 12 months, antibiotic use during the previous 60 days, and drug use in the previous 12 months.

In total, GISP collects between 5,000 and 6,000 isolates per year; although all specimens come from men, the proportion of these men who report being MSM has steadily increased and is now over 30% of GISP participants. The breakpoint MICs for intermediate (decreased) susceptibility and resistance of different antimicrobials are shown in Fig. 2. While GISP monitors resistance to multiple antimicrobials, the major concern now is the development of resistance to ESCs (cefixime and ceftriaxone) and to azithromycin. Susceptibility testing for cefixime began in 1992, was discontinued in GISP in 2007, and was restarted again in 2009. Since 2009, over 90% of isolates have exhibited cefixime MICs of ≤0.03 µg/ml. The percentage of isolates with elevated cefixime MICs (≥0.25 µg/ml) increased from 0.1% in 2006 to 1.4% in 2010 and 2011 and declined to 0.4% in 2013. In 2014, 0.8% of isolates in GISP had reduced susceptibility to cefixime. This percentage was higher in isolates from MSM, with 1.3% that had decreased cefixime susceptibility (118). Susceptibility testing for ceftriaxone began in 1987. Between 2009 and 2013, each year,

Antimicrobial	Minimum Inhibitory Concentration (MIC) range (µg/ml)										
Azithromycin	0.03	0.06	0.125	0.25	0.5	1	2	4	8	16	
Cefixime	0.015	0.03	0.06	0.125	0.25	0.5					
Ceftriaxone	0.008	0.015	0.03	0.06	0.125	0.25	0.5				
Ciprofloxacin	0.015	0.03	0.06	0.125	0.25	0.5	1	2	4	8	16
Penicillin G	0.25	0.5	1	2	4	8	16				
Spectinomycin	128										
Tetracycline	0.25	0.5	1	2	4	8	16				

FIGURE 2 Gonococcal Isolate Surveillance Project (GISP) antimicrobial testing panel with Clinical and Laboratory Standards Institute (CLSI) breakpoints in 2014. Gray = sensitive; yellow = Intermediate; orange/red = resistant.

approximately 90% of isolates exhibited ceftriaxone MICs of ≤0.015 µg/ml. The percentage of GISP isolates that exhibited elevated ceftriaxone MICs, defined as ≥0.125 µg/ml, increased from 0.1% in 2008 to 0.4% in 2011 and decreased to <0.1% in 2013 (http://www.cdc.gov/std/gisp2013/gisp-2013-text-figures-tables.pdf). Susceptibility testing for azithromycin began in 1992. From 2009 to 2013, most isolates had azithromycin MICs of 0.125 to 0.25 µg/ml. The proportion of GISP isolates with azithromycin MICs of ≥2.0 µg/ml varied by year between 0.2% and 0.6% (119). Preliminary data for 2014 suggest that 2.5% of isolates have an MIC of >2 µg/ml for azithromycin, which is clearly cause for concern (unpublished data). The prevalence of resistance to penicillin G, tetracycline, and fluoroquinolones as well as reduced susceptibility to cefixime and azithromycin in *N. gonorrhoeae* in the GISP from 2000 to 2014 is summarized in Fig. 3.

CURRENT TREATMENT FOR GONORRHEA

In clinical practice, antimicrobial treatment of gonorrhea is mostly given empirically, at the first clinical visit, using the recommended antimicrobials in accordance with evidence-based management or treatment guidelines. Because gonorrhea is mostly

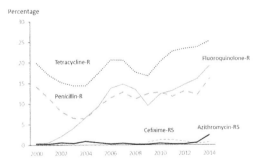

FIGURE 3 Prevalence of resistance in *Neisseria gonorrhoeae* in the U.S. Gonococcal Isolate Surveillance Project (GISP) from 2000 to 2014. R, resistance; RS, reduced susceptibility.

diagnosed based on microscopy of Gram- or methylene blue-stained smears or molecular testing, antimicrobial susceptibility testing is rarely performed and thus not available to the clinician. Furthermore, even if culture and AMR testing are performed, these results are not available at the first clinic visit when treatment is given. As mentioned above, these guidelines are essential to maintain updated recommendations based on quality-assured AMR surveillance data. Traditionally, the first-line antimicrobial therapy should be highly effective, be widely available and affordable, lack toxicity, be a single dose, and (rapidly) cure at least >95% of infected patients (1, 127). However, the evidence base for this cutoff, which was initially stated by the WHO, is limited. Levels of >1% and >3% AMR in high-risk patient groups have also been proposed as cutoffs for changing empirical first-line antimicrobial therapy (127, 128). Ideally, additional criteria, such as gonorrhea prevalence, local epidemiology, diagnostics used, transmission frequency, sexual contact tracing strategies, treatment strategies, and cost, should additionally be taken into account in the decision to change the recommended first-line antimicrobial therapy. Furthermore, an identical cutoff level and recommended treatment regimen(s) will not be the most cost-effective solution in all geographic regions and populations (12, 21, 129).

The antimicrobials used in the United States for the treatment of gonorrhea since the late 1980s can be seen in Fig. 4; note that azithromycin does not appear specifically as it is only recommended as part of dual therapy for gonorrhea. During the last decade, in many geographic regions worldwide, cefixime at one dose of 400 mg orally or ceftriaxone at one dose of 125 to 1,000 mg i.m. or intravenously has been recommended as a first-line empirical antimicrobial monotherapy of gonorrhea (11, 12, 21, 103). However, due to the emergence of *in vitro* resistance, including high-level resistance, to all ESCs as well as clinical treatment fail-

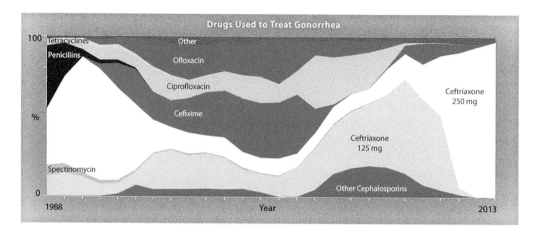

FIGURE 4 Antimicrobials used to treat gonorrhea in the United States from 1988 to 2013. Courtesy of Centers for Disease Control and Prevention (http://www.cdc.gov/std/gisp/gisp2013.htm).

ures using the most potent ESCs, cefixime and ceftriaxone, dual antimicrobial therapy (mainly ceftriaxone at one dose of 250 to 500 mg and azithromycin at one dose of 1 to 2 g, which together additionally eradicate concomitant *Chlamydia trachomatis* infections) and many *Mycoplasma genitalium* infections has been introduced as a first-line empirical therapy for uncomplicated anogenital and pharyngeal gonorrhea treatment in the United States (91), Canada (112), Australia (113), and Europe (2) (Table 2). Adequate clinical data to support the different ceftriaxone and azithromycin doses recommended for the currently circulating gonococcal strains are mainly lacking. The dual antimicrobial treatment regimens have instead been based on early clinical trials, pharmacokinetic/pharmacodynamic simulations (98), *in vitro* AMR surveillance data, predicted trends in AMR emergence, case reports of treatment failures, and expert consultations. In general, these dual antimicrobial treatment regimens are currently highly effective and recommended to be used in all geographic regions where comprehensive, high-quality local AMR surveillance data are lacking or not evidently supporting some other treatment regimen(s).

However, the decreased susceptibility or resistance to ceftriaxone in *N. gonorrhoeae*

has been increasing worldwide, and azithromycin resistance is easily selected and already prevalent in many geographic regions. Furthermore, *N. gonorrhoeae* strains with high-level azithromycin resistance (MIC ≥ 256 µg/ml) have been reported from an increasing number of countries, including Scotland (130), the United Kingdom (80), Ireland (81), Italy (82), Sweden (83), China (85), Australia (84), Argentina (86), Canada (88), and the United States (87). Consequently, the recently introduced dual antimicrobial regimens might not be effective long-term solutions and, most important, are not affordable in many less resourced settings, many of which have the highest burden of gonorrhea. This will significantly limit the mitigation of emergence and spread of gonococcal AMR globally (4, 11, 12, 15, 21).

Ultimately, novel and cost-effective antimicrobials for empirical antimicrobial monotherapy or for inclusion in new dual antimicrobial therapy regimens are essential.

FUTURE TREATMENTS FOR GONORRHEA

Strict adherence to evidence-based treatment guidelines should be the mainstay in the future treatment of gonorrhea. These treatment or management guidelines should be continuously updated using data from quality-assured surveillance of AMR, such as the GISP described above, and ideally also treatment failures. The current dual antimicrobial therapy (ceftriaxone plus azithromycin [2, 91, 112, 113]) is recommended to be used in all countries where appropriate and comprehensive AMR data do not clearly support other recommended treatment regimens. These dual treatment regimens additionally treat concomitant *C. trachomatis* infections and many *M. genitalium* infections.

However, as mentioned above, the currently recommended dual antimicrobial treatment regimen (ceftriaxone plus azithromycin) might not be a long-term solution. Two new dual antimicrobial regimens were recently evaluated for treatment of gonorrhea, that is, gentamicin (one dose of 240 mg i.m.) plus azithromycin (one dose of 2 g orally) and gemifloxacin (one dose of 320 mg orally) plus azithromycin (one dose of 2 g orally) (131). The cure rates were 100% and 99.5%, respectively. However, gastrointestinal side effects were common; e.g., 3.3% and 7.7% of patients, respectively, vomited within 1 h and, accordingly, lost a substantial amount of the given antimicrobial(s) (131). Either of these two regimens might be considered as an alternative treatment option in the presence of ceftriaxone resistance, treatment failure with recommended regimen, or ESC allergy (91).

Clearly, new, cost-effective, and widely accessible antimicrobials for antimicrobial monotherapy or for inclusion in new dual antimicrobial treatment regimens are essential. Spectinomycin is effective for treatment of anogenital gonorrhea, and spectinomycin susceptibility is very high globally, including in South Korea, where it has remained commonly used for treatment (12, 21, 37, 46–48, 50–54, 60, 104, 116, 132, 133). Nevertheless, spectinomycin is not effective against pharyngeal gonorrhea; for example, a 52% eradication rate has been reported (62). In addition, spectinomycin is not available in many geographic settings (2, 12, 91). Additional previously developed antimicrobials suggested for future treatment of gonorrhea include ertapenem (134, 135), fosfomycin (136), and gentamicin. In fact, since 1993, gentamicin has been a recommended first-line treatment (together with doxycycline) in syndromic management in Malawi (11, 12, 15, 37, 115, 131, 137–140). However, all these antimicrobials have shortcomings in their use as first-line therapy for gonorrhea, which have been detailed elsewhere (11, 12, 21, 135, 136, 139, 140). Accordingly, most likely they are primarily options for ESC-resistant gonorrhea, for ESC allergy, and in new dual antimicrobial therapies. A multicenter (*n* = 8), noninferiority, randomized, controlled phase 3 clinical gentamicin trial is also currently running. In this trial, treatment with gentamicin at one dose of 240 mg i.m. plus azithromycin at one dose of 1 g orally is compared to ceftriaxone at one dose of 500 mg i.m. plus azithromycin at one dose of 1 g orally (http://www.research.uhb.nhs.uk/gtog).

During recent years, many derivates or analogues of previously developed and used antimicrobials have also been shown to have high *in vitro* activities against *N. gonorrhoeae* isolates. These include several new fluoroquinolones (141–144), tetracyclines (145, 146), carbapenems (147), macrolides (148, 149), and the lipoglycopeptide dalbavancin (150). These and some additional antimicrobials or therapeutic compounds have been recently reviewed elsewhere (11, 12, 21). The new oral fluoroketolide solithromycin (macrolide family) is most advanced in development. Solithromycin has been shown to have a high *in vitro* activity against *N. gonorrhoeae*, including azithromycin-resistant, ESC-resistant, and multidrug-resistant gonococcal isolates (149). Nevertheless, *N. gonorrhoeae* strains with high-level resistance to azithromycin (MIC ≥ 256 µg/ml) are likely resistant also to solithromycin (MIC = 4 to 32 µg/ml) (149). A minor phase 2 single-center, open-label study has also shown that solithromycin (in single doses of both 1.0 g and 1.2 g orally) is effective for treating uncomplicated gonorrhea (151). Currently, a multicenter, open-label, randomized phase 3 clinical solithromycin trial is running. In this trial, participants with uncomplicated urogenital gonorrhea are treated with solithromycin at one dose of 1 g orally and the control group is treated with the recommended first-line therapy, i.e., ceftriaxone at one dose of 500 mg i.m. plus azithromycin at one dose of 1 g orally (https://clinicaltrials.gov).

Ideally, novel antimicrobials, using new targets or mechanisms of action, should be developed to avoid cross-resistance with any of the previously used antimicrobials. Promisingly, during recent years, several such antimicrobials have been developed and also proven to have a high *in vitro* efficacy against *N. gonorrhoeae* isolates. These include, for example, the new protein synthesis inhibitor pleuromutilin BC-3781 (152), the boron-containing inhibitor AN3365 (153), LpxC inhibitors (154), the species-specific FabI inhibitor MUT056399 (155), and novel bacterial topoisomerase inhibitors with targets different from those of previously used fluoroquinolones, that is, VXc-486 (VT12-008911 [156]) and ETX0914 (AZD0914 [157–159]). The oral spiropyrimidinetrione ETX0914, which also has a novel mode of action (160), is most advanced in development. Initially, a high *in vitro* susceptibility of ETX0914 was verified against a panel of 250 temporally, geographically, and genetically diverse *N. gonorrhoeae* isolates, which included a high proportion of fluoroquinolone-, ESC-, and multidrug-resistant isolates (157). It has now also been shown that ETX0914 susceptibility among 873 contemporary clinical gonococcal isolates from 21 countries in the European Union/European Economic Area countries is exceedingly high, and no ETX0914 resistance has yet been identified (159). Currently, a multicenter, open-label, randomized phase 2 clinical ETX014 trial is running. In this trial, participants with

uncomplicated urogenital gonorrhea are treated ETX0914 (2 g orally), ETX0914 (3 g orally), or, for comparison, ceftriaxone (500 mg i.m.) (https://clinicaltrials.gov).

CONCLUSIONS

Gonorrhea continues to be a worldwide public health problem and is becoming even more so with the emergence of gonococcal strains resistant to most previously or currently used antibiotics. There is every reason to believe that the problem of antibiotic-resistant strains will continue, challenging the effectiveness of clinical treatment regimens. In order to effectively solve this problem, efforts on many levels (Table 3), especially in the areas of new drug development, alternative treatment regimens, continued research on vaccines, genetic point-of-care diagnostics, and AMR testing are essential. In parallel to ongoing research on new antimicrobials to treat gonorrhea, it is important to note that after years of relative stagnation, the quest for a gonococcal vaccine that would protect humans from infection or reduce the severity of disease has been rejuvenated, and target antigens are now being pursued in preclinical vaccine studies (161). Additionally, high-throughput genomics, metabolomics, methylomics, transcriptomics, proteomics, and other novel molecular technologies and approaches will revolutionize future research aimed at improving diagnostics, AMR detection, and vaccine development (161–164). Given the remarkable history of the evolution of AMR displayed by gonococci, how resistance has changed treatment regimens over the past 80 years, the relative dearth of new antimicrobials in the pharmaceutical pipeline that will soon be available in the clinic, and the lack of a vaccine to prevent gonorrhea, there is every reason to be concerned that this sexually transmitted infection will continue to be a major global public health problem in the 21st century.

ACKNOWLEDGMENTS

We thank Robert Kirkcaldy of the Centers for Disease Control and Prevention (Atlanta, GA) for providing Fig. 3 before publication.

Work in the laboratory of M.U. was supported by grants from the Research Committee of Örebro County and the Örebro University Hospital Foundation, Örebro, Sweden. Work in the laboratory of C.D.R. was supported by the CDC (1H25PS004311). Work in the laboratory of W.M.S. was supported by NIH grant R37 AI021150-30 and a VA Merit Award (510 1BX000112-07) from the Biomedical Laboratory Research and Development Service of the Department of Veterans Affairs. W.M.S. is the recipient of a Senior Research Career Scientist Award from the Biomedical Laboratory Research and Development Service of the Department of Veterans Affairs.

The contents of the paper do not represent the views of the Department of Veterans Affairs, the Centers for Disease Control and Prevention, or the U.S. government.

CITATION

Unemo M, del Rio C, Shafer WM. 2016. Antimicrobial resistance expressed by *Neisseria gonorrhoeae*: a major global public health problem in the 21st century. Microbiol Spectrum 4(3):EI10-0009-2015.

REFERENCES

1. **World Health Organization, Department of Reproductive Health and Research.** 2012. *Global Action Plan To Control the Spread and Impact of Antimicrobial Resistance in Neisseria gonorrhoeae.* World Health Organization, Geneva, Switzerland.
2. **Bignell C, Unemo M.** 2013. 2012 European guideline on the diagnosis and treatment of gonorrhoea in adults. *Int J STD AIDS* **24:**85–92.
3. **Cohen MS, Hoffman IF, Royce RA, Kazembe P, Dyer JR, Daly CC, Zimba D, Vernazza PL, Maida M, Fiscus SA, Eron JJ Jr.** 1997. Reduction of concentration of HIV-1 in semen after treatment of urethritis: implications for prevention of sexual transmission of HIV-1. *Lancet* **349:**1868–1873.
4. **Tapsall JW, Ndowa F, Lewis DA, Unemo M.** 2009. Meeting the public health challenge of multidrug- and extensively drug-resistant *Neisseria gonorrhoeae. Expert Rev Anti Infect Ther* **7:**821–834.
5. **Unemo M, Ison C.** 2013. Gonorrhoea. p 21. *In* Unemo M, Ballard R, Ison C, Lewis D, Ndowa F, Peeling R (ed), *Laboratory Diagnosis of Sexually Transmitted Infections, Including Human Immunodeficiency Virus.* World Health Organization, Geneva, Switzerland.
6. **Del Rio C, Stephens DS, Knapp JS, Rice RJ, Schalla WO.** 1989. Comparison of isolates of *Neisseria gonorrhoeae* causing meningitis and report of gonococcal meningitis in a patient with C8 deficiency. *J Clin Microbiol* **27:**1045–1049.
7. **Newman LM, Rowley J, Vander Hoorn S, Wijesooriya NS, Unemo M, Low N, Stevens G, Kiarie J, Temmerman M.** 2015. Global estimates of the prevalence and incidence of four curable sexually transmitted infections in 2012 based on systematic review and global reporting. *PLoS Med* **10**(12):e0143304.
8. **Cámara J, Serra J, Ayats J, Bastida T, Carnicer-Pont D, Andreu A, Ardanuy C.** 2012. Molecular characterization of two high-level ceftriaxone-resistant *Neisseria gonorrhoeae* isolates detected in Catalonia, Spain. *J Antimicrob Chemother* **67:**1858–1860.
9. **Ohnishi M, Golparian D, Shimuta K, Saika T, Hoshina S, Iwasaku K, Nakayama S, Kitawaki J, Unemo M.** 2011. Is *Neisseria gonorrhoeae* initiating a future era of untreatable gonorrhea? Detailed characterization of the first strain with high-level resistance to ceftriaxone. *Antimicrob Agents Chemother* **55:**3538–3545.
10. **Unemo M, Golparian D, Nicholas R, Ohnishi M, Gallay A, Sednaoui P.** 2012. High-level cefixime- and ceftriaxone-resistant *N. gonorrhoeae* in France: novel *penA* mosaic allele in a successful international clone causes treatment failure. *Antimicrob Agents Chemother* **56:**1273–1280.
11. **Unemo M, Nicholas RA.** 2012. Emergence of multidrug-resistant, extensively drug-resistant and untreatable gonorrhea. *Future Microbiol* **7:**1401–1422.
12. **Unemo M, Shafer WM.** 2014. Antimicrobial resistance in *Neisseria gonorrhoeae* in the 21st Century: past, evolution, and future. *Clin Microbiol Rev* **27:**587–613.
13. **Bolan GA, Sparling PF, Wasserheit JN.** 2012. The emerging threat of untreatable gonococcal infection. *N Engl J Med* **366:**485–487.

14. **Ison CA.** 2012. Antimicrobial resistance in sexually transmitted infections in the developed world: implications for rational treatment. *Curr Opin Infect Dis* **25**:73–78.

15. **Unemo M, Shafer WM.** 2011. Antibiotic resistance in *Neisseria gonorrhoeae*: origin, evolution, and lessons learned for the future. *Ann N Y Acad Sci* **1230**:E19–E28.

16. **Whiley DM, Goire N, Lahra MM, Donovan B, Limnios AE, Nissen MD, Sloots TP.** 2012. The ticking time bomb: escalating antibiotic resistance in *Neisseria gonorrhoeae* is a public health disaster in waiting. *J Antimicrob Chemother* **67**:2059–2061.

17. **Groopman J.** 2012. Sex and the superbug—the rise of drug-resistant gonorrhea. *The New Yorker*, New York, NY.

18. **Centers for Disease Control and Prevention.** 2012. *Cephalosporin-Resistant Neisseria gonorrhoeae Public Health Response Plan.* Centers for Disease Control and Prevention, Atlanta, GA.

19. **European Centre for Disease Prevention and Control.** 2012. *Response Plan To Control and Manage the Threat of Multidrug-Resistant Gonorrhoea in Europe.* European Centre for Disease Prevention and Control, Stockholm, Sweden.

20. **Ndowa F, Lusti-Narasimhan M, Unemo M.** 2012. The serious threat of multidrug-resistant and untreatable gonorrhoea: the pressing need for global action to control the spread of antimicrobial resistance, and mitigate the impact on sexual and reproductive health. *Sex Transm Infect* **88**:317–318.

21. **Unemo M.** 2015. Current and future antimicrobial treatment of gonorrhoea—the rapidly evolving *Neisseria gonorrhoeae* continues to challenge. *BMC Infect Dis* **15**:364.

22. **Ashford WA, Golash RG, Henning VG.** 1976. Penicillinase producing *Neisseria gonorrhoeae*. *Lancet* **ii**:657–658.

23. **Phillips I.** 1976. Beta-lactamase producing penicillin-resistant gonococcus. *Lancet* **ii**:656–657.

24. **Morse SA, Johnson SR, Biddle JW, Roberts MC.** 1986. High-level tetracycline resistance in *Neisseria gonorrhoeae* is result of acquisition of streptococcal *tetM* determinant. *Antimicrob Agents Chemother* **30**:664–670.

25. **Nagaev I, Björkman J, Andersson DI, Hughes D.** 2001. Biological cost and compensatory evolution in fusidic acid-resistant *Staphylococcus aureus*. *Mol Microbiol* **40**:433–439.

26. **Rozen DE, McGee L, Levin BR, Klugman KP.** 2007. Fitness costs of fluoroquinolone resistance in *Streptococcus pneumoniae*. *Antimicrob Agents Chemother* **51**:412–416.

27. **Trzcinski K, Thompson CM, Gilbey AM, Dowson CG, Lipsitch M.** 2006. Incremental increase in fitness cost with increased beta-lactam resistance in pneumococci evaluated by competition in an infant rat nasal colonization model. *J Infect Dis* **193**:1296–1303.

28. **Kunz AN, Begum AA, Wu H, D'Ambrozio JA, Robinson JM, Shafer WM, Bash MC, Jerse AE.** 2012. Impact of fluoroquinolone resistance mutations on gonococcal fitness and in vivo selection for compensatory mutations. *J Infect Dis* **205**:1821–1829.

29. **Warner DM, Shafer WM, Jerse AE.** 2008. Clinically relevant mutations that cause derepression of the *Neisseria gonorrhoeae* MtrC-MtrD-MtrE Efflux pump system confer different levels of antimicrobial resistance and in vivo fitness. *Mol Microbiol* **70**:462–478.

30. **Kampmeier RH.** 1983. Introduction of sulfonamide therapy for gonorrhea. *Sex Transm Dis* **10**:81–84.

31. **Dunlop EMC.** 1949. Gonorrhoea and the sulphonamides. *Br J Vener Dis* **25**:81–83.

32. **Fermer C, Kristiansen BE, Sköld O, Swedberg G.** 1995. Sulfonamide resistance in *Neisseria meningitidis* as defined by site-directed mutagenesis could have its origin in other species. *J Bacteriol* **177**:4669–4675.

33. **Johnson SR, Morse SA.** 1988. Antibiotic resistance in *Neisseria gonorrhoeae*: genetics and mechanisms of resistance. *Sex Transm Dis* **15**:217–224.

34. **Swedberg G, Fermér C, Sköld O.** 1993. Point mutations in the dihydropteroate synthase gene causing sulfonamide resistance. *Adv Exp Med Biol* **338**:555–558.

35. **Mahoney JF, Ferguson C, Buchholtz M, van Slyke CJ.** 1943. The use of penicillin sodium in the treatment of sulfonamide-resistant gonorrhea in men. A preliminary report. *Am J Gonorr Vener Dis* **27**:525–528.

36. **Van Slyke CJ, Arnold RC, Buchholtz M.** 1943. Penicillin therapy in sulfonamide-resistant gonorrhea in men. *Am J Public Health Nations Health* **33**:1392–1394.

37. **Lewis DA.** 2010. The gonococcus fights back: is this time a knock out? *Sex Transm Infect* **86**:415–421.

38. **Jaffe HW, Biddle JW, Thornsberry C, Johnson RE, Kaufman RE, Reynolds GH, Wiesner PJ.** 1976. National gonorrhea therapy monitoring study: in vitro antibiotic susceptibility and its correlation with treatment results. *N Engl J Med* **294**:5–9.

39. **Martin JE Jr, Lester A, Price EV, Schmale JD.** 1970. Comparative study of gonococcal

susceptibility to penicillin in the United States, 1955–1969. *J Infect Dis* **122**:459–461.

40. **Reyn A, Korner B, Bentzon MW.** 1958. Effects of penicillin, streptomycin, and tetracycline on *N. gonorrhoeae* isolated in 1944 and in 1957. *Br J Vener Dis* **34**:227–239.

41. **Unemo M, Nicholas RA, Davies C, Jerse A, Shafer WM.** 2013. *Molecular mechanisms of antibiotic resistance expressed by the pathogenic* Neisseria, p 245–268. *In* Genco C, Wetzler L (ed), *Neisseria—Molecular Mechanisms of Pathogenic Neisseria*. Caister Academic Press, London, United Kingdom.

42. **Amies CR.** 1967. Development of resistance of gonococci to penicillin. An eight-year study. *Can Med Ass J* **96**:33–35.

43. **Franks AG.** 1946. Successful combined treatment of penicillin-resistant gonorrhea. *Am J Med Sci* **211**:553–555.

44. **Faruki H, Kohmescher RN, McKinney WP, Sparling PF.** 1985. A community-based outbreak of infection with penicillin-resistant *Neisseria gonorrhoeae* not producing penicillinase (chromosomally mediated resistance). *N Engl J Med* **313**:607–611.

45. **Faruki H, Sparling PF.** 1986. Genetics of resistance in a non-beta-lactamase-producing gonococcus with relatively high-level penicillin resistance. *Antimicrob Agents Chemother* **30**:856–860.

46. **Bala M, Kakran M, Singh V, Sood S, Ramesh V, Members of WHO GASP SEAR Network.** 2013. Monitoring antimicrobial resistance in *Neisseria gonorrhoeae* in selected countries of the WHO South-East Asia Region between 2009 and 2012: a retrospective analysis. *Sex Transm Infect* **89**(Suppl 4):iv28–iv35.

47. **Dillon JA, Trecker MA, Thakur SD, Gonococcal Antimicrobial Surveillance Program Network in Latin America and the Caribbean 1990–2011.** 2013. Two decades of the gonococcal antimicrobial surveillance program in South America and the Caribbean: challenges and opportunities. *Sex Transm Infect* **89**(Suppl 4):iv36–iv41.

48. **Kirkcaldy RD, Kidd S, Weinstock HS, Papp JR, Bolan GA.** 2013. Trends in antimicrobial resistance in *Neisseria gonorrhoeae* in the USA: the Gonococcal Isolate Surveillance Project (GISP), January 2006–June 2012. *Sex Transm Infect* **89**(Suppl 4):iv5–iv10.

49. **Kubanova A, Frigo N, Kubanov A, Sidorenko S, Priputnevich T, Vachnina T, Al-Khafaji N, Polevshikova S, Solomka V, Domeika M, Unemo M.** 2008. National surveillance of antimicrobial susceptibility in *Neisseria gonorrhoeae* in 2005-2006 and recommendations of first-line antimicrobial drugs for gonorrhoea treatment in Russia. *Sex Transm Infect* **84**:285–289.

50. **Lahra MM, Lo YR, Whiley DM.** 2013. Gonococcal antimicrobial resistance in the Western Pacific region. *Sex Transm Infect* **89**(Suppl 4): iv19–iv23.

51. **Martin IM, Hoffmann S, Ison CA, ESSTI Network.** 2006. European Surveillance of Sexually Transmitted Infections (ESSTI): the first combined antimicrobial susceptibility data for *Neisseria gonorrhoeae* in Western Europe. *J Antimicrob Chemother* **58**:587–593.

52. **Ndowa FJ, Francis JM, Machiha A, Faye-Kette H, Fonkoua MC.** 2013. Gonococcal antimicrobial resistance: perspectives from the African region. *Sex Transm Infect* **89** (Suppl 4):iv11–iv15.

53. **Spiteri G, Cole M, Unemo M, Hoffmann S, Ison C, van de Laar M.** 2013. The European Gonococcal Antimicrobial Surveillance Programme (Euro-GASP)—a sentinel approach in the European Union (EU)/European Economic Area (EEA). *Sex Transm Infect* **89**(Suppl 4):iv16–iv18.

54. **Unemo M, Ison CA, Cole M, Spiteri G, van de Laar M, Khotenashvili L.** 2013. Gonorrhoea and gonococcal antimicrobial resistance surveillance networks in the WHO European region, including the independent countries of the former Soviet Union. *Sex Transm Infect* **89**(Suppl 4):iv42–iv46.

55. **Helm RA, Barnhart MM, Seifert HS.** 2007. *pilQ* missense mutations have diverse effects on PilQ multimer formation, piliation, and pilus function in *Neisseria gonorrhoeae*. *J Bacteriol* **189**:3198–3207.

56. **Easmon CS, Forster GE, Walker GD, Ison CA, Harris JR, Munday PE.** 1984. Spectinomycin as initial treatment for gonorrhoea. *Br Med J* **289**:1032–1034.

57. **Judson FN, Ehret JM, Handsfield HH.** 1985. Comparative study of ceftriaxone and spectinomycin for treatment of pharyngeal and anorectal gonorrhea. *JAMA* **253**:1417–1419.

58. **Stolz E, Zwart HG, Michel MF.** 1975. Activity of eight antimicrobial agents in vitro against *N. gonorrhoeae*. *Br J Vener Dis* **51**:257–264.

59. **Boslego JW, Tramont EC, Takafuji ET, Diniega BM, Mitchell BS, Small JW, Khan WN, Stein DC.** 1987. Effect of spectinomycin use on the prevalence of spectinomycin-resistant and penicillinase-producing *Neisseria gonorrhoeae*. *N Engl J Med* **317**:272–278.

60. **Lee H, Unemo M, Kim HJ, Seo Y, Lee K, Chong Y.** 2015. Emergence of decreased susceptibility and resistance to extended-spectrum cephalosporins in *Neisseria gonorrhoeae* in Korea. *J Antimicrob Chemother* **70**:2536–2542.

61. **Lindberg M, Ringertz O, Sandström E.** 1982. Treatment of pharyngeal gonorrhoea due to β-lactamase-producing gonococci. *Br J Vener Dis* **58**:101–104.

62. **Moran JS.** 1995. Treating uncomplicated *Neisseria gonorrhoeae* infections: is the anatomic site of infection important? *Sex Transm Dis* **22**:39–47.

63. **Moran JS, Levine WC.** 1995. Drugs of choice for the treatment of uncomplicated gonococcal infections. *Clin Infect Dis* **20**(Suppl 1):S47–S65.

64. **Galimand M, Gerbaud G, Courvalin P.** 2000. Spectinomycin resistance in *Neisseria* spp. due to mutations in 16S rRNA. *Antimicrob Agents Chemother* **44**:1365–1366.

65. **Unemo M, Fasth O, Fredlund H, Limnios A, Tapsall JW.** 2009. Phenotypic and genetic characterization of the 2008 WHO *Neisseria gonorrhoeae* reference strain panel intended for global quality assurance and quality control of gonococcal antimicrobial resistance surveillance for public health purposes. *J Antimicrob Chemother* **63**:1142–1151.

66. **Unemo M, Golparian D, Skogen V, Olsen AO, Moi H, Syversen G, Hjelmevoll SO.** 2013. *Neisseria gonorrhoeae* strain with high-level resistance to spectinomycin due to a novel resistance mechanism (mutated ribosomal protein S5) verified in Norway. *Antimicrob Agents Chemother* **57**:1057–1061.

67. **Ilina EN, Malakhova MV, Bodoev IN, Oparina NY, Filimonova AV, Govorun VM.** 2013. Mutation in ribosomal protein S5 leads to spectinomycin resistance in *Neisseria gonorrhoeae*. *Front Microbiol* **4**:186.

68. **Tanaka M, Nakayama H, Haraoka M, Saika T.** 2000. Antimicrobial resistance of *Neisseria gonorrhoeae* and high prevalence of ciprofloxacin-resistant isolates in Japan, 1993 to 1998. *J Clin Microbiol* **38**:521–525.

69. **Tanaka M, Kumazawa J, Matsumoto T, Kobayashi I.** 1994. High prevalence of *Neisseria gonorrhoeae* strains with reduced susceptibility to fluoroquinolones in Japan. *Genitourin Med* **70**:90–93.

70. **Berglund T, Unemo M, Olcén P, Giesecke J, Fredlund H.** 2002. One year of *Neisseria gonorrhoeae* isolates in Sweden: the prevalence study of antibiotic susceptibility shows relation to the geographic area of exposure. *Int J STD AIDS* **13**:109–114.

71. **Patrick D, Shaw C, Rekart ML.** 1995. *Neisseria gonorrhoeae* with decreased susceptibility to ciprofloxacin in British Columbia: an imported phenomenon. *Can Common Dis Rep* **21**:137–139.

72. **Su X, Lind I.** 2001. Molecular basis of high-level ciprofloxacin resistance in *Neisseria gonorrhoeae* strains isolated from Denmark from 1995–1998. *Antimicrob Agents Chemother* **45**:117–123.

73. **Iverson CJ, Wang SA, Lee MV, Ohye RG, Trees DL, Knapp JS, Effler PV, O'Connor NP, Levine WC.** 2004. Fluoroquinolone-resistance among *Neisseria gonorrhoeae* isolates in Hawaii, 1990–2000: role of foreign importation and endemic spread. *Sex Transm Dis* **31**:702–708.

74. **Centers for Disease Control and Prevention.** 2004. Increases in fluoroquinolone-resistant *Neisseria gonorrhoeae* among men who have sex with men—United States, 2003, and revised recommendations for gonorrhea treatment, 2004. *MMWR Morb Mortal Wkly Rep* **53**:335–338.

75. **Centers for Disease Control and Preventio.** 2007. Update to CDC's Sexually Transmitted Diseases Treatment Guidelines, 2006: fluoroquinolones no longer recommended for treatment of gonococcal infections. *MMWR Morb Mortal Wkly Rep* **56**:332–336.

76. **Douthwaite S, Champney WS.** 2001. Structures of ketolides and macrolides determine their mode of interaction with the ribosomal target site. *J Antimicrob Chemother* **48**(Suppl T1):1–8.

77. **Dillon JA, Ruben M, Li H, Borthagaray G, Márquez C, Fiorito S, Galarza P, Portilla JL, León L, Agudelo CI, Sanabria OM, Maldonado A, Prabhakar P.** 2006. Challenges in the control of gonorrhea in South America and the Caribbean: monitoring the development of resistance to antibiotics. *Sex Transm Dis* **33**:87–95.

78. **Starnino S, GASP-LAC Working Group, Galarza P, Carvallo ME, Benzaken AS, Ballesteros AM, Cruz OM, Hernandez AL, Carbajal JL, Borthagaray G, Payares D, Dillon JA.** 2012. Retrospective analysis of antimicrobial susceptibility trends (2000-2009) in *Neisseria gonorrhoeae* isolates from countries in Latin America and the Caribbean show evolving resistance to ciprofloxacin, azithromycin and decreased susceptibility to ceftrixone. *Sex Transm Dis* **39**:813–821.

79. **Kubanova A, Frigo N, Kubanov A, Sidorenko S, Lesnaya I, Polevshikova S, Solomka V, Bukanov N, Domeika M, Unemo M.** 2010. The Russian gonococcal antimicrobial susceptibility programme (RU-GASP)—national resistance prevalence in 2007 and 2008, and trends during 2005–2008. *Euro Surveill* **15**(14):19533.

80. **Chisholm SA, Dave J, Ison CA.** 2010. High-level azithromycin resistance occurs in *Neisseria gonorrhoeae* as a result of a single point mutation

in the 23S rRNA genes. *Antimicrob Agents Chemother* **54:**3812–3816.

81. **Lynagh Y, Mac Aogáin M, Walsh A, Rogers TR, Unemo M, Crowley B.** 2015. Detailed characterization of the first high-level azithromycin-resistant *Neisseria gonorrhoeae* cases in Ireland. *J Antimicrob Chemother* **70:**2411–2413.

82. **Starnino S, Stefanelli P, Neisseria gonorrhoeae Italian Study Group.** 2009. Azithromycin-resistant *Neisseria gonorrhoeae* strains recently isolated in Italy. *J Antimicrob Chemother* **63:**1200–1204.

83. **Unemo M, Golparian D, Hellmark B.** 2013. First three *Neisseria gonorrhoeae* isolates with high-level resistance to azithromycin in Sweden: a threat to currently available dual-antimicrobial regimens for treatment of gonorrhea? *Antimicrob Agents Chemother* **58:**624–625.

84. **Stevens K, Zaia A, Tawil S, Bates J, Hicks V, Whiley D, Limnios A, Lahra MM, Howden BP.** 2014. *Neisseria gonorrhoeae* isolates with high-level resistance to azithromycin in Australia. *J Antimicrob Chemother* **70:**1267–1268.

85. **Yuan LF, Yin YP, Dai XQ, Pearline RV, Xiang Z, Unemo M, Chen XS.** 2011. Resistance to azithromycin of *Neisseria gonorrhoeae* isolates from 2 cities in China. *Sex Transm Dis* **38:**764–768.

86. **Galarza PG, Abad R, Canigia LF, Buscemi L, Pagano I, Oviedo C, Vázquez JA.** 2010. New mutation in 23S rRNA gene associated with high level of azithromycin resistance in *Neisseria gonorrhoeae*. *Antimicrob Agents Chemother* **54:**1652–1653.

87. **Katz AR, Komeya AY, Soge OO, MKiaha MI, Lee MV, Wasserman GM, Maningas EV, Whelen AC, Kirkcaldy RD, Shapiro SJ, Bolan GA, Holmes KK.** 2012. *Neisseria gonorrhoeae* with high-level resistance to azithromycin: case report of the first isolate identified in the United States. *Clin Infect Dis* **54:**841–843.

88. **Allen VG, Seah C, Martin I, Melano RG.** 2014. Azithromycin resistance is coevolving with reduced susceptibility to cephalosporins in *Neisseria gonorrhoeae* in Ontario, Canada. *Antimicrob Agents Chemother* **58:**2528–2534.

89. **Young H, Moyes A, McMillan A.** 1997. Azithromycin and erythromycin resistant *Neisseria gonorrhoeae* following treatment with azithromycin. *Int J STD AIDS* **8:**299–302.

90. **Handsfield HH, Dalu ZA, Martin DH, Douglas JM Jr, McCarty JM, Schlossberg D.** 1994. Multicenter trial of single-dose azithromycin vs. ceftriaxone in the treatment of uncomplicated gonorrhea. Azithromycin Gonorrhea Study Group. *Sex Transm Dis* **21:**107–111.

91. **Workowski KA, Bolan GA.** 2015. Sexually transmitted diseases treatment guidelines, 2015. *MMWR Recommend Rep* **64**(RR-03):1–137.

92. **Bignell C, Fitzgerald M.** 2011. UK national guideline for the management of gonorrhoea in adults, 2011. *Int J STD AIDS* **22:**541–547.

93. **Newman LM, Moran JS, Workowski KA.** 2007. Update on the management of gonorrhea in adults in the United States. *Clin Infect Dis* **44**(Suppl 3):S84–S101.

94. **Barry PM, Klausner JD.** 2009. The use of cephalosporins for gonorrhea: the impending problem of resistance. *Expert Opin Pharmacother* **10:**555–577.

95. **Ison CA, Mouton JW, Jones K, Fenton KA, Livermore DM.** 2004. Which cephalosporin for gonorrhoea? *Sex Transm Infect* **80:**386–388.

96. **Akasaka S, Muratani T, Yamada Y, Inatomi H, Takahashi K, Matsumoto T.** 2001. Emergence of cephem- and aztreonam-high-resistant *Neisseria gonorrhoeae* that does not produce beta-lactamase. *J Infect Chemother* **7:**49–50.

97. **Tanaka M, Nakayama H, Tunoe H, Egashira T, Kanayama A, Saika T, Kobayashi I, Naito S.** 2002. A remarkable reduction in the susceptibility of *Neisseria gonorrhoeae* isolates to cephems and the selection of antibiotic regimens for the single-dose treatment of gonococcal infection in Japan. *J Infect Chemother* **8:**81–86.

98. **Chisholm SA, Mouton JW, Lewis DA, Nichols T, Ison CA, Livermore DM.** 2010. Cephalosporin MIC creep among gonococci: time for a pharmacodynamic rethink? *J Antimicrob Chemother* **65:**2141–2148.

99. **Deguchi T, Yasuda M, Yokoi S, Ishida K, Ito M, Ishihara S, Minamidate K, Harada Y, Tei K, Kojima K, Tamaki M, Maeda S.** 2003. Treatment of uncomplicated gonococcal urethritis by double-dosing of 200 mg cefixime at a 6-h interval. *J Infect Chemother* **9:**35–39.

100. **Ito M, Yasuda M, Yokoi S, Ito S, Takahashi Y, Ishihara S, Maeda S, Deguchi T.** 2004. Remarkable increase in central Japan in 2001–2002 of *Neisseria gonorrhoeae* isolates with decreased susceptibility to penicillin, tetracycline, oral cephalosporins, and fluoroquinolones. *Antimicrob Agents Chemother* **48:**3185–3187.

101. **Shimuta K, Watanabe Y, Nakayama S-I, Morita-Ishihara T, Kuroki T, Unemo M, Ohnishi M.** 2015. Emergence and evolution of internationally disseminated cephalosporin-resistant *Neisseria gonorrhoeae* clones from 1995 to 2005 in Japan. *BMC Infect Dis* **15:**378.

102. **Yokoi S, Deguchi T, Ozawa T, Yasuda M, Ito S, Kubota Y, Tamaki M, Maeda S.** 2007. Threat to cefixime treatment for gonorrhea. *Emerg Infect Dis* **13**:1275–1277.

103. **Japanese Society of Sexually Transmitted Infection.** 2011. Gonococcal infection. Sexually transmitted infections, diagnosis and treatment guidelines 2011. *Jpn J Sex Transm Dis* **22** (Suppl 1):52–59 (In Japanese).

104. **Cole MJ, Spiteri G, Jacobsson S, Pitt R, Grigorjev V, Unemo M, Euro-GASP Network.** 2015. Is the tide turning again for cephalosporin resistance in *Neisseria gonorrhoeae* in Europe? Results from the 2013 European surveillance. *BMC Infect Dis* **15**:321.

105. **Hess D, Wu A, Golparian D, Esmaili S, Pandori W, Sena E, Klausner JD, Barry P, Unemo M, Pandori M.** 2012. Genome sequencing of a *Neisseria gonorrhoeae* isolate of a successful international clone with decreased susceptibility and resistance to extended-spectrum cephalosporins. *Antimicrob Agents Chemother* **56**:5633–5641.

106. **Li SY.** 2012. Global transmission of multiple-drug resistant *Neisseria gonorrhoeae* strains refractive to cephalosporin treatment. *J Formos Med Assoc* **111**:463–464.

107. **Martin I, Sawatzky P, Allen V, Hoang L, Lefebvre B, Mina N, Wong T, Gilmour M.** 2012. Emergence and characterization of *Neisseria gonorrhoeae* isolates with decreased susceptibilities to ceftriaxone and cefixime in Canada: 2001–2010. *Sex Transm Dis* **39**:316–323.

108. **Su X, Jiang F Qimuge, Dai X, Sun H, Ye S.** 2007. Surveillance of antimicrobial susceptibilities in *Neisseria gonorrhoeae* in Nanjing, China, 1999–2006. *Sex Transm Dis* **34**:995–999.

109. **Shimuta K, Unemo M, Nakayama S, Morita-Ishihara T, Dorin M, Kawahata T, Ohnishi M.** 2013. Antimicrobial resistance and molecular typing of *Neisseria gonorrhoeae* isolates in Kyoto and Osaka, Japan, 2010 to 2012: intensified surveillance after identification of the first strain (H041) with high-level ceftriaxone resistance. *Antimicrob Agents Chemother* **57**:5225–5232.

110. **Ropp PA, Hu M, Olesky M, Nicholas RA.** 2002. Mutations in *ponA*, the gene encoding penicillin-binding protein 1, and a novel locus, *penC*, are required for high-level chromosomally mediated penicillin resistance in *Neisseria gonorrhoeae*. *Antimicrob Agents Chemother* **46**:769–777.

111. **Zhao S, Duncan M, Tomberg J, Davies C, Unemo M, Nicholas RA.** 2009. Genetics of chromosomally mediated intermediate resistance to ceftriaxone and cefixime in *Neisseria gonorrhoeae*. *Antimicrob Agents Chemother* **53**:3744–3751.

112. **Public Health Agency of Canada.** 2013. *Canadian Guidelines on Sexually Transmitted Infections. Gonococcal Infections Chapter.* Public Health Agency of Canada, Ottawa, Canada. http://www.phac-aspc.gc.ca/std-mts/sti-its/cgsti-ldcits/assets/pdf/section-5-6-eng.pdf. Accessed 22 November 2015.

113. **Australasian Sexual Health Alliance.** *Australian STI Management Guidelines for Use in Primary Care.* Australasian Sexual Health Alliance, Darlinghurst, Australia. http://www.sti.guidelines.org.au/sexually-transmissible-infections/gonorrhoea#management. Accessed 22 November 2015.

114. **Chisholm SA, Unemo M, Quaye N, Johansson E, Cole MJ, Ison CA, Van de Laar MJ.** 2013. Molecular epidemiological typing within the European Gonococcal Antimicrobial Resistance Surveillance Programme reveals predominance of a multidrug-resistant clone. *Euro Surveill* **18**: pii=20358.

115. **Chisholm SA, Quaye N, Cole MJ, Fredlund H, Hoffmann S, Jensen JS, van de Laar MJ, Unemo M, Ison CA.** 2011. An evaluation of gentamicin susceptibility of *Neisseria gonorrhoeae* isolates in Europe. *J Antimicrob Chemother* **66**:592–595.

116. **Cole M, Unemo M, Hoffmann S, Chisholm SA, Ison CA, van de Laar MJ.** 2011. The European gonococcal antimicrobial surveillance programme, 2009. *Euro Surveill* **16**: pii=19995.

117. **Ison CA, Town K, Obi C, Chisholm S, Hughes G, Livermore DM, Lowndes CM, GRASP Collaborative Group.** 2013. Decreased susceptibility to cephalosporins among gonococci: data from the Gonococcal Resistance to Antimicrobials Surveillance Programme (GRASP) in England and Wales, 2007–2011. *Lancet Infect Dis* **13**:762–768.

118. **Kirkcaldy RD, Hook EW III, Soge OO, del Rio C, Kubin G, Zenilman JM, Papp JR.** 2015. Trends in *Neisseria gonorrhoeae* susceptibility to cephalosporins in the United States, 2006–2014. *JAMA* **314**:1869–1871.

119. **Kirkcaldy RD, Soge O, Papp JR, Hook EW III, del Rio C, Kubin G, Weinstock HS.** 2015. Analysis of *Neisseria gonorrhoeae* azithromycin susceptibility in the United States by the Gonococcal Isolate Surveillance Project, 2005 to 2013. *Antimicrob Agents Chemother* **59**:998–1003.

120. **Unemo M, Shipitsyna E, Domeika M.** 2011. Gonorrhoea surveillance, laboratory diagnosis

and antimicrobial susceptibility testing of *Neisseria gonorrhoeae* in 11 countries of the eastern part of the WHO European region. *APMIS* **119**:643–649.

121. **Goire N, Lahra MM, Chen M, Donovan B, Fairley CK, Guy R, Kaldor J, Regan D, Ward J, Nissen MD, Sloots TP, Whiley DM.** 2014. Molecular approaches to enhance surveillance of gonococcal antimicrobial resistance. *Nat Rev Microbiol* **12**:223–229.

122. **Schwarcz SK, Zenilman JM, Schnell D, Knapp JS, Hook EW III, Thompson S, Judson FN, Holmes KK.** 1990. National surveillance of antimicrobial resistance in *Neisseria gonorrhoeae*: the Gonococcal Isolate Surveillance Project. *JAMA* **264**:1413–1417.

123. **Fox KK, del Rio C, Holmes KK, Hook EW III, Judson FN, Knapp JS, Procop GW, Wang SA, Whittington WL, Levine WC.** 2001. Gonorrhea in the HIV era: a reversal in trends among men who have sex with men. *Am J Public Health* **91**:959–964.

124. **Centers for Disease Control and Prevention.** 2007. Update to CDC's Sexually Transmitted Diseases Treatment Guidelines, 2006: fluoroquinolones no longer recommended for treatment of gonococcal infections. *MMWR Morb Mortal Wkly Rep* **56**:332–336.

125. **Workowski KA, Berman S; Centers for Disease Control and Prevention.** 2010. Sexually Transmitted Diseases Treatment Guidelines, 2010. *MMWR Recommend Rep* **59**(RR-12):1–110.

126. **Centers for Disease Control and Prevention.** 2012. Update to CDC's Sexually Transmitted Diseases Treatment Guidelines, 2010: oral cephalosporins no longer a recommended treatment for gonococcal infections. *MMWR Morb Mortal Wkly Rep* **61**:590–594.

127. **World Health Organization.** *Strategies and Laboratory Methods for strengthening Surveillance of Sexually Transmitted Infections.* World Health Organization, Geneva, Switzerland. http://apps.who.int/iris/bitstream/10665/75729/1/9789241504478_eng.pdf. Accessed 22 November 2015.

128. **Centers for Disease Control and Prevention.** 1987. Antibiotic-resistant strains of *Neisseria gonorrhoeae*: policy guidelines for detection, management and control. *MMWR Morb Mortal Wkly Rep* **36**(Suppl 5S):13S.

129. **Roy K, Wang SA, Meltzer MI.** 2005. Optimizing treatment of antimicrobial-resistant *Neisseria gonorrhoeae*. *Emerg Infect Dis* **11**:1265–1273.

130. **Palmer HM, Young H, Winter A, Dave J.** 2008. Emergence and spread of azithromycin-resistant *Neisseria gonorrhoeae* in Scotland. *J Antimicrob Chemother* **62**:490–494.

131. **Kirkcaldy RD, Weinstock HS, Moore PC, Philip SS, Wiesenfeld HC, Papp JR, Kerndt PR, Johnson S, Ghanem KG, Hook EW III.** 2014. The efficacy and safety of gentamicin plus azithromycin and gemifloxacin plus azithromycin as treatment of uncomplicated gonorrhea. *Clin Infect Dis* **59**:1083–1091.

132. **Lee H, Hong SG, Soe Y, Yong D, Jeong SH, Lee K, Chong Y.** 2011. Trends in antimicrobial resistance of *Neisseria gonorrhoeae* isolated from Korean patients from 2000 to 2006. *Sex Transm Dis* **38**:1082–1086.

133. **Olsen B, Pham TL, Golparian D, Johansson E, Tran HK, Unemo M.** 2013. Antimicrobial susceptibility and genetic characteristics of *Neisseria gonorrhoeae* isolates from Vietnam, 2011. *BMC Infect Dis* **13**:40.

134. **Quaye N, Cole MJ, Ison CA.** 2014. Evaluation of the activity of ertapenem against gonococcal isolates exhibiting a range of susceptibilities to cefixime. *J Antimicrob Chemother* **69**:1568–1571.

135. **Unemo M, Golparian D, Limnios A, Whiley D, Ohnishi M, Lahra MM, Tapsall JW.** 2012. In vitro activity of ertapenem vs. ceftriaxone against *Neisseria gonorrhoeae* isolates with highly diverse ceftriaxone MIC values and effects of ceftriaxone resistance determinants—ertapenem for treatment of gonorrhea? *Antimicrob Agents Chemother* **56**:3603–3609.

136. **Hauser C, Hirzberger L, Unemo M, Furrer H, Endimiani A.** 2015. In vitro activity of fosfomycin alone and in combination with ceftriaxone or azithromycin against clinical *Neisseria gonorrhoeae* isolates. *Antimicrob Agents Chemother* **59**:1605–1611.

137. **Brown LB, Krysiak R, Kamanga G, Mapanje C, Kanyamula H, Banda B, Mhango C, Hoffman M, Kamwendo D, Hobbs M, Hosseinipour MC, Martinson F, Cohen MS, Hoffman IF.** 2010. *Neisseria gonorrhoeae* antimicrobial susceptibility in Lilongwe, Malawi, 2007. *Sex Transm Dis* **37**:169–172.

138. **Ross JD, Lewis DA.** 2012. Cephalosporin resistant *Neisseria gonorrhoeae*: time to consider gentamicin? *Sex Transm Infect* **88**:6–8.

139. **Hathorn E, Dhasmana D, Duley L, Ross JD.** 2014. The effectiveness of gentamicin in the treatment of *Neisseria gonorrhoeae*: a systematic review. *Syst Rev* **3**:104.

140. **Dowell D, Kirkcaldy RD.** 2013. Effectiveness of gentamicin for gonorrhea treatment: systematic review and meta-analysis. *Sex Transm Infect* **89**:142–147.

141. **Biedenbach DJ, Turner LL, Jones RN, Farell DJ.** 2012. Activity of JNJ-Q2, a novel fluoroquinolone, tested against *Neisseria gonorrhoeae*, including ciprofloxacin-resistant strains. *Diagn Microbiol Infect Dis* **74:**204–206.

142. **Roberts MC, Remy JM, Longcor JD, Marra A, Sun E, Duffy EM.** 2013. In vitro activity of delafloxacin against *Neisseria gonorrhoeae* clinical isolates. STI & AIDS World Congress 2013, 14 to 17 July, 2013, Vienna, Austria, poster P2.197.

143. **Hamasuna R, Yasuda M, Ishikawa K, Uehara S, Hayami H, Takahashi S, Matsumoto T, Yamamoto S, Minamitani S, Watanabe A, Iwata S, Kaku M, Kadota J, Sunakawa K, Sato J, Hanaki H, Tsukamoto T, Kiyota H, Egawa S, Tanaka K, Arakawa S, Fujisawa M, Kumon H, Kobayashi K, Matsubara A, Naito S, Kuroiwa K, Hirayama H, Narita H, Hosobe T, Ito S, Ito K, Kawai S, Ito M, Chokyu H, Matsumura M, Yoshioka M, Uno S, Monden K, Takayama K, Kaji S, Kawahara M, Sumii T, Kadena H, Yamaguchi T, Maeda S, Nishi S, Nishimura H, Shirane T, Yoh M, Akiyama K, Imai T, Kano M.** 2015. The second nationwide surveillance of the antimicrobial susceptibility of *Neisseria gonorrhoeae* from male urethritis in Japan, 2012-2013. *J Infect Chemother* **21:**340–345.

144. **Kazamori D, Aoi H, Sugimoto K, Ueshima T, Amano H, Itoh K, Kuramoto Y, Yazaki A.** 2014. In vitro activity of WQ-3810, a novel fluoroquinolone, against multidrug-resistant and fluoroquinolone-resistant pathogens. *Int J Antimicrob Agents* **44:**443–449.

145. **Kerstein K, Fyfe C, Sutcliffe JA, Grossman TH.** 2013. Eravacycline (TP-434) is active against susceptible and multidrug-resistant *Neisseria gonorrhoeae*, poster E-1181. Abstr 53rd Intersci Conf Antimicrob Agents Chemother, 10 to 13 September 2013, Denver, CO.

146. **Zhang YY, Zhou L, Zhu DM, Wu PC, Hu FP, Wu WH, Wang F.** 2004. In vitro activities of tigecycline against clinical isolates from Shanghai, China. *Diagn Microbiol Infect Dis* **50:**267–281.

147. **Fujimoto K, Takemoto K, Hatano K, Nakai T, Terashita S, Matsumoto M, Eriguchi Y, Eguchi K, Shimizudani T, Sato K, Kanazawa K, Sunagawa M, Ueda Y.** 2013. Novel carbapenem antibiotics for parenteral and oral applications: in vitro and in vivo activities of 2-aryl carbapenems and their pharmacokinetics in laboratory animals. *Antimicrob Agents Chemother* **57:**697–707.

148. **Jacobsson S, Golparian D, Phan LT, Ohnishi M, Fredlund H, Or YS, Unemo M.** 2015. In

149. **Golparian D, Fernandes P, Ohnishi M, Jensen JS, Unemo M.** 2012. In vitro activity of the new fluoroketolide solithromycin (CEM-101) against a large collection of clinical *Neisseria gonorrhoeae* isolates and international reference strains including those with various high-level antimicrobial resistance—potential treatment option for gonorrhea? *Antimicrob Agents Chemother* **56:**2739–2742.

150. **Koeth LM, Fisher.** 2013. In vitro activity of dalbavancin against *Neisseria gonorrhoeae* and development of a broth microdilution method, poster 255. IDWeek 2013, 2 to 6 October 2013, San Francisco, CA.

151. **Hook EW III, Golden M, Jamieson BD, Dixon PB, Harbison HS, Lowens S, Fernandes P.** 2015. A phase 2 trial of oral solithromycin 1200 mg or 1000 mg as single-dose oral therapy for uncomplicated gonorrhea. *Clin Infect Dis* **61:**1043–1048.

152. **Paukner S, Gruss A, Fritsche TR, Ivezic-Schoenfeld Z, Jones RN.** 2013. In vitro activity of the novel pleuromutilin BC-3781 tested against bacterial pathogens causing sexually transmitted diseases (STD), poster E-1183. Abstr 53rd Intersci Conf Antimicrob Agents Chemother, 10 to 13 September 2013, Denver, CO.

153. **Bouchillon SK, Hoban DJ, Hackel MA, Butler DL, Memarsh P, Alley MRK.** 2010. In vitro activities of AN3365: a novel boron containing protein synthesis inhibitor, and other antimicrobial agents against anaerobes and *Neisseria gonorrhoeae*, poster F1-1640. 50th Intersci Conf Antimicrob Agents Chemother, 12 to 15 September 2010, Boston, MA.

154. **Swanson S, Lee CJ, Liang X, Toone E, Zhou P, Nicholas R.** 2012. LpxC inhibitors as novel therapeutics for treatment of antibiotic-resistant *Neisseria gonorrhoeae*. 18th Int Pathog Neisseria Conf, 9 to 14 September 2012, Wurzburg, Germany, poster p174.

155. **Escaich S, Prouvensier L, Saccomani M, Durant L, Oxoby M, Gerusz V, Moreau F, Vongsouthi V, Maher K, Morrissey I, Soulama-Mouze C.** 2011. The MUT056399 inhibitor of FabI is a new antistaphylococcal compound. *Antimicrob Agents Chemother* **55:**4692–4697.

156. **Jeverica S, Golparian D, Hanzelka B, Fowlie AJ, Maticic M, Unemo M.** 2014. High in vitro

activity of a novel dual bacterial topoisomerase inhibitor of the ATPase activities of GyrB and ParE (VT12-008911) against *Neisseria gonorrhoeae* isolates with various high-level antimicrobial resistance and multidrug resistance. *J Antimicrob Chemother* **69:**1866–1872.

157. **Jacobsson S, Golparian D, Alm RA, Huband M, Mueller J, Jensen JS, Ohnishi M, Unemo M.** 2014. High in vitro activity of the novel spiropyrimidinetrione AZD0914, a DNA gyrase inhibitor, against multidrug resistant *Neisseria gonorrhoeae* isolates suggests a new effective option for oral treatment of gonorrhea. *Antimicrob Agents Chemother* **58:**5585–5588.

158. **Huband MD, Bradford PA, Otterson LG, Basarab GS, Kutschke A, Giacobbe R, Patey SA, Alm RA, Johnstone MR, Potter ME, Miller PF, Mueller JP.** 2015. In vitro antibacterial activity of AZD0914: a new spiropyrimidinetrione DNA gyrase/topoisomerase inhibitor with potent activity against Gram-positive, fastidious Gram-negative, and atypical bacteria. *Antimicrob Agents Chemother* **59:**467–474.

159. **Unemo M, Ringlander J, Wiggins C, Fredlund H, Jacobsson S, Cole M, the European Collaborative Group.** 2015. High in vitro susceptibility to the novel spiropyrimidinetrione ETX0914 (AZD0914) among 873 contemporary clinical *Neisseria gonorrhoeae* isolates in 21 European countries from 2012 to 2014. *Antimicrob Agents Chemother* **59:**5220–5225.

160. **Alm RA, Lahiri SD, Kutschke A, Otterson LG, McLaughlin RE, Whiteaker JD, Lewis LA, Su X, Huband MD, Gardner H, Mueller JP.** 2015. Characterization of the novel DNA gyrase inhibitor AZD0914: low resistance potential and lack of cross-resistance in *Neisseria gonorrhoeae*. *Antimicrob Agents Chemother* **59:**1478–1486.

161. **Jerse AE, Deal CD.** 2013. Vaccine research for gonococcal infections: where are we? *Sex Transm Infect* **89**(Suppl 4)**:**iv63–iv68.

162. **Grad YH, Kirkcaldy RD, Trees D, Dordel J, Harris SR, Goldstein E, Weinstock H, Parkhill J, Hanage WP, Bentley S, Lipsitch M.** 2014. Genomic epidemiology of *Neisseria gonorrhoeae* with reduced susceptibility to cefixime in the USA: a retrospective observational study. *Lancet Infect Dis* **14:**220–226.

163. **Ohnishi M, Unemo M.** 2014. Phylogenomics for drug-resistant *Neisseria gonorrhoeae*. *Lancet Infect Dis* **14:**179–180.

164. **Baarda BI, Sikora AE.** 2015. Proteomics of *Neisseria gonorrhoeae*: the treasure hunt for countermeasures against an old disease. *Front Microbiol* **6:**1190.

Bordetella holmesii: Still Emerging and Elusive 20 Years On

13

LAURE F. PITTET[1] and KLARA M. POSFAY-BARBE[1]

INTRODUCTION

Bordetella holmesii was first described in 1995 by the Centers for Disease Control and Prevention (CDC) (1). The initial 15 strains identified were assigned to the *Bordetella* genus following cellular fatty acid profiles, DNA relatedness studies, 16S rRNA sequencing, and guanine-plus-cytosine (G+C) content analysis. They were originally isolated from cultures of blood from patients from nine different states in the United States, one patient in Switzerland, and one in Saudi Arabia. Initially, *B. holmesii* was described as an agent responsible for bacteremia or other invasive diseases, such as arthritis or endocarditis, particularly in asplenic patients (1, 2). Five years after its first description, a report showed that *B. holmesii* could also cause pertussis-like symptoms in otherwise healthy individuals. Subsequently, it was demonstrated that *B. holmesii* respiratory infections were systematically misdiagnosed as *B. pertussis* because both genomes contain the insertion sequence (IS) targeted by the pertussis diagnostic test, namely, IS481 (3). Following this, several research groups developed discriminative *Bordetella* diagnostic tests (4–8) and retrospectively reanalyzed nasopharyngeal swabs that were *Bordetella* positive in order to determine to what extent this new species was contributing to the

[1]Pediatric Infectious Diseases Unit, Children's Hospital of Geneva, University Hospitals of Geneva, 1211 Geneva 14, Switzerland.
Emerging Infections 10
Edited by W. Michael Scheld, James M. Hughes and Richard J. Whitley
© 2016 American Society for Microbiology, Washington, DC
doi:10.1128/microbiolspec.EI10-0003-2015

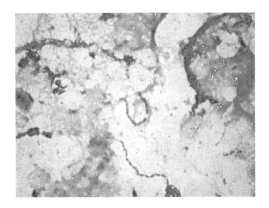

FIGURE 1 **Gram stain of *Bordetella holmesii*. Shown is an optic microscopic study showing colonies of Gram-negative coccobacilli identified as *B. holmesii*. The strain was isolated from a Swiss patient with bacteremia (57). (Courtesy of Stéphane Emonet, University of Geneva, Geneva, Switzerland.)**

increase in pertussis cases worldwide (8–22). Other groups have also conducted prospective studies with a similar objective (22–24). Simultaneously, microbiologists studied further this bacterium by investigating its virulence factors and similarity to other *Bordetella* species (25–30). Its entire genome was published in 2013 (31–33). In parallel, an increasing number of reports of *B. holmesii* infections in a variety of different sites were published (34–61). Nevertheless, *B. holmesii* still remains an underrecognized causative agent for respiratory or invasive infections, partly due to diagnostic difficulties (62). The aim of this chapter is to summarize the current knowledge on *B. holmesii*.

MICROBIOLOGY

Bordetella Genus

The genus *Bordetella* is part of the *Alcaligenaceae* family. It contains 12 species of Gram-negative pleomorphic aerobic bacilli: *B. pertussis*, *B. parapertussis*, and *B. bronchiseptica* (the classical species); *B. avium* and *B. hinzii* (the avian species); and *B. holmesii*, *B. trematum*, *B. petrii*, and *B. ansorpii* (added

in the last 20 years and considered new species). Very recently, *B. bronchialis*, *B. flabilis*, and *B. sputigena* have been isolated from human respiratory specimens (63).

Morphological and Biochemical Characteristics

B. holmesii organisms are predominantly small coccoid and short rods, with rare longer and wider forms (Fig. 1 and 2). Each *Bordetella* species has distinct biochemical characteristics (Table 1). *B. holmesii* differs from the other species because it is nonoxidizing, nonsaccharolytic, urease negative, and not hemolytic on blood agar plates (1). Moreover, it is the only *Bordetella* species that produces brown soluble pigments after 48 h of culture (Fig. 3).

Genome

The genome size of *B. holmesii* is approximately 3.6 Mb, and its G+C content is 63% (33). Cellular fatty acid profiles and genome analyses have demonstrated a strong

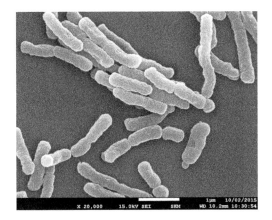

FIGURE 2 **Study of *Bordetella holmesii* by electron microscopy. Shown is a scanning electron microscopy view of a *B. holmesii* strain after 24 h of culture on tryptic soy broth liquid medium (×20,000). The patient is the same as for Fig. 1. (Courtesy of François Barja, University of Geneva, Geneva, Switzerland.)**

TABLE 1 Biochemical characteristics of *Bordetella holmesii* and comparison with other *Bordetella* spp.

Biochemical characteristic	*B. holmesii*	*B. pertussis*	*B. parapertussis*	*B. brochiseptica*	*B. avium*	*B. hinzii*	*B. petrii*	*B. trematum*	*B. ansorpii*
Oxidase	−	+	−	+	+	+	+	−	−
Nitrate reduction	−	−	−	+	−	−	−	+/−	−
Urease	−	−	+	+	−	+/−	−	−	−
Motility	−	−	−	+	+	+	−	+	+
Beta-like hemolysis	−	+	+	−					
Production of brown soluble pigment	+	−	−	−	−	−	−	−	−
Species group	New	Classical	Classical	Classical	Avian	Avian	New	New	New

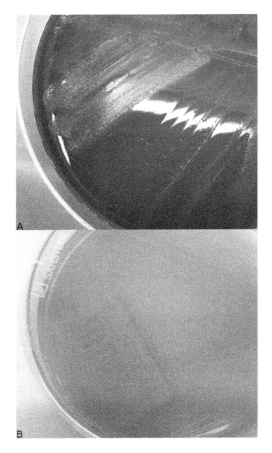

FIGURE 3 Colonies of *B. holmesii* growing on a sheep blood agar plate (A) and producing brown pigments after 48 h of culture on Mueller-Hinton medium (B). The patient is the same as for Fig. 1. (Courtesy of Stéphane Emonet, University of Geneva, Geneva, Switzerland.)

similarity between *B. holmesii* and the avian *Bordetella* species (1, 27, 31–33). However, it is also genetically closely related to the classical *Bordetella* species, which mainly infects mammals (62). Indeed, the 16S rRNA sequences of *B. pertussis* and *B. holmesii* are 99.5% similar (30), and both genomes count several copies of the IS*481* gene (approximately 200 and less than 10 copies, respectively) (4, 64) (Fig. 4). Hence, *B. holmesii* may be originally an avian species that has become pathogenic for humans due to the lateral transfer of genetic material from *B. pertussis* (27) or other bacteria (33). Indeed, Diavatopoulos et al. identified in the genome of *B. holmesii* a 66-kb region highly conserved between *B. pertussis* and *B. holmesii* containing genes primordial for pathogenesis. Analysis shows that this region has likely been transferred from one bacterium to the other (27). Another group found 24 to 114 unique genes in the genome of nine sequenced *B. holmesii* isolates. One of these strains had a gene coding for a residual protein normally found in *Escherichia coli* (33). Thus, all these hypothetic transfers may have contributed to the emergence of *B. holmesii* as a human pathogen. Interestingly, *B. holmesii* isolates of patients with invasive or respiratory infections have identical pulsed-field gel electrophoresis profiles, suggesting that the same strain could cause both types of infections (65).

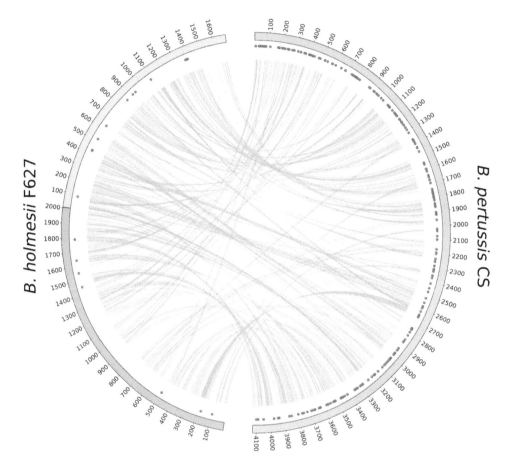

FIGURE 4 Comparison of genome maps of *Bordetella pertussis* and *Bordetella holmesii*. *B. pertussis* strain CS (GenBank accession number CP002695.1) is shown on the right side, and *B. holmesii* strain F627 (GenBank accession number AOEW00000000.1) is shown on the left side. The *B. holmesii* genome is in the form of two individual contigs, as illustrated by the two different shades of green. The grey links indicate sequence similarities at the protein level between the two genomes. Only local gene synteny is observed between the two bacteria. Red dots show the positions of IS*481*, which has 19 occurrences in *B. holmesii* strain F627 and 227 occurrences in *B. pertussis* strain CS. (Figure courtesy of David Hernandez, University of Geneva, Geneva, Switzerland; reproduced from reference 62 with permission.)

Pathogenic Factors

B. pertussis and most other *Bordetella* species produce biologically active components that are regulated by the *bvgAS* two-component system. Gerlach et al. have extensively studied the *bvgAS* system of the new *Bordetella* species and have shown that although there are similarities, *B. holmesii*'s system significantly differs from that of *B. pertussis*. They concluded that *B. holmesii* was therefore more closely related to the avian *Bordetella*,

although certain cytoplasmic signaling domains are functionally interchangeable between *B. pertussis* and *B. holmesii* (26). Regarding the classical pathogenic factors, *B. holmesii* produces a protein highly related to the filamentous hemagglutinin (FHA), an adhesin essential for colonization in other pathogenic *Bordetella* species. FHA expression is tightly regulated by the *bvgAS* locus (28). It also produces lipopolysaccharides, essential components of the outer membrane of Gram-negative bacteria, but its expression is different from that found in other *Bordetella* species. These lipopolysaccharides probably play a role in invasiveness, specifically in the higher invasive potential of *B. holmesii* (25). *B. holmesii* does not produce the pertussis toxin, one of the key pathogenic factors of *B. pertussis* (32, 65, 66). Moreover, the genome of *B. holmesii* lacks most of the other virulence factors implicated in the pathogenicity of *Bordetella* species (e.g., adenylate cyclase toxin, *Bordetella* type II and III secretion systems, pertactin, and fimbriae) (31, 32, 65). It has been found that approximately 400 genes of the *B. holmesii* genome have never been reported previously for any *Bordetella* species. Many of these genes are involved in microbial pathogenicity, e.g., are implicated in transport and detoxification of organic compounds or antibiotics, and it is possible that they have been acquired partly by lateral transfer (33). It remains unknown whether *B. holmesii* has a capsule. If this is the case, its presence could explain to some extent why asplenic patients have an increased risk for *B. holmesii* bacteremia (67).

CLINICAL FEATURES

Pertussis-Like Respiratory Infections

Clinical manifestations of a *B. holmesii* respiratory infection are similar to a pertussis-like disease. They include mild fever, associated with the classical pertussis symptoms of paroxysmal cough, inspiratory whoop, and post-tussive vomiting. The expected duration of the illness and whether it is also divided into the three typical stages of pertussis disease, namely, the catarrhal, paroxysmal, and convalescent periods, is still unknown. However, it is believed that it is similar to a *B. pertussis* infection. In a study comparing 21 cases of *B. holmesii* respiratory infection with 122 cases of *B. pertussis* infection, the authors concluded that the clinical presentation was less severe with *B. holmesii*, as patients presented two or less of the three classical

pertussis symptoms (9). Conversely, Rodgers et al. reported that clinical features were similar in 48 cases of *B. holmesii* respiratory infection and 112 cases of *B. pertussis* (68). However, they found that cough duration was shorter in *B. holmesii* infection, with almost 70% of patients being cough-free 80 days after antibiotic administration (clarithromycin or azithromycin), compared to 30% of patients with *B. pertussis*. This could possibly be explained by the lack of pertussis toxin in *B. holmesii* (68). Neither complications nor deaths have been reported after respiratory infections, but this may reflect a reporting or detection bias. Given the high similarity between *B. holmesii* isolates in respiratory and invasive disease, secondary bloodstream dissemination after a respiratory infection with secondary complications cannot be excluded.

B. pertussis infection in infants correlates with a high mortality and complication rate. The only published report of *B. holmesii* infection of infants younger than 6 months shows no cyanosis or apnea. However, this reassuring information is based on only a very limited (seven) number of patients (69).

Bacteremia

B. holmesii was first reported as an organism causing bacteremia, mainly in immunocompromised individuals. The clinical course is always nonspecific, with mild fever occasionally accompanied by headache, chills, or vomiting (37, 45). Concomitant respiratory symptoms are frequent, suggesting possible secondary blood dissemination. Laboratory assessments are noncontributive; in particular, there is no high lymphocytosis as described for *B. pertussis* respiratory infection. This might be explained also by the lack of pertussis toxin in *B. holmesii*. Although it could be questioned whether *B. holmesii* isolated in patients is the actual cause of infection and not due to infection by another microorganism, growing evidence proves that it is truly pathogenic. In most patients,

B. holmesii was isolated from two or more cultures in blood samples, obtained at different times during the same infectious episode, and was the only microorganism isolated (37). The outcome is usually favorable when the infection is treated with antibiotics, with no fatality reported. However, the presentation can sometimes be severe with secondary infections and even require admission to intensive care (37, 70).

Other Invasive Infections

B. holmesii has been isolated in a variety of body sites, mostly documented in case reports. These have been summarized recently in a review (62) and include cases of pneumonia, endocarditis, pericarditis, meningitis, arthritis, diskitis, and cellulitis. The infection was usually confirmed by using different diagnostic tools, repeated sampling, and, exceptionally, tissue biopsy, suggesting causality. Interestingly, some patients complained of concomitant mild upper respiratory tract symptoms, thus raising the question of whether a primary *B. holmesii* respiratory infection may have further disseminated to a secondary infectious site. Unfortunately, this was investigated only once (56). Although some patients experienced infection relapse, required prolonged treatment, were admitted to the intensive care unit, or even needed a surgical procedure, such as the removal of prosthetic material, outcomes have generally been favorable at the end of the treatment, with no fatality reported (62).

In particular, three cases of pneumonia have been described; two were complicated by pleural effusion (36, 38, 56). One patient had an acute presentation with mediastinal collection, pericarditis, coagulopathy, and pulmonary fibrosis, resulting in a severe restrictive syndrome 6 months later (36, 38). *B. holmesii* has been reported to trigger exacerbation of chronic obstructive pulmonary disease in a 41-year-old woman, requiring intubation and admission to critical care

(2). Endocarditis on both native and prosthetic valves was reported for eight patients (1, 2, 41, 47, 48, 51, 58). Clinical symptoms differed among individuals, ranging from subacute endocarditis to septic shock with acute renal failure. Patients usually required valve replacement. Two additional patients had *B. holmesii* pericarditis; one required more than 2 months of hospital stay (36, 53). Two cases of *B. holmesii* meningitis were reported, one in a 14-year-old girl with anorexia nervosa and the other in a 39-year-old woman with end-stage renal disease secondary to systemic lupus erythematosus. One patient experienced persistent convulsions that required continuous intravenous diazepam and mechanical ventilation (71, 72). Septic arthritis has been reported for patients with both normal and prosthetic knees, followed by the removal of the prosthesis in an immunocompetent 54-year-old woman (1, 46, 60). A case of lumbar diskitis was diagnosed by identification of *B. holmesii* on cultures of both blood and L3-L4 disk biopsy (61). Finally, *B. holmesii* was isolated four times in cultures of blood from a 67-year-old patient receiving rituximab and presenting subsequently with three episodes of cellulitis and one episode of pneumonia. Nasal carriage of *B. holmesii* was also reported later (56).

DIAGNOSIS

Various methods can be used for the detection of *B. holmesii* in clinical specimens. The organism can be cultured if appropriate media are used, such as Bordet-Gengou or Regan-Lowe medium without cephalexin. Its presence can be identified by PCR, whole-cell fatty acid analysis, 16S rRNA analysis, or mass spectrometry (62). In respiratory infections, specimens are collected by either swab, aspiration, or nasopharyngeal wash as for *B. pertussis*, but no study has yet evaluated which sample site yields the best results. *B. holmesii* has been isolated also from blood, tissue biopsy samples, and pleural, articular, and other fluids (62).

Culture

Although culture is frequently used to diagnose *B. holmesii* invasive or respiratory infection, this diagnostic tool is cumbersome, as for all other *Bordetella* species, because of its fastidious growth and low analytical sensitivity (12% to 60%) (7). Specific swabs are required, and rapid transfer to the laboratory is necessary to ensure optimal sensitivity (3, 73). The specimen needs then to be directly plated onto the appropriate medium. If plate inoculation cannot be done rapidly, special transport medium is also required (Regan-Lowe transport medium without cephalexin). Interestingly, it has been demonstrated that the growth of *B. holmesii* is inhibited by cephalexin, an antimicrobial agent widely recommended and used in various *Bordetella* culture media (74). Therefore, recommendations have now changed, and oxacillin or methicillin is now preferred instead of cephalexin to grow *B. holmesii* (75). This intrinsic susceptibility explains also why most laboratories failed to identify *B. holmesii* in nasopharyngeal specimens of patients with pertussis-like symptoms before 2000 (74).

Polymerase Chain Reaction

In 2000, Loeffelholz et al. first reported that the most frequently used technique at that time for the diagnosis of *B. pertussis*, i.e., PCR targeting the IS*481* sequence, was not species specific, as it systematically falsely diagnosed *B. holmesii* respiratory infection as *B. pertussis* (3). This was confirmed by quality control exercises carried out worldwide and showed that only a very few laboratories were able to routinely identify *B. holmesii* (76–78). Indeed, PCR is the most commonly used diagnostic tool when suspecting pertussis given its high sensitivity compared to that of culture (93% sensitivity with the IS*481* target, compared to 15% for culture in a study using an expanded

case definition [79]). Diagnosing infections using PCR has also the advantages of remaining positive later in the course of the disease and of being less affected by antibiotic treatment. However, as no universal recommendations exist, PCR protocols for *B. pertussis* diagnosis differ widely among centers, with each laboratory defining its own assay procedure and detection limit (77, 80, 81). Nevertheless, most laboratories use IS*481* as the target sequence to diagnose *B. pertussis* (77, 81). Since a substantial number of copies of IS*481* is found in the *B. pertussis* genome, the sensitivity of PCR targeting this sequence is greater than that of those using single-copy target sequences (e.g., pertussis toxin) (11). The high sensitivity is at a cost of lower specificity, as few copies of IS*481* are also present in the genome of other *Bordetella* species, such as *B. holmesii* and, occasionally, *B. bronchiseptica* (76, 82). Thus, laboratories aware of this potential false-positive result have decided to perform a second PCR assay on IS*481*-positive specimens using either a *B. pertussis*- or a *B. holmesii*-specific target, or both. However, these other targets are at least 10-fold less sensitive than the IS*481* target, since they are present in fewer copies of the genome. This might lead subsequently to false-negative results (83). A number of potential target sequences have been proposed to increase the diagnosis of *B. pertussis* (*ptx*, IS*1002*, BP*283*, and BP*485*) and *B. holmesii* (*recA*, hIS*1001*, and *bhoE*) (10–12, 84, 85), but there is no recommendation on what is the best PCR diagnostic strategy to use at the present time.

Loop-Mediated Isothermal Amplification Assay

First described by a Japanese group in 2004, the loop-mediated isothermal amplification assay is a novel method that uses a DNA amplification technique and offers a rapid diagnosis of various viral and bacterial infectious diseases. It is usually less expensive and simpler to use than conventional PCR, since it is isothermal and does not require expensive thermocyclers, thus making it a promising method for microbial diagnosis, especially in countries with limited resources. Otsuka et al. developed the first loop-mediated isothermal amplification assay targeting the *recA* gene that successfully detected *B. holmesii* and discriminated it from other *Bordetella* species (86). Although not extensively used, this technique is of potential interest and could increase in the future.

16S Ribosomal RNA

The 16S rRNA sequencing technique is the most frequently used method in the case reports of invasive *B. holmesii* infection (62). Of note, as the sequence obtained in *B. holmesii* is very similar to that of *B. pertussis* (>99% similarity [30]), it is recommended to perform additional sequence analysis for confirmation in a second step, such as detection of *B. holmesii*-specific genes by PCR, for example (27).

Spectrometry

Matrix-assisted laser desorption ionization–time-of-flight mass spectrometry (MALDI-TOF MS) is a soft ionization technique used in mass spectrometry that enables identification of most pathogens retrieved in clinical microbiology (87). Few groups have detected the presence of *B. holmesii* in various clinical specimens by MALDI-TOF MS (51, 54, 59–61). This promising diagnostic tool has the advantage of allowing a rapid and accurate identification of *B. holmesii* in any clinical specimen. However, only a limited number of laboratories have access to this new and expensive technology.

Automated Microbial Identification Devices

Automated microbial identification devices are widely used in clinical microbiology laboratories and enable the rapid and accurate identification of selected medically relevant bacteria. However, reports have highlighted that these devices failed to identify *B. holmesii* or systematically erred, since it was not included in their database (35, 39, 51, 54, 88). For example, Jonckheere et al. (51) and Panagopoulos et al. (88) reported several cases of systematic misidentification of the bacteria as *Acinetobacter* spp. by Vitek2 (bioMérieux Inc., Marcy L'Etoile, France) and API 20 NE gallery (bioMérieux Inc.), respectively.

TREATMENT

No evidence-based recommendations are available regarding the best antibiotic regimen for treating *B. holmesii* infection. Several groups have investigated the *in vitro* susceptibility of *B. holmesii* to various antibiotics using broth microdilution (37), the Epsilometer test (31, 38, 44, 46, 51, 53, 56, 58, 71, 72, 88), automated systems (39, 48), agar dilution (2), and disk diffusion (34, 47, 51, 89). In summary, investigations show that third-generation cephalosporins may not be optimal to treat *B. holmesii* (37). Ceftazidime is probably the best in this class, given its low MICs (2, 39, 51, 88, 89). There are conflicting data on cefotaxime, which is reported as both active (2, 34, 58) and inactive (37, 39, 42, 47, 51, 56, 88) against *B. holmesii*. Resistance to ceftriaxone, cefotaxime, and also trimethoprim-sulfamethoxazole has been reported (42, 56, 71). Concerning macrolides, some data show that erythromycin has a lower activity against *B. holmesii* than *B. pertussis* (1). As for other antimicrobials, carbapenems and fluoroquinolones were effective *in vitro* against *B. holmesii* (37, 53) and are often suggested as the most effective treatment for *B. holmesii* infection (37, 45). As very few data are available on this subject, further microbiological investigations are required to determine the optimal antibiotic treatment and the breakpoints to be used for antimicrobial susceptibility testing of clinical isolates (51).

Respiratory Infections

In cases of *B. holmesii* respiratory infection, most patients are treated as for a *B. pertussis* infection. This happens because the patient has been misdiagnosed as infected with *B. pertussis* or because physicians give empirically the same antimicrobial for any *Bordetella* respiratory infection.

Macrolides are usually the first-choice treatment for a *B. pertussis* infection (75). However, they may not be the best choice for *B. holmesii* (1), and this could become an issue if the distinction between the two species is not made. From both an individual and a public health point of view, it is not clearly established at present whether it is indicated to administer antibiotics to patients with *B. holmesii* respiratory infection. This could probably be discussed on an individual basis for a patient with (or in contact with a person with) an underlying immunocompromised status in order to prevent secondary invasive infections.

Supportive care that is traditionally used in *B. pertussis* infection may also be suitable for *B. holmesii* infections. Examples include avoidance of factors triggering cough, such as physical exercise, cold air, or nasopharyngeal suctioning, as well as maintenance of adequate hydration and nutrition with the use of intravenous fluids and nasogastric feeding if required. Assisted ventilation may be necessary for some severe cases. Other adjunctive treatments, such as bronchodilators, corticosteroids, or antitussive agents, have not been proven to be beneficial in the case of *B. pertussis* infection and should probably not be used either for patients with *B. holmesii* (90).

Bacteremia and Other Invasive Infections

Due to the delayed identification of *B. holmesii*, patients with *B. holmesii* bacteremia or other invasive infections were initially treated empirically with the antibiotics recommended according to the focus of infection. Treatments were sometimes switched later when the microorganism and its antibiotic susceptibility were known. The different antibiotic regimens documented in published case reports have been recently summarized in a review (62). Third-generation cephalosporins, often used empirically in various invasive infections, are not the first-choice antimicrobials for *B. holmesii* (37, 42, 54, 59). Most authors suggest carbapenems and fluoroquinolones, as they are probably the most effective agents against *B. holmesii* (37, 45). Clinicians should also keep in mind that a treatment course of more than 5 to 12 weeks (34, 36, 47, 49) is sometimes required, with some patients experiencing relapse when a shorter antimicrobial course was used (34, 47, 56). Finally, it should be recalled that *B. holmesii* bacteremia has been reported for patients receiving penicillin or trimethoprim-sulfamethoxazole prophylaxis (31, 35, 44, 57).

PREVENTION

Vaccination

As shown by Zhang et al. in an animal model, neither the whole-cell nor the acellular *B. pertussis* vaccine confers protection against *B. holmesii* (17). This observation was confirmed clinically during a *B. pertussis* and *B. holmesii* outbreak in which 60% of patients with a *B. holmesii* respiratory infection had been previously boosted with pertussis vaccine, compared to 44% of the *B. pertussis* cases (68). Since it has been demonstrated that the genes coding for the antigens targeted by the *B. pertussis* acellular vaccine (pertussis toxin, FHA, pertactin, and/or fimbriae, depending on the manufacturer) are absent from the *B. holmesii* genome (32, 34) or immunogenically distinct, antigen-specific immunoglobulins induced by pertussis vaccination will not protect against a *B. holmesii* infection. At the present time, there is no intention to develop a vaccine that induces protection against *B. holmesii*, and this will probably not be necessary in the near future.

Antibiotic Prophylaxis

As the same *B. holmesii* strain could potentially induce both respiratory and invasive disease, postexposure antibiotic prophylaxis may be indicated for individuals particularly at risk of invasive disease, such as asplenic patients. Although macrolides are the first choice for antibioprophylaxis following *B. pertussis* contact, they do not appear to be the best choice in this setting, given their lower activity against *B. holmesii* (1). Penicillins could probably be used as an alternative.

Management Following an Index Case

It is not mandatory to notify a case of *B. holmesii* infection to public health bodies, whereas it is for *B. pertussis* in many countries (91). Misidentification of a case of *B. holmesii* respiratory infection as a pertussis case may result in unnecessary and costly case investigations by public health authorities, including postexposure evaluation and management of contacts of index cases (92). In a hospital setting, droplet precautions should be implemented for a confirmed case of *B. holmesii* infection with respiratory symptoms in order to reduce transmission of the disease (93).

EPIDEMIOLOGY

Transmission and Reservoir

Transmission of respiratory infection is thought to be via droplets, although this has not been extensively investigated. The attack rate among contacts after an index case is unknown. *B. holmesii* carriage may be also suspected, although it is unclear if it is transient or not (48). Incubation time and the inoculum needed for infection are also unknown. Evidence suggests that *B. holmesii* cocirculates with *B. pertussis* (9), as it has been isolated during several pertussis outbreaks (15, 22, 68) and five cases of *B. holmesii* and *B. pertussis* coinfection have been reported (68). The main routes of transmission of *B. holmesii* invasive disease have still to be elucidated. *B. holmesii* strains causing respiratory disease do not seem to differ from strains causing invasive disease, and it can be postulated that secondary blood dissemination can occur following respiratory infection. A few copies of *B. holmesii* have previously been detected in two platelet concentrates, which had been missed by routine bacterial screening (94). *B. holmesii* is believed to be a strictly human pathogen with no recognized animal reservoir. However, this has never been investigated and should be challenged because *B. holmesii* is closely related to the avian *Bordetella* species (27, 30–32, 85, 95).

Prevalence and Incidence

Epidemiological data are lacking, and the prevalence of *B. holmesii* is unclear and probably underestimated, as *B. holmesii* has been recognized as a human pathogen only recently and is challenging to detect. Awareness of *B. holmesii* is increasing, and it seems likely that an increasing number of laboratories will be able to detect it. As reported recently in a laboratory performance exercise, the number of U.S. public health laboratories that are capable of correctly diagnosing *B. holmesii* has increased from 5% to 75% in 2015 (81, 96). However, previous studies have shown that elsewhere, only a very limited number of laboratories were able to distinguish *B. holmesii* from other *Bordetella*: 1/11 (9%) and 1/24 (4%) European laboratories in 2005 and 2013, respectively (76, 77) and 7% of Australian laboratories in 2013 (78).

Studies worldwide have reported that *B. holmesii* could be the causative agent for 0% to 29% of patients with pertussis-like symptoms (6, 9, 10, 14, 15, 19, 20, 62, 68). The highest prevalence was reported in a study conducted during the 2010 Ohio pertussis outbreak, when *B. holmesii* was identified in approximately one-third of the cases of *Bordetella*-confirmed infections and at an even higher proportion in children 11 to 18 years old (45%) (68). All these prevalence studies have been listed in a review (62).

The prevalence of *B. holmesii* can widely differ from one country to another, even when the countries are geographically very close (62). In addition, the organism is more frequently reported between September and March and possibly follows a seasonal pattern (9, 21). At first, *B. holmesii* respiratory infection was identified more frequently in healthy adolescents and young adults (9), but since then, it has been detected in all age groups (19, 97).

Impact of Systematic Misidentification of *B. holmesii* Respiratory Infection as *B. pertussis*

Misdiagnosis of *B. holmesii* respiratory infection as *B. pertussis* affects the epidemiological studies of both species. Although the circulation of *B. holmesii* is low or nonexistent in some areas, one study found that it was present in almost half of the *Bordetella*-positive patients in a certain age group (68). However, given the seemingly high variability in prevalence of *B. holmesii* worldwide, countries should use *Bordetella* species-specific tests at least temporarily to determine whether and to what extent *B. holmesii* contributes to the pertussis cases. The specific diagnosis of *Bordetella* species is important because (i) case investigation required for *B. pertussis* is likely unnecessary for *B. holmesii* (92), (ii) antibioprophylaxis for immunosuppressed or asplenic patients (or persons in contact with them) may be indicated with *B. holmesii* respiratory infection, and (iii) misdiagnosing a *B. holmesii* respiratory infection as a *B. pertussis* breakthrough case following pertussis vaccination modifies the evaluation of the vaccine efficacy.

CONCLUSIONS

B. holmesii is an underdiagnosed emerging organism for which only limited clinical, microbiological, and epidemiological data are available. It has a greater invasive capacity than other *Bordetella* species. Lateral transfer of genetic material of other bacteria has possibly contributed to the emergence of *B. holmesii* as a human pathogen and may enhance its pathogenicity in the future. Hence, increasing awareness and surveillance of this entity are required for both invasive and respiratory infections. Although the optimal treatment for *B. holmesii* is unknown, infection with the organism can be easily diagnosed by PCR, 16S rRNA analysis, or mass spectrometry. Future studies should focus on understanding the epidemiology of *B. holmesii*, including its relation to other *Bordetella* species, establish the full spectrum of its clinical presentation, and determine the best management for patients, depending on the infection site.

ACKNOWLEDGMENTS

We gratefully thank Stéphane Emonet, Patrick Linder, Karl Perron, François Barja, and David Hernandez for the figures, Martine Leplay Fontana for her help in retrieving articles, and Rosemary Sudan for editorial assistance.

CITATION

Pittet LF, Posfay-Barbe KM. 2016. *Bordetella holmesii*: still emerging and elusive 20 years on. Microbiol Spectrum 4(3):EI10-0003-2015.

REFERENCES

1. **Weyant RS, Hollis DG, Weaver RE, Amin MFM, Steigerwalt AG, O'Connor SP, Whitney AM, Daneshvar MI, Moss CW, Brenner DJ.** 1995. *Bordetella holmesii* sp. nov., a new gram-negative species associated with septicemia. *J Clin Microbiol* **33:**1–7.

2. Tang YW, Hopkins MK, Kolbert CP, Hartley PA, Severance PJ, Persing DH. 1998. *Bordetella holmesii*-like organisms associated with septicemia, endocarditis, and respiratory failure. *Clin Infect Dis* 26:389–392.

3. Loeffelholz MJ, Thompson CJ, Long KS, Gilchrist MJR. 2000. Detection of *Bordetella holmesii* using *Bordetella pertussis* IS481 PCR assay. *J Clin Microbiol* 38:467.

4. Reischl U, Lehn N, Sanden GN, Loeffelholz MJ. 2001. Real-time PCR assay targeting IS481 of *Bordetella pertussis* and molecular basis for detecting *Bordetella holmesii*. *J Clin Microbiol* 39:1963–1966.

5. Poddar SK. 2003. Detection and discrimination of *B. pertussis* and *B. holmesii* by real-time PCR targeting IS481 using a beacon probe and probe-target melting analysis. *Mol Cell Probes* 17:91–98.

6. Templeton KE, Scheltinga SA, Van der Zee A, Diederen BMW, Kruijssen AM, Goossens H, Kuijper E, Claas ECJ. 2003. Evaluation of real-time PCR for detection of and discrimination between *Bordetella pertussis*, *Bordetella parapertussis*, and *Bordetella holmesii* for clinical diagnosis. *J Clin Microbiol* 41:4121–4126.

7. Tatti KM, Wu KH, Tondella ML, Cassiday PK, Cortese MM, Wilkins PP, Sanden GN. 2008. Development and evaluation of dual-target real-time polymerase chain reaction assays to detect *Bordetella* spp. *Diagn Microbiol Infect Dis* 61:264–272.

8. Knorr L, Fox JD, Tilley PAG, Ahmed-Bentley J. 2006. Evaluation of real-time PCR for diagnosis of *Bordetella pertussis* infection. *BMC Infect Dis* 6:62.

9. Yih WK, Silva EA, Ida J, Harrington N, Lett SM, George H. 1999. *Bordetella holmesii*-like organisms isolated from Massachusetts patients with pertussis-like symptoms. *Emerg Infect Dis* 5:441–443.

10. Antila M, He Q, De Jong C, Aarts I, Verbakel H, Bruisten S, Keller S, Haanpera M, Makinen J, Eerola E, Viljanen MK, Mertsola J, Van Der Zee A. 2006. *Bordetella holmesii* DNA is not detected in nasopharyngeal swabs from Finnish and Dutch patients with suspected pertussis. *J Med Microbiol* 55:1043–1051.

11. Probert WS, Ely J, Schrader K, Atwell J, Nossoff A, Kwan S. 2008. Identification and evaluation of new target sequences for specific detection of *Bordetella pertussis* by real-time PCR. *J Clin Microbiol* 46:3228–3231.

12. Guthrie JL, Robertson AV, Tang P, Jamieson F, Drews SJ. 2010. Novel duplex real-time PCR assay detects *Bordetella holmesii* in specimens from patients with pertussis-like symptoms in Ontario, Canada. *J Clin Microbiol* 48:1435–1437.

13. Wei Q, Robinson CC, Lovell MA, Hengartner RJ, Kelly KA, Murry KD. 2010. A cautionary tale from Colorado: *Bordetella holmesii* circulates and can lead to false positive results in commonly-used *Bordetella pertussis* PCR. *J Mol Diagn* 12:883.

14. Njamkepo E, Bonacorsi S, Debruyne M, Gibaud SA, Guillot S, Guiso N. 2011. Significant finding of *Bordetella holmesii* DNA in nasopharyngeal samples from French patients with suspected pertussis. *J Clin Microbiol* 49:4347–4348.

15. Kamiya H, Otsuka N, Ando Y, Odaira F, Yoshino S, Kawano K, Takahashi H, Nishida T, Hidaka Y, Toyoizumi-Ajisaka H, Shibayama K, Kamachi K, Sunagawa T, Taniguchi K, Okabe N. 2012. Transmission of *Bordetella holmesii* during pertussis outbreak, Japan. *Emerg Infect Dis* 18:1166–1169.

16. Rodgers LE, Cohn A, Martin S, Clark T, Budd J, A Terranella, S Mandal, L McGlone, A Emanuel, L Tondella, L Pawloski, K Tatti, M Marcon, K Spicer, A Leber, R Iyer, D Salamon, N Tucker, C Hicks, M DiOrio, E Koch, LeMaile-Williams M. 2012. *Bordetella holmesii* epidemiology during an outbreak of pertussis-like illness—Ohio, 2010-2011, p 86. *In* 61st Annu Epidemic Intelligence Service (EIS) Conf, 18 April 2012. Centers for Disease Control and Prevention, Atlanta, GA.

17. Zhang X, Weyrich LS, Lavine JS, Karanikas AT, Harvill ET. 2012. Lack of cross-protection against *Bordetella holmesii* after pertussis vaccination. *Emerg Infect Dis* 18:1771–1779.

18. Cox HC, Jacob K, Whiley DM, Bletchly C, Nimmo GR, Nissen MD, Sloots TP. 2013. Further evidence that the IS481 target is suitable for real-time PCR detection of *Bordetella pertussis*. *Pathology* 45:202–203.

19. Bottero D, Griffith MM, Lara C, Flores D, Pianciola L, Gaillard ME, Mazzeo M, Zamboni MI, Spoleti MJ, Anchart E, Ruggeri D, Sorhouet C, Fiori S, Galas M, Tondella ML, Hozbor DF. 2013. *Bordetella holmesii* in children suspected of pertussis in Argentina. *Epidemiol Infect* 141:714–717.

20. Pittet LF, Emonet S, Francois P, Bonetti EJ, Schrenzel J, Hug M, Altwegg M, Siegrist CA, Posfay-Barbe KM. 2014. Diagnosis of whooping cough in Switzerland: differentiating *Bordetella pertussis* from *Bordetella holmesii* by polymerase chain reaction. *PLoS One* 9:e88936.

21. Spicer KB, Salamon D, Cummins C, Leber A, Marcon MJ. 2014. Occurrence of three *Bordetella* species during an outbreak of cough

Illness in Ohio: epidemiology, clinical features, laboratory findings, and antimicrobial susceptibility. *Pediatr Infect Dis J* **33**:e162–e167.

22. **Miranda C, Wozniak A, Castillo C, Geoffroy E, Zumaran C, Porte L, Roman JC, Potin M, Garcia P.** 2013. Presence of *Bordetella holmesii* in an outbreak of pertussis in Chile. *Rev Chilena Infectol* **30**:237–243. (In Spanish.)

23. **Zouari A, Smaoui H, Brun D, Njamkepo E, Sghaier S, Zouari E, Felix R, Menif K, Ben Jaballah N, Guiso N, Kechrid A.** 2012. Prevalence of *Bordetella pertussis* and *Bordetella parapertussis* infections in Tunisian hospitalized infants: results of a 4-year prospective study. *Diagn Microbiol Infect Dis* **72**:303–317.

24. **Dinu S, Guillot S, Dragomirescu CC, Brun D, Lazar S, Vancea G, Ionescu BM, Gherman MF, Bjerkestrand AF, Ungureanu V, Guiso N, Damian M.** 2014. Whooping cough in South-East Romania: a 1-year study. *Diagn Microbiol Infect Dis* **78**:302–306.

25. **van den Akker WM.** 1998. Lipopolysaccharide expression within the genus *Bordetella*: influence of temperature and phase variation. *Microbiology* **144**(Part 6):1527–1535.

26. **Gerlach G, Janzen S, Beier D, Gross R.** 2004. Functional characterization of the BvgAS two-component system of *Bordetella holmesii*. *Microbiology* **150**:3715–3729.

27. **Diavatopoulos DA, Cummings CA, Van Der Heide HGJ, Van Gent M, Liew S, Relman DA, Mooi FR.** 2006. Characterization of a highly conserved island in the otherwise divergent *Bordetella holmesii* and *Bordetella pertussis* genomes. *J Bacteriol* **188**:8385–8394.

28. **Link S, Schmitt K, Beier D, Gross R.** 2007. Identification and regulation of expression of a gene encoding a filamentous hemagglutinin-related protein in *Bordetella holmesii*. *BMC Microbiol* **7**:100.

29. **Horvat A, Gross R.** 2009. Molecular characterization of the BvgA response regulator of *Bordetella holmesii*. *Microbiol Res* **164**:243–252.

30. **Gross R, Keidel K, Schmitt K.** 2010. Resemblance and divergence: the "new" members of the genus *Bordetella*. *Med Microbiol Immunol* **199**:155–163.

31. **Planet PJ, Narechania A, Hymes SR, Gagliardo C, Huard RC, Whittier S, Della-Latta P, Ratner AJ.** 2013. *Bordetella holmesii*: initial genomic analysis of an emerging opportunist. *Pathog Dis* **67**:132–135.

32. **Tatti KM, Loparev VN, Ranganathanganakammal S, Changayil S, Frace M, Weil MR, Sammons S, Maccannell D, Mayer LW, Tondella ML.** 2013. Draft genome sequences of *Bordetella holmesii* strains from blood (F627)

and nasopharynx (H558). *Genome Announc* **1**:e0005613.

33. **Harvill ET, Goodfield LL, Ivanov Y, Smallridge WE, Meyer JA, Cassiday PK, Tondella ML, Brinkac L, Sanka R, Kim M, Losada L.** 2014. Genome sequences of nine *Bordetella holmesii* strains isolated in the United States. *Genome Announc* **2**:e00438-14. doi:10.1128/genomeA.00438-14.

34. **Njamkepo E, Delisle F, Hagege I, Gerbaud G, Guiso N.** 2000. *Bordetella holmesii* isolated from a patient with sickle cell anemia: analysis and comparison with other *Bordetella holmesii* isolates. *Clin Microbiol Infect* **6**:131–136.

35. **Greig JR, Gunda SS, Kwan JTC.** 2001. *Bordetella holmesii* bacteraemia in an individual on haemodialysis. *Scand J Infect Dis* **33**:716–717.

36. **Russell FM, Davis JM, Whipp MJ, Janssen PH, Ward PB, Vyas JR, Starr M, Sawyer SM, Curtis N.** 2001. Severe *Bordetella holmesii* infection in a previously healthy adolescent confirmed by gene sequence analysis. *Clin Infect Dis* **33**:129–130.

37. **Shepard CW, Daneshvar MI, Kaiser RM, Ashford DA, Lonsway D, Patel JB, Morey RE, Jordan JG, Weyant RS, Fischer M.** 2004. *Bordetella holmesii* bacteremia: a newly recognized clinical entity among asplenic patients. *Clin Infect Dis* **38**:799–804.

38. **Dorbecker C, Licht C, Korber F, Plum G, Haefs C, Hoppe B, Seifert H.** 2007. Community-acquired pneumonia due to *Bordetella holmesii* in a patient with frequently relapsing nephrotic syndrome. *J Infect* **54**:e203–e205.

39. **Lam MC, Verity R, Tyrrell GJ, Arent R, Nigrin J, Forgie SE.** 2008. Gram-negative bacteremia and asplenia in a well 15-year-old girl. *Can J Infect Dis Med Microbiol* **19**:391–392.

40. **McCavit TL, Grube S, Revell P, Quinn CT.** 2008. *Bordetella holmesii* bacteremia in sickle cell disease. *Pediatr Blood Cancer* **51**:814–816.

41. **Clare S, Ahmed T, Singh R, Gough S.** 2010. *Bordetella holmesii*: a rare cause of bacterial endocarditis in a post-splenectomy patient. *BMJ Case Rep.* doi:10.1136/bcr.11.2009.2459.

42. **Monnier S, Therby A, Couzon B, Doucet-Populaire F, Greder-Belan A.** 2010. *Bordetella holmesii* bacteremia in a 26-year-old patient with sickle cell disease. *Med Mal Infect* **40**:299–301.

43. **Abouanaser S, Srigley J, Wilcox L, Johnstone J.** 2011. Prosthetic joint infection caused by *Bordetella holmesii*. *Can J Infect Dis Med Microbiol* **22**:22A.

44. **Barrado L, Barrios M, Sanz F, Chaves F.** 2011. *Bordetella holmesii* bacteremia in a child with

sickle cell disease. *Enfermed Infecc Microbiol Clin* **29:**779–780.

45. **Kanji J, Gee S, Ahmed-Bentley J, Lee MC, Nigrin J, Verity R, Solomon N.** 2011. *Bordatella holmesii* bacteremia in Northern Alberta: a 5-year case review. *Can J Infect Dis Med Microbiol* **22:**22A.

46. **Moissenet D, Leverger G, Merens A, Bonacorsi S, Guiso N, Vu-Thien H.** 2011. Septic arthritis caused by *Bordetella holmesii* in an adolescent with chronic haemolytic anaemia. *J Med Microbiol* **60:**1705–1707.

47. **Bassetti M, Nicco E, Roberto Giacobbe D, Marchese A, Coppo E, Barbieri R, Viscoli C.** 2012. *Bordetella holmesii* endocarditis in a patient with systemic lupus erythematous treated with immunosuppressive agents. *J Chemother* **24:**240–242.

48. **Bush LM, Davidson E, Daugherty J.** 2012. *Bordetella holmesii* prosthetic valve endocarditis: a case report and review. *Infect Dis Clin Pract* **20:**248–253.

49. **Chambaraud T, Dickson Z, Ensergueix G, Barraud O, Essig M, Lacour C, Allard J, Bocquentin F, Aldigier JC, Rerolle JP.** 2012. *Bordetella holmesii* bacteremia in a renal transplant recipient: emergence of a new pathogen. *Transpl Infect Dis* **14:**E134–E136.

50. **de Nobrega R, Kotecha K.** 2012. *Bordetella holmesii* in asplenic patients: a new pathogen? *Arch Dis Child* **97:**A89–A90.

51. **Jonckheere S, De Baere T, Schroeyers P, Soetens O, De Bel A, Surmont I.** 2012. Prosthetic valve endocarditis caused by *Bordetella holmesii*, an *Acinetobacter* look-alike. *J Med Microbiol* **61:**874–877.

52. **Livovsky DM, Leibowitz D, Hidalgo-Grass C, Temper V, Salameh S, Korem M.** 2012. *Bordetella holmesii* meningitis in an asplenic patient with systemic lupus erythematosus. *J Med Microbiol* **61:**1165–1167.

53. **Nei T, Hyodo H, Sonobe K, Dan K, Saito R.** 2012. First report of infectious pericarditis due to *Bordetella holmesii* in an adult patient with malignant lymphoma. *J Clin Microbiol* **50:**1815–1817.

54. **van Balen T, Nieman AE, Hermans MH, Schneeberger PM, de Vries E.** 2012. *Bordetella holmesii* meningitis in a 12-year-old anorectic girl. *Pediatr Infect Dis J* **31:**421–422.

55. **Katsukawa C, Kushibiki C, Nishito A, Nishida R, Kuwabara N, Kawahara R, Otsuka N, Miyaji Y, Toyoizumi-Ajisaka H, Kamachi K.** 2013. Bronchitis caused by *Bordetella holmesii* in a child with asthma misdiagnosed as mycoplasmal infection. *J Infect Chemother* **19:**534–537.

56. **Nguyen LB, Epelboin L, Gabarre J, Lecso M, Guillot S, Bricaire F, Caumes E, Guiso N.** 2013. Recurrent *Bordetella holmesii* bacteremia and nasal carriage in a patient receiving rituximab. *Emerg Infect Dis* **19:**1703–1705.

57. **Pittet LF, Emonet S, Ansari M, Girardin E, Schrenzel J, Siegrist C-A, Posfay-Barbe KM.** 2013. *Bordetella holmesii* bacteremia in a child with nephroblastoma. *Swiss Med Wkly* **143:**50S.

58. **Soloaga R, Carrion N, Almuzara M, Barberis C, Pidone J, Guelfand L, Vay C.** 2013. *Bordetella holmesii* endocarditis in an asplenic patient. *Rev Argent Microbiol* **45:**86–88.

59. **Stoddard JM.** 2013. A case of *Bordetella holmesii* endocarditis in an asplenic pediatric patient. *Clin Lab Sci* **26:**171–174.

60. **Abouanaser SF, Srigley JA, Nguyen T, Dale SE, Johnstone J, Wilcox L, Jamieson F, Rawte P, Pernica JM.** 2013. *Bordetella holmesii*: n emerging cause of septic arthritis. *J Clin Microbiol* **51:**1313–1315.

61. **Fishbain JT, Riederer K, Sawaf H, Mody R.** 2015. Invasive *Bordetella holmesii* infections. *Infect Dis* **47:**65–68.

62. **Pittet LF, Emonet S, Schrenzel J, Siegrist CA, Posfay-Barbe KM.** 2014. *Bordetella holmesii*: an under-recognised *Bordetella* species. *Lancet Infect Dis* **14:**510–519.

63. **Vandamme PA, Peeters C, Cnockaert M, Inganas E, Falsen E, Moore ER, Nunes OC, Manaia CM, Spilker T, LiPuma JJ.** 2015. *Bordetella bronchialis* sp. nov., *Bordetella flabilis* sp. nov. and *Bordetella sputigena* sp. nov., isolated from human respiratory specimens, and reclassification of *Achromobacter sediminum* (Zhang et al. 2014) as *Verticia sediminum* gen. nov., comb. nov. *Int J Syst Evol Microbiol*. doi:10.1099/ijsem.0.000473.

64. **Tizolova A, Guiso N, Guillot S.** 2013. Insertion sequences shared by *Bordetella* species and implications for the biological diagnosis of pertussis syndrome. *Eur J Clin Microbiol Infect Dis* **32:**89–96.

65. **Bouchez V, Guiso N.** 2013. *Bordetella holmesii*: comparison of two isolates from blood and a respiratory sample. *Adv Infect Dis* **3:**123–133.

66. **Gerlach G, von Wintzingerode F, Middendorf B, Gross R.** 2001. Evolutionary trends in the genus *Bordetella*. *Microbes Infect* **3:**61–72.

67. **Di Sabatino A, Carsetti R, Corazza GR.** 2011. Post-splenectomy and hyposplenic states. *Lancet* **378:**86–97.

68. **Rodgers L, Martin SW, Cohn A, Budd J, Marcon M, Terranella A, Mandal S, Salamon D, Leber A, Tondella ML, Tatti K, Spicer K, Emanuel A, Koch E, McGlone L, Pawloski L,**

Lemaile-Williams M, Tucker N, Iyer R, Clark TA, Diorio M. 2013. Epidemiologic and laboratory features of a large outbreak of pertussis-like illnesses associated with co-circulating *Bordetella holmesii* and *Bordetella pertussis*—Ohio, 2010-2011. *Clin Infect Dis* **56:** 322–331.

69. Bottero D, Griffith MM, Lara C, Flores D, Pianciola L, Gaillard ME, Mazzeo M, Zamboni MI, Spoleti MJ, Anchart E, Ruggeri D, Sorhouet C, Fiori S, Galas M, Tondella ML, Hozbor DF. 2013. *Bordetella holmesii* in children suspected of pertussis in Argentina. *Epidemiol Infect* **141:**714–717.

70. Tartof SY, Gounder P, Weiss D, Lee L, Cassiday PK, Clark TA, Briere EC. 2014. *Bordetella holmesii* bacteremia cases in the United States, April 2010–January 2011. *Clin Infect Dis* **58:**e39–e43.

71. van Balen T, Nieman AE, Hermans MHA, Schneeberger PM, de Vries E. 2012. *Bordetella holmesii* meningitis in a 12-year old anorectic girl. *Pediatr Infect Dis J* **31:**421–422.

72. Livovsky DMM, Leibowitz D, Hidalgo-Grass C, Temper V, Salameh S, Korem M. 2012. Bordetella holmesii meningitis in an asplenic patient with systemic lupus erythematosus. *J Med Microbiol* **61:**1165–1167.

73. Centers for Disease Control and Prevention. 2007. Outbreaks of respiratory illness mistakenly attributed to pertussis—New Hampshire, Massachusetts, and Tennessee, 2004–2006. *MMWR Morb Mortal Wkly Rep* **56:**837–842.

74. Mazengia E, Silva EA, Peppe JA, Timperi R, George H. 2000. Recovery of *Bordetella holmesii* from patients with pertussis-like symptoms: use of pulsed-field gel electrophoresis to characterize circulating strains. *J Clin Microbiol* **38:**2330–2333.

75. Mattoo S, Cherry JD. 2005. Molecular pathogenesis, epidemiology, and clinical manifestations of respiratory infections due to *Bordetella pertussis* and other *Bordetella* subspecies. *Clin Microbiol Rev* **18:**326–382.

76. Muyldermans G, Soetens O, Antoine M, Bruisten S, Vincart B, Doucet-Populaire F, Fry NK, Olcen P, Scheftel JM, Senterre JM, Van Der Zee A, Riffelmann M, Pierard D, Lauwers S. 2005. External quality assessment for molecular detection of *Bordetella pertussis* in European laboratories. *J Clin Microbiol* **43:**30–35.

77. Dalby T, Fry NK, Krogfelt KA, Jensen JS, He Q. 2013. Evaluation of PCR methods for the diagnosis of pertussis by the European surveillance network for vaccine-preventable diseases (EUVAC.NET). *Eur J Clin Microbiol Infect Dis* **32:**1285–1289.

78. McIntyre PB, Sintchenko V. 2013. The "how" of PCR testing for *Bordetella pertussis* depends on the "why." *Clin Infect Dis* **56:**332–334.

79. Loeffelholz MJ, Thompson CJ, Long KS, Gilchrist MJ. 1999. Comparison of PCR, culture, and direct fluorescent-antibody testing for detection of *Bordetella pertussis*. *J Clin Microbiol* **37:**2872–2876.

80. Faulkner A, Skoff T, Martin S, Cassiday P, Tondella ML, Liang J, Ejigiri OG. 2011. *Manual for the Surveillance of Vaccine-Preventable Diseases*. Centers for Disease Control and Prevention, Atlanta, GA.

81. Tatti KM, Martin SW, Boney KO, Brown K, Clark TA, Tondella ML. 2013. Qualitative assessment of pertussis diagnostics in United States laboratories. *Pediatr Infect Dis J* **32:** 942–945.

82. Register KB, Sanden GN. 2006. Prevalence and sequence variants of IS*481* in *Bordetella bronchiseptica*: implications for IS*481*-based detection of *Bordetella pertussis*. *J Clin Microbiol* **44:**4577–4583.

83. Sloan LM, Hopkins MK, Mitchell PS, Vetter EA, Rosenblatt JE, Harmsen WS, Cockerill FR, Patel R. 2002. Multiplex lightcycler PCR assay for detection and differentiation of *Bordetella pertussis* and *Bordetella parapertussis* in nasopharyngeal specimens. *J Clin Microbiol* **40:**96–100.

84. Tatti KM, Sparks KN, Boney KO, Tondella ML. 2011. Novel multitarget real-time PCR assay for rapid detection of *Bordetella* species in clinical specimens. *J Clin Microbiol* **49:**4059–4066.

85. Mooi FR, Bruisten S, Linde I, Reubsaet F, Heuvelman K, van der Lee S, King AJ. 2012. Characterization of *Bordetella holmesii* isolates from patients with pertussis-like illness in the Netherlands. *FEMS Immunol Med Microbiol* **64:** 289–291.

86. Otsuka N, Yoshino S, Kawano K, Toyoizumi-Ajisaka H, Shibayama K, Kamachi K. 2012. Simple and specific detection of *Bordetella holmesii* by using a loop-mediated isothermal amplification assay. *Microbiol Immunol* **56:**486–489.

87. Seng P, Drancourt M, Gouriet F, La Scola B, Fournier PE, Rolain JM, Raoult D. 2009. Ongoing revolution in bacteriology: routine identification of bacteria by matrix-assisted laser desorption ionization time-of-flight mass spectrometry. *Clin Infect Dis* **49:**543–551.

88. Panagopoulos MI, Jean MS, Brun D, Guiso N, Bekal S, Ovetchkine P, Tapiero B. 2010. *Bordetella holmesii* bacteremia in asplenic children: report of four cases initially misidentified

as *Acinetobacter lwoffii*. *J Clin Microbiol* **48:** 3762–3764.

89. **Lindquist SW, Weber DJ, Mangum ME, Hollis DG, Jordan J.** 1995. *Bordetella holmesii* sepsis in an asplenic adolescent. *Pediatr Infect Dis J* **14:**813–815.

90. **Wang K, Bettiol S, Thompson MJ, Roberts NW, Perera R, Heneghan CJ, Harnden A.** 2014. Symptomatic treatment of the cough in whooping cough. *Cochrane Database Syst Rev* **9:**CD003257.

91. **Tan T, Dalby T, Forsyth K, Halperin SA, Heininger U, Hozbor D, Plotkin S, Ulloa-Gutierrez R, von Konig CH.** 2015. Pertussis across the globe: recent epidemiologic trends from 2000–2013. *Pediatr Infect Dis J* **34:**e222–32. doi:10.1097/INF.0000000000000795.

92. **Weber DJ, Miller MB, Brooks RH, Brown VM, Rutala WA.** 2010. Healthcare worker with "pertussis": consequences of a false-positive polymerase chain reaction test result. *Infect Control Hosp Epidemiol* **31:**306–307.

93. **Siegel JD, Rhinehart E, Jackson M, Chiarello L, Health Care Infection Control Practices Advisory Committee.** 2007. 2007 guideline for isolation precautions: preventing transmission of infectious agents in health care settings. *Am J Infect Control* **35:**S65–S164.

94. **Thibault L, Nolin M, Jacques A, Daoud H, De Grandmont M, Delage G.** 2012. Bacterial contamination of platelet concentrates: implication of negative culture when retesting the blood product after a positive result with the BacT/ALERT 3D. *Transfusion* **52:**201A.

95. **Pittet LF, Posfay-Barbe KM.** 2015. *Bordetella holmesii* infection: current knowledge and a vision for future research. *Expert Rev Anti Infect Ther* **13:**965–971.

96. **Williams MM, Taylor TH Jr, Warshauer DM, Martin MD, Valley AM, Tondella ML.** 2015. Harmonization of *Bordetella pertussis* real-time PCR diagnostics in the United States in 2012. *J Clin Microbiol* **53:**118–123.

97. **Miranda C, Porte L, Garcia P.** 2012. *Bordetella holmesii* in nasopharyngeal samples from Chilean patients with suspected *Bordetella pertussis* infection. *J Clin Microbiol* **50:**1505.

14

Cronobacter spp.

BRIAN P. BLACKWOOD[1] and CATHERINE J. HUNTER[1]

INTRODUCTION

The genus *Cronobacter* consists of a group of opportunistic Gram-negative pathogens associated with severe and potentially life-threatening medical diseases. Until fairly recently, the *Cronobacter* genus was thought to be a single species known as *Enterobacter sakazakii* (1–3). However, in 2007, the genus *Cronobacter* was formally named as a member of the *Enterobacteriaceae* family (4). Through new identification techniques and genomic sequencing, we have since learned a great deal about the bacteria that make up this genus (5, 6). Now, 10 individual species have been identified (2, 7, 8). These bacteria have been found in a wide range of environments, including water, food, and soil (9). In the clinical setting, *Cronobacter* spp. have been isolated in feces, sputum, blood, bone marrow, and cerebrospinal fluid (6, 10).

These bacteria are associated with neonatal diseases, including necrotizing enterocolitis (NEC), meningitis, and sepsis (11). Additionally, in the elderly population, *Cronobacter* has been linked to cases of urosepsis and bacteremia (2). Despite a better understanding of this genus, the pathophysiology behind its infections is not well known, and few virulence factors have been identified.

This chapter outlines the history behind the epidemiology of the genus *Cronobacter*. We analyze how our understanding of these bacteria has changed

[1]Ann and Robert H. Lurie Children's Hospital of Chicago, Chicago, IL 60611.
Emerging Infections 10
Edited by W. Michael Scheld, James M. Hughes and Richard J. Whitley
© 2016 American Society for Microbiology, Washington, DC
doi:10.1128/microbiolspec.EI10-0002-2015

over time. Additionally, we highlight the clinical significance these opportunistic bacteria have for both the neonatal and elderly patient populations as well as the treatment of the associated infections.

CLASSIFICATION, EPIDEMIOLOGY, AND ENVIRONMENTAL SOURCES

Cronobacter spp. are Gram-negative, non-spore-forming, motile rods (Fig. 1) (9). The initial *Cronobacter* infection was reported in 1961 by Urmenyi and Franklin (12). At that time, it was thought to be yellow-pigmented *Enterobacter cloacae*. It was not until 1980 that species status was given when the bacterium was named *Enterobacter sakazakii* (1). It was then another 28 years before *Enterobacter sakazakii* was accurately described as the genus *Cronobacter*, a member of the family *Enterobacteriaceae* (1–4).

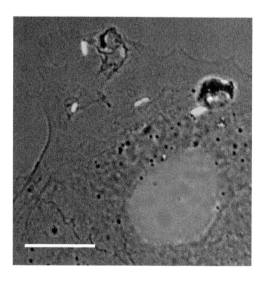

FIGURE 1 Image is taken at magnification of ×100 with z-stack under fluorescein isothiocyanate, 4′,6-diamidino-2-phenylindole (DAPI), and differential interference contrast channels. *Cronobacter sakazakii* has been cloned with green fluorescent protein expression and is shown in green; the nucleus is stained with DAPI and shown in blue. *C. sakazakii* can be seen to permeabilize the cell (Caco-2). Scale bar is 15 μm.

Advances in culture and measuring techniques have allowed us to gain a better understanding of the *Cronobacter* spp. The use of 16S ribosomal rRNA genes, *hsp60* sequencing, and polyphasic analysis was responsible for truly shedding light on the fact that *Enterobacter sakazakii* isolates were actually unique species (5, 13, 14). DNA-DNA hybridization and phenotyping confirmed these findings (15). Multilocus sequence typing (MLST) and analysis (MLSA) using housekeeping genes (*atpD, fusA, glnS, gltB, gyrB, infB,* and *ppsA*) have allowed us to see how truly diverse this genus really is (8, 16–18).

As a result of the MLST and MLSA, we know that *Cronobacter* evolved over the last 40 million years, and it is estimated that *Cronobacter sakazakii* and *C. malonaticus* became unique species approximately 11 million to 23 million years ago (9, 19). Today, the genus contains 10 different species, including *C. sakazakii, C. malonaticus, C. turicensis, C. universalis, C. dublinensis, C. muytjensii, C. condimenti, C. pulveris, C. helveticus,* and *C. zurichensis* (2, 7, 8). The more clinically relevant bacteria can be divided into two groups. Group 1 contains *C. sakazakii* and *C. malonaticus,* and these two species form the majority of clinical isolates (2). Group 2 contains *C. turicensis* and *C. universalis,* which are reported less frequently. The other six species are primarily environmental commensals and appear to be of little clinical significance (2).

The natural environment of *Cronobacter* spp. is not completely clear, but species have been found in a variety of environments, including water, soil, and plants. Additionally, these bacteria have been detected in both raw and fresh animal and vegetable products. They have also been found in processed and prepared foods that include powdered milk substitutes, processed cheeses, meats, spices, and herbs (20–23). Cockroaches, flies, and rats have been identified as potential sources of contamination as well (24–26).

Cronobacter is not typically found in the mammalian intestinal tract, and there has to date been only one report of it being isolated from the human vagina (27). This makes vertical transmission unlikely. *Cronobacter*-contaminated powder infant formula (PIF), which led to clinical disease, became a popular topic of both scientific and lay conversation (22, 28). Outbreaks of neonatal infections, specifically NEC and meningitis, have been linked directly to contaminated PIF (Fig. 2) (29). Early studies of powdered breast milk substitutes found 141 breast milk substitutes from 35 different countries to be contaminated with *Cronobacter* spp. (30).

In more recent years, *Cronobacter* isolates have continued to be found in formula and weaning foods (24). *C. sakazakii* has demonstrated its remarkable tolerance to desiccation and temperature extremes, being able to withstand temperatures as high as 60°C and as low as 4°C (31–34). This thermoresistance has allowed *C. sakazakii* to survive standard manufacturing processes. The Food and Agriculture Organization and the World Health Organization have, as a result, produced specific recommendations for PIF to be reconstituted with hot water at a temperature of >70°C in order to help reduce bacterial load and infection rates (35–38).

CLINICAL ASSOCIATIONS

There have been many cases reported of *Cronobacter*-related infections, and many of these were reported as outbreaks (3, 37–40). *Cronobacter* is associated with infections in neonates and infants, as well as infections in the elderly (2).

Cronobacter is most known clinically for its association with neonatal infections, including NEC, meningitis, and sepsis (39, 41, 42). There are estimated rates of *Cronobacter* neonatal infections in the United States of 1 per 100,000 infants, 8.7 to 9.4 per 100,000 low-birth-weight infants, and 1 per 10.660 very-low-birth-weight infants (2, 3, 37, 38, 43). In fact, the sentinel *Cronobacter* case in 1961 was a case of neonatal meningitis (1). Previously thought to be as high as 80%, the rate of mortality from microbiologically confirmed cases of *Cronobacter* has been found to be 26.9% (40, 44).

NEC is the most common gastrointestinal emergency in neonates. It occurs in up to 5% of all neonatal ICU admissions, and nearly 10,000 infants are diagnosed with this disease each year in the United States (45). NEC is a multifactorial disease and has been associated with many different pathologic bacteria, including *Cronobacter* spp., but no one bacterium has been identified as being more involved in the pathogenesis than any other bacteria (2, 46–48). Furthermore, the actual role of *Cronobacter* in the pathogenesis of the disease remains unknown (2). The only consistent risk factors identified in this patient population have been prematurity and a history of formula feeding (11, 45, 49). These patients have transmural inflammation and necrosis of both the large and small bowel, which often requires abdominal drainage or

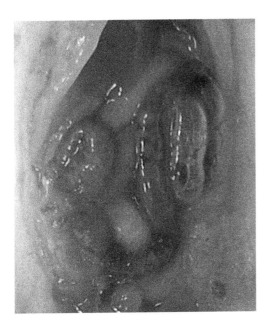

FIGURE 2 **Rat pups fed formula contaminated with *C. sakazakii* have findings resembling neonatal NEC. The rat pup bowel is dilated, and pneumatosis can be clearly seen in the bowel wall.**

surgical resection of the infected bowel. Those infants that survive the disease have significant long-term morbidities, including growth delay, short-gut syndrome, and neurodevelopmental syndromes (50–53).

Cronobacter is also associated with neonatal meningitis. This disease process has an extremely poor clinical outcome, with an approximate mortality rate of 42% (2, 3). It usually manifests in infants that are born at full gestational age, and it occurs in the first few days of life (2, 44). *Cronobacter*-associated meningitis causes ventriculitis, brain abscesses, brain cysts, cerebral infarcts, and late development of hydrocephalus, requiring ventriculoperitoneal shunt placement (54–56). Those patients that survive the disease can suffer from mental and/or physical developmental delay and quadriplegia (2, 57).

While not to the same degree as in the neonates, *Cronobacter* infections also affect the elderly. In the United States, there are approximately 3.93 *Cronobacter*-related cases per 100,000 people (58). In adults, *Cronobacter* spp. have been associated with bacteremia, splenic abscesses, osteomyelitis, pneumonia, wound infections, conjunctivitis, and urinary tract infections (2, 59–61). Reports indicate that older and immunocompromised adults seem to be at an increased risk of *Cronobacter* infection (2, 59).

PATHOGENESIS AND VIRULENCE

The pathogenesis and virulence of *Cronobacter*-related infections are an area of active research (3, 62, 63). Genome sequencing has allowed for potential virulence factors to be identified (64). Of the 4,392 genes identified in *Cronobacter sakazakii*, 223 appear to be related to virulence (6). The encoded proteins have been shown to be associated specifically with acid transport, phosphotransferase systems, and pilus assembly as well as both toxin and antitoxin transport systems (3, 65).

One of the best-characterized virulence factors to date is outer membrane protein A

(OmpA). This virulence factor is encoded by the *ompA* gene, and it has been noted to be required, not only by *Cronobacter* but also by *Escherichia coli* K1, for binding and invading the endothelial cells of the brain, leading to meningitis (66–68). *Cronobacter* has also been shown to produce an endotoxin-like compound which aids in its translocation across both the blood-brain barrier in the central nervous system and the intestinal epithelial barrier in the gut. Additionally, this toxin seems to work similarly to lipopolysaccharide in that it induces an inflammatory response secondary to Toll-like receptor 4 activation (69, 70).

With regard to oral inoculation, it appears as though *Cronobacter* adheres to the intestinal epithelial cells, causing breakdown of the intestinal epithelial barrier and producing an inflammatory response (3). The inflammatory cascade, inducible nitric oxide synthase, and interleukin-6, all activated by *Cronobacter*, then cause downstream effects, such as apoptosis (46, 62, 71). *Cronobacter* then breaks through the barrier, gaining access to the bloodstream and causing sepsis or meningitis in the susceptible host. Evidence suggests that *Cronobacter* virulence factors may also help resist complement-mediated killing and can even alter the host immune response, in effect allowing these bacteria to hide from the host's immune system (71, 72).

ANTIBIOTIC SUSCEPTIBILITY

Antibiotic treatment is essential in the care of a patient with a confirmed *Cronobacter* infection. The traditional antibiotic regimen for *Cronobacter* spp. was ampicillin in combination with either gentamicin or chloramphenicol (57). However, like many bacteria in our current age, *Cronobacter* spp. have developed resistance to these antibiotics (57, 73). There is a discrepancy in the literature as to how *Cronobacter* resistance occurs and whether or not these bacteria produce beta-lactamases. There have been studies that report beta-lactamase production in nearly all identified *Cronobacter* spp., while others report finding no beta-lactamase production (57, 74, 75). To date, *Cronobacter* isolates have been found to be resistant to not only ampicillin but also most first- and second-generation cephalosporins (23, 57). As a result, it has been suggested that carbapenems or third-generation cephalosporins be used with an aminoglycoside or trimethoprim-sulfamethoxazole (57). This treatment has been relatively successful for *Cronobacter*-related infections, but antibiotic resistance appears to be increasing (57, 76).

CONCLUSION

In conclusion, the once-misnamed genus now known as *Cronobacter* represents a group of opportunistic Gram-negative bacteria associated with severe and potentially life-threatening infections. *Cronobacter*-related sepsis, meningitis, and NEC are terrible diseases of the neonate, with poor long-term prognoses. Additionally, these bacteria are associated with less severe, yet still debilitating, infections in the elderly and immunocompromised.

Although we have achieved a significant improvement in our understanding of *Cronobacter* since it was first discovered, we still do not completely understand the environment, pathogenesis, virulence, or treatment of the genus *Cronobacter*, and these represent areas of future investigation.

CITATION

Blackwood BP, Hunter CJ. 2016. *Cronobacter* spp. Microbiol Spectrum 4(3):EI10-0002-2015.

REFERENCES

1. **Farmer JJ III, Davis BR, Hickman-Brenner FW, McWhorter A, Huntley-Carter GP,** **Asbury MA, Riddle C, Wathen-Grady HG, Elias C, Fanning GR, Steigerwalt AG, O'Hara CM, Morris GK, Smith PB, Brenner DJ.** 1985. Biochemical identification of new species and biogroups of *Enterobacteriaceae* isolated from clinical specimens. *J Clin Microbiol* **21:**46–76.

2. **Holy O, Forsythe S.** 2014. *Cronobacter* spp. as emerging causes of healthcare-associated infection. *J Hosp Infect* **86:**169–177.

3. **Hunter CJ, Bean JF.** 2013. *Cronobacter*: an emerging opportunistic pathogen associated with neonatal meningitis, sepsis and necrotizing enterocolitis. *J Perinatol* **33:**581–585.

4. **Iversen C, Mullane N, McCardell B, Tall BD, Lehner A, Fanning S, Stephan R, Joosten H.** 2008. *Cronobacter* gen. nov., a new genus to accommodate the biogroups of *Enterobacter sakazakii*, and proposal of *Cronobacter sakazakii* gen. nov., comb. nov., *Cronobacter malonaticus* sp. nov., *Cronobacter turicensis* sp. nov., *Cronobacter muytjensii* sp. nov., *Cronobacter dublinensis* sp. nov., *Cronobacter* genomospecies 1, and of three subspecies, *Cronobacter dublinensis* subsp. *dublinensis* subsp. nov., *Cronobacter dublinensis* subsp. *lausannensis* subsp. nov. and *Cronobacter dublinensis* subsp. *lactaridi* subsp. nov. *Int J Syst Evol Microbiol* **58:**1442–1447.

5. **Iversen C, Druggan P, Schumacher S, Lehner A, Feer C, Gschwend K, Joosten H, Stephan R.** 2008. Development of a novel screening method for the isolation of "*Cronobacter*" spp. (*Enterobacter sakazakii*). *Appl Environ Microbiol* **74:**2550–2553.

6. **Kucerova E, Clifton SW, Xia XQ, Long F, Porwollik S, Fulton L, Fronick C, Minx P, Kyung K, Warren W, Fulton R, Feng D, Wollam A, Shah N, Bhonagiri V, Nash WE, Hallsworth-Pepin K, Wilson RK, McClelland M, Forsythe SJ.** 2010. Genome sequence of *Cronobacter sakazakii* BAA-894 and comparative genomic hybridization analysis with other *Cronobacter* species. *PLoS One* **5:**e9556.

7. **Brady C, Cleenwerck I, Venter S, Coutinho T, De Vos P.** 2013. Taxonomic evaluation of the genus *Enterobacter* based on multilocus sequence analysis (MLSA): proposal to reclassify *E. nimipressuralis* and *E. amnigenus* into *Lelliottia* gen. nov. as *Lelliottia nimipressuralis* comb. nov. and *Lelliottia amnigena* comb. nov., respectively, *E. gergoviae* and *E. pyrinus* into *Pluralibacter* gen. nov. as *Pluralibacter gergoviae* comb. nov. and *Pluralibacter pyrinus* comb. nov., respectively, *E. cowanii, E. radicincitans, E. oryzae* and *E. arachidis* into *Kosakonia* gen. nov. as *Kosakonia cowanii* comb. nov., *Kosakonia radicincitans* comb. nov., *Kosakonia oryzae* comb. nov. and *Kosakonia arachidis* comb. nov.,

respectively, and *E. turicensis, E. helveticus* and *E. pulveris* into *Cronobacter* as *Cronobacter zurichensis* nom. nov., *Cronobacter helveticus* comb. nov. and *Cronobacter pulveris* comb. nov., respectively, and emended description of the genera *Enterobacter* and *Cronobacter. Syst Appl Microbiol* **36:**309–319.

8. **Joseph S, Cetinkaya E, Drahovska H, Levican A, Figueras MJ, Forsythe SJ.** 2012. *Cronobacter condimenti* sp. nov., isolated from spiced meat, and *Cronobacter universalis* sp. nov., a species designation for *Cronobacter* sp. genomospecies 1, recovered from a leg infection, water and food ingredients. *Int J Syst Evol Microbiol* **62:**1277–1283.

9. **Joseph S, Desai P, Ji Y, Cummings CA, Shih R, Degoricija L, Rico A, Brzoska P, Hamby SE, Masood N, Hariri S, Sonbol H, Chuzhanova N, McClelland M, Furtado MR, Forsythe SJ.** 2012. Comparative analysis of genome sequences covering the seven *Cronobacter* species. *PLoS One* **7:**e49455.

10. **Gurtler JB, Kornacki JL, Beuchat LR.** 2005. *Enterobacter sakazakii*: a coliform of increased concern to infant health. *Int J Food Microbiol* **104:**1–34.

11. **Hunter CJ, Petrosyan M, Ford HR, Prasadarao NV.** 2008. *Enterobacter sakazakii*: an emerging pathogen in infants and neonates. *Surg Infect (Larchmt)* **9:**533–539.

12. **Urmenyi AM, Franklin AW.** 1961. Neonatal death from pigmented coliform infection. *Lancet* **i:**313–315.

13. **Iversen C, Lancashire L, Waddington M, Forsythe S, Ball G.** 2006. Identification of *Enterobacter sakazakii* from closely related species: the use of artificial neural networks in the analysis of biochemical and 16S rDNA data. *BMC Microbiol* **6:**28.

14. **Iversen C, Waddington M, On SL, Forsythe S.** 2004. Identification and phylogeny of *Enterobacter sakazakii* relative to *Enterobacter* and *Citrobacter* species. *J Clin Microbiol* **42:**5368–5370.

15. **Iversen C, Lehner A, Mullane N, Bidlas E, Cleenwerck I, Marugg J, Fanning S, Stephan R, Joosten H.** 2007. The taxonomy of *Enterobacter sakazakii*: proposal of a new genus *Cronobacter* gen. nov. and descriptions of *Cronobacter sakazakii* comb. nov. *Cronobacter sakazakii* subsp. *sakazakii*, comb. nov., *Cronobacter sakazakii* subsp. *malonaticus* subsp. nov., *Cronobacter turicensis* sp. nov., *Cronobacter muytjensii* sp. nov., *Cronobacter dublinensis* sp. nov. and *Cronobacter* genomospecies 1. *BMC Evol Biol* **7:**64.

16. **Baldwin A, Loughlin M, Caubilla-Barron J, Kucerova E, Manning G, Dowson C, Forsythe S.** 2009. Multilocus sequence typing of *Cronobacter sakazakii* and *Cronobacter malonaticus* reveals stable clonal structures with clinical significance which do not correlate with biotypes. *BMC Microbiol* **9:**223.

17. **Joseph S, Forsythe SJ.** 2012. Insights into the emergent bacterial pathogen *Cronobacter* spp., generated by multilocus sequence typing and analysis. *Front Microbiol* **3:**397.

18. **Kuhnert P, Korczak BM, Stephan R, Joosten H, Iversen C.** 2009. Phylogeny and prediction of genetic similarity of *Cronobacter* and related taxa by multilocus sequence analysis (MLSA). *Int J Food Microbiol* **136:**152–158.

19. **Joseph S, Sonbol H, Hariri S, Desai P, McClelland M, Forsythe SJ.** 2012. Diversity of the *Cronobacter* genus as revealed by multilocus sequence typing. *J Clin Microbiol* **50:**3031–3039.

20. **Friedemann M.** 2007. *Enterobacter sakazakii* in food and beverages (other than infant formula and milk powder). *Int J Food Microbiol* **116:**1–10.

21. **Baumgartner A, Grand M, Liniger M, Iversen C.** 2009. Detection and frequency of *Cronobacter* spp. (*Enterobacter sakazakii*) in different categories of ready-to-eat foods other than infant formula. *Int J Food Microbiol* **136:**189–192.

22. **Kandhai MC, Reij MW, Gorris LG, Guillaume-Gentil O, van Schothorst M.** 2004. Occurrence of *Enterobacter sakazakii* in food production environments and households. *Lancet* **363:**39–40.

23. **Kim K, Jang SS, Kim SK, Park JH, Heu S, Ryu S.** 2008. Prevalence and genetic diversity of *Enterobacter sakazakii* in ingredients of infant foods. *Int J Food Microbiol* **122:**196–203.

24. **Chap J, Jackson P, Siqueira R, Gaspar N, Quintas C, Park J, Osaili T, Shaker R, Jaradat Z, Hartantyo SH, Abdullah Sani N, Estuningsih S, Forsythe SJ.** 2009. International survey of *Cronobacter sakazakii* and other *Cronobacter* spp. in follow up formulas and infant foods. *Int J Food Microbiol* **136:**185–188.

25. **Hamilton JV, Lehane MJ, Braig HR.** 2003. Isolation of *Enterobacter sakazakii* from midgut of *Stomoxys calcitrans. Emerg Infect Dis* **9:**1355–1356.

26. **Pava-Ripoll M, Pearson RE, Miller AK, Ziobro GC.** 2012. Prevalence and relative risk of *Cronobacter* spp., *Salmonella* spp., and *Listeria monocytogenes* associated with the body surfaces and guts of individual filth flies. *Appl Environ Microbiol* **78:**7891–7902.

27. **Chenu JW, Cox JM.** 2009. *Cronobacter* ('*Enterobacter sakazakii*'): current status and future prospects. *Lett Appl Microbiol* **49:**153–159.

28. **Pan Z, Cui J, Lyu G, Du X, Qin L, Guo Y, Xu B, Li W, Cui Z, Zhao C.** 2014. Isolation and

molecular typing of *Cronobacter* spp. in commercial powdered infant formula and follow-up formula. *Foodborne Pathog Dis* **11:**456–461.

29. **Clark NC, Hill BC, O'Hara CM, Steingrimsson O, Cooksey RC.** 1990. Epidemiologic typing of *Enterobacter sakazakii* in two neonatal nosocomial outbreaks. *Diagn Microbiol Infect Dis* **13:**467–472.

30. **Muytjens HL, Roelofs-Willemse H, Jaspar GH.** 1988. Quality of powdered substitutes for breast milk with regard to members of the family *Enterobacteriaceae*. *J Clin Microbiol* **26:**743–746.

31. **Alvarez-Ordonez A, Begley M, Hill C.** 2012. Polymorphisms in rpoS and stress tolerance heterogeneity in natural isolates of *Cronobacter sakazakii*. *Appl Environ Microbiol* **78:**3975–3984.

32. **Arku B, Fanning S, Jordan K.** 2011. Heat adaptation and survival of *Cronobacter* spp. (formerly *Enterobacter sakazakii*). *Foodborne Pathog Dis* **8:**975–981.

33. **Walsh D, Molloy C, Iversen C, Carroll J, Cagney C, Fanning S, Duffy G.** 2011. Survival characteristics of environmental and clinically derived strains of *Cronobacter sakazakii* in infant milk formula (IMF) and ingredients. *J Appl Microbiol* **110:**697–703.

34. **Al-Nabulsi AA, Osaili TM, Al-Holy MA, Shaker RR, Ayyash MM, Olaimat AN, Holley RA.** 2009. Influence of desiccation on the sensitivity of *Cronobacter* spp. to lactoferrin or nisin in broth and powdered infant formula. *Int J Food Microbiol* **136:**221–226.

35. **Chen PC, Zahoor T, Oh SW, Kang DH.** 2009. Effect of heat treatment on *Cronobacter* spp. in reconstituted, dried infant formula: preparation guidelines for manufacturers. *Lett Appl Microbiol* **49:**730–737.

36. **Edelson-Mammel SG, Buchanan RL.** 2004. Thermal inactivation of *Enterobacter sakazakii* in rehydrated infant formula. *J Food Prot* **67:**60–63.

37. **World Health Organization, Food and Agriculture Organization of the United Nations.** 2004. *Enterobacter sakazakii and Other Microorganisms in Powdered Infant Formula: Meeting Report.* World Health Organization, Geneva, Switzerland.

38. **World Health Organization, Food and Agriculture Organization of the United Nations.** 2006. *Enterobacter sakazakii and Salmonella in Powdered Infant Formula: Meeting Report.* World Health Organization, Geneva, Switzerland.

39. **Caubilla-Barron J, Hurrell E, Townsend S, Cheetham P, Loc-Carrillo C, Fayet O, Prere MF, Forsythe SJ.** 2007. Genotypic and phenotypic analysis of *Enterobacter sakazakii* strains from an outbreak resulting in fatalities in a neonatal intensive care unit in France. *J Clin Microbiol* **45:**3979–3985.

40. **Friedemann M.** 2009. Epidemiology of invasive neonatal *Cronobacter* (*Enterobacter sakazakii*) infections. *Eur J Clin Microbiol Infect Dis* **28:** 1297–1304.

41. **Giovannini M, Verduci E, Ghisleni D, Salvatici E, Riva E, Agostoni C.** 2008. *Enterobacter sakazakii*: an emerging problem in paediatric nutrition. *J Int Med Res* **36:**394–399.

42. **Mullane NR, Whyte P, Wall PG, Quinn T, Fanning S.** 2007. Application of pulsed-field gel electrophoresis to characterise and trace the prevalence of *Enterobacter sakazakii* in an infant formula processing facility. *Int J Food Microbiol* **116:**73–81.

43. **Stoll BJ, Hansen N, Fanaroff AA, Lemons JA.** 2004. *Enterobacter sakazakii* is a rare cause of neonatal septicemia or meningitis in VLBW infants. *J Pediatr* **144:**821–823.

44. **Bowen AB, Braden CR.** 2006. Invasive *Enterobacter sakazakii* disease in infants. *Emerg Infect Dis* **12:**1185–1189.

45. **Hunter CJ, Podd B, Ford HR, Camerini V.** 2008. Evidence vs experience in neonatal practices in necrotizing enterocolitis. *J Perinatol* **28** (Suppl 1):S9–S13.

46. **Emami CN, Petrosyan M, Giuliani S, Williams M, Hunter C, Prasadarao NV, Ford HR.** 2009. Role of the host defense system and intestinal microbial flora in the pathogenesis of necrotizing enterocolitis. *Surg Infect (Larchmt)* **10:**407–417.

47. **Grishin A, Papillon S, Bell B, Wang J, Ford HR.** 2013. The role of the intestinal microbiota in the pathogenesis of necrotizing enterocolitis. *Semin Pediatr Surg* **22:**69–75.

48. **Peter CS, Feuerhahn M, Bohnhorst B, Schlaud M, Ziesing S, von der Hardt H, Poets CF.** 1999. Necrotising enterocolitis: is there a relationship to specific pathogens? *Eur J Pediatr* **158:**67–70.

49. **Holman RC, Stoll BJ, Clarke MJ, Glass RI.** 1997. The epidemiology of necrotizing enterocolitis infant mortality in the United States. *Am J Public Health* **87:**2026–2031.

50. **Blakely ML, Lally KP, McDonald S, Brown RL, Barnhart DC, Ricketts RR, Thompson WR, Scherer LR, Klein MD, Letton RW, Chwals WJ, Touloukian RJ, Kurkchubasche AG, Skinner MA, Moss RL, Hilfiker ML, NEC Subcommittee of the NICHD Neonatal Research Network.** 2005. Postoperative outcomes of extremely low birth-weight infants with necrotizing enterocolitis or isolated intestinal perforation: a prospective cohort study by the NICHD Neonatal Research Network. *Ann Surg* **241:**984–989; discussion, 989–994.

51. **Salhab WA, Perlman JM, Silver L, Sue Broyles R.** 2004. Necrotizing enterocolitis and neuro-developmental outcome in extremely low birth weight infants <1000 g. *J Perinatol* **24:**534–540.

52. **Schulzke SM, Deshpande GC, Patole SK.** 2007. Neurodevelopmental outcomes of very low-birth-weight infants with necrotizing enterocolitis: a systematic review of observational studies. *Arch Pediatr Adolesc Med* **161:**583–590.

53. **Vohr BR, Wright LL, Dusick AM, Mele L, Verter J, Steichen JJ, Simon NP, Wilson DC, Broyles S, Bauer CR, Delaney-Black V, Yolton KA, Fleisher BE, Papile LA, Kaplan MD.** 2000. Neurodevelopmental and functional outcomes of extremely low birth weight infants in the National Institute of Child Health and Human Development Neonatal Research Network, 1993-1994. *Pediatrics* **105:**1216–1226.

54. **Bar-Oz B, Preminger A, Peleg O, Block C, Arad I.** 2001. *Enterobacter sakazakii* infection in the newborn. *Acta Paediatr* **90:**356–358.

55. **Burdette JH, Santos C.** 2000. *Enterobacter sakazakii* brain abscess in the neonate: the importance of neuroradiologic imaging. *Pediatr Radiol* **30:**33–34.

56. **Gallagher PG, Ball WS.** 1991. Cerebral infarctions due to CNS infection with *Enterobacter sakazakii*. *Pediatr Radiol* **21:**135–136.

57. **Lai KK.** 2001. *Enterobacter sakazakii* infections among neonates, infants, children, and adults. Case reports and a review of the literature. *Medicine (Baltimore)* **80:**113–122.

58. **Patrick ME, Mahon BE, Greene SA, Rounds J, Cronquist A, Wymore K, Boothe E, Lathrop S, Palmer A, Bowen A.** 2014. Incidence of *Cronobacter* spp. infections, United States, 2003–2009. *Emerg Infect Dis* **20:**1520–1523.

59. **Healy B, Cooney S, O'Brien S, Iversen C, Whyte P, Nally J, Callanan JJ, Fanning S.** 2010. *Cronobacter* (*Enterobacter sakazakii*): an opportunistic foodborne pathogen. *Foodborne Pathog Dis* **7:**339–350.

60. **See KC, Than HA, Tang T.** 2007. *Enterobacter sakazakii* bacteraemia with multiple splenic abscesses in a 75-year-old woman: a case report. *Age Ageing* **36:**595–596.

61. **Gosney MA, Martin MV, Wright AE, Gallagher M.** 2006. *Enterobacter sakazakii* in the mouths of stroke patients and its association with aspiration pneumonia. *Eur J Intern Med* **17:**185–188.

62. **Hunter CJ, Singamsetty VK, Chokshi NK, Boyle P, Camerini V, Grishin AV, Upperman JS, Ford HR, Prasadarao NV.** 2008. *Enterobacter sakazakii* enhances epithelial cell injury by inducing apoptosis in a rat model of necrotizing enterocolitis. *J Infect Dis* **198:**586–593.

63. **Richardson AN, Lambert S, Smith MA.** 2009. Neonatal mice as models for *Cronobacter sakazakii* infection in infants. *J Food Prot* **72:**2363–2367.

64. **Stephan R, Lehner A, Tischler P, Rattei T.** 2011. Complete genome sequence of *Cronobacter turicensis* LMG 23827, a food-borne pathogen causing deaths in neonates. *J Bacteriol* **193:**309–310.

65. **Yan QQ, Condell O, Power K, Butler F, Tall BD, Fanning S.** 2012. *Cronobacter* species (formerly known as *Enterobacter sakazakii*) in powdered infant formula: a review of our current understanding of the biology of this bacterium. *J Appl Microbiol* **113:**1–15.

66. **Nair MK, Venkitanarayanan K, Silbart LK, Kim KS.** 2009. Outer membrane protein A (OmpA) of *Cronobacter sakazakii* binds fibronectin and contributes to invasion of human brain microvascular endothelial cells. *Foodborne Pathog Dis* **6:**495–501.

67. **Prasadarao NV.** 2002. Identification of *Escherichia coli* outer membrane protein A receptor on human brain microvascular endothelial cells. *Infect Immun* **70:**4556–4563.

68. **Singamsetty VK, Wang Y, Shimada H, Prasadarao NV.** 2008. Outer membrane protein A expression in *Enterobacter sakazakii* is required to induce microtubule condensation in human brain microvascular endothelial cells for invasion. *Microb Pathog* **45:**181–191.

69. **Pagotto FJ, Nazarowec-White M, Bidawid S, Farber JM.** 2003. *Enterobacter sakazakii*: infectivity and enterotoxin production in vitro and in vivo. *J Food Prot* **66:**370–375.

70. **Townsend S, Caubilla Barron J, Loc-Carrillo C, Forsythe S.** 2007. The presence of endotoxin in powdered infant formula milk and the influence of endotoxin and *Enterobacter sakazakii* on bacterial translocation in the infant rat. *Food Microbiol* **24:**67–74.

71. **Emami CN, Mittal R, Wang L, Ford HR, Prasadarao NV.** 2011. Recruitment of dendritic cells is responsible for intestinal epithelial damage in the pathogenesis of necrotizing enterocolitis by *Cronobacter sakazakii*. *J Immunol* **186:**7067–7079.

72. **Franco AA, Kothary MH, Gopinath G, Jarvis KG, Grim CJ, Hu L, Datta AR, McCardell BA, Tall BD.** 2011. Cpa, the outer membrane protease of *Cronobacter sakazakii*, activates plasminogen and mediates resistance to serum bactericidal activity. *Infect Immun* **79:**1578–1587.

73. **Muytjens HL, Zanen HC, Sonderkamp HJ, Kollee LA, Wachsmuth IK, Farmer JJ III.** 1983. Analysis of eight cases of neonatal meningitis and sepsis due to *Enterobacter sakazakii*. *J Clin Microbiol* **18:**115–120.

74. **Block C, Peleg O, Minster N, Bar-Oz B, Simhon A, Arad I, Shapiro M.** 2002. Cluster of neonatal infections in Jerusalem due to unusual biochemical variant of *Enterobacter sakazakii. Eur J Clin Microbiol Infect Dis* **21:**613–616.

75. **Stock I, Wiedemann B.** 2002. Natural antibiotic susceptibility of *Enterobacter amnigenus,* *Enterobacter cancerogenus, Enterobacter gergoviae* and *Enterobacter sakazakii* strains. *Clin Microbiol Infect* **8:**564–578.

76. **Burgos JM, Ellington BA, Varela MF.** 2005. Presence of multidrug-resistant enteric bacteria in dairy farm topsoil. *J Dairy Sci* **88:**1391–1398.

Clostridium difficile Infection

15

JAE HYUN SHIN,[1] ESTEBAN CHAVES-OLARTE,[2] and CIRLE A. WARREN[1]

PATHOPHYSIOLOGY

The primary virulence factors that are known to cause clinical disease in *Clostridium difficile* infection (CDI) are the two large toxins: TcdA (toxin A; 308 kDa) and TcdB (toxin B; 270 kDa) (1). Both toxins are glucosyltransferases that inactivate Rho, Rac, and Cdc42 and result in actin condensation and subsequent cytoskeletal changes, apoptosis, and cell death of target cells. These toxins also induce an intense inflammatory response characterized by infiltration of inflammatory cells, especially neutrophils; activation of submucosal neurons; secretion of cytokines, chemokines, and arachidonic acid metabolites; and production of substance P and reactive oxygen intermediates (1, 2). We have published previously that mediators of inflammation such as COX2 and angiotensin II, inflammatory cytokines such as interleukin-8 (IL-8), and immune cells such as neutrophils are significantly elevated in intestinal loops treated with TcdA (3–5). Similarly, we see in our patients' histopathology mucosal disruption, intense inflammatory cell infiltration, and thick fibrinous exudates of degenerating cells (pseudomembranes), which are the hallmarks of pseudomembranous colitis (PMC) (6) (Fig. 1). Increased fecal

[1]Department of Medicine, Division of Infectious Disease and International Health, University of Virginia, Charlottesville, VA 22908; [2]Centro de Investigación en Enfermedades Tropicales, Facultad de Microbiología, Universidad de Costa Rica, Costa Rica.

Emerging Infections 10
Edited by W. Michael Scheld, James M. Hughes and Richard J. Whitley
© 2016 American Society for Microbiology, Washington, DC
doi:10.1128/microbiolspec.EI10-0007-2015

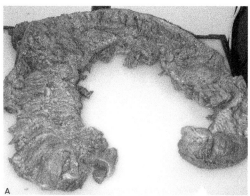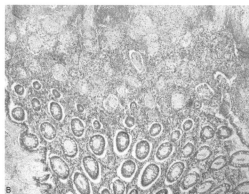

FIGURE 1 (A) Gross pathology of pseudomembranous colitis. (B) Histopathology of pseudomembranous colitis.

lactoferrin, IL-1β, and IL-8 were observed in patients with CDI (7). The link between glucosylation of the small GTPases and induction of the inflammatory cascade is unclear. This raises the possibility that the host inflammatory response is not a direct effect of the toxins on intracellular signaling but a concerted response by the cells surrounding the "intoxicated" cell to the changes that occurred in the latter.

In addition to TcdA and TcdB, some epidemic strains harbor an additional toxin known as binary toxin or CDT (8). However, the role of this toxin in the pathophysiology of CDI is still being debated. There is considerable variation in the sequence and activity of Tcds among different strains. For instance, the epidemic strain NAP1/027 encodes for a TcdB with an enhanced ability to penetrate, and thus intoxicate, target cells due to variations in the receptor binding and autoprocessing domains (9, 10). Furthermore, the presence of TcdA-negative strains in different locations has been consistently reported. Strikingly, all these strains encode for a variant TcdB with variations in the catalytic N-terminal domain that result in a different set of small GTPases being modified (11). The impact of this differential pattern of modified small GTPases in the pathophysiology of CDI is currently unknown, but it is certainly interesting that these TcdA-

negative strains are fully virulent. In humans, CDI is predominantly a localized disease in the colon, although the spectrum of disease may range from asymptomatic infection to severe diarrhea associated with PMC, sepsis, and even death. Even in severe disease, extracolonic infection and bacteremia are very rare (12). However, an intense systemic inflammatory response is observed where patients present with fever, leukocytosis, and even leukemoid reactions (13).

EPIDEMIOLOGY

CDIs have been extensively studied in high-income countries such as the United States and European countries such as the United Kingdom, France, and The Netherlands. In contrast, regions encompassing low- and middle-income countries such as Latin America in general show a lack of information on these diseases. Several reasons might account for this relatively small amount of knowledge on the impact of CDIs. These infectious diseases mainly affect a population that has access to good health care systems with the economic capability to support expensive treatments for chronic diseases (e. g., antibiotics, chemotherapy, and immunosuppressants, among others). The relationship between access to health care and CDI incidence has been recently put forward in an elegant study indicating that racial differences, directly relating to health care access, account for significant differences in CDI incidence rates (14). This study concluded that CDI represents a deviation from the paradigm that increased health care access is associated with less morbidity. If this concept is applied to a global scale, it can be hypothesized that low- and middle-income countries with budget limitations in their health care systems would generate a decreased number of *C. difficile* target populations in comparison to high-income countries. This would then result in less CDI incidence in low- and middle-income countries. In addition, the relatively expensive and technically challenging procedures required for the diagnosis of CDIs and the molecular characterization of circulating *C. difficile* would also play a role in the lack of information available about this nosocomial infectious disease in low- and middle-income countries.

North America and Europe

In the past decade, the incidence rates of CDI and fulminant *C. difficile* colitis have increased in the United States (15–17), Canada (18–20), and Europe (21, 22). The rising rates and severity of CDI were attributed to strains characterized as "group BI" by restriction endonuclease analysis, as North American pulse-field type "NAP1" by pulse-field gel electrophoresis, as ribotype 027 (BI/NAP1/027), and as toxinotype III (23). More recently, other strains such as PCR ribotypes 001, 017, and 078 were identified in certain outbreaks and severe cases of CDI (24–28). Although typically seen in older adults exposed to antibiotics in health care settings, community-associated CDI in younger populations—including children and pregnant women—and cases with no previous exposure to antibiotics have also now been noted (29–32). Advanced age remains the critical risk factor for severe disease, recurrence, and mortality (33, 34).

Latin America

Most of the studies in Argentina, Brazil, Mexico, Chile, and Costa Rica have been performed in hospitalized adult populations being treated for various chronic conditions. Whereas hospitalized populations have been the main objective of these studies, community-acquired CDI prevalence rates were found to range from 18.7 to 30% (24, 25). Several studies have focused on antibiotic-associated diarrhea (26, 27), whereas others have addressed the impact of CDIs in specific hospitalized populations, such as those with immunosuppressive disorders or hematologic and hematopoietic stem cell transplantation patients (28, 35). Several CDI diagnostic tests have been used, including technically challenging strategies such as toxigenic culture and cell cytotoxic assays (24, 36), but most of the studies were based on enzyme immunoassay (EIA) detection of *C. difficile* toxins (26–35). *C. difficile* has been found to cause antibiotic-associated diarrhea and diarrhea in nosocomial settings in as low as 8.3 to up to 38.5% of cases (26, 36, 37). Similar to North America and Europe, advanced age (mean age ranging from 65 to 72.9 years) appears to be an important risk factor for CDI in these regions (24, 38). A study conducted in Mexico identified H_2 blockers, advanced age, prior hospitalization within 12 weeks of diagnosis, prior use of cephalosporins and fluoroquinolones, extended hospital stay, and antimicrobial use before diagnosis as significant risk factors for the development of CDI (39). The role of CDI in the community setting is less well documented. A case report of a community-acquired CDI caused by the epidemic NAP1/027 strain in an 18-month-old child has been published (40). The presence of toxigenic *C. difficile* has been reported in retail meats, dogs, and South American coati, suggesting these as sources and possible reservoirs for community-acquired CDI (41–43). However, these few studies do not shed light on the real impact of *C. difficile* in the induction of diarrhea in ambulatory patients.

Several attempts have been made to characterize the molecular feature of the strains circulating in the region and to define their virulence potential. Of particular interest due to its global circulation is the report of the presence of the epidemic NAP1/BI/027 strain. In Latin America, this strain was initially reported in Costa Rica and was described as a major participant during an outbreak in a tertiary hospital in 2009 (44). This epidemic strain harbored all the molecular determinants recognized in other reports such as resistance to fluoroquinolones, deletion in *tcdC*, and presence of the binary toxin. Recent analysis by whole-genome sequencing has indicated that the NAP1/BI/027 strain circulating in Costa Rica belongs to the FQR2 epidemic lineage, which is spread more widely and is associated with outbreaks in the United Kingdom, continental Europe, and Australia (45; C. Rodriguez, personal communication). In addition to the presence of the NAP1/BI/027 strain in Costa Rica, this epidemic variant has recently been reported in countries separated by thousands of kilometers such as Mexico, Panama, and Chile, demonstrating the distribution of this epidemic strain throughout the continent (46–48).

In all these studies, the molecular hallmarks of NAP1/BI/027 strains (*tcdC* deletion, presence of binary toxin, fluoroquinolone resistance) have been detected. In a study of 719 isolates of *C. difficile* from 45 hospitals in Chile, 79% of the strains were found to be of the epidemic variant, reinforcing the notion of the ability of this strain to have an epidemic character and potentially displace local circulating strains (47). Another interesting genotype reported was of the TcdA-negative, TcdB-positive *C. difficile* strain belonging to ribotype 017/toxinotype VIII. The annual percentage of this particular genotype went from 7.7% in 2000 to 92% in 2004 in an Argentinean general hospital (49). *C. difficile* strains belonging to ribotypes 014 and 106, the latter found previously in the United Kingdom, have also been reported

(35, 43). Autochthonous *C. difficile* strains have also been described. Of particular interest is a variant described as responsible, together with an epidemic NAP1/BI/027 strain, of causing an outbreak in a tertiary hospital in Costa Rica (44). This strain belongs to a previously undescribed NAP type called NAPCR1 and had virulent behavior comparable to that of cocirculating NAP1/BI/027 epidemic strains. In addition, it shared with these epidemic strains molecular determinants such as deletions in *tcdC*, the presence of binary toxin, and resistance to fluoroquinolones due to mutations in *gyrA*, but unlike the epidemic strains, it did not overproduce TcdA or TcdB (50).

Asia

A review of epidemiology of CDI in Asia is inevitably linked to discussion of TcdA-negative, TcdB-positive variant strains, the most commonly reported ribotypes being 017 and 018 (51).

East Asia

Despite interest in *C. difficile* and different molecular techniques to type them, there has been only one recent study on the epidemiology of CDI in Japan. Honda et al. found in a retrospective study of a tertiary regional referral center that the incidence at 3.31 cases per 10,000 patient-days is slightly lower than North America or Europe at 4.1 to 9.8 cases per 10,000 patient-days. However, 30-day all-cause mortality reached 15%, and 51.6% of patients met criteria for severe CDI, rates which were all higher than those seen in other countries (52). This may be due to a low index of suspicion leading to diagnosing only patients with severe illnesses. Multiple typing techniques have been employed to characterize the strains. Several ribotyping studies have indicated predominance of ribotype "smz" over the past decade (53, 54). Ribotype smz is recognized internationally as ribotype 018, which is one of the TcdA-negative, TcdB-positive strains (55).

Ribotype 027, a recently epidemic strain in North America and Europe, has been reported only occasionally (54).

There have been multiple studies on the epidemiology and molecular characteristics of *C. difficile* in South Korea. A country-wide survey of 17 tertiary hospitals from 2004 to 2008 showed an incidence of CDI that increased from 1.7 cases per 1,000 adult admissions to 2.7 cases per 1,000 adult admissions (56). A large proportion of the CDI cases in South Korea are caused by TcdA-negative, TcdB-positive strains as demonstrated in multiple studies (57, 58). In a retrospective survey of six tertiary care hospitals in South Korea between 2000 and 2005, the prevalence of TcdA-negative, TcdB-positive strains grew from less than 7% before 2002 to a peak of 50.3% in 2004 (57). In another study evaluating the cause of PMC in a tertiary care hospital between 2004 and 2005 it was found that TcdA-negative, TcdB-positive strains caused 50.9% of PMC cases (58). Ribotypes 017 and 018 were predominantly TcdA-negative, TcdB-positive strains based on different molecular studies (51, 59). Ribotypes 027 and 078, more common in North America and Europe were also reported, with 078 being the most common binary-toxin positive strain (51).

CDI is not part of the diagnostic testing for diarrhea in hospitals in mainland China, and hence there is a paucity of epidemiologic studies looking at the incidence of CDI in the hospitalized patients in China (60, 61). In a study of diarrheal samples in hospitalized patients who were treated with antibiotics, 21/70 (30%) were positive for *C. difficile* by culture (60). Consistent with studies in Japan and Korea, the predominant PCR ribotype was 017 (48%), followed by 046 (14%) and 012 (14%); strains of the epidemic PCR ribotypes 027 and 078 were not observed (60). Another study looking at diarrheal stool in hospitalized patients showed 31/111 stools (28%) positive for *C. difficile* by PCR (61). The authors of this study noted that since CDI is not tested for as part of diagnostic work-ups,

it is possible that CDI is an underrecognized problem in China.

In Taiwan, reports of CDI have appeared only quite recently. Of stools tested for CDI, 5.3% came back positive in one retrospective study, while another retrospective study showed an incidence of 42.6 cases per 100,000 patient-days, or 3.4 cases per 1,000 discharges, comparable to reports from North America (62, 63). An analysis of 110 isolates from 2002 to 2007 showed 70 isolates that were TcdA and TcdB positive, while 40 isolates were TcdA-negative, TcdB-positive (64). Interestingly, the TcdA-negative, TcdB-positive strains were initially higher, making up 73.3% of all isolates in 2004, but decreased to 23.9% in 2007, while TcdA-positive, TcdB-positive strains increased in numbers (64). Ribotype 027 strain was not found in Taiwan until recently, when three isolated cases were reported (65–67).

A retrospective study in Hong Kong showed that 12.5% of patients tested were positive for *C. difficile*, but only 5.9% were positive for toxin production (68). In terms of ribotyping, 70% of isolates were of a pattern not represented by 23 of the most internationally common ribotypes, with a further 11.6% being nontypable (55). Ribotype 002 was the predominant strain, representing 9.4% of the isolates (68). Another surveillance study showed 5.1% of the stools positive for *C. difficile* by cytotoxic assay (69). Cheng et al. also found that while testing for CDI increased, the prevalence of CDI-positive cases remained constant (23). The first and only case of CDI from a ribotype 027 strain was identified in the same study (69).

Southeast Asia

There are few reports from Southeast Asia on CDI. In the Philippines, a recent study demonstrated underestimation of CDI by showing that while historically patients with colitis were presumed to be infected with *Entamoeba histolytica*, 43.6% of the stools were positive for *C. difficile*, compared to 25.6% which were positive for *E. histolytica*

(70). Since the first-line treatment for both is metronidazole, the outcome would be indistinguishable between the two pathogens. Toxin assays on stool samples from patients with antibiotic-associated diarrheas at a tertiary hospital in northeastern Malaysia showed 13.7% prevalence (71). No ribotyping or other molecular analysis has been reported on Malaysian or Philippine *C. difficile* isolates. A study of diarrhea in children identified *C. difficile* in 1.3% of stool samples tested in both hospital and community settings in Jakarta, Indonesia (72). A molecular study of isolates from Indonesia showed that five of eight isolates were ribotype 017/toxinotype VIII (73).

There have been multiple studies evaluating the prevalence of *C. difficile* in the stool of pediatric and adult patients in Thailand, but the prevalence of positive stools varied widely from 14.3 to 52.2% between studies, which may be related to the differences in method of detection (cytotoxicity assay versus toxin A EIA) (74, 75). Since 2000, more studies have been performed on patients admitted with antibiotic-associated diarrhea. A retrospective study in 2003 showed *C. difficile* isolated in 18.6% of diarrheal stool specimens, all of which were positive for both *tcdA* and *tcdB* by PCR, with only one *tcdA*-negative, *tcdB*-negative result (76). A more recent study in 2012 showed even higher prevalence of 26.9% of stool specimens, with mortality due to *C. difficile* reported to be 6.4% (76).

There are few reports on the epidemiology and clinical behavior of *C. difficile* in Singapore. An earlier report indicated a percentage of isolation of this nosocomial pathogen of 9.6% in samples processed for its detection (77). Another study indicated an incidence of 3.2 cases per 1,000 admissions, occurring mainly in renal and hematology patients. From all the isolates, 11.8% corresponded to TcdA-negative strains (78). Interestingly, a decrease in the incidence of CDI was detected in the period of 2006–2008 despite an increase in the use of carbapenems

and fluoroquinolones (79). The hypervirulent strain NAP1/027 was detected and reported in 2011 (80). However, the antibiotic resistance pattern of this strain was more compatible with historic isolates, indicating that it probably does not correspond to the epidemic strain of global distribution.

South Asia

CDI was detected in India first in 1986 by toxin detection and culture from Nehru Hospital (81). A subsequent prospective study in a hospital in Delhi in 1999 showed CDI in 15.2% of hospitalized patients with antibiotic-associated diarrhea as detected by culture and toxin A EIA (82). Analysis of antibiotic-associated diarrhea in the same institution in 2009 revealed a similar incidence of 12.1% of patients being positive for *C. difficile* and deaths in 23% of the cases (83). Multiple studies have documented the presence of *C. difficile* in stool of patients with antibiotic-associated diarrhea, with incidences ranging between 11 to 17% (84, 85). Molecular epidemiology of *C. difficile* strains in India is not currently known. A study in the 1990s in Bangladesh found that only 13/814 children admitted to the hospital with diarrhea had stool positive for *C. difficile* by cell cytotoxin assay (86).

Australia

In Australia, CDIs have been associated with the use of cephalosporins since the 1980s. Indeed, a decrease in the use of third-generation cephalosporins has been observed to be followed by a concomitant decrease of CDIs (87). A survey in 48 microbiology laboratories carried out between 2009 and 2010 indicated that most laboratories screened stools by EIA. This study determined an overall mean incidence of 25.6 per 100,000 population (88). As in other parts of the world, CDI incidence is increasing in Australia and thus so is its impact on health care and the economy. A prospective study carried out between 2011 and 2012 in 450 public hospitals covering all the Australian states revealed that the increases in rates were notable in hospital-identified CDI, hospital-associated CDI, and community-associated CDI (89). *C. difficile* positivity in clinical samples increased from 5.9% in 2003 to 18.8% in 2012 in one study (90). In another study in 2011, CDIs were identified to be the third-most-costly complications in hospitalized patients in Australia, behind only complications associated with procedures related to endocrine or metabolic disorders and multidrug-resistent *Staphylococcus aureus* infections (91). A comprehensive survey in two tertiary care hospitals in Australia determined that 53.8% of CDIs were hospital onset disease, whereas 28.8% were community-onset and health care facility–associated disease, and only 7.5% were community-associated disease (92). In addition, severe disease was reported in 40% of the cases, but the 30-day mortality rate was low at only 2.5% (92).

A global study comparing the strains circulating in North America, Europe, and Australia as detected by restriction endonuclease analysis and PCR ribotyping was performed on 894 isolates (93). From those, ribotype 027 was the most common isolate in North America and some European countries but not in Australia. Instead, ribotypes circulating in Australia corresponded to strains rarely found in other developed countries. A study of 274 samples screened for toxigenic *C. difficile* determined a prevalence of the infection of 9.8%, of which the most frequent ribotypes were 014 and 052 (94). In other analyses the predominant ribotypes were 014 (24.3%), 020 (5.7%), 056 (5.7%), and 070 (5.7%) (92), while in yet another analysis of 474 isolates collected in 2013, the most frequent ribotypes were 014 (29.8%) and 002 (15.9%). Epidemic ribotype 027 was not identified, and small numbers of virulent ribotype 078 were found (95). In Queensland, the most common ribotypes were 002 (22.9%), 014 (13.3%), and 244 (8.4%) (96). The ribotype 244 strain had a single deletion in the *tcdC* gene and was positive for binary toxin and found to be closely related to ribotype 027 epidemic strains by whole-genome sequencing. This strain was associated with a more severe disease and a higher mortality rate (97, 98). Thus, strain 244 represents an autochthonous strain in Australia, with an increased virulence potential probably related to its genomic closeness to epidemic NAP1/027 strains.

TcdA-negative strains reported elsewhere have also been found in Australia. In a study of 817 human clinical isolates from all Australian states, 9 (1.1%) were found to be TcdA negative. Of those, six were positive for binary toxin. These TcdA-negative strains belonged to seven different ribotypes. Among these ribotypes, 017, a common genotype found in TcdA-negative strains, was seen in only two strains (99). The epidemic strain NAP1/BI/027 was not reported in Australia until 2009, when it was isolated from a patient who was infected in the United States (100). The first recognized case of the epidemic *C. difficile* strain acquired in Australia was not reported until 2011 (101). So far, the prevalence of the NAP1/BI/027 genotype is low in Australia and has not been able to displace other common ribotypes. Among 477 cases of *C. difficile* between 2010 and 2011 reported by the Victorian Health Care infection surveillance system, only 2.3% corresponded to the hypervirulent strains (102).

Africa

South Africa has published the most reports on CDI. A random sampling of stool specimens at the University of Venda between 2004 and 2005 evaluating 322 stool specimens showed toxigenic *C. difficile* in 11.4% of all diarrheal stool samples (103). There was also an outbreak reported in 2008 in a tertiary hospital in Pretoria during which time 17.2% of all diarrheal stools were positive for *C. difficile* toxin (104). A more recent study reported *C. difficile* as the most frequently detected pathogen (16% of cases) in patients with diarrhea at a tertiary care center in the 21- to 87-year-old age range (105).

There are few published studies on CDI in other African countries, and the published studies have had a focus on evaluating patients with HIV infection. The earlier studies in the 1990s evaluating chronic diarrhea in HIV-infected patients in Zambia and Kenya showed that 0% of diarrheal stools were positive with *C. difficile* (106, 107). More recent studies evaluating HIV-infected patients with diarrhea suggest increasing prevalence of CDI in this population (108, 109). A study of HIV patients in Zimbabwe reported a prevalence of 8.6% in diarrheal stools (109). In Nigeria, CDI prevalence was 14% for hospitalized HIV-negative patients and 43% for hospitalized HIV-infected patients with diarrhea (108).

CLINICAL PRESENTATION

CDI may present without any symptoms, with varying degrees of diarrhea, or with sepsis to fulminant colitis leading to death. Severe disease is particularly notable in the elderly. Several factors have been reported to increase the risk of acquisition of CDI (Table 1).

Risk Factors for Symptomatic Infection

Antibiotic exposure is the most common predisposing factor in the development of CDI. Historically, clindamycin has been the

TABLE 1 Risk factors associated with acquisition of *Clostridium difficile*

Colonization	Infection
Recent hospitalization (within 2–3 months) (114, 212)	Advanced age (212)
	Antibiotic use (111, 113, 212)
	Colonization (114)
Cancer chemotherapy (212)	Proton pump inhibitor use (212)
	Enteral feeding (213)
	Gastrointestinal surgery (214)
	Obesity (214)
	Cancer chemotherapy (212)

first agent to be associated with severe diarrhea (21% of those receiving the antibiotic) and PMC (seen in 50% of those with diarrhea) (110). Most antibiotics have been implicated, but the most common agents include penicillins, cephalosporins, and fluoroquinolones. In a meta-analysis of antimicrobial usage in community-acquired CDI, clindamycin (odds ratio [OR] = 20.43) carried the greatest risk of community-acquired CDI, followed by fluoroquinolones (OR = 5.65), cephalosporins (OR = 4.47), penicillins (OR = 3.25), macrolides (OR = 2.55), and sulfonamides/trimethoprim (OR = 1.84) (111). In health care settings, the role of antibiotics is difficult to ascertain because of confounding variables associated with patients in these settings (112). However, it appears that cephalosporins, clindamycin, carbapenems, trimethoprim/sulfonamides, fluoroquinolones, and penicillin combinations are associated with hospital-acquired CDI (113).

Initial acquisition of *C. difficile* spores invariably precedes infection. In a systematic review of 19 studies that examined colonization in patients on hospital admission, the pooled prevalence of toxigenic *C. difficile* carriage was about 8% (range 0 to 24%) (114). The risk of CDI for colonized patients was significantly higher at 21.8% compared to 3.4% in noncolonized patients. Hospitalization in the previous 3 months and no previous antibiotic exposure, proton pump inhibitor (PPI) use, or history of CDI was associated with higher risk of colonization. While health care facilities appear to be a major source of *C. difficile* transmission (presumably from asymptomatic and symptomatic patients) (115, 116), a recent study of symptomatic patients with CDI in health care settings or in the community in the United Kingdom found that 45% of the isolates were genetically distinct from previous health care– or community-related cases, indicating the presence of genetically diverse sources, including asymptomatic carriers in both settings (117). *C. difficile* spores may be acquired through the contaminated skin or environment of both asymptomatic and symptomatic carriers (118–120). Skin contamination in infected patients persists even after resolution of diarrhea (121).

Advanced age increases the risk for developing CDI as documented in multiple studies. Studies in the 1990s and 2000s in North America when the dramatic increase in CDI cases occurred showed a significant increase in the age group 65 or older and a population incidence more than 5-fold higher than the other age groups (15, 20). In a more recent survey of hospital stays for CDI in U.S. hospitals in 2009, the rate of CDI was 1,554 per 100,000 population for patients 65 or older compared to 138 per 100,000 in the rest of the age groups (122).

Advanced age is also a risk factor for worse outcome from CDI. Mortality has been found to be significantly higher with older age (19, 123). Even when controlling for comorbidity burden, Pépin et al. demonstrated that 30-day and 1-year mortality increased with older age, especially above the age of 75 (124). The death registry from 2008 also showed that 92% of deaths from CDI occurred in people age 65 and over (125). In a more recent study of the burden of CDI in the United States in 2011, it was found that while people 65 and older made up 57% of estimated total CDI cases, the deaths from CDI in this age group made up 83% of the total estimated deaths from CDI (126). In a study of 336 patients with stool positive for *C. difficile* in Brigham and Women's Hospital in 2004 and 2005, the odds ratio for severe disease was 3.35 for ages 70 and older (127). Increased risk for recurrence of CDI in people 65 and older was seen in multiple studies, with the chance of recurrence ranging from 2 to 10 times more likely in this age group, depending on the study (128, 129).

Symptoms and Signs

The clinical manifestations of infection with toxin-producing strains of *C. difficile* range from symptomless carriage to mild or moderate diarrhea to fulminant and sometimes fatal PMC (130–132). Symptoms of CDI usually begin soon after colonization, with a median time to onset of 2 to 3 days (119). *C. difficile* diarrhea may be associated with the passage of mucus or occult blood in the stool, but melena or hematochezia are rare. Fever, cramping, abdominal discomfort, and peripheral leukocytosis are common (131). In one study, 24.7% of patients had mild, self-limiting disease, 35.6% had moderately severe disease, and 39.7% had prolonged symptoms (130). In addition, 8.2% of patients had fulminant colitis with severe inflammation and pseudomembrane formation necessitating emergency colectomy in half of these patients (130). Extraintestinal manifestations, such as arthritis or bacteremia, are very rare (131). *C. difficile* ileitis or pouchitis has also been rarely recognized in patients who have previously undergone a total colectomy (for complicated CDI or some other indication) (133). Patients with severe disease may develop a colonic ileus or toxic dilatation and present with abdominal pain and distension but with minimal or no diarrhea (130–132). Complications of severe *C. difficile* colitis include dehydration, electrolyte disturbances, hypoalbuminemia, toxic megacolon, bowel perforation, hypotension, renal failure, systemic inflammatory response syndrome, sepsis, and death (130–132).

Severity of Disease: White Blood Cell Count (WBC), Creatinine, Complicated versus Uncomplicated

The following criteria for defining severity of CDI were adapted from the Infectious Diseases Society of America (IDSA) and Society for Healthcare Epidemiology of America clinical practice guidelines (131). Mild or moderate CDI is defined by a WBC of 15,000 cells/ml or lower and serum creatinine level less than 1.5 times the premorbid level (131). Severe CDI is with WBC of 15,000 cells/ml or higher or a serum creatinine level greater than or equal to 1.5 times the premorbid level (131). Severe complicated CDI refers to cases with hypotension or shock, ileus, or megacolon (131). The distinctions are made to guide the choice of therapy. In a retrospective study evaluating patients with CDI in Brigham and Women's Hospital, maximum WBC of >20,000 cells/ml, maximum serum creatinine level of >2 mg/dl, minimum serum albumin level of <2.5 g/dl, ileus or small bowel obstruction, and abnormal abdominal computed tomography image were all independent risk factors for severe outcome as defined by death within 30 days after onset, more than one ICU admission, colectomy, or intestinal perforation in which CDI was a major contributor (127). In other studies as well, the peak WBC and peak serum creatinine level are predictive of complicated CDI (20). Other experts and practice guidelines consider age, body temperature, comorbidities, serum albumin, serum lactate, and other factors in defining disease severity in CDI (134–136).

Mortality

In a review of patients admitted to a single tertiary center with an urban population in the United States from 2006 to 2011, 30-day overall mortality was 12.9% for hospital-associated CDI and 13.8% for community-associated CDI, which was a decrease from 2006 to 2008, when the mortality was 17.0% and 17.1%, respectively (137). Through multivariate analysis, age, WBC, and albumin level at the time of diagnosis were all associated with the 30-day mortality (137). For attributable mortality, a pooled mortality of 5.99% was calculated from the published literature up to 2010 (138). When studies before 2000 were excluded to reflect the recent trend since the emergence of the epidemic NAP1/BI/027 strain, the mortality went up to 8.03% (138).

Recurrent Disease

CDI is particularly difficult to treat due to its high rate of relapse. In a review of patients treated in Quebec, the proportion of patients who had at least one relapse was 28.8% in patients treated with metronidazole and 27.7% in patients treated with vancomycin (129). A more recent study in 2015 indicated a first relapse rate of 13.5% in community-associated CDI and 20.9% in health care–acquired CDI (126). Risk factors for recurrence included age 65 or older, severe or fulminant underlying illness as determined by the Horn index, additional antibiotic use after discontinuation of metronidazole or vancomycin therapy for the initial CDI episode, and low serum antitoxin A IgG concentration (129, 139).

DIAGNOSIS

Diagnosis of CDI is a field with significant recent advances as reflected in the difference between the IDSA practice guidelines and current practice in many health care facilities. For example, when the guidelines were written in 2010, PCR was still considered not to have enough evidence to be included in the recommendations (131).

Diagnostic Methods

Two conventional microbiologic laboratory methods are considered the reference standards for testing of *C. difficile*: toxigenic culture and cell culture cytotoxicity assay. Toxigenic culture consists of culture on selective media followed by *in vitro* toxin detection to determine the toxigenicity of the isolated strain (140). In cell culture cytotoxicity assay, stool filtrates are inoculated onto a monolayer of a cell culture, which is then observed for a toxin-induced cytopathic effect (rounding of the cells) after 24 and 48 hours. To determine the specificity of the cytopathic effect, neutralization with an antiserum (*Clostridium sordellii* antitoxin or *C. difficile* antitoxin) is executed (140). These reference methods have a longer turnaround time, as well as requiring specific laboratory facilities and technical expertise, such as anaerobic cultures and cell cultures. As a result, many laboratories have started utilizing newer techniques.

The newer techniques are rapid and easy to perform. One technique is EIA, which can detect the presence of *C. difficile* by detecting the enzyme glutamate dehydrogenase (GDH), which is abundantly produced by *C. difficile*. EIA can also be used to detect the presence of *C. difficile* toxins A and B (140). Multiple assays are available, some of which combine both GDH and toxin EIA. Another technique is real-time PCR to detect the presence of *C. difficile* by detecting the toxin B gene (*tcdB*) (140).

All of the above techniques have limitations. According to the IDSA practice guidelines, culture is the gold standard but is not clinically practical because of its slow turnaround time, and while EIA is rapid, it is less sensitive and is thus a suboptimal approach for diagnosis (131). Limitations of the methods are closely related to their targets.

Toxigenic culture, GDH EIA, and PCR all detect the presence of *C. difficile* in the stool. These methods of detection have higher sensitivity compared to methods designed to detect the production of toxins but may identify clinically nonsignificant cases such as colonization without CDI or even the presence of nontoxigenic *C. difficile* in the case of the GDH EIA, since GDH is present in both toxigenic and nontoxigenic *C. difficile*. An early study from 1986 showed that patients with positive cytotoxicity assay results had worse outcomes and indicators of severity (141). Recently, a multicenter study of CDI evaluated both reference methods, toxigenic culture and cytotoxicity assay, on 12,420 diarrheal stool samples sent to four diagnostic laboratories, the largest study to date (142). In this study the case fatality rate was higher for patients with positive cytotoxicity assay compared to patients with positive toxigenic culture but negative cytotoxicity assay. The patients with stool only positive for toxigenic culture had a similar case fatality rate as patients with a negative culture.

However, cell culture cytotoxicity assay and toxin EIA, which are designed to detect only the production of toxins, will identify only clinically meaningful cases of CDI that definitely need to be treated but have lower sensitivity compared to the previous methods, and there have been concerns about underdiagnosis of CDI. In the study referenced above, the sensitivity and specificity of four commercial CDI tests were also measured against the two reference standards (142). Toxin EIA has sensitivity ranging from 45.6 to 57.8% when compared to toxigenic culture and 66.9 to 83.2% even when compared to cytotoxicity assay.

Testing Strategy

The current IDSA/Society for Healthcare Epidemiology of America recommendation for diagnosis of CDI is to do toxigenic culture, but this has been noted to be impractical due to the need for anaerobic culturing capacity and turnaround time (131). Another strategy is a two-step method that uses GDH EIA for initial screening and then cell cytotoxicity assay or toxigenic culture as the confirmatory test (131). A recent guideline in the *American Journal of Gastroenterology* recommends nucleic acid amplification (PCR) as a stand-alone test or a two-step method with GDH EIA for initial screening (136). However, as demonstrated by Planche et al., PCR is not an appropriate stand-alone test due to its low positive predictive value (142). Planche et al. recommend as an alternative testing strategy similar to one recommended by the IDSA, a two-step test using GDH EIA followed by toxin EIA or toxin EIA followed by PCR (142).

A testing strategy that is agreed upon by different guidelines is the need to test for CDI only in unformed stool (131, 136). This is due to the high rate of asymptomatic colonization of patients with *C. difficile* ranging as high as 59 to 94% on admission to the hospital based on some studies (115, 119). With such high rates of asymptomatic colonization, the question of testing and diagnosis in appropriate clinical settings becomes very important. Additionally, it has been found that restricting the samples tested to unformed stool does not decrease the sensitivity of the test (143).

In conclusion, with very high rates of asymptomatic colonization, only patients with an appropriate clinical picture and loose, unformed stool should be tested for CDI. Patients with ileus from toxic megacolon should be tested with rectal swab (144). For the laboratory testing strategy, there currently is not a consensus among different societies, but a two-step approach using a combination of GDH EIA, toxin EIA, or PCR may yield the best positive and negative predictive values.

MANAGEMENT

Management approaches for CDI may include targeting bacteria (antibiotics), toxins (antibodies, binders), host response (modulating inflammation), or microbiota (preservation or restoration), and in fulminant cases or where nonsurgical approaches fail, colectomy or other less invasive procedures. The choice of approach depends on the severity of illness, previous history of the disease, and host factors. Various international professional societies and experts have published management guidelines (131, 134–136). There have been significant advances in drug and biological research and developments in the treatment of CDI, although the current standard of care is still the administration of anti–*C. difficile* antibiotics (Table 2). The challenges continue to be disease prevention in the susceptible host and prevention, and treatment of recurrences and management of fulminant cases.

Antibacterial Agents

Discontinuation of the offending antibiotics to allow the normal intestinal flora to recover

TABLE 2 Emerging trends in the management of *Clostridium difficile* infection

Goal	Approach
Prevention of CDI	Vaccines
	Probiotics
Treatment of initial CDI	Anti–*C. difficile* antibiotics
Prevention of recurrence	Addition of antitoxin agent to anti–*C. difficile* antibiotics
	Nontoxigenic *C. difficile* posttreatment with anti–*C. difficile* antibiotics
Prevention or treatment of multiple recurrences	Fecal microbiota transplantation
Management of fulminant colitis	Surgery: less invasive approach vs. colectomy

is the ideal treatment for CDI. However, in cases where there is high infection burden and/or a need for continuing antibiotic treatment for another infection, an antimicrobial agent targeting *C. difficile* is often required. Unfortunately, nearly all antibiotics, including those specific for *C. difficile* have the potential to further disrupt the intestinal microbiota, delay recovery of colonization resistance, and predispose to another CDI.

Metronidazole

Oral preparations of metronidazole were widely used for CDI in the 1990s because of observed equivalence in efficacy with vancomycin, cost advantage, and concerns about the spread of vancomycin-resistant enterococci. Metronidazole was the recommended drug for CDI, with vancomycin reserved for severe and potentially life-threatening infection, unresponsiveness to metronidazole, or when oral metronidazole could not be used (145, 146). With the emergence of the epidemic strain of *C. difficile*, BI/NAP1/027/ III, treatment failures with metronidazole have increasingly been reported (129, 147). Recent data from clinical trials have shown that vancomycin is superior to metronidazole, especially for severe disease (148, 149).

Intravenous (i.v.) metronidazole is usually empirically added to oral or rectal vancomycin for complicated severe disease. A recent retrospective observational study in a single institution has shown that in patients who were admitted to an intensive care unit, the receipt of combination treatment with i.v. metronidazole with either oral or rectal vancomycin was significantly associated with improved mortality (150). In this study, patients on combination therapy had more renal disease, hypoalbuminemia, leukocytosis, and fever. Administration of i.v. metronidazole alone is not recommended. In a prospective cohort study comparing oral metronidazole, i.v. metronidazole, and oral vancomycin for mild CDI, administration of i.v. metronidazole alone was observed to be associated with increased mortality (151).

Vancomycin

Vancomycin is the first FDA-approved drug for CDI. Soon after the identification of toxigenic *C. difficile* as the cause of antibiotic-associated PMC, the efficacy of oral vancomycin against PMC and postoperative diarrhea was tested in a small randomized controlled trial (152). Among 44 patients randomized to 5 days of either 125 mg of vancomycin or placebo taken orally, 16 patients had very high titers of neutralizable toxin and 12 had PMC by sigmoidoscopy and biopsy. After treatment, fecal toxin was undetectable and PMC was cured when treated with vancomycin in eight of nine patients with high toxin levels and six of seven patients with PMC compared to five of seven patients with high toxins and one of five patients with PMC in those who received placebo. A later study showed that oral vancomycin doses of 125 mg and 500 mg are equally efficacious in resolving diarrhea secondary to antibiotic-associated *C. difficile* colitis (153). Indeed, fecal levels of vancomycin at 125 mg every 6 hours are above the MIC_{90} for *C. difficile* (152, 154). Although vancomycin quickly became the standard of treatment, metronidazole was noted to be as effective for CDI in the 1980s (155). Metronidazole was preferred by clinicians because it was cheaper and theoretically less likely to promote colonization with vancomycin-

resistant enterococci (156). However, more recent randomized, controlled trials have shown that vancomycin is superior to metronidazole for severe disease (148, 149), and most experts now recommend it as the drug of choice for severe disease (131, 134, 135). Although there is not sufficient evidence of efficacy, vancomycin delivered by rectal enema or intracolonic administration has also been used in cases when oral administration is not possible and in the presence of complicated severe disease (157, 158). Vancomycin at pulsed or tapering doses has been recommended for treatment of recurrent episodes of CDI (159).

Fidaxomicin

Fidaxomicin is the only other FDA-approved drug for CDI. Two multicenter, randomized, noninferiority trials that enrolled a total of 1,164 patients from Europe, Canada, and the United States were conducted to compare the efficacy of fidaxomicin with vancomycin (160, 161). Both phase 3 trials revealed that fidaxomicin at 200 mg two times a day is noninferior in treating acute CDI and superior in preventing recurrent disease when compared to vancomycin at 125 mg four times a day, both given for 10 days. The lower recurrence rates noted in the fidaxomicin group may be secondary to the persistence of major microbiome components in patients treated with the new agent, compared to vancomycin, which was associated with 2- to 4-fold decreases of the *Bacteroides/Prevotella* groups (162). It appears that protection from recurrence was conferred by fidaxomicin in both relapse and reinfection (163). However, decreased cure rates and increased recurrences were noted in both fidaxomicin- and vancomycin-treated participants who were infected with isolates of the BI strain by restriction endonuclease analysis (164). Indeed, the advantage of fidaxomicin in preventing recurrences is lost in infections caused by the prevalent epidemic strain, BI/NAP1/027. In animal studies, we have shown that pretreatment with fidaxomicin, just as with vancomycin, increases susceptibility to initial infection and is as likely to cause recurrent disease in mice (165). Although fidaxomicin is an alternative drug to vancomycin in patients with severe CDI, no data are available on its efficacy in severe complicated or life-threatening disease.

Antitoxin

The pathogenesis of CDI is predominantly toxin-mediated, and thus, strategies that neutralize or block toxins are logical approaches. Interestingly, although in animal models antitoxins appear to ameliorate disease, the benefits in humans only involve reduction of recurrent CDI.

Monoclonal antibodies

The results of a phase 2, randomized, double-blind, placebo-controlled study investigating two neutralizing, human monoclonal antibodies against *C. difficile* toxins A and B were promising (166). Both antibodies were given as a single infusion (each antibody at 10 mg per kg of body weight) in patients (still with diarrhea) receiving either metronidazole or vancomycin. Among 200 participants equally divided into antibody and placebo groups, the rate of recurrence of CDI was lower in the treatment group (7% versus 25%; $p < 0.001$). The recurrence rates were even lower in those participants with the epidemic BI/NAP1/027 (8% versus 29%; $p = 0.06$) or with a history of previous CDI (7% versus 38%; $p = 0.006$). However, the duration and severity of diarrhea and length of hospital stay were not reduced by the monoclonal antibodies. Subgroup analyses suggested that subjects who are hospitalized, are older, have severe underlying comorbidities, and have severe CDI may not respond as well to treatment. Two phase 3 studies were recently completed: one investigated the effect of each monoclonal antibody and their combination on CDI recurrence (MODIFY I), and the other investigated the effect of the monoclonal antibody against TcdB compared with the

two monoclonal antibodies combined on CDI recurrence (MODIFY II). Preliminary results presented at two international conferences indicate that the monoclonal antibody to TcdB (bezlotoxumab), and not to TcdA (actoxumab), when given with standard of care, significantly decreased *C. difficile* recurrence at 12-week follow-up (16.5% versus placebo 26.6%; $p < 0.0001$). Combination treatment with both monoclonal antibodies did not confer additional benefit (215).

Tolevamer

Tolevamer is a high molecular weight, soluble polymer of styrenesulfonate that binds and neutralizes *C. difficile* toxins *in vitro* (167). A phase 2 study in patients with mild to moderate disease showed a dose response for tolevamer with 3- or 6-g daily doses, with the 6-g dose considered to be noninferior to vancomycin administered at 500 mg per day because of a <1-day difference in median time to resolution of diarrhea (tolevamer at 2.5 days compared to vancomycin at 2 days) (168). Because of these promising initial studies, 2 identical, phase 3, multicenter, randomized, double-blind, active-controlled studies in 91 sites in the United States and Canada and 109 sites in Europe, Australia, and Canada were conducted (149). Unfortunately, the clinical success of tolevamer (given as a loading dose of 9 g followed by 3 g every 8 hours) was found to be inferior to both metronidazole (375 mg every 6 hours) and vancomycin (125 mg every 6 hours). In the pooled analyses, 44.2% of 534 patients who received tolevamer, compared to 72.7% of 278 receiving metronidazole and 81% of 259 receiving vancomycin, attained clinical success. Clinical success appeared to decrease further with increasing severity of disease. Interestingly, recurrence rates were significantly higher in both the metronidazole and vancomycin groups compared to tolevamer (23% and 20.6%, respectively, compared to 4.5%), although the authors warned that this advantage may have been secondary to selection bias and the predominantly mild disease in clinical responders. The roles of pathogen clearance and perturbation of the microbiomes have been implicated to explain the outcomes of treatments in these subjects (169).

It is unclear if combination treatment with tolevamer and a *C. difficile* antibiotic may be beneficial in preventing recurrences. However, there may be issues about binding of the antibiotic, and in addition, the effect of the latter may abrogate the flora-preserving advantage of the toxin binder.

Immunoglobulin (IG)

The benefit of i.v. IG in the treatment of recurrent CDI or severe CDI has not been studied systematically. Anecdotal evidence of efficacy has been reported in few case reports and case series (170). The doses, number of times administered, and intervals between doses have been variable. A retrospective study in Pittsburgh of 18 *C. difficile*–infected subjects receiving i.v. IG pair-matched by baseline characteristics and severity of CDI with 61 subjects not receiving i.v. IG did not show any differences in all-cause mortality, colectomies, and length of stay. Inconsistencies in the effect of i.v. IG on clinical outcomes may be secondary to the unpredictable presence of antitoxin antibodies in the general population (171).

Bacteriotherapy

Perturbation of the intestinal microbiota is the critical factor for the development of CDI. Vancomycin or metronidazole treatment of asymptomatic infection has only led to recurrent and prolonged clostridial shedding (172). Consistent with these findings is the observation that the risk of recurrence in humans increases from 24% in individuals with one episode of CDI to up to 64.7% in those with prior recurrences (and, therefore, consequent CDI treatments) (159). Restoration of the disrupted intestinal microbiota by either defined organisms or an undefined microbial community has re-emerged as a strategy to break the cycle of CDI-antibiotics-CDI.

Fecal microbiota transplant

Transfer of fecal suspension from a "healthy" donor to a patient with CDI or fecal microbiota transplantation (FMT) is the most direct way of restoring the intestinal flora homeostasis. The earliest documentation of FMT use for gastrointestinal disease was reported to be in the fourth (Dong-jin dynasty) and sixth (Ming dynasty) centuries A.D. (173). FMT, mostly through rectal enema, has been used since the 1950s for PMC. Since toxigenic *C. difficile* was discovered to be the pathogen involved in PMC, succeeding reports of success were published in case reports, case series, and other observational studies in the 1980s and onward (174, 175). The overall rate of symptom resolution after FMT was around 90%, with a trend toward higher clinical resolution after lower gastrointestinal FMT route (174–176). A randomized controlled trial compared FMT using nasoduodenal tube with two control groups (177). FMT was performed after 4 to 5 days of oral vancomycin (500 mg four times daily), while control groups received the same amount of vancomycin for 14 days. In the FMT group, 81% of patients achieved resolution of symptoms at 3 months compared with 31% and 23% of the vancomycin and vancomycin plus bowel lavage control groups, respectively ($p < 0.001$ for FMT versus both control groups). The trial was prematurely terminated because of the unexpected extremely low response rates in the control groups.

Another randomized controlled trial comparing FMT via colonoscopy with oral vancomycin at 125 mg four times daily for 10 days followed by 125 to 500 mg/day every 2 to 3 days for at least 3 weeks showed similar findings. In the FMT group, 18 of 20 patients (90%) had symptom resolution compared with 5 of 19 (26%) patients in the vancomycin control ($p < 0.0001$). This study was terminated after a 1-year interim analysis. While most studies have administered fecal suspension via a nasogastric or nasoduodenal route, rectal enema, or colonoscopy, oral administration using encapsulated fecal material is emerging as an option for FMT. An open-label, single-arm study was conducted to determine the efficacy of oral, capsulized, frozen feces among 20 patients with at least three episodes of mild to moderate CDI and failure of a prolonged tapering course of vancomycin or at least two episodes of severe CDI requiring hospitalization (178). Patients received 15 capsules on 2 consecutive days and were followed for up to 6 months. Resolution of diarrhea was achieved in 70% of patients after one FMT, and after another FMT for the nonresponders, in 90% of all patients. No serious adverse events attributed to the capsule-based FMT were observed. Regardless of route of administration, FMT appears to be effective in patients who have recurrent CDI.

Although FMT has been used for decades now, there remain concerns about its efficacy for severe, complicated CDI, safety in the immunocompromised hosts, and long-term safety of transfusing undefined donor feces to a recipient. An observational study examined the efficacy and safety of FMT in elderly patients with recurrent, severe and complicated CDI (179). In this study, patients were age 65 years or older. Severe CDI was defined by albumin <3 g/dl, WBC >15,000/×l, and/or abdominal tenderness. Complicated CDI was defined by the occurrence of one or more of the following as a consequence of CDI: admission to the intensive care unit, altered mental status, hypotension, fever >38.5°C, ileus, WBC <2,000 or >30,000/×l, lactate >2.2 mmol/liter, or evidence of end-organ damage. Primary cure (resolution of CDI symptoms after initial FMT with no recurrence in the subsequent 12 weeks) in recurrent, severe, and complicated CDI was 82%, 91%, and 66%, respectively. In a small study of 17 patients, of whom 76.4% had severe and complicated CDI, primary and secondary cure rates were reported to be 88% and

94%, respectively (179). In a retrospective study of 80 immunocompromised patients (75 adult and 5 pediatric), the primary and secondary cure rates were noted to be 78% and 89%, respectively (180). The immunocompromised state was reported as HIV/AIDS (3), solid organ transplant (19), malignancy (7), immunosuppressive therapy for inflammatory bowel disease (36), and other medical conditions (15). It appears that in select patients with either severe or complicated CDI or who are immunocompromised, FMT is effective, although some patients may require repeat FMT to achieve resolution of disease.

The efficacy of FMT, as well as potential long-term effects of other components of the donor stool, have driven interest in defining the microbial community that confers protection from recurrent CDI. Investigators from Ontario, Canada, have isolated 33 species from purified bacterial cultures from a single healthy donor and administered the bacterial preparation, via colonoscopy, to two patients with recurrent CDI to "RePOOPulate" their gut (181). Both patients achieved normal bowel pattern within 2 to 3 days after the procedure and remained symptom-free at 6-month follow-up. Bacterial rRNA analyses of the recipient stools at 6 months revealed persistence of donor bacteria. Commercial products either for oral or rectal enema delivery of defined bacterial spores or microbiota suspension, respectively, are currently being tested in clinical trials.

Probiotics

Multiple small studies performed on various probiotics have been reported, and meta-analyses or systematic reviews of these studies have shown some association of probiotic use with prevention of *C. difficile*–associated diarrhea (182, 183). Two of the most common probiotic species studied in small clinical trials are *Lactobacillus acidophilus* and *Bifidobacterium* spp. In six previously published small studies (sample sizes ranged from 40 to 437) of *L. acidophilus* and/or *Bifidobacterium bifidum* containing probiotics, the relative risk ratio associated with treatment ranged from 0.21 to 0.40 (184–189). Recently, a multicenter, randomized, double-blind, placebo-controlled study tested the efficacy of a high-dose probiotic preparation containing two strains each of *L. acidophilus* and *Bifidobacterium* (*B. bifidum* and *Bifidobacterium lactis*) in patients age ≥65 years who were exposed to one or more oral or parenteral antibiotics (181, 190). One group of subjects (1,493) were randomly assigned to the treatment group, and 1,488 were assigned to the placebo group; 1,470 and 1,471, respectively, were included in the analyses of primary endpoints. Antibiotic-associated diarrhea (AAD) occurred in 10.8% of subjects in the probiotic group and 10.4% of the placebo group (p = 0.71), while CDI occurred in 0.8% and 1.2% of the probiotic and placebo groups, respectively (p = 0.35). It is unclear whether the low incidence of CDI in the European study (Wales and England) may have influenced the results, but based on this well-powered study, the lactobacilli- and bifidobacteria-containing preparations were not effective in the prevention of either AAD or CDI.

Nontoxigenic *C. difficile* (NTCD)

In hamsters, prior colonization with nontoxigenic *C. difficile* provided protection from subsequent colonization and disease with toxigenic strains (191). Following this observation in animals, two patients with relapsing CDI after treatment with metronidazole and vancomycin were reported to respond to a defined NTCD given orally in three doses (192). Indeed, NTCD has been shown to colonize asymptomatic patients in the hospital, suggesting that the presence of the bacteria may protect against development of symptomatic infection (193). Different strains of NTCD have been tested and have been shown to prevent mortality from CDI in hamsters (194, 195). Spores of one of the strains used in animal studies (VP20621/M3)

were then tested in healthy subjects (196). VP20621 was found to be well tolerated and colonized the gastrointestinal tract of subjects pretreated with vancomycin. Persistent colonization was detected in stools of 44% of the subjects on days 21 to 28. A phase 2, randomized, double-blind, placebo-controlled, dose-ranging study was conducted among 173 participants age 18 years or older (at least one-third were ≥65 years old) with a diagnosis of CDI (first episode or first recurrence) successfully treated with metronidazole, oral vancomycin, or both at 44 centers in the United States, Canada, and Europe (197). Participants received NTCD-M3 at 10^4 spores daily for 7 days, 10^7 spores daily for 7 days, 10^7 spores daily for 14 days, or placebo for 14 days. Of the participants who received treatment, 69% had stools colonized with NTCD-M3. Recurrence of CDI occurred in 30% of the placebo group and 11% of the NTCD-M3 groups combined (odds ratio, 0.28; 95% CI, 0.11 to 0.69; p = 0.006). The lowest recurrence rate was 5%, which was noted in subjects who received 10^7 spores daily for 7 days. Recurrence was 2% versus 31% in subjects who were colonized versus those who were not colonized by NTCD-M3, respectively (p < 0.001). The results of this phase 2 study suggest that colonization with NTCD reduces CDI recurrence.

Surgical Interventions

Removal of the diseased intestinal tissue (colectomy) is considered in those that have failed medical therapy or have fulminant colitis. The overall rates for colectomies remain low, but in some centers, the emergence of the epidemic strain of *C. difficile* has been associated with increased rates of colectomies for severe CDI (16, 198). In Pittsburgh, Pennsylvania, 1.1% of patients with nosocomial CDI from 1989 to 1999 and 10.3% from 2000 to 2001 underwent colectomy. Because of the condition of the patients and the degree of disease severity, the procedure is usually associated with very high mortality.

Colectomy

Indications for surgery include fulminant colitis with shock and multiorgan failure, toxic megacolon, perforation, peritonitis, and failure of medical treatment (199). Partial (segmental) or total colectomy with end ileostomy is the most common surgical procedure performed for fulminant colitis. Subtotal or total abdominal colectomy with end ileostomy is the procedure of choice because other procedures (segmental resection, defunctioning stoma, nontherapeutic laparotomy) are associated with high rates of reoperation and mortality (200). When indicated, surgery appears to be most beneficial in patients who are 65 years or older, immunocompetent, with WBC of $\geq 20 \times 10^9/$ liter and lactate level of 2.2 to 4.9 mmol/liter (199, 201). Risk factors for poor outcomes include age ≥ 75, immunosuppression, WBC of $\geq 50 \times 10^9/$liter, lactate level of ≥ 5 mmol/liter, mental status change, and delay in timing (201–203). Delayed surgical intervention has been associated with high mortality rates (33, 204), although a recent retrospective study suggested that a shorter time between diagnosis and surgery (median time 2 versus 3 days, $p = 0.009$) correlates with postsurgical mortality (205). The authors of the latter study mentioned improved medical treatment as the reason for their unexpected findings, although it is unclear whether patients who underwent early surgery were sicker than those who did not. Mortality rates from surgery for CDI were reported to range from 30 to 80% in the 1990s and 34 to 57% in the 2000s (199). Although deaths after surgery appear to be high, mortality from fulminant colitis without surgical intervention is almost 100%.

Diverting loop ileostomy with lavage

In an attempt to preserve the colon and avoid morbidity and mortality associated with aggressive surgical interventions, a minimally invasive procedure involving diverting loop ileostomy with colonic lavage has been described (206). In this procedure, an ileostomy is created, through which antegrade colonic lavage and colonic enemas with vancomycin are administered. Compared to a historical control of age-, sex-, and disease severity–matched patients who underwent colectomy, postoperative death was lower (19%) in those who had diverting ileostomy, compared to 50% of the control group ($p = 0.006$). Recurrence rates were not reported in these patients.

Vaccine

Because of the increasing incidence, morbidity, mortality, and health care cost from CDI, immunization to prevent the disease itself would be ideal. Active immunization has been successful in controlling and even eradicating some infectious diseases. Human data suggest that an adequate humoral response to *C. difficile* toxins is associated with either asymptomatic colonization or decreased recurrence (128, 207). Several vaccine candidates— toxoid-based, recombinant toxin-based peptide, DNA-based, and surface protein antigens —are in development, but most are in the preclinical stage (208). A few vaccines are in varying stages of clinical studies.

A partially purified toxoid A and B vaccine has been found to be safe and immunogenic in 30 healthy adults (209). In this study, $\geq 90\%$ of the subjects developed serum antibody responses to both toxins. In a follow-up pilot study, three patients with multiple episodes of CDI and on prolonged treatment with oral vancomycin were given the toxoid preparation intramuscularly on days 0, 7, 28, and 56 (210). Two of the three patients had increased serum IgG levels to both toxins (IgG against TcdB several-fold higher than IgG against TcdA). All three patients stopped vancomycin after the vaccination, and no recurrence was observed at 6-month follow-up. A highly purified version of the toxoid was tested in 50 healthy adults (18 to 55 years old) and

48 elderly (≥65 years old) volunteers in a phase 1 study (211). The vaccine (2 μg, 10 μg, or 50 μg) or placebo was given on days 0, 28, and 56. Seroconversion for TcdA was 100% in the younger age group, while 100% conversion was achieved only in the elderly group receiving the highest dose. Seroconversion for TcdB was lower in all groups. IgG levels remained high in the younger volunteers and was declining in the older volunteers at day 236. Two phase 2 trials recently completed testing the vaccine in middle-aged to elderly individuals at risk (NCT01230957) and subjects with first-episode CDI (NCT00772343), and a phase 3 trial is underway to evaluate the efficacy of the vaccine to prevent primary (first episode) CDI in up to 15,000 participants in 17 countries (NCT 01887912). Other vaccine candidates that have recently completed a phase 1 study include a genetically and chemically modified full-length TcdA and B (NCT01706367) and a recombinant fusion protein, IC84 (NCT01296386). No results have been published yet on these recently concluded phase 1 and 2 studies.

CONCLUSIONS

CDI continues to be a major health care problem in North America, Canada, and Europe and is now being recognized as a significant cause of morbidity in other parts of the world as well. Community-associated onset and infections in children and otherwise healthy adults are emerging, but advanced age remains a key risk factor in the acquisition of severe disease. Nonantimicrobial approaches such as use of monoclonal antibodies, nontoxigenic *C. difficile*, FMT, and less invasive surgery are novel interventions that may change management and outcomes of CDI.

CITATION

Shin JH, Chaves-Olarte E, Warren CA. 2016. *Clostridium difficile* infection. Microbiol Spectrum 4(3):EI10-0007-2015.

REFERENCES

1. **Voth DE, Ballard JD.** 2005. *Clostridium difficile* toxins: mechanism of action and role in disease. *Clin Microbiol Rev* **18**:247–263.

2. **Sun X, Savidge T, Feng H.** 2010. The enterotoxicity of *Clostridium difficile* toxins. *Toxins (Basel)* **2**:1848–1880.

3. **Alcantara C, Stenson WF, Steiner TS, Guerrant RL.** 2001. Role of inducible cyclooxygenase and prostaglandins in *Clostridium difficile* toxin A-induced secretion and inflammation in an animal model. *J Infect Dis* **184**:648–652.

4. **Alcantara CS, Jin X-H, Brito GAC, Carneiro-Filho BA, Barrett LJ, Carey RM, Guerrant RL.** 2005. Angiotensin II subtype 1 receptor blockade inhibits *Clostridium difficile* toxin A-induced intestinal secretion in a rabbit model. *J Infect Dis* **191**:2090–2096.

5. **Warren CA, Calabrese GM, Li Y, Pawlowski SW, Figler RA, Rieger J, Ernst PB, Linden J, Guerrant RL.** 2012. Effects of adenosine A_2A receptor activation and alanyl-glutamine in *Clostridium difficile* toxin-induced ileitis in rabbits and cecitis in mice. *BMC Infect Dis* **12**:13.

6. **Guerrant RL, Walker DH, Weller PF (ed).** 2011. *Tropical Infectious Diseases: Principles, Pathogens and Practice*, 3rd ed. Saunders/Elsevier, Edinburgh, Scotland.

7. **Steiner TS, Flores CA, Pizarro TT, Guerrant RL.** 1997. Fecal lactoferrin, interleukin-1beta, and interleukin-8 are elevated in patients with severe *Clostridium difficile* colitis. *Clin Diagn Lab Immunol* **4**:719–722.

8. **Schwan C, Stecher B, Tzivelekidis T, van Ham M, Rohde M, Hardt W-D, Wehland J, Aktories K.** 2009. *Clostridium difficile* toxin CDT induces formation of microtubule-based protrusions and increases adherence of bacteria. *PLoS Pathog* **5**:e1000626. doi:10.1371/journal.ppat.1000626.

9. **Lanis JM, Barua S, Ballard JD.** 2010. Variations in TcdB activity and the hypervirulence of emerging strains of *Clostridium difficile*. *PLoS Pathog* **6**:e1001061. doi:10.1371/journal.ppat.1001061.

10. **Lanis JM, Heinlen LD, James JA, Ballard JD.** 2013. *Clostridium difficile* 027/BI/NAP1 encodes a hypertoxic and antigenically variable form of TcdB. *PLoS Pathog* **9**:e1003523. doi:10.1371/journal.ppat.1003523.

11. **Chaves-Olarte E, Löw P, Freer E, Norlin T, Weidmann M, von Eichel-Streiber C, Thelestam M.** 1999. A novel cytotoxin from *Clostridium difficile* serogroup F is a functional hybrid between two other large clostridial cytotoxins. *J Biol Chem* **274**:11046–11052.

12. **Mattila E, Arkkila P, Mattila PS, Tarkka E, Tissari P, Anttila V-J.** 2013. Extraintestinal *Clostridium difficile* infections. *Clin Infect Dis* **57:**e148–e153.

13. **Wanahita A, Goldsmith EA, Marino BJ, Musher DM.** 2003. *Clostridium difficile* infection in patients with unexplained leukocytosis. *Am J Med* **115:**543–546.

14. **Mao EJ, Kelly CR, Machan JT.** 2015. Racial differences in *Clostridium difficile* infection rates are attributable to disparities in health care access. *Antimicrob Agents Chemother* **59:**6283–6287.

15. **McDonald LC, Owings M, Jernigan DB.** 2006. *Clostridium difficile* infection in patients discharged from US short-stay hospitals, 1996-2003. *Emerg Infect Dis* **12:**409–415.

16. **Muto CA, Pokrywka M, Shutt K, Mendelsohn AB, Nouri K, Posey K, Roberts T, Croyle K, Krystofiak S, Patel-Brown S, Pasculle AW, Paterson DL, Saul M, Harrison LH.** 2005. A large outbreak of *Clostridium difficile*-associated disease with an unexpected proportion of deaths and colectomies at a teaching hospital following increased fluoroquinolone use. *Infect Control Hosp Epidemiol* **26:**273–280.

17. **Zilberberg MD, Shorr AF, Kollef MH.** 2008. Increase in adult *Clostridium difficile*-related hospitalizations and case-fatality rate, United States, 2000-2005. *Emerg Infect Dis* **14:**929–931.

18. **Labbé A-C, Poirier L, Maccannell D, Louie T, Savoie M, Béliveau C, Laverdière M, Pépin J.** 2008. *Clostridium difficile* infections in a Canadian tertiary care hospital before and during a regional epidemic associated with the BI/NAP1/027 strain. *Antimicrob Agents Chemother* **52:**3180–3187.

19. **Loo VG, Poirier L, Miller MA, Oughton M, Libman MD, Michaud S, Bourgault A-M, Nguyen T, Frenette C, Kelly M, Vibien A, Brassard P, Fenn S, Dewar K, Hudson TJ, Horn R, René P, Monczak Y, Dascal A.** 2005. A predominantly clonal multi-institutional outbreak of *Clostridium difficile*-associated diarrhea with high morbidity and mortality. *N Engl J Med* **353:**2442–2449.

20. **Pépin J, Valiquette L, Alary M-E, Villemure P, Pelletier A, Forget K, Pépin K, Chouinard D.** 2004. *Clostridium difficile*-associated diarrhea in a region of Quebec from 1991 to 2003: a changing pattern of disease severity. *CMAJ* **171:**466–472.

21. **Kuijper EJ, Coignard B, Tüll P.** 2006. ESCMID Study Group for *Clostridium difficile*, EU Member States, European Centre for Disease Prevention and Control. Emergence of *Clostridium difficile*-associated disease in North America and Europe. *Clin Microbiol Infect* **12**(Suppl 6):2–18.

22. **Kuijper EJ, Barbut F, Brazier JS, Kleinkauf N, Eckmanns T, Lambert ML, Drudy D, Fitzpatrick F, Wiuff C, Brown DJ, Coia JE, Pituch H, Reichert P, Even J, Mossong J, Widmer AF, Olsen KE, Allerberger F, Notermans DW, Delmée M, Coignard B, Wilcox M, Patel B, Frei R, Nagy E, Bouza E, Marin M, Akerlund T, Virolainen-Julkunen A, Lyytikäinen O, Kotila S, Ingebretsen A, Smyth B, Rooney P, Poxton IR, Monnet DL.** 2008. Update of *Clostridium difficile* infection due to PCR ribotype 027 in Europe, 2008. *Euro Surveill* **13:**18942.

23. **McDonald LC, Killgore GE, Thompson A, Owens RC, Jr, Kazakova SV, Sambol SP, Johnson S, Gerding DN.** 2005. An epidemic, toxin gene-variant strain of *Clostridium difficile*. *N Engl J Med* **353:**2433–2441.

24. **Fernandez Canigia L, Nazar J, Arce M, Dadamio J, Smayevsky J, Bianchini H.** 2001. *Clostridium difficile* diarrhea: frequency of detection in a medical center in Buenos Aires, Argentina. *Rev Argent Microbiol* **33:**101–107. [In Spanish.]

25. **Souza Dias MB, Yamashiro J, Borrasca VL, Stempliuk VA, Araújo MRE, Costa SF, Levin AS.** 2010. Pseudo-outbreak of *Clostridium difficile* associated diarrhea (CDAD) in a tertiary-care hospital. *Rev Inst Med Trop Sao Paulo* **52:**133–137.

26. **Zumbado-Salas R, Gamboa-Coronado MM, Rodríguez-Cavallini E, Chaves-Olarte E.** 2008. *Clostridium difficile* in adult patients with nosocomial diarrhea in a Costa Rican hospital. *Am J Trop Med Hyg* **79:**164–165.

27. **Lopardo G, Morfin-Otero R, Moran-Vazquez II, Noriega F, Zambrano B, Luxemburger C, Foglia G, Rivas EE.** 2015. Epidemiology of *Clostridium difficile*: a hospital-based descriptive study in Argentina and Mexico. *Braz J Infect Dis* **19:**8–14.

28. **Spadão F, Gerhardt J, Guimarães T, Dulley F, Almeida JN, Jr, Batista MV, Shikanai-Yasuda MA, Levin AS, Costa SF.** 2014. Incidence of diarrhea by *Clostridium difficile* in hematologic patients and hematopoietic stem cell transplantation patients: risk factors for severe forms and death. *Rev Inst Med Trop Sao Paulo* **56:**325–331.

29. **Dumyati G, Stevens V, Hannett GE, Thompson AD, Long C, Maccannell D, Limbago B.** 2012. Community-associated *Clostridium difficile* infections, Monroe County, New York, USA. *Emerg Infect Dis* **18:**392–400.

30. **Khanna S, Pardi DS, Aronson SL, Kammer PP, Orenstein R, St Sauver JL, Harmsen WS, Zinsmeister AR.** 2012. The epidemiology of

community-acquired *Clostridium difficile* infection: a population-based study. *Am J Gastroenterol* **107:**89–95.

31. **Pai S, Aliyu SH, Enoch DA, Karas JA.** 2012. Five years experience of *Clostridium difficile* infection in children at a UK tertiary hospital: proposed criteria for diagnosis and management. *PLoS One* **7:**e51728. doi:10.1371/journal.pone.0051728.

32. **Sandora TJ, Fung M, Flaherty K, Helsing L, Scanlon P, Potter-Bynoe G, Gidengil CA, Lee GM.** 2011. Epidemiology and risk factors for *Clostridium difficile* infection in children. *Pediatr Infect Dis J* **30:**580–584.

33. **Sailhamer EA, Carson K, Chang Y, Zacharias N, Spaniolas K, Tabbara M, Alam HB, DeMoya MA, Velmahos GC.** 2009. Fulminant *Clostridium difficile* colitis: patterns of care and predictors of mortality. *Arch Surg* **144:**433–439; discussion 439–440.

34. **Zilberberg MD, Shorr AF, Micek ST, Doherty JA, Kollef MH.** 2009. *Clostridium difficile*-associated disease and mortality among the elderly critically ill. *Crit Care Med* **37:**2583–2589.

35. **Balassiano IT, Miranda KR, Boente RF, Pauer H, Oliveira ICM, Santos-Filho J, Amorim ELT, Caniné GA, Souza CF, Gomes MZR, Ferreira EO, Brazier JS, Domingues RMCP.** 2009. Characterization of *Clostridium difficile* strains isolated from immunosuppressed inpatients in a hospital in Rio de Janeiro, Brazil. *Anaerobe* **15:**61–64.

36. **Legaria MC, Lumelsky G, Rosetti S.** 2003. *Clostridium difficile*-associated diarrhea from a general hospital in Argentina. *Anaerobe* **9:**113–116.

37. **Pires RN, Monteiro AA, Carneiro LC, Baethgen LF, Tavares R, Lincho CS, Park S, Perlin D, Rodrigues Filho EM, Pasqualotto AC.** 2014. *Clostridium difficile* infection in Brazil: a neglected problem? *Am J Infect Control* **42:**459–460.

38. **Balassiano IT, Dos Santos-Filho J, de Oliveira MPB, Ramos MC, Japiassu AM, Dos Reis AM, Brazier JS, de Oliveira Ferreira E, Domingues RMCP.** 2010. An outbreak case of *Clostridium difficile*-associated diarrhea among elderly inpatients of an intensive care unit of a tertiary hospital in Rio de Janeiro, Brazil. *Diagn Microbiol Infect Dis* **68:**449–455.

39. **Camacho-Ortiz A, Ponce-de-León A, Sifuentes-Osornio J.** 2009. *Clostridum difficile* associated disease in Latin America. *Gac Med Mex* **145:**223–229. [In Spanish.]

40. **Quesada-Gómez C, Vargas P, López-Ureña D, Gamboa-Coronado MM, Rodríguez-Cavillini E.** 2012. Community-acquired *Clostridium difficile* NAP1/027-associated diarrhea in an eighteen month old child. *Anaerobe* **18:**581–583.

41. **Quesada-Gómez C, Mulvey MR, Vargas P, Gamboa-Coronado MM, Rodríguez C, Rodríguez-Cavillini E.** 2013. Isolation of a toxigenic and clinical genotype of *Clostridium difficile* in retail meats in Costa Rica. *J Food Prot* **76:**348–351.

42. **Silva ROS, Santos RLR, Pires PS, Pereira LC, Pereira ST, Duarte MC, de Assis RA, Lobato FCF.** 2013. Detection of toxins A/B and isolation of *Clostridium difficile* and *Clostridium perfringens* from dogs in Minas Gerais, Brazil. *Braz J Microbiol* **44:**133–137.

43. **Silva ROS, Ribeiro de Almeida L, Oliveira Junior CA, de Magalhães Soares DF, Pereira PLL, Rupnik M, Lobato FCF.** 2014. Carriage of *Clostridium difficile* in free-living South American coati (*Nasua nasua*) in Brazil. *Anaerobe* **30:**99–101.

44. **Quesada-Gómez C, Rodríguez C, Gamboa-Coronado MM, Rodríguez-Cavallini E, Du T, Mulvey MR, Villalobos-Zúñiga M, Boza-Cordero R.** 2010. Emergence of *Clostridium difficile* NAP1 in Latin America. *J Clin Microbiol* **48:**669–670.

45. **He M, Miyajima F, Roberts P, Ellison L, Pickard DJ, Martin MJ, Connor TR, Harris SR, Fairley D, Bamford KB, D'Arc S, Brazier J, Brown D, Coia JE, Douce G, Gerding D, Kim HJ, Koh TH, Kato H, Senoh M, Louie T, Michell S, Butt E, Peacock SJ, Brown NM, Riley T, Songer G, Wilcox M, Pirmohamed M, Kuijper E, Hawkey P, Wren BW, Dougan G, Parkhill J, Lawley TD.** 2013. Emergence and global spread of epidemic healthcare-associated *Clostridium difficile*. *Nat Genet* **45:**109–113.

46. **López-Ureña D, Quesada-Gómez C, Miranda E, Fonseca M, Rodríguez-Cavillini E.** 2014. Spread of epidemic *Clostridium difficile* NAP1/027 in Latin America: case reports in Panama. *J Med Microbiol* **63:**322–324.

47. **Aguayo C, Flores R, Lévesque S, Araya P, Ulloa S, Lagos J, Hormazabal JC, Tognarelli J, Ibáñez D, Pidal P, Duery O, Olivares B, Fernández J.** 2015. Rapid spread of *Clostridium difficile* NAP1/027/ST1 in Chile confirms the emergence of the epidemic strain in Latin America. *Epidemiol Infect* **143:**3069–3073.

48. **Camacho-Ortiz A, López-Barrera D, Hernández-García R, Galván-De Los Santos AM, Flores-Treviño SM, Llaca-Díaz JM, Maldonado-Garza HJ, Bosques-Padilla FJ, Garza-González E.** 2015. First report of *Clostridium difficile* NAP1/027 in a Mexican hospital.

PLoS One **10**:e0122627. doi:10.1371/journal.pone.0122627.

49. **Goorhuis A, Legaria MC, van den Berg RJ, Harmanus C, Klaassen CHW, Brazier JS, Lumelsky G, Kuijper EJ.** 2009. Application of multiple-locus variable-number tandem-repeat analysis to determine clonal spread of toxin A-negative *Clostridium difficile* in a general hospital in Buenos Aires, Argentina. *Clin Microbiol Infect* **15**:1080–1086.

50. **Quesada-Gómez C, López-Ureña D, Acuña-Amador L, Villalobos-Zúñiga M, Du T, Freire R, Guzmán-Verri C, del Mar Gamboa-Coronado M, Lawley TD, Moreno E, Mulvey MR, de Castro Brito GA, Rodríguez-Cavallini E, Rodríguez C, Chaves-Olarte E.** 2015. Emergence of an outbreak-associated *Clostridium difficile* variant with increased virulence. *J Clin Microbiol* **53**:1216–1226.

51. **Kim H, Jeong SH, Roh KH, Hong SG, Kim JW, Shin M-G, Kim M-N, Shin HB, Uh Y, Lee H, Lee K.** 2010. Investigation of toxin gene diversity, molecular epidemiology, and antimicrobial resistance of *Clostridium difficile* isolated from 12 hospitals in South Korea. *Korean J Lab Med* **30**:491–497.

52. **Honda H, Yamazaki A, Sato Y, Dubberke ER.** 2014. Incidence and mortality associated with *Clostridium difficile* infection at a Japanese tertiary care center. *Anaerobe* **25**:5–10.

53. **Kato H, Kato N, Watanabe K, Yamamoto T, Suzuki K, Ishigo S, Kunihiro S, Nakamura I, Killgore GE, Nakamura S.** 2001. Analysis of *Clostridium difficile* isolates from nosocomial outbreaks at three hospitals in diverse areas of Japan. *J Clin Microbiol* **39**:1391–1395.

54. **Sawabe E, Kato H, Osawa K, Chida T, Tojo N, Arakawa Y, Okamura N.** 2007. Molecular analysis of *Clostridium difficile* at a university teaching hospital in Japan: a shift in the predominant type over a five-year period. *Eur J Clin Microbiol Infect Dis* **26**:695–703.

55. **Collins DA, Hawkey PM, Riley TV.** 2013. Epidemiology of *Clostridium difficile* infection in Asia. *Antimicrob Resist Infect Control* **2**:21.

56. **Kim YS, Han DS, Kim YH, Kim WH, Kim JS, Kim HS, Kim HS, Park YS, Song HJ, Shin SJ, Yang SK, Ye BD, Eun CS, Lee KM, Lee SH, Jang BI, Jung SA, Cheon JH, Choi CH, Huh KC.** 2013. Incidence and clinical features of *Clostridium difficile* infection in Korea: a nationwide study. *Epidemiol Infect* **141**:189–194.

57. **Shin B-M, Kuak EY, Yoo HM, Kim EC, Lee K, Kang J-O, Whang DH, Shin J-H.** 2008. Multicentre study of the prevalence of toxigenic *Clostridium difficile* in Korea: results of a retrospective study 2000-2005. *J Med Microbiol* **57**:697–701.

58. **Shin B-M, Kuak EY, Yoo SJ, Shin WC, Yoo HM.** 2008. Emerging toxin A-B+ variant strain of *Clostridium difficile* responsible for pseudomembranous colitis at a tertiary care hospital in Korea. *Diagn Microbiol Infect Dis* **60**:333–337.

59. **Kim J, Kang JO, Pai H, Choi TY.** 2012. Association between PCR ribotypes and antimicrobial susceptibility among *Clostridium difficile* isolates from healthcare-associated infections in South Korea. *Int J Antimicrob Agents* **40**:24–29.

60. **Hawkey PM, Marriott C, Liu WE, Jian ZJ, Gao Q, Ling TKW, Chow V, So E, Chan R, Hardy K, Xu L, Manzoor S.** 2013. Molecular epidemiology of *Clostridium difficile* infection in a major Chinese hospital: an under-recognized problem in Asia? *J Clin Microbiol* **51**:3308–3313.

61. **Galaydick J, Xu Y, Sun L, Landon E, Weber SG, Sun D, Zhou J, Sherer R.** 2015. Seek and you shall find: prevalence of *Clostridium difficile* in Wuhan, China. *Am J Infect Control* **43**:301–302.

62. **Chung C-H, Wu C-J, Lee H-C, Yan J-J, Chang C-M, Lee N-Y, Chen P-L, Lee C-C, Hung Y-P, Ko W-C.** 2010. *Clostridium difficile* infection at a medical center in southern Taiwan: incidence, clinical features and prognosis. *J Microbiol Immunol Infect* **43**:119–125.

63. **Lai C-C, Lin S-H, Tan C-K, Liao C-H, Huang Y-T, Hsueh P-R.** 2014. Clinical manifestations of *Clostridium difficile* infection in a medical center in Taiwan. *J Microbiol Immunol Infect* **47**:491–496.

64. **Chia J-H, Lai H-C, Su L-H, Kuo A-J, Wu T-L.** 2013. Molecular epidemiology of *Clostridium difficile* at a medical center in Taiwan: persistence of genetically clustering of A$^-$B$^+$ isolates and increase of A$^+$B$^+$ isolates. *PLoS One* **8**:e75471. doi:10.1371/journal.pone.0075471.

65. **Hung Y-P, Cia C-T, Tsai B-Y, Chen P-C, Lin H-J, Liu H-C, Lee J-C, Wu Y-H, Tsai P-J, Ko W-C.** 2015. The first case of severe *Clostridium difficile* ribotype 027 infection in Taiwan. *J Infect* **70**:98–101.

66. **Lai M-J, Chiueh T-S, Huang Z-Y, Lin J-C.** 2015. The first *Clostridium difficile* ribotype 027 strain isolated in Taiwan. *J Formos Med Assoc Taiwan* **115**:210–212.

67. **Liao T-L, Lin C-F, Chiou C-S, Shen G-H, Wang J.** 2015. *Clostridium difficile* PCR ribotype 027 emerges in Taiwan. *Jpn J Infect Dis* **68**:338–340.

68. **Cheng VCC, Yam WC, Lam OTC, Tsang JLY, Tse EYF, Siu GKH, Chan JFW, Tse H, To**

KKW, Tai JWM, Ho PL, Yuen KY. 2011. *Clostridium difficile* isolates with increased sporulation: emergence of PCR ribotype 002 in Hong Kong. *Eur J Clin Microbiol Infect Dis* **30:**1371–1381.

69. Cheng VCC, Yam WC, Chan JFW, To KKW, Ho PL, Yuen KY. 2009. *Clostridium difficile* ribotype 027 arrives in Hong Kong. *Int J Antimicrob Agents* **34:**492–493.

70. Warren CA, Labio E, Destura R, Sevilleja JE, Jamias JD, Daez MLO. 2012. *Clostridium difficile* and *Entamoeba histolytica* infections in patients with colitis in the Philippines. *Trans R Soc Trop Med Hyg* **106:**424–428.

71. Hassan SA, Othman N, Idris FM, Abdul Rahman Z, Maning N, Abdul Rahman R, Tiong CG. 2012. Prevalence of *Clostridium difficile* toxin in diarhoeal stool samples of patients from a tertiary hospital in North Eastern Penisular Malaysia. *Med J Malaysia* **67:**402–405.

72. Oyofo BA, Subekti D, Tjaniadi P, Machpud N, Komalarini S, Setiawan B, Simanjuntak C, Punjabi N, Corwin AL, Wasfy M, Campbell JR, Lesmana M. 2002. Enteropathogens associated with acute diarrhea in community and hospital patients in Jakarta, Indonesia. *FEMS Immunol Med Microbiol* **34:**139–146.

73. Rupnik M, Kato N, Grabnar M, Kato H. 2003. New types of toxin A-negative, toxin B-positive strains among *Clostridium difficile* isolates from Asia. *J Clin Microbiol* **41:**1118–1125.

74. Thamlikitkul V, Danpakdi K, Chokloikaew S. 1996. Incidence of diarrhea and *Clostridium difficile* toxin in stools from hospitalized patients receiving clindamycin, beta-lactams, or nonantibiotic medications. *J Clin Gastroenterol* **22:**161–163.

75. Wongwanich S, Ramsiri S, Vanasin B, Khowsaphit P, Tantipatayangkul P, Phanurai R. 1990. *Clostridium difficile* associated disease in Thailand. *Southeast Asian J Trop Med Public Health* **21:**367–372.

76. Putsathit P, Kiratisin P, Ngamwongsatit P, Riley TV. 2015. *Clostridium difficile* infection in Thailand. *Int J Antimicrob Agents* **45:**1–7.

77. Kumarasinghe G, Lim YS, Chow C, Bassett DC. 1992. Prevalence of bacterial agents of diarrhoeal disease at the National University Hospital, Singapore and their resistance to antimicrobial agents. *Trop Geogr Med* **44:**229–232.

78. Koh TH, Tan AL, Tan ML, Wang G, Song KP. 2007. Epidemiology of *Clostridium difficile* infection in a large teaching hospital in Singapore. *Pathology* **39:**438–442.

79. Hsu L-Y, Tan TY, Koh TH, Kwa AL, Krishnan P, Tee NW, Jureen R. 2011. Decline in *Clostridium difficile*-associated disease rates in Singapore public hospitals, 2006 to 2008. *BMC Res Notes* **4:**77.

80. Lim PL, Ling ML, Lee HY, Koh TH, Tan AL, Kuijper EJ, Goh SS, Low BS, Ang LP, Harmanus C, Lin RT, Krishnan P, James L, Lee CE. 2011. Isolation of the first three cases of *Clostridium difficile* polymerase chain reaction ribotype 027 in Singapore. *Singapore Med J* **52:**361–364.

81. Ayyagari A, Sharma P, Venkateswarlu, Mehta S, Agarwal KC. 1986. Prevalence of *Clostridium difficile* in pseudomembranous and antibiotic-associated colitis in north India. *J Diarrhoeal Dis Res* **4:**157–160.

82. Dhawan B, Chaudhry R, Sharma N. 1999. Incidence of *Clostridium difficile* infection: a prospective study in an Indian hospital. *J Hosp Infect* **43:**275–280.

83. Joshy L, Chaudhry R, Dhawan B. 2009. Detection and characterization of *Clostridium difficile* from patients with antibiotic-associated diarrhoea in a tertiary care hospital in North India. *J Med Microbiol* **58:**1657–1659.

84. Niyogi SK, Bhattacharya SK, Dutta P, Naik TN, De SP, Sen D, Saha MR, Datta D, Nair GB, Mitra U, Rasaily R, and Chandra Pal S. 1991. Prevalence of *Clostridium difficile* in hospitalised patients with acute diarrhoea in Calcutta. *J Diarrhoeal Dis Res* **9:**16–19.

85. Ingle M, Deshmukh A, Desai D, Abraham P, Joshi A, Rodrigues C, Mankeshwar R. 2011. Prevalence and clinical course of *Clostridium difficile* infection in a tertiary-care hospital: a retrospective analysis. *Indian J Gastroenterol* **30:**89–93.

86. Albert MJ, Faruque AS, Faruque SM, Sack RB, Mahalanabis D. 1999. Case-control study of enteropathogens associated with childhood diarrhea in Dhaka, Bangladesh. *J Clin Microbiol* **37:**3458–3464.

87. Thomas C, Stevenson M, Williamson DJ, Riley TV. 2002. *Clostridium difficile*-associated diarrhea: epidemiological data from Western Australia associated with a modified antibiotic policy. *Clin Infect Dis* **35:**1457–1462.

88. Ferguson JK, Cheng AC, Gilbert GL, Gottlieb T, Korman T, McGregor A, Richards M, Roberts S, Robson J, Van Gessel H, Riley TV. 2011. *Clostridium difficile* laboratory testing in Australia and New Zealand: national survey results and Australasian Society for Infectious Diseases recommendations for best practice. *Pathology* **43:**482–487.

89. Slimings C, Armstrong P, Beckingham WD, Bull AL, Hall L, Kennedy KJ, Marquess J, McCann R, Menzies A, Mitchell BG, Richards MJ, Smollen PC, Tracey L, Wilkinson IJ,

Wilson FL, Worth LJ, Riley TV. 2014. Increasing incidence of *Clostridium difficile* infection, Australia, 2011-2012. *Med J Aust* **200:**272–276.

90. Furuya-Kanamori L, Robson J, Soares Magalhães RJ, Yakob L, McKenzie SJ, Paterson DL, Riley TV, Clements ACA. 2014. A population-based spatio-temporal analysis of *Clostridium difficile* infection in Queensland, Australia over a 10-year period. *J Infect* **69:**447–455.

91. Jackson T, Nghiem HS, Rowell D, Jorm C, Wakefield J. 2011. Marginal costs of hospital-acquired conditions: information for priority-setting for patient safety programmes and research. *J Health Serv Res Policy* **16:**141–146.

92. Foster NF, Collins DA, Ditchburn SL, Duncan CN, van Schalkwyk JW, Golledge CL, Keed ABR, Riley TV. 2014. Epidemiology of *Clostridium difficile* infection in two tertiary-care hospitals in Perth, Western Australia: a cross-sectional study. *New Microbes New Infect* **2:**64–71.

93. Cheknis AK, Sambol SP, Davidson DM, Nagaro KJ, Mancini MC, Hidalgo-Arroyo GA, Brazier JS, Johnson S, Gerding DN. 2009. Distribution of *Clostridium difficile* strains from a North American, European and Australian trial of treatment for *C. difficile* infections: 2005-2007. *Anaerobe* **15:**230–233.

94. Wilson R, Beerbaum P, Giglio S. 2015. Community and hospital acquired *Clostridium difficile* in South Australia: ribotyping of isolates and a comparison of laboratory detection methods. *Lett Appl Microbiol* **60:**33–36.

95. Knight DR, Giglio S, Huntington PG, Korman TM, Kotsanas D, Moore CV, Paterson DL, Prendergast L, Huber CA, Robson J, Waring L, Wehrhahn MC, Weldhagen GF, Wilson RM, Riley TV. 2015. Surveillance for antimicrobial resistance in Australian isolates of *Clostridium difficile*, 2013-14. *J Antimicrob Chemother* **70:**2992–2999.

96. Huber CA, Hall L, Foster NF, Gray M, Allen M, Richardson LJ, Robson J, Vohra R, Schlebusch S, George N, Nimmo GR, Riley TV, Paterson DL. 2014. Surveillance snapshot of *Clostridium difficile* infection in hospitals across Queensland detects binary toxin producing ribotype UK 244. *Commun Dis Intell Q Rep* **38:**E279–E284.

97. Lim SK, Stuart RL, Mackin KE, Carter GP, Kotsanas D, Francis MJ, Easton M, Dimovski K, Elliott B, Riley TV, Hogg G, Paul E, Korman TM, Seemann T, Stinear TP, Lyras D, Jenkin GA. 2014. Emergence of a ribotype 244 strain of *Clostridium difficile* associated with severe disease and related to the epidemic ribotype 027 strain. *Clin Infect Dis* **58:**1723–1730.

98. Eyre DW, Tracey L, Elliott B, Slimings C, Huntington PG, Stuart RL, Korman TM, Kotsiou G, McCann R, Griffiths D, Fawley WN, Armstrong P, Dingle KE, Walker AS, Peto TE, Crook DW, Wilcox MH, Riley TV. 2015. Emergence and spread of predominantly community-onset *Clostridium difficile* PCR ribotype 244 infection in Australia, 2010 to 2012. *Euro Surveill* **20:**21059. http://www.eurosurveillance.org/ViewArticle.aspx?ArticleId=21059.

99. Elliott B, Squire MM, Thean S, Chang BJ, Brazier JS, Rupnik M, Riley TV. 2011. New types of toxin A-negative, toxin B-positive strains among clinical isolates of *Clostridium difficile* in Australia. *J Med Microbiol* **60:**1108–1111.

100. Riley TV, Thean S, Hool G, Golledge CL. 2009. First Australian isolation of epidemic *Clostridium difficile* PCR ribotype 027. *Med J Aust* **190:**706–708.

101. Richards M, Knox J, Elliott B, Mackin K, Lyras D, Waring LJ, Riley TV. 2011. Severe infection with *Clostridium difficile* PCR ribotype 027 acquired in Melbourne, Australia. *Med J Aust* **194:**369–371.

102. Bull AL, Worth LJ, Richards MJ. 2012. Implementation of standardised surveillance for *Clostridium difficile* infections in Australia: initial report from the Victorian Healthcare Associated Infection Surveillance System. *Intern Med J* **42:**715–718.

103. Samie A, Obi CL, Franasiak J, Archbald-Pannone L, Bessong PO, Alcantara-Warren C, Guerrant RL. 2008. PCR detection of *Clostridium difficile* triose phosphate isomerase (tpi), toxin A (tcdA), toxin B (tcdB), binary toxin (cdtA, cdtB), and tcdC genes in Vhembe District, South Africa. *Am J Trop Med Hyg* **78:**577–585.

104. Lekalakala MR, Lewis E, Hoosen AA. 2010. *Clostridium difficile* infections in a tertiary hospital: value of surveillance. *J Hosp Infect* **75:**328–329.

105. Kullin B, Meggersee R, D'Alton J, Galvao B, Rajabally N, Whitelaw A, Bamford C, Reid SJ, Abratt VR. 2015. Prevalence of gastrointestinal pathogenic bacteria in patients with diarrhoea attending Groote Schuur Hospital, Cape Town, South Africa. *S Afr Med J* **105:**121–125.

106. Mwachari C, Batchelor BI, Paul J, Waiyaki PG, Gilks CF. 1998. Chronic diarrhoea among HIV-infected adult patients in Nairobi, Kenya. *J Infect* **37:**48–53.

107. Zulu I, Kelly P, Mwansa J, Veitch A, Farthing MJ. 2000. Contrasting incidence of *Clostridium difficile* and other enteropathogens in AIDS

patients in London and Lusaka. *Trans R Soc Trop Med Hyg* **94:**167–168.

108. **Onwueme K, Fadairo Y, Idoko L, Onuh J, Alao O, Agaba P, Lawson L, Ukomadu C, Idoko J.** 2011. High prevalence of toxinogenic *Clostridium difficile* in Nigerian adult HIV patients. *Trans R Soc Trop Med Hyg* **105:**667–669.

109. **Simango C, Uladi S.** 2014. Detection of *Clostridium difficile* diarrhoea in Harare, Zimbabwe. *Trans R Soc Trop Med Hyg* **108:**354–357.

110. **Tedesco FJ, Barton RW, Alpers DH.** 1974. Clindamycin-associated colitis. A prospective study. *Ann Intern Med* **81:**429–433.

111. **Deshpande A, Pasupuleti V, Thota P, Pant C, Rolston DDK, Sferra TJ, Hernandez AV, Donskey CJ.** 2013. Community-associated *Clostridium difficile* infection and antibiotics: a meta-analysis. *J Antimicrob Chemother* **68:**1951–1961.

112. **Pakyz AL, Moczygemba LR, Wang H, Stevens MP, Edmond MB.** 2015. An evaluation of the association between an antimicrobial stewardship score and antimicrobial usage. *J Antimicrob Chemother* **70:**1588–1591.

113. **Slimings C, Riley TV.** 2014. Antibiotics and hospital-acquired *Clostridium difficile* infection: update of systematic review and meta-analysis. *J Antimicrob Chemother* **69:**881–891.

114. **Zacharioudakis IM, Zervou FN, Pliakos EE, Ziakas PD, Mylonakis E.** 2015. Colonization with toxinogenic *C. difficile* upon hospital admission, and risk of infection: a systematic review and meta-analysis. *Am J Gastroenterol* **110:**381–390, quiz 391.

115. **Clabots CR, Johnson S, Olson MM, Peterson LR, Gerding DN.** 1992. Acquisition of *Clostridium difficile* by hospitalized patients: evidence for colonized new admissions as a source of infection. *J Infect Dis* **166:**561–567.

116. **Curry SR, Muto CA, Schlackman JL, Pasculle AW, Shutt KA, Marsh JW, Harrison LH.** 2013. Use of multilocus variable number of tandem repeats analysis genotyping to determine the role of asymptomatic carriers in *Clostridium difficile* transmission. *Clin Infect Dis* **57:**1094–1102.

117. **Eyre DW, Cule ML, Wilson DJ, Griffiths D, Vaughan A, O'Connor L, Ip CLC, Golubchik T, Batty EM, Finney JM, Wyllie DH, Didelot X, Piazza P, Bowden R, Dingle KE, Harding RM, Crook DW, Wilcox MH, Peto TEA, Walker AS.** 2013. Diverse sources of *C. difficile* infection identified on whole-genome sequencing. *N Engl J Med* **369:**1195–1205.

118. **Kim K-H, Fekety R, Batts DH, Brown D, Cudmore M, Silva J Jr, Waters D.** 1981. Isolation of *Clostridium difficile* from the environment and contacts of patients with antibiotic-associated colitis. *J Infect Dis* **143:**42–50.

119. **McFarland LV, Mulligan ME, Kwok RY, Stamm WE.** 1989. Nosocomial acquisition of *Clostridium difficile* infection. *N Engl J Med* **320:**204–210.

120. **Dubberke ER, Reske KA, Noble-Wang J, Thompson A, Killgore G, Mayfield J, Camins B, Woeltje K, McDonald JR, McDonald LC, Fraser VJ.** 2007. Prevalence of *Clostridium difficile* environmental contamination and strain variability in multiple health care facilities. *Am J Infect Control* **35:**315–318.

121. **Bobulsky GS, Al-Nassir WN, Riggs MM, Sethi AK, Donskey CJ.** 2008. *Clostridium difficile* skin contamination in patients with *C. difficile*-associated disease. *Clin Infect Dis* **46:**447–450.

122. **Lucado J, Gould C, Elixhauser A.** 2012. *Clostridium difficile* infections (CDI) in hospital stays, 2009. Statistical brief 124. Healthcare Cost and Utilization Project (HCUP) Statistical Briefs [Internet]. Agency for Health Care Policy and Research, Rockville, MD. http://www.ncbi.nlm.nih.gov/books/NBK92613/.

123. **Miller M, Gravel D, Mulvey M, Taylor G, Boyd D, Simor A, Gardam M, McGeer A, Hutchinson J, Moore D, Kelly S.** 2010. Health care-associated *Clostridium difficile* infection in Canada: patient age and infecting strain type are highly predictive of severe outcome and mortality. *Clin Infect Dis* **50:**194–201.

124. **Pépin J, Valiquette L, Cossette B.** 2005. Mortality attributable to nosocomial *Clostridium difficile*-associated disease during an epidemic caused by a hypervirulent strain in Quebec. *CMAJ* **173:**1037–1042.

125. **Miniño AM, Murphy SL, Xu J, Kochanek KD.** 2011. Deaths: final data for 2008. *Natl Vital Stat Rep* **59:**1–126.

126. **Lessa FC, Mu Y, Bamberg WM, Beldavs ZG, Dumyati GK, Dunn JR, Farley MM, Holzbauer SM, Meek JI, Phipps EC, Wilson LE, Winston LG, Cohen JA, Limbago BM, Fridkin SK, Gerding DN, McDonald LC.** 2015. Burden of *Clostridium difficile* infection in the United States. *N Engl J Med* **372:**825–834.

127. **Henrich TJ, Krakower D, Bitton A, Yokoe DS.** 2009. Clinical risk factors for severe *Clostridium difficile*-associated disease. *Emerg Infect Dis* **15:**415–422.

128. **Kyne L, Warny M, Qamar A, Kelly CP.** 2001. Association between antibody response to toxin A and protection against recurrent *Clostridium difficile* diarrhoea. *Lancet* **357:**189–193.

129. **Pepin J, Alary M-E, Valiquette L, Raiche E, Ruel J, Fulop K, Godin D, Bourassa C.** 2005. Increasing risk of relapse after treatment of

Clostridium difficile colitis in Quebec, Canada. *Clin Infect Dis* **40:**1591–1597.

130. **Kyne L, Merry C, O'Connell B, Kelly A, Keane C, O'Neill D.** 1999. Factors associated with prolonged symptoms and severe disease due to *Clostridium difficile*. *Age Ageing* **28:**107–113.

131. **Cohen SH, Gerding DN, Johnson S, Kelly CP, Loo VG, McDonald LC, Pepin J, Wilcox MH, Society for Healthcare Epidemiology of America, Infectious Diseases Society of America.** 2010. Clinical practice guidelines for *Clostridium difficile* infection in adults: 2010 update by the Society for Healthcare Epidemiology of America (SHEA) and the Infectious Diseases Society of America (IDSA). *Infect Control Hosp Epidemiol* **31:**431–455.

132. **Kelly CP, Pothoulakis C, LaMont JT.** 1994. *Clostridium difficile* colitis. *N Engl J Med* **330:**257–262.

133. **Freiler JF, Durning SJ, Ender PT.** 2001. *Clostridium difficile* small bowel enteritis occurring after total colectomy. *Clin Infect Dis.* **33:**1429–1431.

134. **Cheng AC, Ferguson JK, Richards MJ, Robson JM, Gilbert GL, McGregor A, Roberts S, Korman TM, Riley TV, Australasian Society for Infections Diseases.** 2011. Australasian Society for Infectious Diseases guidelines for the diagnosis and treatment of *Clostridium difficile* infection. *Med J Aust* **194:**353–358.

135. **Debast SB, Bauer MP, Kuijper EJ, European Society of Clinical Microbiology and Infectious Diseases.** 2014. European Society of Clinical Microbiology and Infectious Diseases: update of the treatment guidance document for *Clostridium difficile* infection. *Clin Microbiol Infect* **20**(Suppl 2)**:**1–26.

136. **Surawicz CM, Brandt LJ, Binion DG, Ananthakrishnan AN, Curry SR, Gilligan PH, McFarland LV, Mellow M, Zuckerbraun BS.** 2013. Guidelines for diagnosis, treatment, and prevention of *Clostridium difficile* infections. *Am J Gastroenterol* **108:**478–498, quiz 499.

137. **Feuerstadt P, Das R, Brandt LJ.** 2014. The evolution of urban *C. difficile* infection (CDI): CDI in 2009-2011 is less severe and has better outcomes than CDI in 2006-2008. *Am J Gastroenterol* **109:**1265–1276.

138. **Karas JA, Enoch DA, Aliyu SH.** 2010. A review of mortality due to *Clostridium difficile* infection. *J Infect* **61:**1–8.

139. **Hu MY, Katchar K, Kyne L, Maroo S, Tummala S, Dreisbach V, Xu H, Leffler DA, Kelly CP.** 2009. Prospective derivation and validation of a clinical prediction rule for recurrent *Clostridium difficile* infection. *Gastroenterology* **136:**1206–1214.

140. **Planche T, Wilcox MH.** 2015. Diagnostic pitfalls in *Clostridium difficile* infection. *Infect Dis Clin North Am* **29:**63–82.

141. **Gerding DN, Olson MM, Peterson LR, Teasley DG, Gebhard RL, Schwartz ML, Lee JT, Jr.** 1986. *Clostridium difficile*-associated diarrhea and colitis in adults. A prospective case-controlled epidemiologic study. *Arch Intern Med* **146:**95–100.

142. **Planche TD, Davies KA, Coen PG, Finney JM, Monahan IM, Morris KA, O'Connor L, Oakley SJ, Pope CF, Wren MW, Shetty NP, Crook DW, Wilcox MH.** 2013. Differences in outcome according to *Clostridium difficile* testing method: a prospective multicentre diagnostic validation study of *C difficile* infection. *Lancet Infect Dis* **13:**936–945.

143. **Berrington A, Settle CD.** 2007. Which specimens should be tested for *Clostridium difficile* toxin? *J Hosp Infect* **65:**280–282.

144. **Kundrapu S, Sunkesula VCK, Jury LA, Sethi AK, Donskey CJ.** 2012. Utility of perirectal swab specimens for diagnosis of *Clostridium difficile* infection. *Clin Infect Dis* **55:**1527–1530.

145. **Gerding DN, Johnson S, Peterson LR, Mulligan ME, Silva J, Jr.** 1995. *Clostridium difficile*-associated diarrhea and colitis. *Infect Control Hosp Epidemiol* **16:**459–477.

146. **Am J Health Syst Pharm.** 1998. ASHP therapeutic position statement on the preferential use of metronidazole for the treatment of *Clostridium difficile*-associated disease. *Am J Health Syst Pharm* **55:**1407–1411.

147. **Musher DM, Aslam S, Logan N, Nallacheru S, Bhaila I, Borchert F, Hamill RJ.** 2005. Relatively poor outcome after treatment of *Clostridium difficile* colitis with metronidazole. *Clin Infect Dis* **40:**1586–1590.

148. **Zar FA, Bakkanagari SR, Moorthi KMLST, Davis MB.** 2007. A comparison of vancomycin and metronidazole for the treatment of *Clostridium difficile*-associated diarrhea, stratified by disease severity. *Clin Infect Dis* **45:**302–307.

149. **Johnson S, Louie TJ, Gerding DN, Cornely OA, Chasan-Taber S, Fitts D, Gelone SP, Broom C, Davidson DM, Polymer Alternative for CDI Treatment (PACT) investigators.** 2014. Vancomycin, metronidazole, or tolevamer for *Clostridium difficile* infection: results from two multinational, randomized, controlled trials. *Clin Infect Dis* **59:**345–354.

150. **Rokas KEE, Johnson JW, Beardsley JR, Ohl CA, Luther VP, Williamson JC.** 2015. The addition of intravenous metronidazole to oral vancomycin is associated with improved mortality in critically ill patients with *Clostridium difficile* infection. *Clin Infect Dis* **61:**934–941.

151. **Wenisch JM, Schmid D, Kuo H-W, Allerberger F, Michl V, Tesik P, Tucek G, Laferl H, Wenisch C.** 2012. Prospective observational study comparing three different treatment regimes in patients with *Clostridium difficile* infection. *Antimicrob Agents Chemother* **56:**1974–1978.

152. **Keighley MR, Burdon DW, Arabi Y, Williams JA, Thompson H, Youngs D, Johnson M, Bentley S, George RH, Mogg GA.** 1978. Randomised controlled trial of vancomycin for pseudomembranous colitis and postoperative diarrhoea. *BMJ* **2:**1667–1669.

153. **Fekety R, Silva J, Kauffman C, Buggy B, Deery HG.** 1989. Treatment of antibiotic-associated *Clostridium difficile* colitis with oral vancomycin: comparison of two dosage regimens. *Am J Med* **86:**15–19.

154. **Gonzales M, Pepin J, Frost EH, Carrier JC, Sirard S, Fortier L-C, Valiquette L.** 2010. Faecal pharmacokinetics of orally administered vancomycin in patients with suspected *Clostridium difficile* infection. *BMC Infect Dis* **10:**363.

155. **Teasley DG, Gerding DN, Olson MM, Peterson LR, Gebhard RL, Schwartz MJ, Lee JT, Jr.** 1983. Prospective randomised trial of metronidazole versus vancomycin for *Clostridium-difficile*-associated diarrhoea and colitis. *Lancet* **2:**1043–1046.

156. **Gerding DN.** 1997. Is there a relationship between vancomycin-resistant enterococcal infection and *Clostridium difficile* infection? *Clin Infect Dis* **25**(Suppl 2):S206–S210.

157. **Apisarnthanarak A, Razavi B, Mundy LM.** 2002. Adjunctive intracolonic vancomycin for severe *Clostridium difficile* colitis: case series and review of the literature. *Clin Infect Dis* **35:**690–696.

158. **Kim PK, Huh HC, Cohen HW, Feinberg EJ, Ahmad S, Coyle C, Teperman S, Boothe H.** 2013. Intracolonic vancomycin for severe *Clostridium difficile* colitis. *Surg Infect (Larchmt)* **14:**532–539.

159. **McFarland LV, Elmer GW, Surawicz CM.** 2002. Breaking the cycle: treatment strategies for 163 cases of recurrent *Clostridium difficile* disease. *Am J Gastroenterol* **97:**1769–1775.

160. **Louie TJ, Miller MA, Mullane KM, Weiss K, Lentnek A, Golan Y, Gorbach S, Sears P, Shue Y-K, OPT-80-003 Clinical Study Group.** 2011. Fidaxomicin versus vancomycin for *Clostridium difficile* infection. *N Engl J Med* **364:**422–431.

161. **Cornely OA, Crook DW, Esposito R, Poirier A, Somero MS, Weiss K, Sears P, Gorbach S, OPT-80-004 Clinical Study Group.** 2012. Fidaxomicin versus vancomycin for infection with *Clostridium difficile* in Europe, Canada, and the USA: a double-blind, non-inferiority, randomised controlled trial. *Lancet Infect Dis* **12:**281–289.

162. **Louie TJ, Cannon K, Byrne B, Emery J, Ward L, Eyben M, Krulicki W.** 2012. Fidaxomicin preserves the intestinal microbiome during and after treatment of *Clostridium difficile* infection (CDI) and reduces both toxin reexpression and recurrence of CDI. *Clin Infect Dis* **55**(Suppl 2):S132–S142.

163. **Eyre DW, Babakhani F, Griffiths D, Seddon J, Del Ojo Elias C, Gorbach SL, Peto TEA, Crook DW, Walker AS.** 2014. Whole-genome sequencing demonstrates that fidaxomicin is superior to vancomycin for preventing reinfection and relapse of infection with *Clostridium difficile*. *J Infect Dis* **209:**1446–1451.

164. **Petrella LA, Sambol SP, Cheknis A, Nagaro K, Kean Y, Sears PS, Babakhani F, Johnson S, Gerding DN.** 2012. Decreased cure and increased recurrence rates for *Clostridium difficile* infection caused by the epidemic *C. difficile* BI strain. *Clin Infect Dis* **55:**351–357.

165. **Warren CA, van Opstal EJ, Riggins MS, Li Y, Moore JH, Kolling GL, Guerrant RL, Hoffman PS.** 2013. Vancomycin treatment's association with delayed intestinal tissue injury, clostridial overgrowth, and recurrence of *Clostridium difficile* infection in mice. *Antimicrob Agents Chemother* **57:**689–696.

166. **Lowy I, Molrine DC, Leav BA, Blair BM, Baxter R, Gerding DN, Nichol G, Thomas WD, Jr, Leney M, Sloan S, Hay CA, Ambrosino DM.** 2010. Treatment with monoclonal antibodies against *Clostridium difficile* toxins. *N Engl J Med* **362:**197–205.

167. **Hinkson PL, Dinardo C, DeCiero D, Klinger JD, Barker RH, Jr.** 2008. Tolevamer, an anionic polymer, neutralizes toxins produced by the BI/027 strains of *Clostridium difficile*. *Antimicrob Agents Chemother* **52:**2190–2195.

168. **Louie TJ, Peppe J, Watt CK, Johnson D, Mohammed R, Dow G, Weiss K, Simon S, John JF, Jr, Garber G, Chasan-Taber S, Davidson DM, Tolevamer Study Investigator Group.** 2006. Tolevamer, a novel nonantibiotic polymer, compared with vancomycin in the treatment of mild to moderately severe *Clostridium difficile*-associated diarrhea. *Clin Infect Dis* **43:**411–420.

169. **Louie TJ, Byrne B, Emery J, Ward L, Krulicki W, Nguyen D, Wu K, Cannon K.** 2015. Differences of the fecal microflora with *Clostridium difficile* therapies. *Clin Infect Dis* **60**(Suppl 2):S91–S97.

170. **Abougergi MS, Kwon JH.** 2011. Intravenous immunoglobulin for the treatment of *Clostridium difficile* infection: a review. *Dig Dis Sci* **56:**19–26.

171. Viscidi R, Laughon BE, Yolken R, Bo-Linn P, Moench T, Ryder RW, Bartlett JG. 1983. Serum antibody response to toxins A and B of *Clostridium difficile*. *J Infect Dis* 148:93–100.

172. Johnson S, Homann SR, Bettin KM, Quick JN, Clabots CR, Peterson LR, Gerding DN. 1992. Treatment of asymptomatic *Clostridium difficile* carriers (fecal excretors) with vancomycin or metronidazole. A randomized, placebo-controlled trial. *Ann Intern Med* 117:297–302.

173. Zhang F, Luo W, Shi Y, Fan Z, Ji G. 2012. Should we standardize the 1,700-year-old fecal microbiota transplantation? *Am J Gastroenterol.* 107:1755.

174. Gough E, Shaikh H, Manges AR. 2011. Systematic review of intestinal microbiota transplantation (fecal bacteriotherapy) for recurrent *Clostridium difficile* infection. *Clin Infect Dis* 53:994–1002.

175. Kassam Z, Lee CH, Yuan Y, Hunt RH. 2013. Fecal microbiota transplantation for *Clostridium difficile* infection: systematic review and meta-analysis. *Am J Gastroenterol* 108:500–508.

176. Youngster I, Sauk J, Pindar C, Wilson RG, Kaplan JL, Smith MB, Alm EJ, Gevers D, Russell GH, Hohmann EL. 2014. Fecal microbiota transplant for relapsing *Clostridium difficile* infection using a frozen inoculum from unrelated donors: a randomized, open-label, controlled pilot study. *Clin Infect Dis* 58:1515–1522.

177. van Nood E, Vrieze A, Nieuwdorp M, Fuentes S, Zoetendal EG, de Vos WM, Visser CE, Kuijper EJ, Bartelsman JFWM, Tijssen JGP, Speelman P, Dijkgraaf MGW, Keller JJ. 2013. Duodenal infusion of donor feces for recurrent *Clostridium difficile*. *N Engl J Med* 368:407–415.

178. Youngster I, Russell GH, Pindar C, Ziv-Baran T, Sauk J, Hohmann EL. 2014. Oral, capsulized, frozen fecal microbiota transplantation for relapsing *Clostridium difficile* infection. *JAMA* 312:1772–1778.

179. Agrawal M, Aroniadis OC, Brandt LJ, Kelly C, Freeman S, Surawicz C, Broussard E, Stollman N, Giovanelli A, Smith B, Yen E, Trivedi A, Hubble L, Kao D, Borody T, Finlayson S, Ray A, Smith R. 2015. The long-term efficacy and safety of fecal microbiota transplant for recurrent, severe, and complicated *Clostridium difficile* infection in 146 elderly individuals. *J Clin Gastroenterol.* [Epub ahead of print.]

180. Kelly CR, Ihunnah C, Fischer M, Khoruts A, Surawicz C, Afzali A, Aroniadis O, Barto A, Borody T, Giovanelli A, Gordon S, Gluck M, Hohmann EL, Kao D, Kao JY, McQuillen DP, Mellow M, Rank KM, Rao K, Ray A, Schwartz MA, Singh N, Stollman N, Suskind DL, Vindigni SM, Youngster I, Brandt L. 2014. Fecal microbiota transplant for treatment of *Clostridium difficile* infection in immunocompromised patients. *Am J Gastroenterol* 109:1065–1071.

181. Petrof EO, Gloor GB, Vanner SJ, Weese SJ, Carter D, Daigneault MC, Brown EM, Schroeter K, Allen-Vercoe E. 2013. Stool substitute transplant therapy for the eradication of *Clostridium difficile* infection: 'RePOOPulating' the gut. *Microbiome* 1:3.

182. Johnston BC, Ma SSY, Goldenberg JZ, Thorlund K, Vandvik PO, Loeb M, Guyatt GH. 2012. Probiotics for the prevention of *Clostridium difficile*-associated diarrhea: a systematic review and meta-analysis. *Ann Intern Med* 157:878–888.

183. Goldenberg JZ, Ma SSY, Saxton JD, Martzen MR, Vandvik PO, Thorlund K, Guyatt GH, Johnston BC. 2013. Probiotics for the prevention of *Clostridium difficile*-associated diarrhea in adults and children. *Cochrane Database Syst Rev* 5:CD006095.

184. Beausoleil M, Fortier N, Guénette S, L'ecuyer A, Savoie M, Franco M, Lachaine J, Weiss K. 2007. Effect of a fermented milk combining *Lactobacillus acidophilus* Cl1285 and *Lactobacillus casei* in the prevention of antibiotic-associated diarrhea: a randomized, double-blind, placebo-controlled trial. *Can J Gastroenterol* 21:732–736.

185. Gao XW, Mubasher M, Fang CY, Reifer C, Miller LE. 2010. Dose-response efficacy of a proprietary probiotic formula of *Lactobacillus acidophilus* CL1285 and *Lactobacillus casei* LBC80R for antibiotic-associated diarrhea and *Clostridium difficile*-associated diarrhea prophylaxis in adult patients. *Am J Gastroenterol* 105:1636–1641.

186. Plummer S, Weaver MA, Harris JC, Dee P, Hunter J. 2004. *Clostridium difficile* pilot study: effects of probiotic supplementation on the incidence of *C. difficile* diarrhoea. *Int Microbiol* 7:59–62.

187. Sampalis J, Psaradellis E, Rampakakis E. 2010. Efficacy of BIO K+ CL1285 in the reduction of antibiotic-associated diarrhea: a placebo controlled double-blind randomized, multi-center study. *Arch Med Sci* 6:56–64.

188. Safdar N, Barigala R, Said A, McKinley L. 2008. Feasibility and tolerability of probiotics for prevention of antibiotic-associated diarrhoea in hospitalized US military veterans. *J Clin Pharm Ther* 33:663–668.

189. Wenus C, Goll R, Loken EB, Biong AS, Halvorsen DS, Florholmen J. 2008. Prevention of antibiotic-associated diarrhoea by a fermented probiotic milk drink. *Eur J Clin Nutr* 62:299–301.

190. **Allen SJ, Wareham K, Wang D, Bradley C, Hutchings H, Harris W, Dhar A, Brown H, Foden A, Gravenor MB, Mack D.** 2013. Lactobacilli and bifidobacteria in the prevention of antibiotic-associated diarrhoea and *Clostridium difficile* diarrhoea in older inpatients (PLACIDE): a randomised, double-blind, placebo-controlled, multicentre trial. *Lancet* **382:**1249–1257.

191. **Borriello SP, Barclay FE.** 1985. Protection of hamsters against *Clostridium difficile* ileocaecitis by prior colonisation with non-pathogenic strains. *J Med Microbiol* **19:**339–350.

192. **Seal D, Borriello SP, Barclay F, Welch A, Piper M, Bonnycastle M.** 1987. Treatment of relapsing *Clostridium difficile* diarrhoea by administration of a non-toxigenic strain. *Eur J Clin Microbiol* **6:**51–53.

193. **Shim JK, Johnson S, Samore MH, Bliss DZ, Gerding DN.** 1998. Primary symptomless colonisation by *Clostridium difficile* and decreased risk of subsequent diarrhoea. *Lancet* **351:**633–636.

194. **Sambol SP, Merrigan MM, Tang JK, Johnson S, Gerding DN.** 2002. Colonization for the prevention of *Clostridium difficile* disease in hamsters. *J Infect Dis* **186:**1781–1789.

195. **Merrigan MM, Sambol SP, Johnson S, Gerding DN.** 2003. Prevention of fatal *Clostridium difficile*-associated disease during continuous administration of clindamycin in hamsters. *J Infect Dis* **188:**1922–1927.

196. **Villano SA, Seiberling M, Tatarowicz W, Monnot-Chase E, Gerding DN.** 2012. Evaluation of an oral suspension of VP20621, spores of nontoxigenic *Clostridium difficile* strain M3, in healthy subjects. *Antimicrob Agents Chemother* **56:**5224–5229.

197. **Gerding DN, Meyer T, Lee C, Cohen SH, Murthy UK, Poirier A, Van Schooneveld TC, Pardi DS, Ramos A, Barron MA, Chen H, Villano S.** 2015. Administration of spores of nontoxigenic *Clostridium difficile* strain M3 for prevention of recurrent *C. difficile* infection: a randomized clinical trial. *JAMA* **313:**1719–1727.

198. **Kasper AM, Nyazee HA, Yokoe DS, Mayer J, Mangino JE, Khan YM, Hota B, Fraser VJ, Dubberke ER, Centers for Disease Control and Prevention Epicenters Program.** 2012. A multicenter study of *Clostridium difficile* infection-related colectomy, 2000–2006. *Infect Control Hosp Epidemiol* **33:**470–476.

199. **Jaber MR, Olafsson S, Fung WL, Reeves ME.** 2008. Clinical review of the management of fulminant clostridium difficile infection. *Am J Gastroenterol* **103:**3195–3203, quiz 3204.

200. **Bhangu A, Nepogodiev D, Gupta A, Torrance A, Singh P, West Midlands Research Collab-** orative. 2012. Systematic review and meta-analysis of outcomes following emergency surgery for *Clostridium difficile* colitis. *Br J Surg* **99:**1501–1513.

201. **Lamontagne F, Labbé A-C, Haeck O, Lesur O, Lalancette M, Patino C, Leblanc M, Laverdière M, Pépin J.** 2007. Impact of emergency colectomy on survival of patients with fulminant *Clostridium difficile* colitis during an epidemic caused by a hypervirulent strain. *Ann Surg* **245:**267–272.

202. **Dallal RM, Harbrecht BG, Boujoukas AJ, Sirio CA, Farkas LM, Lee KK, Simmons RL.** 2002. Fulminant *Clostridium difficile*: an underappreciated and increasing cause of death and complications. *Ann Surg* **235:**363–372.

203. **Byrn JC, Maun DC, Gingold DS, Baril DT, Ozao JJ, Divino CM.** 2008. Predictors of mortality after colectomy for fulminant *Clostridium difficile* colitis. *Arch Surg* **143:**150–154.

204. **Synnott K, Mealy K, Merry C, Kyne L, Keane C, Quill R.** 1998. Timing of surgery for fulminating pseudomembranous colitis. *Br J Surg* **85:**229–231.

205. **Clanton J, Fawley R, Haller N, Daley T, Porter J, Paranjape C, Bonilla H.** 2014. Patience is a virtue: an argument for delayed surgical intervention in fulminant *Clostridium difficile* colitis. *Am Surg* **80:**614–619.

206. **Neal MD, Alverdy JC, Hall DE, Simmons RL, Zuckerbraun BS.** 2011. Diverting loop ileostomy and colonic lavage: an alternative to total abdominal colectomy for the treatment of severe, complicated *Clostridium difficile* associated disease. *Ann Surg* **254:**423–427, discussion 427–429.

207. **Kyne L, Warny M, Qamar A, Kelly CP.** 2000. Asymptomatic carriage of *Clostridium difficile* and serum levels of IgG antibody against toxin A. *N Engl J Med* **342:**390–397.

208. **Leuzzi R, Adamo R, Scarselli M.** 2014. Vaccines against *Clostridium difficile*. *Hum Vaccin Immunother* **10:**1466–1477.

209. **Kotloff KL, Wasserman SS, Losonsky GA, Thomas W, Jr, Nichols R, Edelman R, Bridwell M, Monath TP.** 2001. Safety and immunogenicity of increasing doses of a *Clostridium difficile* toxoid vaccine administered to healthy adults. *Infect Immun* **69:**988–995.

210. **Sougioultzis S, Kyne L, Drudy D, Keates S, Maroo S, Pothoulakis C, Giannasca PJ, Lee CK, Warny M, Monath TP, Kelly CP.** 2005. *Clostridium difficile* toxoid vaccine in recurrent *C. difficile*-associated diarrhea. *Gastroenterology* **128:**764–770.

211. **Greenberg RN, Marbury TC, Foglia G, Warny M.** 2012. Phase I dose finding studies

of an adjuvanted *Clostridium difficile* toxoid vaccine. *Vaccine* **30:**2245–2249.

212. **Loo VG, Bourgault A-M, Poirier L, Lamothe F, Michaud S, Turgeon N, Toye B, Beaudoin A, Frost EH, Gilca R, Brassard P, Dendukuri N, Béliveau C, Oughton M, Brukner I, Dascal A.** 2011. Host and pathogen factors for *Clostridium difficile* infection and colonization. *N Engl J Med* **365:**1693–1703.

213. **Bliss DZ, Johnson S, Savik K, Clabots CR, Willard K, Gerding DN.** 1998. Acquisition of *Clostridium difficile* and *Clostridium difficile*-associated diarrhea in hospitalized patients receiving tube feeding. *Ann Intern Med* **129:** 1012–1019.

214. **Bishara J, Farah R, Mograbi J, Khalaila W, Abu-Elheja O, Mahamid M, Nseir W.** 2013. Obesity as a risk factor for *Clostridium difficile* infection. *Clin Infect Dis* **57:**489–493.

215. **Wilcox M, Gerding D, Poxton I, Kelly C, Nathan R, Cornely O, Rahav G, Lee C, Eves K, Pedley A, Tipping R, Guris D, Kartsonis N, Dorr MB.** 2015. Bezlotoxumab alone and with actoxumab for prevention of recurrent *Clostridium difficile* infection in patients on standard of care antibiotics: Integrated results of two Phase 3 studies (MODIFY I and MODIFY II). International Conference on Antimicrobial Agents and Chemotherapy. San Diego, CA.

16

Emerging Tick-Borne Bacterial Pathogens

TAHAR KERNIF,[1,2] HAMZA LEULMI,[1,3] DIDIER RAOULT,[1] and
PHILIPPE PAROLA[1]

INTRODUCTION

Ticks are obligate hematophagous arthropods that are considered to be the second most common vectors of pathogens after the mosquitoes that cause diseases in humans (1). Two families of ticks are capable of transmitting a broad range of pathogens (2): *Ixodidae* (hard ticks) currently comprise over 700 species worldwide (3), and *Argasidae* (soft ticks) comprise roughly 200 species (4). A vast number of novel tick-related microorganisms and tick-borne disease agents have been identified in the past 20 years, and more are being described due to several factors, from the curiosity of clinicians faced with unusual clinical syndromes to new tools used by microbiologists and entomologists (5). Borrelioses, ehrlichioses, anaplasmosis, and tick-borne rickettsial diseases are some of the emerging diseases that have been described throughout the world in recent years. In certain cases, the microorganism has been identified from ticks before its causal relationship with a disease is established; examples of new pathogens associated with human infections

[1]Aix Marseille Université, Unité de Recherche sur les Maladies Infectieuses Transmissibles et Emergentes (URMITE), UM63, CNRS 7278, IRD 198, Inserm 1095, Faculté de Médecine, 13385 Marseille cedex 5, France; [2]Institut Pasteur d'Algérie, Algiers, Algeria; [3]Ecole Nationale Supérieure Vétérinaire d'Alger, El Aliya Alger, Algérie.

Emerging Infections 10
Edited by W. Michael Scheld, James M. Hughes and Richard J. Whitley
© 2016 American Society for Microbiology, Washington, DC
doi:10.1128/microbiolspec.EI10-0012-2016

TABLE 1 Tick-borne spotted fever group *Rickettsiae* agents of human diseases and new data published in the last 2 years

Rickettsia species or strain	Year of first microbiological documentation of human cases[a]	Comments (including related diseases)	Geographical distribution	New data published (2013–2015)
Rickettsia aeschlimannii	2002	Spotted fever	Sub-Saharan Africa	
		Spotted fever	Europe	Infection in a man from Greece (23)
		No human cases, identified in ticks in Kazakhstan and Israel	Asia	
		Detected in humans in Tunisia and Algeria and in ticks in Algeria, Morocco, Tunisia, and Egypt	North Africa	
Rickettsia africae	1992	African tick-bite fever	Sub-Saharan Africa	
		Imported from Africa to the West Indies during early 1800s; currently established in Guadeloupe, St. Kitts, Nevis, Dominica, U.S. Virgin Islands, Montserrat, St. Lucia, Martinique, and Antigua; causes eschar-associated illness, with clinical cases reported from Guadeloupe	North and Central America	
		African tick bite fever	Pacific islands	
		No human cases reported from Asia; identified in ticks in Turkey	Asia	
		No human cases; detected in dromedary ticks in sub-Saharan Algeria and Egypt	North Africa	
Rickettsia australis	1946	Queensland tick typhus	Australia	
Rickettsia strain Atlantic rainforest or Bahia	2010	Genetically related to *Rickettsia parkeri*, *R. africae*, and *Rickettsia sibirica*. Two nonfatal cases reported in Brazil; symptoms include rash, eschar, and lymphadenopathy	South America	Named *R. parkeri*–like agent and reported in ticks from Colombia (44) and Argentina (45)
Rickettsia conorii caspia	1991	Astrakhan fever	Europe	
		Astrakhan fever	Sub-Saharan Africa	
R. conorii conorii	1932	Mediterranean spotted fever	Europe	
		Mediterranean spotted fever Human cases reported and detected in brown ticks in all of North Africa	North Africa	New genotype isolated in a skin biopsy from Tunisia (33)
		Mediterranean spotted fever	Sub-Saharan Africa	
		Asiatic part of Turkey	Asia	
R. conorii indica	2001	Indian tick typhus	Europe, Asia	
R. conorii israelensis	1971	Israeli tick typhus	Europe, Asia	
			North Africa	

Species	Year		Distribution	Notes
		Israeli tick-bite fever Two cases of Israeli spotted fever from Sfax city confirmed by detection of rickettsia in skin biopsy specimens		New genotype isolated in human from Tunisia (33)
Rickettsia heilongjiangensis	1992	Far-Eastern spotted fever in Russia, China, Korea, and Japan	Asia	
Rickettsia helvetica	1999	Serologically-only confirmed cases in Laos and Thailand; in *Ixodes* ticks in Japan and Turkey	Asia	
			Europe	
		No human cases; detected in *Ixodes* spp. in Algeria and Morocco	North Africa	
Rickettsia honei	1992	Flinders Island spotted fever	Asia, Australia, and Pacific	
		Spotted fever identical to Flinders Island spotted fever in Australia	Asia	
R. honei strain "marmionii"	2003	Australian spotted fever	Australia	
Rickettsia japonica	1985	Japanese spotted fever in Japan and Korea	Asia	
"*Rickettsia kellyi*"		A single case reported from India, several amplicons from patients are referenced in GenBank	Asia	
Rickettsia massiliae	2005	Recognized pathogen in other countries and detected in brown dog ticks in Arizona and California; no confirmed human cases in United States	North and Central America	
		One case reported in a patient in Spain, recently arrived from Argentina; also reported infecting *Rickettsia sanguineus* in Argentina	South America	
		Spotted fever	Europe	An imported case in Greece (20)
		Spotted fever	Sub-Saharan Africa	
		Identified in ticks in Israel	Asia	
		No human cases detected in *Rhipicephalus* spp. in Morocco, Algeria, and Tunisia	North Africa	
Rickettsia monacensis	2007	Spotted fever (first clinical description 2007)	Europe	
		Found only in ticks in Turkey		
		No human cases; identified in *Ixodes* spp. in Tunisia, Algeria, and Morocco	North Africa	
R. parkeri	2004	Southeastern United States; causes a mild, eschar-associated rickettsiosis; despite the occurrence of *Amblyomma maculatum* in Central America, no confirmed cases have been reported from that region	North and Central America	

(Continued on next page)

TABLE 1 Tick-borne spotted fever group *Rickettsiae* agents of human diseases and new data published in the last 2 years (*Continued*)

Rickettsia species or strain	Year of first microbiological documentation of human cases[a]	Comments (including related diseases)	Geographical distribution	New data published (2013–2015)
		Causes spotted fever in Uruguay and Argentina; symptoms include rash, eschar, and lymphadenopathy; no fatal cases reported; also reported infecting ticks in Brazil and Bolivia	South America	
			Europe	Confirmed case in Spain in a traveler from Uruguay (28)
"*Rickettsia philipii*" (364D)	2008	California; causes a relatively mild, eschar-associated illness; only a few recognized cases	North and Central America	
Rickettsia raoultii	2006 Named in 2008	SENLAT: scalp eschar and neck lymphadenopathy (old TIBOLA/DEBONEL)	Europe	
		Identified in *Dermacentor* spp. ticks in North Asia; in *Haemaphysalis* and *Amblyomma* ticks in South Asia	Asia	Two human cases in China (25)
		No human cases; identified in *Dermacentor* spp. in Morocco	North Africa	
Rickettsia rickettsii	1906	Causes Rocky Mountain spotted fever, the most severe rickettsiosis in the world; occurs sporadically and infrequently in ticks throughout Canada, the United States, Mexico, Costa Rica, and Panama	North and Central America	Fatal Rocky Mountain spotted fever case with coinfection by *Streptococcus pyogenes* (32)
		Also causes Brazilian spotted fever; reported in Argentina, Brazil, and Colombia; current case fatality 20–40%	South America	The phylogeography of various genotypes of *R. rickettsii*, associated with fatal RMSF from six countries exists independently of the distribution of a particular tick vector (136)
R. sibirica mongolitimonae	1996	Lymphangitis-associated rickettsiosis	Europe	Two additional cases reported in France (22, 30) and in two immunocompetent adults from Spain (29); coinfection with *R. conorii* in a human patient from Spain (31)
		Lymphangitis-associated rickettsiosis	Sub-Saharan Africa	
		A type strain isolated in China; no cases from Asia are reported; identified in Israel.	Asia	
		One human case	North Africa	

R. sibirica sibirica	1946	Siberian tick typhus in Russia, China, and Mongolia	Asia	**One case with subspecies *sibirica* BJ-90 in China** (24)
Rickettsia slovaca	1997	SENLAT (TIBOLA/DEBONEL)	Europe	One human case in Portugal (21) and another in Greece (26)
		No human cases in Asia; identified in Russia and China SENLAT (TIBOLA DEBONEL) No human cases; detected in *Dermacentor* ticks from Algeria and Morocco	Asia North Africa	
Rickettsia tamurae	2011	A case was reported from Japan and Laos	Asia	
Candidatus Rickettsia tarasevichiae	2013		Asia	Genome sequenced by Sentausa (137) Human cases in China with different symptoms: fever, asthenia, anorexia, nausea, headache, eschar, and lymphadenopathy (36)

*a*Documentation by one and/or several techniques: culture, molecular tools, animal or human inoculation, serology

include *Candidatus* Neoehrlichia mikurensis (*C. N. mikurensis*), *Borrelia miyamotoi*, and some *Rickettsia* species (6–8). In contrast, other emerging tick-borne diseases such as ehrlichiosis are caused by "*Ehrlichia muris–like*," or EML, agents, with cases being identified first and the correlation with tick bites being recognized later (9). In this chapter, we focus on the bacterial agents and diseases that have been recognized in the past three years and refer to major recent reviews of other recognized infections, diagnosis, and treatment aspects.

EMERGING TICK-BORNE RICKETTSIOSES

Tick-borne rickettsioses are caused by obligate intracellular bacteria belonging to the spotted fever group (SFG) of the genus *Rickettsia*, the most significant genus within the family *Rickettsiaceae* and order *Rickettsiales*. Clinical signs may include fever and a rash that can be maculopapular (such as in most cases of Rocky Mountain spotted fever [RMSF], Mediterranean spotted fever, and many other SFG rickettsioses), vesicular (such as in many cases of African tick bite fever), purpuric in severe cases, or absent. The typical inoculation eschar at the tick bite site is a hallmark of many SFG rickettsioses but may be absent, as in RMSF. These diseases can be mild, severe, or even fatal. A major review of tick-borne rickettsioses and tick-borne-associated rickettsias recognized throughout the world was published in 2013 (Table 1) (6). Here, we describe recent publications since then and present some more rickettsias that have been associated with human infections since that time.

Recent Reports on Tick-Borne Rickettsioses

Tick-borne rickettsioses are presented in Table 1 and include older diseases such as RMSF, caused by *Rickettsia rickettsii*, and Mediterranean spotted fever, caused by

Rickettsia conorii, as well as more recently described diseases. Among these, cases of African tick bite fever continue to be regularly reported in travelers, and its agent, *Rickettsia africae*, continues to be detected in many areas in ticks from sub-Saharan Africa (10–17) as well as Israel (18, 19). Also, new data and new human cases of tick-borne rickettsioses have been recently reported, including infections caused by *R. rickettsii*, *Rickettsia sibirica sibirica*, the agent of Siberian tick typhus, and emerging infections caused by *Rickettsia aeschlimannii*, *Rickettsia massiliae*, *Rickettsia parkeri*, *Rickettsia raoultii*, *R. sibirica mongolitimonae*, and *Rickettsia slovaca* (20–30). Also, a coinfection with *R. sibirica mongolitimonae* and *R. conorii* was reported in a human patient from Spain (31). A case of coinfection caused by *R. rickettsii* and *Streptococcus pyogenes* has been reported as a fatal case of RMSF (32). New *Rickettsia* spotted fever strain genotypes, *R. conorii* subsp. *conorii*, and *R. conorii* subsp. *israelensis*, were found in humans and ticks from Tunisia (33).

Candidatus Rickettsia tarasevichiae

Between 2003 and 2005, a novel rickettsial agent, *C.* Rickettsia tarasevichiae, was reported in *Ixodes persulcatus* ticks collected in various regions of Russia, including the southern Urals and Siberia (34, 35). This bacterium was identified as an emerging pathogen causing human infection 10 years later (36). Human cases of *C.* Rickettsia tarasevichiae were reported in northeastern China when the DNA of this pathogen was magnified from the blood and eschars of patients. All five patients had a recent tick bite, and they were hospitalized with different symptoms: fever, asthenia, anorexia, nausea, headache, eschar, and lymphadenopathy. One patient died after a coma, renal dysfunction, and respiratory acidosis (36). *C.* Rickettsia tarasevichiae is spread across a wide region, from Estonia to Japan, but it demonstrates a high rate of sequence homology between sequences of the partial citrate synthase *gltA* and outer membrane protein *ompA* genes from different regions (37). Although several authors incriminated *I. persulcatus* as the main vector for a new *Rickettsia* species, *C.* Rickettsia tarasevichiae, it will be interesting to investigate if this *Rickettsia* species could infect the sympatric tick species such as *Ixodes ricinus* (37, 38).

Rickettsia sp. Atlantic Rainforest Strain or Bahia Strain

In 2009 and 2010, two cases characterized by mild fever, inoculation eschar, and lymphadenopathy and very similar to the disease caused by *R. parkeri* were reported in São Paulo and Bahia, Brazil respectively (39). Both cases were confirmed to be caused by a new rickettsial agent and a recognized SFG rickettsia, Atlantic rainforest strain or Bahia strain, very closely related to *R. parkeri*, *R. africae*, and *R. sibirica* (6). In 2010, the *Amblyomma ovale* ticks collected in Atlantic rainforests in the state of São Paulo, Brazil, were the presumed vectors transmitting the Atlantic rainforest strain to humans (40). Subsequently, in the state of Santa Catarina in southern Brazil, *Amblyomma aureolatum* and *Rhipicephalus sanguineus* ticks collected from domestic and wild animals were also found to be infected by this novel bacterial strain (41). Recently, an epidemiological study was performed around the index case in an Atlantic rainforest reserve in the Peruibe municipality of southeastern Brazil. This survey revealed that *A. ovale* was the most abundant tick species, with a 12.9% infection rate by the Atlantic rainforest strain, and incriminated *A. ovale* as the main vector for this strain (42). In contrast, secondary epidemiological evidence found that the spotted fever in the state of Santa Catarina, Brazil, was caused by *Rickettsia* sp. Atlantic rainforest strain and transmitted to humans by either *A. ovale* or *A. aureolatum* (43). Subsequently, this *Rickettsia* strain was identified and isolated in *A. ovale* ticks in the Antioquia and Córdoba provinces of Colombia, the first report of this *Rickettsia* sp. outside Brazil (44). More recently, one study revealed the presence of rickettsial DNA of the pathogenic *Rickettsia* sp. Atlantic rainforest strain in *Amblyomma dubitatum* ticks from northeastern Argentina (45). It is possible that the occurrence of SFG rickettsia caused by the Atlantic rainforest strain (*R. parkeri*–like agent) is much broader than currently thought.

EHRLICHIOSES, ANAPLASMOSIS, AND NEOEHRLICHIOSIS

Members of the rickettsial family, *Anaplasmataceae*, are intracellular alpha-1 proteobacteria that multiply within membrane-bound vacuoles in the cytoplasm of eukaryotic cells (46). According to the current classification, the family *Anaplasmataceae* comprises the genera *Anaplasma*, *Ehrlichia*, *Aegyptianella*, *Neorickettsia*, and *Wolbachia*, as well as two candidate genera, "*Candidatus* Neoehrlichia" and "*Candidatus* Xenohaliotis" (47–50).

Most cases of human tick-borne ehrlichioses and anaplasmosis are caused by *Ehrlichia chaffeensis* and *A. phagocytophilum* (51–54), and with a smaller impact, by *Ehrlichia ewingii* (50, 55, 56). Others species of *Anaplasma* or *Ehrlichia*, including veterinary pathogens, have been suspected to cause human diseases, including *Ehrlichia canis* (57, 58), *Ehrlichia ruminantium* (59, 60), *Anaplasma ovis* (61, 62), *Anaplasma platys* (63–66), and the "Panola Mountain *Ehrlichia*" (67). In the United States, two passive surveillance systems have reported many cases of undetermined human ehrlichiosis and anaplasmosis because evidence to the species level was unavailable (53). These undetermined agents might already be causing human disease in the United States and elsewhere. Three agents have emerged in the past few years: EML (9, 68), *A. capra* (69), and *C. N. mikurensis* (49, 70).

EML "Wisconsin"

In 2009, an unnamed *Ehrlichia* species was detected among four patients in Minnesota and Wisconsin (9) presenting with fever, fatigue, and headache. In the same study, DNA from this organism was also detected in at least 17 of 697 *Ixodes scapularis* ticks collected by dragging a fabric flag across vegetation at or near the residences of patients in Wisconsin and Minnesota (9). Genetic analyses revealed that this new *Ehrlichia* species is closely related to *E. muris*, which is considered to be a murine pathogenic agent found in different ticks of the *I. persulcatus* complex extending from Eastern Europe to Japan (50, 71–73). Exact taxonomic placement of this organism cannot yet be determined, but it can be referred to as an EML agent (68, 74). Between 2007 and 2013, blood samples from 69 patients tested by PCR were positive for the *groEL* gene for the EML pathogen. Those patients came from five states: Indiana (1), Michigan (1), Minnesota (33), North Dakota (3), and Wisconsin (31). However, all patients were exposed to ticks in Minnesota or Wisconsin. Clinical presentation is similar to human anaplasmosis and human monocytic ehrlichiosis, and the most common symptoms are fever, malaise, thrombocytopenia, and lymphopenia (68). More recently, one study was performed on blood from small mammals and white-tailed deer in the same area where EML agents in humans and ticks were previously reported. DNA of the EML agent was detected in two *Peromyscus leucopus* mice, the same animal that is a carrier for *A. phagocytophilum* in this region (74).

A. capra

Li and colleagues have detected a new species of *Anaplasma* when monitoring *Anaplasma* species infections among goats (*Capra aegagrus hircus*) from northern China from 2012 to 2013. In 2015, they sought this new species in patients with a history of tick bites and who lived in areas where it had been identified in ticks and goats. To their surprise, this new *Anaplasma* species was identified in 28 patients and has been provisionally named "*Anaplasma capra*" (69). This new pathogenic *Anaplasma* species has different morphological characteristics from other *Anaplasma* species such as *A. phagocytophilum*, including difficulties in detection in peripheral blood smears. The *A. capra* DNA was amplified and sequenced, and 27 patients had serological evidence of infection. All patients developed different clinical manifestations, including fever, headache, malaise, dizziness, myalgia, and chills. Other symptoms were observed including rash or eschar, lymphadenopathy, gastrointestinal symptoms, and stiff neck. In addition, *A. capra* was also identified in *I. persulcatus* ticks collected at the same time as the patient samples from the region in which the infected patients lived. Finally, one patient had neurological complications, suggesting that *A. capra* could pose a substantial threat to public health.

C. N. mikurensis

The history of the discovery of *C. N. mikurensis* started in the late 1990s when the initially named *Ehrlichia*-like species belonging to the family *Anaplasmataceae* was described in *Ixodes ovatus* in Japan (48). Later, *C. N. mikurensis* was detected in engorged *I. ricinus* ticks collected from roe deer in The Netherlands, and it was then named after Corrie Schot as the "Schottivariant" (75). Similar DNA sequences were detected in *I. ricinus* and *I. persulcatus* ticks from Baltic countries (76). The bacteria detected in *Rattus norvegicus* rats in China was named *Ehrlichia* sp. "Rattus strain" (77). The first information on the ultrastructure of this organism as well as its phylogenetic analysis became available in 2004 when the sequencing of the agent in laboratory rats led to its description as the new species *C. N. mikurensis* (48). Further findings of the

microorganism in *I. ricinus* were reported from other European countries (78–83). *C. N. mikurensis* was also isolated from *Ixodes frontalis* ticks which fed on one migratory bird (84).

The first evidence of *C. N. mikurensis* pathogenicity for humans was identified in the blood samples of febrile patients in various European countries and China (8, 85–89). It has also been found in one dog in Germany (90). Infection with *C. N. mikurensis* results mainly in fever, headache, and malaise. Most patients described in Europe suffered from autoimmune disorders, unlike the patients in China, who were immunocompetent (49, 91, 92). However, the first asymptomatic cases in immunocompetent humans were reported in Europe (93). Several studies have identified the DNA of *C. N. mikurensis* in questing or host-attached *I. ricinus* in Europe (94–98). *C. N. mikurensis* has been detected in 6 rodent species in Europe and 10 in Asia (49) and in the first nonrodent host, the northern white-breasted hedgehog (*Erinaceus roumanicus*) (99). This finding raised the question of the role of animals other than rodents in the ecology of *C. N. mikurensis*.

EMERGING TICK-BORNE BORRELIOSES

The genus *Borrelia* is a group consisting of helical-shaped, motile bacteria within the phylum *Spirochetes*, which are known agents of two groups of human diseases: Lyme disease (100) and relapsing fever (100, 101). Recent advances in molecular and biotechnological methods have significantly increased the number of *Borrelia* species and also those associated with ticks (5). Lyme disease is caused by members of the *Borrelia burgdorferi sensu lato* complex transmitted by *Ixodes* ticks in North America and Eurasia (102). In addition to *B. burgdorferi sensu stricto*, *B. burgdorferi*, *Borrelia afzelii*, *Borrelia garinii*, *Borrelia valaisiana*, *Borrelia spielmanii*, and *Borrelia bissettii* have been recently associated with Lyme disease (103). The relapsing fever group comprises diverse zoonotic agents transmitted through the bite of soft ticks of the genus *Ornithodoros*, which are responsible for recurrent fevers associated with spirochetemia (104). Recently, new relapsing fever, tick-borne borrelias were discovered, namely *B. miyamotoi* (105), along with several new uncultured borrelia such as *Candidatus* Borrelia algerica (106), unrecognized *Borrelia* spp. *Amblyomma* and *Rhipicephalus* ticks in Ethiopia (107), an "uncultured *Borrelia merionesi*" in Morocco (108), and an unnamed new species in *Ornithodoro porcinus* ticks in Tanzania (109).

B. miyamotoi

Recently, several relapsing fever *Borrelia* spp. have been found to be hosted by hard ticks (101). These include *Borrelia lonestari*, a possible cause of southern tick-associated rash illness (110), which is transmitted by *Amblyomma americanum* (111); *Borrelia theileri*, the agent of bovine borreliosis, transmitted by *Boophilus microplus* and *Rhipicephalus geigyi* in Mali (112); and *B. miyamotoi*. Interestingly, *B. miyamotoi* has been associated with *Ixodes* ticks, such as agents of Lyme borreliosis and human granulocytic anaplasmosis (113, 114). The rate of *B. miyamotoi* infection in *Ixodes* ticks (*I. persulcatus*, *I. scapularis*, *Ixodes pacificus*, *Ixodes dentatus*, and *I. ricinus*) in Europe, Asia, and North America ranges between 0.5 and 5% (105, 114–117). Knowledge about the geographic distribution of *B. miyamotoi* is fragmentary, but it is likely to be similar to that of Lyme disease (118). After its first discovery in Japan in 1995 (105), *B. miyamotoi* was detected in the United States (114, 119) and Canada (120). In Europe, the first report of *B. miyamotoi*–like *Borrelia* in *I. ricinus* was in Sweden (115). Subsequently, *B. miyamotoi* (or *B. miyamotoi*–like *Borrelia* or relapsing fever–like *Borrelia*) has been detected at low rates throughout Europe, namely, in

Germany (121), Ireland (122), The Czech Republic (119), Sweden, The Netherlands (123), Estonia (124), Poland (125), France (126), Denmark (127), Belgium (123), England (128), Hungary (129), and Norway (130). Recently, there have been several reports concluding that *B. miyamotoi* may be a new pathogen of human infections (104, 131–134).

The first human cases of *B. miyamotoi* infection were reported in Russia in 2011 (7). More recently, human infections have been described in the United States (133) and Europe (132). Case reports from Russia, the United States, and Europe describe the clinical manifestation of *B. miyamotoi* infection as an influenza-like illness with fever (7), viral-like illness (118), or symptoms similar to those due to anaplasmosis (131). A potentially severe complication of *B. miyamotoi* infection is meningoencephalitis; two case reports from immunocompromised patients infected with *B. miyamotoi* in America and Europe were described as a severe manifestation of the disease (104, 118, 132). However, the full clinical picture of a *B. miyamotoi* infection has yet to be properly described. The most common clinical manifestations are fever, headache, fatigue, chills, myalgia, arthralgia, and nausea (118). Furthermore, validated diagnostic tools to verify human infection of *B. miyamotoi* are still lacking.

Uncultured and New Borrelia spp.

Recently, several new *Borrelia* spp. were identified in ticks mainly from Africa. A *Borrelia* sp. was detected in *Rhipicephalus* ticks from Ethiopia (107), an uncultured *B. merionesi* was identified in *Ornithodoros* ticks in Morocco (108), and an unnamed new species was found in *O. porcinus* ticks in Tanzania (109).

In Algeria, a new *Borrelia* sp. was described, named *Candidatus* Borrelia algerica. Initially, this *Borrelia* sp. was detected by qPCR targeting the 16S rRNA and confirmed by performing multispacer sequence typing. The result showed a 97% similarity with

Borrelia crocidurae, *Borrelia duttonii*, and *Borrelia recurrentis*. The *in silico* comparison with *Borrelia hispanica* and *B. garinii* showed similarity of 94% and 89%, respectively. These results point to a new *Borrelia* sp. named *B. algerica* (106). This *Borrelia* sp. was detected in blood from a patient with prolonged fever, but the full spectrum of symptoms remains to be defined. Recently, in Asia, a relapsing fever group *Borrelia* sp. similar to *B. lonestari* was found among wild sika deer (*Cervus nippon yesoensis*) and *Haemaphysalis* spp. ticks in Hokkaido, Japan (135). In conclusion, some of these newly identified *Borrelia* spp. are readily linked to human infection, while others are not yet known to cause human disease (5).

CONCLUSIONS

Tick-borne infections have presented a paradigm for emerging infectious diseases, with new agents described in recent years. It would not be surprising that the list of tick-borne bacterial pathogens causing disease in humans expands in the near future due to increased tick exposure combined with the current public health focus on these diseases and improvements in detection methods (5). Many *Rickettsiaceae*, *Anaplasmataceae*, and *Borrelia* were first identified in ticks before being found to be human pathogens. Such entomological searches for additional pathogens in arthropods remain key to the future discovery of tick-borne bacterial infections in humans.

ACKNOWLEDGMENTS

This work was carried out with the support of the A*MIDEX project (#ANR-11-IDEX-0001-02) funded by the French Government's Investissements d'Avenir program, managed by the French National Research Agency (ANR).

T. Kernif and H. Leulmi contibuted equally to this chapter.

CITATION

Kernif T, Leulmi H, Raoult R, Parola P. 2016. Emerging tick-borne bacterial pathogens. Microbiol Spectrum 4(3):EI10-0012-2016.

REFERENCES

1. **Parola P, Raoult D.** 2001. Ticks and tickborne bacterial diseases in humans: an emerging infectious threat. *Clin Infect Dis* **32:**897–928.
2. **Estrada-Peña A.** 2015. Ticks as vectors: taxonomy, biology and ecology. *Rev Sci Tech* **34:**53–65.
3. **Guglielmone AA, Nava S.** 2014. Names for *Ixodidae* (*Acari: Ixodoidea*): valid, synonyms, *incertae sedis*, *nomina dubia*, *nomina nuda*, *lapsus*, incorrect and suppressed names—with notes on confusions and misidentifications. *Zootaxa* **3767:**1–256.
4. **Horak IG, Camicas JL, Keirans JE.** 2002. The *Argasidae, Ixodidae* and *Nuttalliellidae* (*Acari: Ixodida*): a world list of valid tick names. *Exp Appl Acarol* **28:**27–54.
5. **Tijsse-Klasen E, Koopmans MP, Sprong H.** 2014. Tick-borne pathogen: reversed and conventional discovery of disease. *Front Public Health* **2:**73.
6. **Parola P, Paddock CD, Socolovschi C, Labruna MB, Mediannikov O, Kernif T, Abdad MY, Stenos J, Bitam I, Fournier PE, Raoult D.** 2013. Update on tick-borne rickettsioses around the world: a geographic approach. *Clin Microbiol Rev* **26:**657–702.
7. **Platonov AE, Karan LS, Kolyasnikova NM, Makhneva NA, Toporkova MG, Maleev VV, Fish D, Krause PJ.** 2011. Humans infected with relapsing fever spirochete *Borrelia miyamotoi*, Russia. *Emerg Infect Dis* **17:**1816–1823.
8. **Welinder-Olsson C, Kjellin E, Vaht K, Jacobsson S, Wenneras C.** 2010. First case of human "*Candidatus* Neoehrlichia mikurensis" infection in a febrile patient with chronic lymphocytic leukemia. *J Clin Microbiol* **48:**1956–1959.
9. **Pritt BS, Sloan LM, Johnson DK, Munderloh UG, Paskewitz SM, McElroy KM, McFadden JD, Binnicker MJ, Neitzel DF, Liu G, Nicholson WL, Nelson CM, Franson JJ, Martin SA, Cunningham SA, Steward CR, Bogumill K, Bjorgaard ME, Davis JP, McQuiston JH, Warshauer DM, Wilhelm MP, Patel R, Trivedi VA, Eremeeva ME.** 2011. Emergence of a new pathogenic *Ehrlichia* species, Wisconsin and Minnesota, 2009. *N Engl J Med* **365:**422–429.

10. **Kumsa B, Socolovschi C, Raoult D, Parola P.** 2015. Spotted fever group rickettsiae in ixodid ticks in Oromia, Ethiopia. *Ticks Tick Borne Dis* **6:**8–15.

11. **Lorusso V, Gruszka KA, Majekodunmi A, Igweh A, Welburn SC, Picozzi K.** 2013. *Rickettsia africae* in *Amblyomma variegatum* ticks, Uganda and Nigeria. *Emerg Infect Dis* **19:**1705–1707.

12. **Maina AN, Jiang J, Omulo SA, Cutler SJ, Ade F, Ogola E, Feikin DR, Njenga MK, Cleaveland S, Mpoke S, Ng'ang'a Z, Breiman RF, Knobel DL, Richards AL.** 2014. High prevalence of *Rickettsia africae* variants in *Amblyomma variegatum* ticks from domestic mammals in rural western Kenya: implications for human health. *Vector Borne Zoonotic Dis* **14:**693–702.

13. **Nakao R, Qiu Y, Igarashi M, Magona JW, Zhou L, Ito K, Sugimoto C.** 2013. High prevalence of spotted fever group *Rickettsiae* in *Amblyomma variegatum* from Uganda and their identification using sizes of intergenic spacers. *Ticks Tick Borne Dis* **4:**506–512.

14. **Nakao R, Qiu Y, Salim B, Hassan SM, Sugimoto C.** 2015. Molecular detection of *Rickettsia africae* in *Amblyomma variegatum* collected from Sudan. *Vector Borne Zoonotic Dis* **15:**323–325.

15. **Sambou M, Faye N, Bassene H, Diatta G, Raoult D, Mediannikov O.** 2014. Identification of rickettsial pathogens in ixodid ticks in northern Senegal. *Ticks Tick Borne Dis* **5:**552–556.

16. **Yssouf A, Socolovschi C, Kernif T, Temmam S, Lagadec E, Tortosa P, Parola P.** 2014. First molecular detection of *Rickettsia africae* in ticks from the Union of the Comoros. *Parasit Vectors* **7:**444.

17. **Zammarchi L, Farese A, Trotta M, Amantini A, Raoult D, Bartoloni A.** 2014. *Rickettsia africae* infection complicated with painful sacral syndrome in an Italian traveller returning from Zimbabwe. *Int. J Infect Dis* **29:**194–196.

18. **Kleinerman G, Baneth G, Mumcuoglu KY, van Straten M, Berlin D, Apanaskevich DA, Abdeen Z, Nasereddin A, Harrus S.** 2013. Molecular detection of *Rickettsia africae, Rickettsia aeschlimannii,* and *Rickettsia sibirica mongolitimonae* in camels and *Hyalomma* spp. ticks from Israel. *Vector Borne Zoonotic Dis* **13:**851–856.

19. **Waner T, Keysary A, Eremeeva ME, Din AB, Mumcuoglu KY, King R, Atiya-Nasagi Y.** 2014. *Rickettsia africae* and *Candidatus* Rickettsia barbariae in ticks in Israel. *Am J Trop Med Hyg* **90:**920–922.

20. **Chochlakis D, Bongiorni C, Partalis N, Tselentis Y, Psaroulaki A.** 2015. Possible *Rickettsia massiliae* infection in Greece: an imported case. *Jpn J Infect Dis.* [Epub ahead of print.] doi:10.7883/yoken.JJID.2015.195.

21. **de Sousa R, Pereira BI, Nazareth C, Cabral S, Ventura C, Crespo P, Marques N, da Cunha S.** 2013. *Rickettsia slovaca* infection in humans, Portugal. *Emerg Infect Dis* **19:**1627–1629.

22. **Gaillard E, Socolovschi C, Fourcade C, Lavigne JP, Raoult D, Sotto A.** 2015. A case of severe sepsis with disseminated intravascular coagulation during *Rickettsia sibirica mongolitimonae* infection. *Med Mal Infect* **45:**57–59. [In French.]

23. **Germanakis A, Chochlakis D, Angelakis E, Tselentis Y, Psaroulaki A.** 2013. *Rickettsia aeschlimannii* infection in a man, Greece. *Emerg Infect Dis* **19:**1176–1177.

24. **Jia N, Jiang JF, Huo QB, Jiang BG, Cao WC.** 2013. *Rickettsia sibirica* subspecies *sibirica* BJ-90 as a cause of human disease. *N Engl J Med* **369:**1176–1178.

25. **Jia N, Zheng YC, Ma L, Huo QB, Ni XB, Jiang BG, Chu YL, Jiang RR, Jiang JF, Cao WC.** 2014. Human infections with *Rickettsia raoultii,* China. *Emerg Infect Dis* **20:**866–868.

26. **Kostopoulou V, Chochlakis D, Kanta C, Katsanou A, Rossiou K, Rammos A, Papadopoulos SF, Katsarou T, Tselentis Y, Psaroulaki A, Boukas C.** 2015. A case of human infection by *Rickettsia slovaca* in Greece. *Jpn J Infect Dis.* [Epub ahead of print.] doi:10.7883/yoken.JJID.2015.194.

27. **Nelson R.** 2015. Rocky Mountain spotted fever in Native Americans. *Lancet Infect Dis* **15:**1013–1014.

28. **Portillo A, Garcia-Garcia C, Sanz MM, Santibanez S, Venzal JM, Oteo JA.** 2013. A confirmed case of *Rickettsia parkeri* infection in a traveler from Uruguay. *Am J Trop Med Hyg* **89:**1203–1205.

29. **Pulido-Perez A, Gomez-Recuero L, Lozano-Masdemont B, Suarez-Fernandez R.** 2015. *Rickettsia sibirica mongolitimonae* infection in two immunocompetent adults. *Enferm Infecc Microbiol Clin* **33:**635–636. [In Spanish.]

30. **Solary J, Socolovschi C, Aubry C, Brouqui P, Raoult D, Parola P.** 2014. Detection of *Rickettsia sibirica mongolitimonae* by using cutaneous swab samples and quantitative PCR. *Emerg Infect Dis* **20:**716–718.

31. **Nogueras MM, Roson B, Lario S, Sanfeliu I, Pons I, Anton E, Casanovas A, Segura F.** 2015. Coinfection with "*Rickettsia sibirica subsp. mongolotimonae*" and *Rickettsia conorii* in a human patient: a challenge for molecular diagnosis tools. *J Clin Microbiol* **53:**3057–3062.

32. **Raczniak GA, Kato C, Chung IH, Austin A, McQuiston JH, Weis E, Levy C, Carvalho MG,**

Mitchell A, Bjork A, Regan JJ. 2014. Case report: co-infection of *Rickettsia rickettsii* and *Streptococcus pyogenes*: is fatal Rocky Mountain spotted fever underdiagnosed? *Am J Trop Med Hyg* **91**:1154–1155.

33. Znazen A, Khrouf F, Elleuch N, Lahiani D, Marrekchi C, M'Ghirbi Y, Ben JM, Bouattour A, Hammami A. 2013. Multispacer typing of *Rickettsia* isolates from humans and ticks in Tunisia revealing new genotypes. *Parasit Vectors* **6**:367.

34. Shpynov S, Fournier PE, Rudakov N, Raoult D. 2003. "*Candidatus* Rickettsia tarasevichiae" in *Ixodes persulcatus* ticks collected in Russia. *Ann N Y Acad Sci* **990**:162–172.

35. Shpynov SN, Rudakov NV, Fournier PE, Raoult D. 2005. Detection of a new species of *Rickettsiae* in the ticks of *Ixodes persulcatus* in Russia. *Med Parazitol (Mosk)* (**2**):6–9. [In Russian.]

36. Jia N, Zheng YC, Jiang JF, Ma L, Cao WC. 2013. Human infection with *Candidatus* Rickettsia tarasevichiae. *N Engl J Med* **369**:1178–1180.

37. Katargina O, Geller J, Ivanova A, Varv K, Tefanova V, Vene S, Lundkvist A, Golovljova I. 2015. Detection and identification of *Rickettsia* species in *Ixodes* tick populations from Estonia. *Ticks Tick Borne Dis* **6**:689–694.

38. Igolkina YP, Rar VA, Yakimenko VV, Malkova MG, Tancev AK, Tikunov AY, Epikhina TI, Tikunova NV. 2015. Genetic variability of *Rickettsia* spp. in *Ixodes persulcatus/Ixodes trianguliceps* sympatric areas from Western Siberia, Russia: identification of a new *Candidatus* Rickettsia species. *Infect Genet Evol* **34**:88–93.

39. Spolidorio MG, Labruna MB, Mantovani E, Brandao PE, Richtzenhain LJ, Yoshinari NH. 2010. Novel spotted fever group *Rickettsiosis*, Brazil. *Emerg Infect Dis* **16**:521–523.

40. Sabatini GS, Pinter A, Nieri-Bastos FA, Marcili A, Labruna MB. 2010. Survey of ticks (*Acari*: *Ixodidae*) and their rickettsia in an Atlantic rain forest reserve in the state of São Paulo, Brazil. *J Med Entomol* **47**:913–916.

41. Medeiros AP, Souza AP, Moura AB, Lavina MS, Bellato V, Sartor AA, Nieri-Bastos FA, Richtzenhain LJ, Labruna MB. 2011. Spotted fever group *Rickettsia* infecting ticks (*Acari*: *Ixodidae*) in the state of Santa Catarina, Brazil. *Mem Inst Oswaldo Cruz* **106**:926–930.

42. Szabó MP, Pinter A, Labruna MB. 2013. Ecology, biology and distribution of spotted-fever tick vectors in Brazil. *Front Cell Infect Microbiol* **3**:27.

43. Barbieri AR, Filho JM, Nieri-Bastos FA, Souza JC Jr, Szabo MP, Labruna MB. 2014. Epide-miology of *Rickettsia* sp. strain Atlantic rain-forest in a spotted fever-endemic area of southern Brazil. *Ticks Tick Borne Dis* **5**:848–853.

44. Londono AF, Diaz FJ, Valbuena G, Gazi M, Labruna MB, Hidalgo M, Mattar S, Contreras V, Rodas JD. 2014. Infection of *Amblyomma ovale* by *Rickettsia* sp. strain Atlantic rainforest, Colombia. *Ticks Tick Borne Dis* **5**:672–675.

45. Monje LD, Nava S, Eberhardt AT, Correa AI, Guglielmone AA, Beldomenico PM. 2015. Molecular detection of the human pathogenic *Rickettsia* sp. strain Atlantic rainforest in *Amblyomma dubitatum* ticks from Argentina. *Vector Borne Zoonotic Dis* **15**:167–169.

46. Dumler JS, Barbet AF, Bekker CP, Dasch GA, Palmer GH, Ray SC, Rikihisa Y, Rurangirwa FR. 2001. Reorganization of genera in the families *Rickettsiaceae* and *Anaplasmataceae* in the order *Rickettsiales*: unification of some species of *Ehrlichia* with *Anaplasma*, *Cowdria* with *Ehrlichia* and *Ehrlichia* with *Neorickettsia*, descriptions of six new species combinations and designation of *Ehrlichia equi* and 'HGE agent' as subjective synonyms of *Ehrlichia phagocytophila*. *Int J Syst Evol Microbiol* **51**:2145–2165.

47. Friedman CS, Andree KB, Beauchamp KA, Moore JD, Robbins TT, Shields JD, Hedrick RP. 2000. '*Candidatus* Xenohaliotis californiensis', a newly described pathogen of abalone, *Haliotis* spp., along the west coast of North America. *Int J Syst Evol Microbiol* **50**:847–855.

48. Kawahara M, Rikihisa Y, Isogai E, Takahashi M, Misumi H, Suto C, Shibata S, Zhang C, Tsuji M. 2004. Ultrastructure and phylogenetic analysis of '*Candidatus* Neoehrlichia mikurensis' in the family *Anaplasmataceae*, isolated from wild rats and found in *Ixodes ovatus* ticks. *Int J Syst Evol Microbiol* **54**:1837–1843.

49. Silaghi C, Beck R, Oteo JA, Pfeffer M, Sprong H. 2015. *Neoehrlichiosis*: an emerging tick-borne zoonosis caused by *Candidatus* Neoehrlichia mikurensis. *Exp Appl Acarol* **68**:279–297.

50. Rar V, Golovljova I. 2011. *Anaplasma*, *Ehrlichia*, and "*Candidatus* Neoehrlichia" bacteria: pathogenicity, biodiversity, and molecular genetic characteristics, a review. *Infect Genet Evol* **11**:1842–1861.

51. Atif FA. 2015. *Anaplasma marginale* and *Anaplasma phagocytophilum*: *Rickettsiales* pathogens of veterinary and public health significance. *Parasitol Res* **114**:3941–3957.

52. Rikihisa Y. 2015. Molecular pathogenesis of *Ehrlichia chaffeensis* infection. *Annu Rev Microbiol* **69**:283–304.

53. Dahlgren FS, Heitman KN, Behravesh CB. 2015. Undetermined human ehrlichiosis and

anaplasmosis in the United States, 2008-2012: a catch-all for passive surveillance. *Am J Trop Med Hyg* pii:15-0691.

54. **Kocan KM, de la Fuente J, Cabezas-Cruz A.** 2015. The genus *Anaplasma*: new challenges after reclassification. *Rev Sci Tech* **34:**577–586.

55. **Ismail N, Bloch KC, McBride JW.** 2010. Human ehrlichiosis and anaplasmosis. *Clin Lab Med* **30:**261–292.

56. **Heitman KN, Dahlgren FS, Drexler NA, Massung RF, Behravesh CB.** 2015. Increasing incidence of ehrlichiosis in the United States: a summary of national surveillance of *Ehrlichia chaffeensis* and *Ehrlichia ewingii* infections in the United States, 2008-2012. *Am J Trop Med Hyg* **94:**52–60.

57. **Perez M, Rikihisa Y, Wen B.** 1996. *Ehrlichia canis*-like agent isolated from a man in Venezuela: antigenic and genetic characterization. *J Clin Microbiol* **34:**2133–2139.

58. **Perez M, Bodor M, Zhang C, Xiong Q, Rikihisa Y.** 2006. Human infection with *Ehrlichia canis* accompanied by clinical signs in Venezuela. *Ann N Y Acad Sci* **1078:**110–117.

59. **Allsopp BA.** 2015. Heartwater: *Ehrlichia ruminantium* infection. *Rev Sci Tech* **34:**557–568.

60. **Allsopp MT, Louw M, Meyer EC.** 2005. *Ehrlichia ruminantium*: an emerging human pathogen. *S Afr Med J* **95:**541.

61. **Chochlakis D, Ioannou I, Tselentis Y, Psaroulaki A.** 2010. Human anaplasmosis and *Anaplasma ovis* variant. *Emerg Infect Dis* **16:**1031–1032.

62. **Hosseini-Vasoukolaei N, Oshaghi MA, Shayan P, Vatandoost H, Babamahmoudi F, Yaghoobi-Ershadi MR, Telmadarraiy Z, Mohtarami F.** 2014. Anaplasma infection in ticks, livestock and human in Ghaemshahr, Mazandaran province, Iran. *J Arthropod Borne Dis* **8:**204–211.

63. **Arraga-Alvarado C, Montero-Ojeda M, Bernardoni A, Anderson BE, Parra O.** 1996. Human ehrlichiosis: report of the 1st case in Venezuela. *Invest Clin* **37:**35–49. [In Spanish.]

64. **Arraga-Alvarado C, Palmar M, Parra O, Salas P.** 1999. Fine structural characterisation of a *Rickettsia*-like organism in human platelets from patients with symptoms of ehrlichiosis. *J Med Microbiol* **48:**991–997.

65. **Breitschwerdt EB, Hegarty BC, Qurollo BA, Saito TB, Maggi RG, Blanton LS, Bouyer DH.** 2014. Intravascular persistence of *Anaplasma platys*, *Ehrlichia chaffeensis*, and *Ehrlichia ewingii* DNA in the blood of a dog and two family members. *Parasit Vectors* **7:**298.

66. **Maggi RG, Mascarelli PE, Havenga LN, Naidoo V, Breitschwerdt EB.** 2013. Co-infec-

tion with *Anaplasma platys*, *Bartonella henselae* and *Candidatus* Mycoplasma haematoparvum in a veterinarian. *Parasit Vectors* **6:**103.

67. **Reeves WK, Loftis AD, Nicholson WL, Czarkowski AG.** 2008. The first report of human illness associated with the Panola Mountain *Ehrlichia* species: a case report. *J Med Case Rep* **2:**139.

68. **Johnson DK, Schiffman EK, Davis JP, Neitzel DF, Sloan LM, Nicholson WL, Fritsche TR, Steward CR, Ray JA, Miller TK, Feist MA, Uphoff TS, Franson JJ, Livermore AL, Deedon AK, Theel ES, Pritt BS.** 2015. Human infection with *Ehrlichia muris*-like pathogen, United States, 2007-2013. *Emerg Infect Dis* **21:**1794–1799.

69. **Li H, Zheng YC, Ma L, Jia N, Jiang BG, Jiang RR, Huo QB, Wang YW, Liu HB, Chu YL, Song YD, Yao NN, Sun T, Zeng FY, Dumler JS, Jiang JF, Cao WC.** 2015. Human infection with a novel tick-borne *Anaplasma* species in China: a surveillance study. *Lancet Infect Dis* **15:**663–670.

70. **Wenneras C.** 2015. Infections with the tick-borne bacterium *Candidatus* Neoehrlichia mikurensis. *Clin Microbiol Infect* **21:**621–630.

71. **Eremeeva ME, Oliveira A, Robinson JB, Ribakova N, Tokarevich NK, Dasch GA.** 2006. Prevalence of bacterial agents in *Ixodes persulcatus* ticks from the Vologda province of Russia. *Ann N Y Acad Sci* **1078:**291–298.

72. **Rar VA, Fomenko NV, Dobrotvorsky AK, Livanova NN, Rudakova SA, Fedorov EG, Astanin VB, Morozova OV.** 2005. Tickborne pathogen detection, Western Siberia, Russia. *Emerg Infect Dis* **11:**1708–1715.

73. **Spitalská E, Boldis V, Kostanová Z, Kocianová E, Stefanidesová K.** 2008. Incidence of various tick-borne microorganisms in rodents and ticks of central Slovakia. *Acta Virol* **52:**175–179.

74. **Castillo CG, Eremeeva ME, Paskewitz SM, Sloan LM, Lee X, Irwin WE, Tonsberg S, Pritt BS.** 2015. Detection of human pathogenic *Ehrlichia muris*-like agent in *Peromyscus leucopus*. *Ticks Tick Borne Dis* **6:**155–157.

75. **Schouls LM, Van De Pol I, Rijpkema SG, Schot CS.** 1999. Detection and identification of ehrlichia, *Borrelia burgdorferi* sensu lato, and *Bartonella* species in Dutch *Ixodes ricinus* ticks. *J Clin Microbiol* **37:**2215–2222.

76. **Alekseev AN, Dubinina HV, Van De Pol I, Schouls LM.** 2001. Identification of *Ehrlichia* spp. and *Borrelia burgdorferi* in *Ixodes* ticks in the Baltic regions of Russia. *J Clin Microbiol* **39:**2237–2242.

77. **Pan H, Liu S, Ma Y, Tong S, Sun Y.** 2003. *Ehrlichia*-like organism gene found in small

mammals in the suburban district of Guangzhou of China. *Ann N Y Acad Sci* **990:**107–111.

78. **Lommano E, Bertaiola L, Dupasquier C, Gern L.** 2012. Infections and coinfections of questing *Ixodes ricinus* ticks by emerging zoonotic pathogens in Western Switzerland. *Appl Environ Microbiol* **78:**4606–4612.

79. **Potkonjak A, Gutierrez R, Savic S, Vracar V, Nachum-Biala Y, Jurisic A, Kleinerman G, Rojas A, Petrovic A, Baneth G, Harrus S.** 2016. Molecular detection of emerging tick-borne pathogens in Vojvodina, Serbia. *Ticks Tick Borne Dis* **7:**199–203.

80. **Sanogo YO, Parola P, Shpynov S, Camicas JL, Brouqui P, Caruso G, Raoult D.** 2003. Genetic diversity of bacterial agents detected in ticks removed from asymptomatic patients in northeastern Italy. *Ann N Y Acad Sci* **990:**182–190.

81. **Silaghi C, Woll D, Mahling M, Pfister K, Pfeffer M.** 2012. Candidatus Neoehrlichia mikurensis in rodents in an area with sympatric existence of the hard ticks *Ixodes ricinus* and *Dermacentor reticulatus*, Germany. *Parasit Vectors* **5:**285.

82. **Venclikova K, Mendel J, Betasova L, Blazejova H, Jedlickova P, Strakova P, Hubalek Z, Rudolf I.** 2016. Neglected tick-borne pathogens in the Czech Republic, 2011-2014. *Ticks Tick Borne Dis* **7:**107–112.

83. **Von Loewenich FD, Stumpf G, Baumgarten BU, Röllinghoff M, Dumler JS, Bogdan C.** 2003. Human granulocytic ehrlichiosis in Germany: evidence from serological studies, tick analyses, and a case of equine ehrlichiosis. *Ann N Y Acad Sci* **990:**116–117.

84. **Movila A, Alekseev AN, Dubinina HV, Toderas I.** 2013. Detection of tick-borne pathogens in ticks from migratory birds in the Baltic region of Russia. *Med Vet Entomol* **27:**113–117.

85. **Fehr JS, Bloemberg GV, Ritter C, Hombach M, Lüscher TF, Weber R, Keller PM.** 2010. Septicemia caused by tick-borne bacterial pathogen Candidatus Neoehrlichia mikurensis. *Emerg Infect Dis* **16:**1127–1129.

86. **Li H, Jiang JF, Liu W, Zheng YC, Huo QB, Tang K, Zuo SY, Liu K, Jiang BG, Yang H, Cao WC.** 2012. Human infection with Candidatus Neoehrlichia mikurensis, China. *Emerg Infect Dis* **18:**1636–1639.

87. **Maurer FP, Keller PM, Beuret C, Joha C, Achermann Y, Gubler J, Bircher D, Karrer U, Fehr J, Zimmerli L, Bloemberg GV.** 2013. Close geographic association of human neoehrlichiosis and tick populations carrying "Candidatus Neoehrlichia mikurensis" in eastern Switzerland. *J Clin Microbiol* **51:**169–176.

88. **Pekova S, Vydra J, Kabickova H, Frankova S, Haugvicova R, Mazal O, Cmejla R, Hardekopf DW, Jancuskova T, Kozak T.** 2011. Candidatus Neoehrlichia mikurensis infection identified in 2 hematooncologic patients: benefit of molecular techniques for rare pathogen detection. *Diagn Microbiol Infect Dis* **69:**266–270.

89. **von Loewenich FD, Geissdorfer W, Disque C, Matten J, Schett G, Sakka SG, Bogdan C.** 2010. Detection of "Candidatus Neoehrlichia mikurensis" in two patients with severe febrile illnesses: evidence for a European sequence variant. *J Clin Microbiol* **48:**2630–2635.

90. **Diniz PP, Schulz BS, Hartmann K, Breitschwerdt EB.** 2011. "Candidatus Neoehrlichia mikurensis" infection in a dog from Germany. *J Clin Microbiol* **49:**2059–2062.

91. **Moniuszko A, Dunaj J, Czupryna P, Zajkowska J, Pancewicz S.** 2015. Neoehrlichiosis—a new tick-borne disease: is there a threat in Poland? *Przegl Epidemiol* **69:**23–26, 131–133.

92. **Grankvist A, Moore ER, Svensson SL, Pekova S, Bogdan C, Geissdorfer W, Grip-Linden J, Brandstrom K, Marsal J, Andreasson K, Lewerin C, Welinder-Olsson C, Wenneras C.** 2015. Multilocus sequence analysis of clinical "Candidatus Neoehrlichia mikurensis" strains from Europe. *J Clin Microbiol* **53:**3126–3132.

93. **Welc-Faleciak R, Sinski E, Kowalec M, Zajkowska J, Pancewicz SA.** 2014. Asymptomatic "Candidatus Neoehrlichia mikurensis" infections in immunocompetent humans. *J Clin Microbiol* **52:**3072–3074.

94. **Derdakova M, Vaclav R, Pangracova-Blanarova L, Selyemova D, Koci J, Walder G, Spitalska E.** 2014. Candidatus Neoehrlichia mikurensis and its co-circulation with *Anaplasma phagocytophilum* in *Ixodes ricinus* ticks across ecologically different habitats of Central Europe. *Parasit Vectors* **7:**160.

95. **Hornok S, Meli ML, Gonczi E, Hofmann-Lehmann R.** 2013. First evidence of Candidatus Neoehrlichia mikurensis in Hungary. *Parasit Vectors* **6:**267.

96. **Jahfari S, Fonville M, Hengeveld P, Reusken C, Scholte EJ, Takken W, Heyman P, Medlock JM, Heylen D, Kleve J, Sprong H.** 2012. Prevalence of *Neoehrlichia mikurensis* in ticks and rodents from North-west Europe. *Parasit Vectors* **5:**74.

97. **Szekeres S, Claudia CE, Rigo K, Majoros G, Jahfari S, Sprong H, Foldvari G.** 2015. Candidatus Neoehrlichia mikurensis and *Anaplasma phagocytophilum* in natural rodent and tick communities in Southern Hungary. *Ticks Tick Borne Dis* **6:**111–116.

98. Labbe SL, Tolf C, Larsson S, Wilhelmsson P, Salaneck E, Jaenson TG, Lindgren PE, Olsen B, Waldenstrom J. 2015. *Candidatus* Neoehrlichia mikurensis in ticks from migrating birds in Sweden. *PLoS One* **10:**e0133250. doi:10.1371/journal.pone.0133250.

99. Földvári G, Jahfari S, Rigó K, Jablonszky M, Szekeres S, Majoros G, Tóth M, Molnár V, Coipan EC, Sprong H. 2014. *Candidatus* Neoehrlichia mikurensis and *Anaplasma phagocytophilum* in urban hedgehogs. *Emerg Infect Dis* **20:**496–498.

100. Stanek G, Wormser GP, Gray J, Strle F. 2012. Lyme borreliosis. *Lancet* **379:**461–473.

101. Wagemakers A, Staarink PJ, Sprong H, Hovius JW. 2015. *Borrelia miyamotoi*: a widespread tick-borne relapsing fever spirochete. *Trends Parasitol* **31:**260–269.

102. Koedel U, Fingerle V, Pfister HW. 2015. Lyme neuroborreliosis: epidemiology, diagnosis and management. *Nat Rev Neurol* **11:**446–456.

103. Schutzer SE, Fraser-Liggett CM, Qiu WG, Kraiczy P, Mongodin EF, Dunn JJ, Luft BJ, Casjens SR. 2012. Whole-genome sequences of *Borrelia bissettii*, *Borrelia valaisiana*, and *Borrelia spielmanii*. *J Bacteriol* **194:**545–546.

104. Gugliotta JL, Goethert HK, Berardi VP, Telford SR III. 2013. Meningoencephalitis from *Borrelia miyamotoi* in an immunocompromised patient. *N Engl J Med* **368:**240–245.

105. Fukunaga M, Takahashi Y, Tsuruta Y, Matsushita O, Ralph D, McClelland M, Nakao M. 1995. Genetic and phenotypic analysis of *Borrelia miyamotoi* sp. nov., isolated from the ixodid tick *Ixodes persulcatus*, the vector for Lyme disease in Japan. *Int J Syst Bacteriol* **45:**804–810.

106. Fotso FA, Angelakis E, Mouffok N, Drancourt M, Raoult D. 2015. Blood-borne *Candidatus* Borrelia algerica in a patient with prolonged fever in Oran, Algeria. *Am J Trop Med Hyg* **93:**1070–1073.

107. Kumsa B, Socolovschi C, Raoult D, Parola P. 2015. New *Borrelia* species detected in ixodid ticks in Oromia, Ethiopia. *Ticks Tick Borne Dis* **6:**401–407.

108. Trape JF, Diatta G, Arnathau C, Bitam I, Sarih M, Belghyti D, Bouattour A, Elguero E, Vial L, Mane Y, Balde C, Prugnolle F, Chauvancy G, Mahe G, Granjon L, Duplantier JM, Durand P, Renaud F. 2013. The epidemiology and geographic distribution of relapsing fever borreliosis in West and North Africa, with a review of the *Ornithodoros erraticus* complex (*Acari: Ixodida*). *PLoS One* **8:**e78473. doi:10.1371/journal.pone.0078473.

109. Mitani H, Talbert A, Fukunaga M. 2004. New World relapsing fever *Borrelia* found in *Ornithodoros porcinus* ticks in central Tanzania. *Microbiol Immunol* **48:**501–505.

110. James AM, Liveris D, Wormser GP, Schwartz I, Montecalvo MA, Johnson BJ. 2001. *Borrelia lonestari* infection after a bite by an *Amblyomma americanum* tick. *J Infect Dis* **183:**1810–1814.

111. Rich SM, Armstrong PM, Smith RD, Telford SR III. 2001. Lone star tick-infecting borreliae are most closely related to the agent of bovine borreliosis. *J Clin Microbiol* **39:**494–497.

112. McCoy BN, Maiga O, Schwan TG. 2014. Detection of *Borrelia theileri* in *Rhipicephalus geigyi* from Mali. *Ticks Tick Borne Dis* **5:**401–403.

113. Barbour AG, Bunikis J, Travinsky B, Hoen AG, Diuk-Wasser MA, Fish D, Tsao JI. 2009. Niche partitioning of *Borrelia burgdorferi* and *Borrelia miyamotoi* in the same tick vector and mammalian reservoir species. *Am J Trop Med Hyg* **81:**1120–1131.

114. Scoles GA, Papero M, Beati L, Fish D. 2001. A relapsing fever group spirochete transmitted by *Ixodes scapularis* ticks. *Vector Borne Zoonotic Dis* **1:**21–34.

115. Fraenkel CJ, Garpmo U, Berglund J. 2002. Determination of novel *Borrelia* genospecies in Swedish *Ixodes ricinus* ticks. *J Clin Microbiol* **40:**3308–3312.

116. Hamer SA, Hickling GJ, Keith R, Sidge JL, Walker ED, Tsao JI. 2012. Associations of passerine birds, rabbits, and ticks with *Borrelia miyamotoi* and *Borrelia andersonii* in Michigan, U.S.A. *Parasit Vectors* **5:**231.

117. Mun J, Eisen RJ, Eisen L, Lane RS. 2006. Detection of a *Borrelia miyamotoi* sensu lato relapsing-fever group spirochete from *Ixodes pacificus* in California. *J Med Entomol* **43:**120–123.

118. Krause PJ, Fish D, Narasimhan S, Barbour AG. 2015. *Borrelia miyamotoi* infection in nature and in humans. *Clin Microbiol Infect* **21:**631–639.

119. Crowder CD, Carolan HE, Rounds MA, Honig V, Mothes B, Haag H, Nolte O, Luft BJ, Grubhoffer L, Ecker DJ, Schutzer SE, Eshoo MW. 2014. Prevalence of *Borrelia miyamotoi* in *Ixodes* ticks in Europe and the United States. *Emerg Infect Dis* **20:**1678–1682.

120. DiBernardo A, Cote T, Ogden NH, Lindsay LR. 2014. The prevalence of *Borrelia miyamotoi* infection, and co-infections with other *Borrelia* spp. in *Ixodes scapularis* ticks collected in Canada. *Parasit Vectors* **7:**183.

121. Richter D, Schlee DB, Matuschka FR. 2003. Relapsing fever-like spirochetes infecting European vector tick of Lyme disease agent. *Emerg Infect Dis* **9:**697–701.

122. **Pichon B, Rogers M, Egan D, Gray J.** 2005. Blood-meal analysis for the identification of reservoir hosts of tick-borne pathogens in Ireland. *Vector Borne Zoonotic Dis* **5:**172–180.

123. **Cochez C, Heyman P, Heylen D, Fonville M, Hengeveld P, Takken W, Simons L, Sprong H.** 2015. The presence of *Borrelia miyamotoi*, a relapsing fever spirochaete, in questing *Ixodes ricinus* in Belgium and in The Netherlands. *Zoonoses Public Health* **62:**331–333.

124. **Geller J, Nazarova L, Katargina O, Jarvekulg L, Fomenko N, Golovljova I.** 2012. Detection and genetic characterization of relapsing fever spirochete *Borrelia miyamotoi* in Estonian ticks. *PLoS One* **7:**e51914. doi:10.1371/journal. pone.0051914.

125. **Kiewra D, Stanczak J, Richter M.** 2014. *Ixodes ricinus* ticks (*Acari, Ixodidae*) as a vector of *Borrelia burgdorferi* sensu lato and *Borrelia miyamotoi* in Lower Silesia, Poland: preliminary study. *Ticks Tick Borne Dis* **5:**892–897.

126. **Vayssier-Taussat M, Moutailler S, Michelet L, Devillers E, Bonnet S, Cheval J, Hebert C, Eloit M.** 2013. Next generation sequencing uncovers unexpected bacterial pathogens in ticks in western Europe. *PLoS One* **8:**e81439. doi:10.1371/journal.pone.0081439.

127. **Michelet L, Delannoy S, Devillers E, Umhang G, Aspan A, Juremalm M, Chirico J, van der Wal FJ, Sprong H, Boye Pihl TP, Klitgaard K, Bødker R, Fach P, Moutailler S.** 2014. High-throughput screening of tick-borne pathogens in Europe. *Front Cell Infect Microbiol* **4:**103.

128. **Hansford KM, Fonville M, Jahfari S, Sprong H, Medlock JM.** 2015. *Borrelia miyamotoi* in host-seeking *Ixodes ricinus* ticks in England. *Epidemiol Infect* **143:**1079–1087.

129. **Szekeres S, Coipan EC, Rigo K, Majoros G, Jahfari S, Sprong H, Foldvari G.** 2015. Eco-epidemiology of *Borrelia miyamotoi* and Lyme borreliosis spirochetes in a popular hunting and recreational forest area in Hungary. *Parasit Vectors* **8:**309.

130. **Kjelland V, Rollum R, Korslund L, Slettan A, Tveitnes D.** 2015. *Borrelia miyamotoi* is wide-spread in *Ixodes ricinus* ticks in southern Norway. *Ticks Tick Borne Dis* **6:**516–521.

131. **Chowdri HR, Gugliotta JL, Berardi VP, Goethert HK, Molloy PJ, Sterling SL, Telford SR.** 2013. *Borrelia miyamotoi* infection presenting as human granulocytic anaplasmosis: a case report. *Ann Intern Med* **159:**21–27.

132. **Hovius JW, de Wever B, Sohne M, Brouwer MC, Coumou J, Wagemakers A, Oei A, Knol H, Narasimhan S, Hodiamont CJ, Jahfari S, Pals ST, Horlings HM, Fikrig E, Sprong H, van Oers MH.** 2013. A case of meningoencephalitis by the relapsing fever spirochaete *Borrelia miyamotoi* in Europe. *Lancet* **382:**658.

133. **Krause PJ, Narasimhan S, Wormser GP, Rollend L, Fikrig E, Lepore T, Barbour A, Fish D.** 2013. Human *Borrelia miyamotoi* infection in the United States. *N Engl J Med* **368:**291–293.

134. **Telford SR III, Goethert HK, Molloy PJ, Berardi VP, Chowdri HR, Gugliotta JL, Lepore TJ.** 2015. *Borrelia miyamotoi* disease: neither lyme disease nor relapsing fever. *Clin Lab Med* **35:**867–882.

135. **Lee K, Takano A, Taylor K, Sashika M, Shimozuru M, Konnai S, Kawabata H, Tsubota T.** 2014. A relapsing fever group *Borrelia* sp. similar to *Borrelia lonestari* found among wild sika deer (*Cervus nippon yesoensis*) and *Haemaphysalis* spp. ticks in Hokkaido, Japan. *Ticks Tick Borne Dis* **5:**841–847.

136. **Paddock CD, Denison AM, Lash RR, Liu L, Bollweg BC, Dahlgren FS, Kanamura CT, Angerami RN, Pereira dos Santos FC, Brasil MR, Karpathy SE.** 2014. Phylogeography of *Rickettsia rickettsii* genotypes associated with fatal Rocky Mountain spotted fever. *Am J Trop Med Hyg* **91:**589–597.

137. **Sentausa E, El Karkouri K, Michelle C, Caputo A, Raoult D, Fournier PE.** 2014. Genome sequence of *Rickettsia tamurae*, a recently detected human pathogen in Japan. *Genome Announc* **2:**e00838-14. doi:10.1128/genomeA.00838-14.

17

Bordetella pertussis

DELMA J. NIEVES[1] and ULRICH HEININGER[2]

INTRODUCTION

Pertussis is a highly contagious acute respiratory illness classically known as "whooping cough" because of its characteristic cough. The majority of cases are caused by *Bordetella pertussis*, with some caused by *B. parapertussis* (1, 2). Pertussis is a vaccine-preventable disease that was a major cause of childhood morbidity and mortality during the first half of the 20th century. Following worldwide implementation of pertussis vaccination, cases declined significantly (3) (Fig. 1). However, it was never fully eliminated, and epidemic peaks continued on a cycle of every 2 or 3 to 5 years. In the past several years, even countries with generally high immunization rates in early childhood have experienced a rise in pertussis cases. In 2014, the World Health Organization (WHO) reported 139,786 cases of pertussis in spite of an estimated global 86% diphtheria-tetanus-pertussis (DTP) vaccine coverage with three doses (4). In 2013 and 2014, there were 28,639 and 32,791, respectively yearly reported cases of pertussis in the United States, which makes pertussis the most prominent emerging vaccine-preventable disease in this country. Of those cases involving patients 6 months to 6 years of age, 42% had a DTaP vaccination history of 3 or more doses, 6% had 1 or 2 doses, 8% had none, and

[1]Pediatric Infectious Diseases, CHOC Children's, Orange, CA 92868; [2]Universitäts-Kinderspital beider Basel (UKBB), CH-4031 Basel, Switzerland.

Emerging Infections 10
Edited by W. Michael Scheld, James M. Hughes and Richard J. Whitley
© 2016 American Society for Microbiology, Washington, DC
doi:10.1128/microbiolspec.EI10-0008-2015

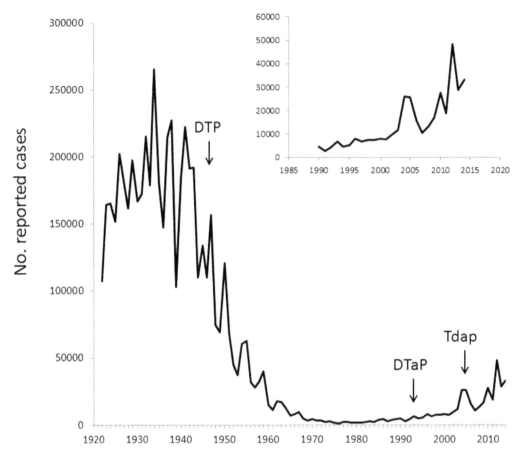

FIGURE 1 Reported pertussis cases from the National Notifiable Disease Surveillance System, United States, 1922 to 2014. The inset show cases from 1990 to 2014. Data for 1950 to 2013 were obtained from the Centers for Disease Control and Prevention National Notifiable Diseases Surveillance System. Data for 1922 to 1949 were obtained from passive reports to the U.S. Public Health Service. DTP, diphtheria and tetanus toxoids combined with whole-cell pertussis vaccine; DTaP, diphtheria and tetanus toxoids and acellular pertussis vaccine; Tdap, reduced-dose acellular pertussis vaccine combined with tetanus and diphtheria toxoids. Figure adapted with permission from reference 272.

44% had an unknown vaccination status (5). In 2014, there were more than 10,000 reported cases of pertussis in California alone. The greatest morbidity and mortality associated with pertussis infection occur in young infants, particularly those under 3 months of age, often requiring hospitalization in an intensive care setting (6, 7). With this upsurge in pertussis, much more has been learned about the organism, the vaccines available, and the variability of illness presentation. This complex disease has promoted many public health actions aimed at reducing the spread of *Bordetella pertussis*, specifically to the fragile neonate, at risk of much worse disease than older age groups and of high mortality.

THE ORGANISM

Bordetella is a Gram-negative, pleomorphic, aerobic coccobacillus. The genus *Bordetella* consists of nine species, four of which are known to cause human respiratory illness (*B. pertussis*, *B. parapertussis*, *B. bronchiseptica*, and *B. holmesii*). *B. pertussis*, first isolated in 1906 by Bordet and Gengou, causes 86% to 95% of whooping cough cases (2, 8–10). It is slow growing and fastidious and infects only humans (2). *B. parapertussis*, first isolated in the 1930s, has been recovered from sheep as well as humans with usually a milder pertussis-like illness than that caused by *B. pertussis* (11, 12). *B. bronchiseptica*, identified in 1910, has rarely been isolated from humans with a pertussis-like cough illness but is normally enzootic in pigs (atrophic rhinitis), dogs (kennel cough), cats, rabbits (snuffles), rodents, and other animals (13–20). *B. holmesii*, first isolated in 1983, is an occasional cause of pertussis-like illness in humans (21, 22).

Virulence Factors and Pathogenesis

B. pertussis contains ~3,121 proteins, many of which are antigenic or biologically active (2). Fimbriae (FIM) are protein projections on the surface of *B. pertussis* which are highly immunogenic and appear to function as adhesins (23–26). Antibody to FIM appears to be important in protection (27, 28). Filamentous hemagglutinin (FHA) is a component of the cell wall of all *Bordetella* spp. (2, 29–37). It is highly immunogenic and is the dominant attachment factor for *Bordetella* in animal model systems (2, 38, 39). FHA is a component of most diphtheria, tetanus, and acellular component pertussis combination (DTaP and Tdap) vaccines; however, it is not clear if antibody to FHA offers protection from disease (27, 28). Pertactin (PRN) is an outer membrane protein of *B. pertussis* that allows it to resist neutrophil-mediated clearance (2, 30, 40–44). Some DTaP vaccines containing PRN in addition to pertussis toxin (PT) and FHA were shown to be more effective than those without (2, 45–47). Anti-PRN antibodies appear to help phagocytosis of *B. pertussis* by host immune cells (44). PT is a critical factor related to mortality in young infants and is unique to *B. pertussis*. PT is responsible for leukocytosis with lymphocytosis seen in *B. pertussis*

infections in unimmunized individuals. Leukocytosis is a major risk factor for severe disease in unprotected infants (2, 31).

Adenylate cyclase toxin is an extracytoplasmic enzyme that impairs host immune cell function by enabling *B. pertussis* to evade nitric oxide killing in macrophages (37, 48–52). Dermonecrotic toxin is a cytoplasmic protein which causes skin necrosis in laboratory animals (53). Tracheal cytotoxin causes local damage to respiratory epithelium in hamster tracheal organ cultures and in cultured hamster tracheal epithelial cells (54, 55). The type III secretion system allows *Bordetella* to translocate effector proteins directly into the plasma membrane or cytoplasm of host cells (56, 57). The lipopolysaccharide (LPS) of *B. pertussis* is similar to the endotoxins of other Gram-negative bacteria and may act as an adhesin (2, 31, 32, 58). It is a major cause of reactions to whole-cell pertussis vaccines (59). Antibody to LPS may lead to reduced colonization (60).

The exact mechanism of pathogenesis in human disease is not fully understood. Infection is initiated in the respiratory tract by the attachment of *B. pertussis* organisms to the cilia of ciliated epithelial cells (26). PT appears to be the major causative factor in deaths in young infants (61–63). PT inhibits G proteins, leading to leukocytosis with lymphocytosis. Extreme leukocytosis, most commonly seen in young infants with pertussis, may result in obstruction of small pulmonary vessels and lead to severe pulmonary hypertension (62). It is also possible that the inhibition of G proteins in other organ cells, such as of the lungs or heart, is the cause of death (61, 63). Tracheal cytotoxin, dermonecrotic toxin, and adenylate cyclase toxin all have been implicated in animal experiments as contributors to local tissue damage in the respiratory tract (31, 53, 55).

The cause of the hallmark paroxysmal cough of disease caused by *B. pertussis* infection is unknown, but bradykinin may play a role (64). During *B. pertussis* infection, bradykinin production is increased, bradykinin has a prolonged half-life in the airways, and responsiveness to bradykinin reception activation is increased. Bradykinin activates sensory nerves implicated in cough.

Various antibodies (agglutinins, hemagglutination-inhibiting antibodies, and bactericidal antibodies) develop after human infection with *B. pertussis* (1). Following infection, IgA, IgE, IgG, and IgM have been shown by enzyme-linked immunosorbent assay (ELISA) to develop in the blood against many of the specific proteins of *B. pertussis* (65–67). With the exception of IgA antibodies, these antibodies also develop in various amounts after immunization. However, lifelong protection does not occur with infection or immunization, leaving the host susceptible for continued reinfection with *B. pertussis* (68–83). The combination and concentrations of antibody needed to confer immunity are not well understood (84). In a nested household contact study looking at the roles of IgG antibodies to PT, FHA, PRN, and FIM 2 in children at the time of household exposure to *B. pertussis*, it was shown that geometric mean values for antibody to PT, PRN, and FIM 2 were higher in uninfected persons than in infected persons; however, in the classification tree and regression analyses, only antibodies against PRN contributed significantly to protection (27). Similarly, a Swedish study found that higher values for antibody to PRN and FIM 2/3 correlated with protection (28). However, some children get pertussis in spite of large amounts of antibody to either or both PRN and FIM (76, 85). Data from studies suggested that high values for antibody to PT may have a blocking effect on the protective effect of antibody to PRN and perhaps FIM (86, 87).

Cell-mediated immune function is altered by *B. pertussis* infection, sometimes depressed and at other times augmented (88). Studies with humans demonstrate a cellular immune response shortly after natural infection with *B. pertussis*, with PT, FHA, and PRN preferentially inducing the synthesis of TH1 cells (89). Immunization with a whole-cell pertus-

sis vaccine resulted in a TH1 response, whereas the response to acellular vaccines is more heterogeneous and involves both TH1 and TH2 cells. Persistent memory T and B cells and anamnestic antibody responses are important in long-term immunity (90).

CLINICAL SYNDROME

Bordetella pertussis Infections

The typical presentation of pertussis is seen in unimmunized children (less frequently in adolescents and adults) and is a three-stage illness: catarrhal, paroxysmal, and convalescent (91). The duration of illness is typically 6 to 12 weeks but sometimes longer. Symptoms develop after an average incubation period of 7 to 10 days (range, 5 to 28 days). The catarrhal phase of disease is a nonspecific, mild clinical syndrome which lasts from 1 to 2 weeks. Nasal congestion, rhinorrhea, lacrimation with conjunctival injection, malaise, mild sore throat, and mild cough similar to a common cold are seen. Fever is not common and if present may suggest a secondary infection. Pertussis is often not suspected during this early phase. It is then followed by worsening cough, and the paroxysmal stage begins. The respiratory secretions are most infectious during the catarrhal stage, but transmission is most efficient during the first 3 weeks after the cough onset. The paroxysmal phase usually lasts 2 to 6 weeks. The paroxysms are repetitive series of 5 to 10 or more forceful coughs during a single expiration, followed by a sudden inspiratory effort leading to the characteristic whoop. Posttussive vomiting is a common phenomenon. Between attacks, the patient appears relatively well. As the illness progresses, episodes of cough paroxysms usually increase in frequency and severity, particularly at night. The convalescent stage, which usually lasts 1 to 12 weeks, is characterized by a decreasing frequency and severity of coughing episodes, whooping, and vomiting. During the recovery period, superimposed viral respiratory infections can trigger a recurrence of paroxysms. Patients with classic pertussis caused by primary infection have leukocytosis associated with lymphocytosis.

However, the clinical presentation in older children, adolescents, and adults can be nonspecific, especially in immunized or partially immune hosts, and can include coryza and cough without the characteristic whoop, making diagnosis and appropriate treatment quite challenging. Several studies have found that from 12% to >30% of persons with acute illness with cough of at least 1 to 2 weeks' duration have evidence of *B. pertussis* infection, while in those with classic pertussis symptoms, such as paroxysmal cough, whoop, and posttussive vomiting, the rate varies from 21 to 86% (2, 69, 71, 84, 91–103). Nonpurulent coryza, lack of fever, and the lack of leukocytosis with lymphocytosis are often found. Also important in pertussis in adults is the occurrence of sweating episodes between paroxysms of coughing. While complications of pertussis in adolescents and adults are less common than in young children, hospitalization can be required and pneumonia and seizures do occur (2). Increased intrathoracic pressure during severe cough episodes can cause pneumothorax (4%), epistaxis, subconjunctival hemorrhage, subdural hematoma, hernia, rectal prolapse, urinary incontinence (28%), rib fracture (4%), and cough syncope (6%) (104). In addition, herniated intervertebral disc, hearing loss, angina attacks, carotid artery dissection, and encephalopathy have been described (2, 69, 91, 92, 97).

Pertussis in neonates and young infants is a unique experience with much higher concern for associated morbidity and mortality risk (2, 91, 105). The spectrum of clinical manifestations varies by age, immunization status, and the presence or absence of transplacentally acquired antibody (106–111). A review of 6 clinical studies looking at characteristics of pertussis in young infants mostly in the first 3 months of life which encompassed over 250 hospitalized babies diagnosed with pertussis found that cough (89 to 100%), apnea (49 to 58%), supplemental oxygen need (59 to 100%), mechanical ventilation (27 to 100%), and pulmonary hypertension (11 to 39%) were notable (105). Most deaths resulting from *B. pertussis* infection occur in neonates and early infancy. The case fatality rate of pertussis in neonates is 1 to 3% (61, 63, 106, 109, 112–122). From 1997 through 2000, 8,276 cases of pertussis were reported to occur in infants in the United States, with 59% leading to hospitalization (123). Eleven percent had pneumonia, 1% had seizures, 0.2% had encephalopathy, and 0.7% died. Eighty-seven percent of these infant cases occurred before 6 months of age. Pertussis in infants less than 6 months of age can present with apnea without the typical cough (124). Seizures can be seen in association with apnea and is thought to be caused by the induced hypoxia. Severe pulmonary hypertension is a relatively common problem in pertussis, especially seen in the first 4 months of life (61, 62, 114, 125–132). Disease severity and mortality correlate directly with the white blood cell (WBC) count and, in particular, the number of lymphocytes (62, 106, 107, 109, 111, 117, 125, 127, 129, 132). WBC counts in the range of 30,000 to more than 100,000 cells/mm^3 are common findings. A California Department of Public Health study looking at 31 infants ≤90 days of age with pertussis who were admitted to pediatric intensive care units has provided useful information relating to risk factors for pulmonary hypertension and death (61). Infants with pulmonary hypertension or who died had higher WBC counts (>30,000 cells/mm^3), had more rapid pulse (>170) and respiratory rates (>70), and were more likely to have pneumonia than those who did not have pulmonary hypertension or die. Pulmonary hypertension and death were associated with a rapidly rising WBC count.

Coinfections with respiratory viruses (respiratory syncytial virus, adenovirus, and influenza viruses) and respiratory bacterial pathogens (*Streptococcus pneumoniae* and *Haemophilus influenzae*) are dependent on local epidemiology and do not necessarily contribute to severity of pertussis (62, 106, 113, 120, 133–140).

A large multicenter study in Australia of defined predictors of disease severity in hospitalized children during an epidemic indicated that an age of <2 months, fever of >37.5°C at presentation, history of premature birth, and identified coinfection were independently associated with severe disease as defined by a pertussis severity score (141). Zamir et al. in Jerusalem also looked for risk markers and vaccination among reported pertussis cases in children under 1 year old (142). They found that low birth weight and high birth order (4th and above) were independent risk markers. Male gender and low socioeconomic status were more frequent among cases. The majority of hospitalized patients were under 4 months of age. However, Heininger and Burckhardt argued that high rates of concomitant infections from these and several other studies are probably explained by the fact that they were detected during respiratory virus outbreaks and in specific patient groups, mainly young children (140).

Shojaei et al. performed a retrospective study to compare clinical and laboratory findings between hospitalized infants with confirmed versus clinical pertussis disease and found that whoop and apnea as well as leukocytosis ($\geq$16,000 WBCs/mm^3) and lymphocytosis ($\geq$11,000 WBCs/mm^3) were more frequently seen in confirmed pertussis cases (143). Those with confirmed pertussis had longer hospital stays and were more likely to require pediatric intensive care. Other studies also have found that whoop is more common in culture-positive than in culture-negative cases (144).

Berger et al. described 127 children hospitalized with critical pertussis and again found the worse severity of illness in patients under 3 months of age (145). Eighty-three percent of patients were under 3 months of age. The median WBC counts were significantly higher in those requiring mechanical ventilation (35,200/mm^3 versus 26,100/mm^3), those with pulmonary hypertension (68,400/mm^3 versus 25,100/mm^3), and nonsurvivors (66,300/mm^3 versus 26,100/mm^3).

Sudden infant death syndrome (SIDS) has been noted in association with *B. pertussis* infection, but whether a cause-and-effect relationship exists is not clear (116, 118, 146, 147). Using PCR, *B. pertussis* DNA was found in nasopharyngeal specimens from 9 (18%) of 51 infants who had sudden, unexpected deaths (116). In a subsequent study, specimens were collected for PCR from 254 infants who experienced sudden, unexplained deaths and from 441 healthy matched controls (146). The rate of PCR-positive results in the sudden-death cases was 5.1%, and that in the controls was 5.3%. In a careful follow-up histopathologic study with unique immunohistochemical staining of specimens from a subset of these fatal cases, no evidence of specific *B. pertussis* pulmonary infection or pathologic features were found (148).

Aside from prevention of disease, early detection can make a difference in outcomes. However, early and/or presenting symptoms in neonates are not often obvious, especially since presenting symptoms of pertussis can overlap with symptoms of viral illness. So, the clinician must have a high suspicion for testing for pertussis and perhaps a low threshold for treating once appropriate testing has been sent. A study comparing hospitalized patients under 3 months of age with confirmed pertussis versus respiratory syncytial virus or influenza virus indicated several features that should alert clinicians to pertussis, including paroxysmal cough, posttussive emesis, lack of congestion, and lack of fever (139).

OTHER *BORDETELLA* INFECTIONS

Bordetella parapertussis

B. parapertussis infection in children can range from atypical respiratory disease to mild or typical pertussis (2). Studies comparing *B. pertussis* and *B. parapertussis* cough etiologies show that *B. parapertussis* infection can have a very significant cough illness with paroxysms but usually is less severe in terms of apnea, cyanosis, whoop, and posttussive emesis (9, 149). Concomitant infections with *B.pertussis* and *B. parapertussis* may occur (150–152).

During the period from 2008 to 2010, clinical specimens from 9 states in the United States were tested by PCR for *B. pertussis* and *B. parapertussis* in a commercial laboratory (10). Of the positive samples, 13.9% were identified as containing *B. parapertussis*. The *B. parapertussis*-positive samples had no seasonal periodicity, whereas the *B. pertussis* positives peaked between weeks 22 and 38 each year.

Bordetella bronchiseptica

B. bronchiseptica causes respiratory infections in at least 18 different mammals (32). Most notable are atrophic rhinitis in pigs, kennel cough (rhinotracheitis) in dogs, and bronchopneumonia in rabbits and other laboratory animals. Otherwise healthy children who became infected with *B. bronchiseptica* after being exposed to farm animals or pets usually had pertussis-like illnesses (2).

Occasional infections in humans have been noted during the last 40 years, with the majority occurring in immunocompromised adults, including patients with AIDS (15, 153–155). Respiratory infections have ranged from mild upper respiratory illnesses to pneumonia. In patients with AIDS, the pneumonia frequently is cavitary. Sinusitis and bronchitis also occur.

Bordetella holmesii

B. holmesii has been isolated from nasopharyngeal specimens from patients with pertussis-like illnesses in the United States, France, Canada, and the Netherlands (156–158). The incidence of pertussis-like illness due to *B. holmesii* is unknown.

EPIDEMIOLOGY

Transmission of bordetellae is thought to occur by respiratory droplets from a coughing patient that directly infect a susceptible host or contaminate surfaces that then act as fomites of disease to a host who autoinoculates infection (31). Transmissibility is greatest early in the illness, that is, during the catarrhal and early paroxysmal phases.

B. pertussis is an extremely infectious organism, with an estimated 12 to 17 secondary cases produced by a typical primary case in an entirely susceptible population (86, 159, 160). Attack rates in susceptible household contacts range from 70 to 100% (1, 31). In the prevaccine era in the United States, the average attack rate of reported pertussis was 157 per 100,000 population (1). With the introduction and widespread use of whole-cell pertussis vaccines, the attack rate of reported pertussis in the United State fell dramatically, to a rate of between 0.5 and 1.0 per 100,000 population from 1976 to 1982. Then, from 1982 to 2012, the attack rate curve shifted modestly upward and reached 15.2 per 100,000 in 2012 (161). Pertussis epidemics in the prevaccine era occurred at 2- to 5-year intervals, and these cycles have continued in the vaccine era (162, 163).

In the prevaccine era, the majority of cases were seen in 1- to 9-year-olds (<1 year, 7.5%; 1 to 4 years, 41.1%; 5 to 9 years, 46.0%; 10 to 14 years, 4.1%; and 15 years and older, 0.9%.) (91, 164). Following widespread pediatric immunization in the United States, a marked reduction in reported cases of pertussis was seen, as well as a major shift in the percentages by age category, with the majority of illness from 1978 to 1981 being seen in young children (<1 year, 53.5%; 1 to 4 years, 26.5%; 5 to 9 years, 8.2%; 10 to 14 years, 5.4%; and 15 years or older, 6.5%) (91). In contrast, U.S. data for 2010 revealed the following age proportions for cases: younger than 1 year, 15%; 1 to 6 years, 22%; 7 to 10 years, 18%; 10 to 19 years, 20%; and 20 years or older, 25%. Hence, pertussis in adolescents and adults is comparatively frequent and thereby an important source of *B. pertussis* infection of unimmunized or partially immunized children (165).

Multiple studies have demonstrated that the source of infection in infants usually is a family member (84, 110, 113, 166–168). In a study of 616 infant cases, the source was identified in 43% (167). A family member was the source 75% of the time, and the mother was the most common source (32%). Of the source persons, 56% were adults and 20% were 10 to 19 years of age. In studies of household contacts, asymptomatic infections in family members are common occurrences (84, 169, 170). Deen et al. (84) found that 52 (46%) of 114 household contacts who remained well had laboratory evidence of *B. pertussis* infection. In another study, 21 of 399 healthy infants who were controls in a study of SIDS had PCR-positive nasopharyngeal samples (146). In a study at one hospital during the California pertussis epidemic of 2009-2010, 32 infants under 3 months of age were hospitalized with pertussis, and household coughing contacts were reported for 24 out of the 32 patients with pertussis (75%); the patient's mother was the primary contact for 10 patients (42%), and a sibling was the contact for 11 patients (46%) (139). In recent years, a shift in the most common source of infant pertussis infection from mothers to siblings has been observed in the United States (171). Among 1,306 cases of pertussis in infants, a source of infection was identified in 569, and of these, 35.5% were siblings, 20.6% were mothers, and 10.0% were fathers.

DIAGNOSIS

Differential Diagnosis

Other agents besides *B. pertussis* which can cause pertussis-like symptoms include other *Bordetella* species, adenovirus, respiratory syncytial virus, bocavirus, other respiratory viruses, *Mycoplasma pneumoniae*, *Chlamydia pneumoniae*, *Mycobacterium tuberculosis*, and endemic fungi. In addition, sinusitis, gastroesophageal reflex, aspirated foreign body, asthma, bacterial pneumonia, and cystic fibrosis also should be considered as differential diagnoses for a prolonged cough (2, 104). In typical pertussis, however, the clinical diagnosis should be apparent based on the paroxysmal cough with posttussive vomiting and whooping and lack of significant fever. However, the cause of the illness can be *B. pertussis, B. parapertussis, B. holmesii*, and perhaps *B. bronchiseptica*. The presence of leukocytosis with lymphocytosis in a child with a cough illness or the presence of apnea in an infant is a strong indication that the illness is caused by *B. pertussis* and not a different *Bordetella* sp. (9).

Specific Diagnosis

Growth of *B. pertussis* or other *Bordetella* spp. on appropriate culture media confirms the diagnosis. However, by demonstrating the presence of specific antibodies and, more commonly, by PCR techniques, the diagnosis can also be reached. *Bordetella* spp. can be recovered from nasopharyngeal specimens, with the highest probability of isolation within the first 3 weeks of cough (91, 144, 172). In classic disease in children, the culture will be positive in approximately 80% of cases if the specimen is obtained within 2 weeks of the onset of cough and antibiotics have not been administered previously (67, 144).

Since the late 1980s, numerous PCR assays with primers derived from many different chromosomal regions have been developed for the diagnosis of *B. pertussis, B. parapertussis, B. holmesii*, and *B. bronchiseptica* infections, and they have been evaluated in multiple studies by comparison with culture and clinically typical pertussis (85, 96, 173–190). PCR has the advantage of having much higher sensitivity than that of conventional culture. At present, the most commonly used primers for the diagnosis of pertussis include IS481 and IS1001 (2, 10, 180, 188). False-positive results are a potential problem with the use of PCR for establishing the diagnosis of pertussis (191, 192).

Diagnosis of *B. pertussis* with the use of ELISA can be helpful in cases where culture or PCR detection is suboptimal, such as with illness duration of >3 weeks or prior antibiotic use (2). Natural infection with *B. pertussis* is followed by a rise in serum concentrations of IgA, IgG, and IgM antibodies to specific antigens (anti-PT and anti-FHA) of the organism (66, 67, 99, 193–197). Primary immunization induces mainly IgM and IgG, but not IgA, antibodies. Serologic testing for *B. pertussis* infection in the clinical setting is not well standardized but is widely available in Europe and North America (96). Demonstration of a significant increase in antibody values between acute-phase and convalescent-phase serum specimens serves as proof of acute infection. Alternatively, a single serum specimen can be used to demonstrate recent infection (71, 84, 99, 103, 198). *B. parapertussis* infection induces cross-reacting antibodies to *B. pertussis* FHA; therefore, use of this antigen alone cannot differentiate *B. pertussis* from *B. parapertussis* infection (196, 199). Not all infected persons develop antibody responses to PT. In children, approximately 25% lack an adequate response, as do approximately 10% of adolescents and adults (196).

Today in clinical practice, the laboratory diagnosis of pertussis should be approached as follows. In all cases in which the cough illness is of less than 2 weeks' duration in adolescents and adults or 3 weeks' duration in children, a nasopharyngeal specimen should be obtained for culture or PCR. In adults who have had cough for more than 2 weeks' duration, single-serum ELISA is the preferred method provided they have not been immunized against pertussis in the previous 12 months (96). This method also can be used for children if they have not been immunized within a year. Serology plays no role in diagnosing pertussis in infants <6 months of age due to interfering maternal antibodies. At present, many commercial laboratories offer single-serum diagnostic tests for *B. pertussis*, and almost all the offered tests lack specificity. Any test that employs the whole organism is fraught with false-positive results. Tests that report specific IgM antibodies also are unreliable. The greatest sensitivity and specificity for the serologic diagnosis of *B. pertussis* infection are achieved by ELISA or an ELISA-like test with the measurement of IgG and IgA antibodies to PT. Single high values of IgG or IgA antibodies to PT are indicative of infection (2).

TREATMENT

Antibiotics

Antibiotic therapy for confirmed cases and prophylaxis for close contacts is recommended (200). Early treatment of pertussis with recommended antimicrobials may ameliorate the severity and reduce the duration of clinical symptoms, eliminate *B. pertussis* from the nasopharynx, shorten the period of infectivity, and thereby reduce the risk of secondary spread to susceptible individuals. Starting treatment after 3 weeks of paroxysmal cough does little to change the cough illness in the affected individual but accelerates time to culture negativity and decreases spread to others (201).

Several antibiotics have *in vitro* efficacy against *B. pertussis* (202–205). The first choice for treatment since the 1970s has been oral erythromycin; it ameliorates the symptoms if it is given early during the course of the illness and eliminates the organism from the nasopharynx within a few days, thereby shortening the period of contagiousness (203). The dose for children is 40 to 50 mg/kg (of body weight)/day given every 6 (to 8) h for 14 days. A 7-day course of erythromycin estolate was shown in a large study in Canada to be as efficacious as 14 days of treatment (206).

The newer macrolides azithromycin (10 mg/kg on day 1 and 5 mg/kg on days 2 to 5 as a single dose for 5 days for children) and clarithromycin (15 to 20 mg/kg/day in two divided doses for 7 days for children) also can be expected to be effective (200, 205). Although rare, the use of erythromycin in young infants is associated with hypertrophic pyloric stenosis, so parents need to be educated about the symptoms of this potential risk (207–209). Because of this risk, the Centers for Disease Control and Prevention (CDC) and several European authorities recommend treating neonates with azithromycin rather than erythromycin (205, 210). Trimethoprim-sulfamethoxazole can be used as an alternative agent in those who cannot tolerate erythromycin (211). Table 1 shows the CDC's published recommended antimicrobial treatment and postexposure prophylaxis for pertussis by age group. Erythromycin resistance, macrolide resistance, and fluoroquinolone resistance have rarely been found (137, 212–215). No significant macrolide resistance is suspected at this time, but with fewer centers using culture methods for diagnosis, we may not identify emerging resistance patterns quickly any longer.

Patients infected with *B. parapertussis* and *B. holmesii* also can be treated with macrolides, but *B. bronchiseptica* usually is resistant to erythromycin, so alternative therapy is necessary (2). *B. bronchiseptica* strains usually are sensitive to aminoglycosides, extended-spectrum penicillins, tetracyclines, quinolones, and trimethoprim-sulfamethoxazole.

Supportive Care

In addition to antibiotic therapy, supportive care is a mainstay of pertussis management, especially in hospitalized patients. This includes proper hydration and nutrition as well

TABLE 1 Recommended antimicrobial treatment and postexposure prophylaxis for pertussis, by age group

Age group	Primary agents			Alternate agent, TMP-SMZ[a]
	Azithromycin	Erythromycin	Clarithromycin	
<1 mo	Recommended agent. 10 mg/kg per day in a single dose for 5 days (limited safety data available)	Not preferred. Associated with infantile hypertrophic pyloric stenosis. Use if azithromycin is unavailable; 40–50 mg/kg per day in 4 divided doses for 14 days	Not recommended (safety data unavailable)	Contraindications for infants ages <2 mo (risk for kernicterus)
1–5 mo	10 mg/kg per day in a single dose for 5 days	40–50 mg/kg per day in 4 divided doses for 14 days	15 mg/kg per day in 2 divided doses for 7 days	Contraindicated at age <2 mo. For infants aged >2 mo, TMP at 8 mg/kg per day and SMZ at 40 mg/kg per day in 2 divided doses for 14 days
Infants (aged >6 mo) and children	10 mg/kg in a single dose on day 1 and then 5 mg/kg per day (maximum: 500 mg) on days 2–5	40–50 mg/kg per day (maximum: 2 g per day) in 4 divided doses for 14 days	15 mg/kg per day in 2 divided doses (maximum: 1 g per day) for 7 days	TMP at 8 mg/kg per day and SMZ at 40 mg/kg per day in 2 divided doses for 14 days
Adults	500 mg in a single dose on day 1 then 250 mg per day on days 2–5	2 g per day in 4 divided doses for 14 days	1 g per day in 2 divided doses for 7 days	TMP at 320 mg per day and SMZ at 1,600 mg per day in 2 divided doses for 14 days

[a]Trimethoprim-sulfamethoxazole (TMP-SMZ) can be used as an alternate to macrolides in patients aged ≥2 months who are allergic to macrolides, who cannot tolerate macrolides, or who are infected with a rare macrolide-resistant strain of *Bordetella pertussis*.

as avoidance of factors that provoke coughing attacks. In the hospital, gentle suction to remove secretions and well-humidified oxygen may be required, particularly for infants with pneumonia and significant respiratory distress. In severe infections, assisted ventilation may be necessary.

Infants who develop severe pulmonary hypertension and develop respiratory and cardiovascular failure respond poorly to vasodilators and frequently require extracorporeal membrane oxygenation. Data suggest that refractory pulmonary hypertension results from the extreme leukocytosis with lymphocytosis; hence, WBC-reducing measures such as exchange transfusion (ET) could be life-saving (61, 127, 129, 216–218). ET may be better than leukofiltration because it potentially also removes circulating PT, which inhibits other G proteins that might also contribute to cardiac or pulmonary failure, in addition to reducing the WBC count.

However, data on the effectiveness of ET are lacking. A retrospective analysis of 10 young infants in California (2005 to 2011) indicated that 5 died and 5 survived (218). All infants had WBC counts of $\geq 62,000$ cells/mm^3, and all were intubated. Nine of the 10 had pneumonia. The median WBC count among fatal cases was 76,000/mm^3, and it was 82,000/mm^3 among cases with survivors. All five infants who died had pulmonary hypertension, shock/hypotension, and pneumonia; four of five had organ failure; three of five received extracorporeal membrane oxygenation; and none had seizures.

A literature review revealed limited further data on ET, but the conclusion was that WBC reduction was most successful when done early in the course of a complicated illness, as in patients already suffering significant complications, presumably very little could change the course of illness. In our opinion, ET for management of very severe pertussis in young infants is a biologically sound procedure and the decision for ET should be based on the early appearance of pneumonia, the presence of pulmonary hy-

pertension, and the rapidity in the rise of the WBC count (145, 218, 219).

The use of corticosteroids in the treatment of pertussis has received attention (220, 221). Cortisone treatment in the murine model of pertussis increased the mortality rate (222). In a study by Roberts and associates (223), dexamethasone treatment did not shorten the course of hospitalization compared with that for untreated controls.

The use of salbutamol has also been suggested as having some value, but no benefit was noted in three studies reviewed by Bettiol and coworkers (220, 224). Pillay and Swingler (225) reviewed the symptomatic treatment of pertussis and found no statistically significant benefit for the use of diphenhydramine, dexamethasone, or salbutamol.

PREVENTION

Immunization

Whole-cell vaccines (DTwP)

The first pertussis vaccines were developed in the 1920s, and effective vaccines have enjoyed worldwide use since the late 1940s (1, 2, 31). From 1943 to 1976, a 150-fold reduction in the pertussis attack rate was noted in association with widespread childhood pertussis immunization in the United States. However, concerns for association with SIDS and "vaccine encephalopathy" led to avoidance of a whole-cell pertussis component in diphtheria-tetanus- pertussis combination vaccines (DTwP) in many countries. The connection with SIDS or "vaccine encephalopathy" with DTwP has been refuted since (2, 91, 226). However, DTwP immunization is associated with many local and systemic side effects (redness and induration at the injection site, fever, drowsiness, fretfulness, vomiting, anorexia, and persistent crying), high-pitched unusual crying in 0.1%, convulsions in 0.06%, and hypotonic-hyporesponsive episodes in 0.06% (59).

Acellular Vaccines (DTaP and Tdap)

The adverse reactions associated with whole-cell pertussis component vaccines led to the development of acellular pertussis component combination (DTaP) vaccines, which were less frequently associated with adverse events but were also associated with reduced effectiveness. Research in the 1970s showed that three *B. pertussis* antigens (PT, FHA, and LPS) were liberated into the medium during culture and that these antigens could be concentrated and separated by density gradient centrifugation (31, 227, 228). This finding allowed for the development and production of acellular vaccines with minimal or no LPS and different amounts of PT, FHA, FIM 2, and PRN (228–231). Efficacy trials showed that three- and four-component vaccines (containing PRN and FIM as well as PT and FHA) had greater efficacy than PT or PT-FHA vaccines (2, 91, 232). Currently, two vaccines are routinely used in the United States and throughout much of the world. Because DTaP vaccines do not contain LPS, they are less reactogenic than DTwP vaccines. Temporally related persistent crying, hypotonic-hyporesponsive episodes, and seizures were rare events after receipt of immunization with DTaP vaccines in the efficacy trials (91, 232, 233).

In ~2005, two acellular pertussis component, diphtheria, and tetanus toxoid vaccines (Tdap vaccines) became available for use in adolescents and adults (234–239). Both vaccines elicit vigorous antibody responses to the antigens that they contain after a single dose.

DTaP vaccines were adopted for routine use in infants and young children in many countries in the late 1990s, and the use of DTwP vaccines was discontinued. In many of the same countries, Tdap vaccines have been put into routine use in preadolescents and adolescents and are selectively used in adults.

Immunization schedules, recommendations, and contraindications

Although there are many different schedules in use throughout the world for both DTaP and DTP vaccines, the most frequently used schedules in infants are a primary series at 6, 10, and 14 weeks (expanded program on immunization by the WHO) and 2, 4, and 6 months. In the United States and some other countries, booster doses of DTaP are given during the first half of the second year of life and at 4 to 6 years of age. Other primary schedules used in some countries rely on 2 doses in the first year of life (given at 2 and 4 or 3 and 5 months of age) followed by a third dose at 11 or 12 months of age.

Tdap schedules vary considerably throughout the world and are also changing. The most common recommendation is for universal immunization of preadolescents and adolescents and the selective immunization of adults. Various "cocooning" programs have been or are being established (240–247). These programs include immunization of mothers-to-be during the 2nd or 3rd trimester of pregnancy, postpartum immunization of the mother who was not immunized during pregnancy, and immunization of the father, grandparents, and siblings (cocooning strategy).

In July 2010, the California Department of Public Health recommended use of Tdap vaccine in pregnant women (248). In June 2011, the Advisory Committee on Immunization Practices (ACIP) recommended Tdap vaccine after 20 weeks of pregnancy for those who previously had not received Tdap (240). Pregnant women were immunized after delivery, prior to discharge from the hospital. Munoz et al. showed that maternal vaccination during pregnancy is associated with significantly higher levels of pertussis antibodies (including antibody to PT) at birth and at 2 months, both in mothers and in infants (249). Antibody to PT prevents all but mild illness in children (250). Antibody to the A subunit of PT in the sera of young infants born to pregnant women vaccinated during pregnancy prevents severe leukocytosis with lymphocytosis in these infants (2).

Due to waning antibody, current recommendations are to immunize again with each subsequent pregnancy. In 2012, the ACIP voted to recommend use of Tdap during every pregnancy (251). Based on antibody kinetic studies, maternal anti-pertussis antibodies are short lived, repeat vaccines are safe and well tolerated, and vaccinating during the third trimester (optimally at weeks 30 to 32 of pregnancy) would provide the highest antibody transfer and protection to the newborn (252–259).

Moreover, one recent study showed lower median cord blood PT, FHA, and PRN IgG antibody values in 20 infants with PCR-confirmed pertussis before 6 months of age than for 80 age-matched control infants (10.5 versus 13.5 IU/ml for anti-PT, 14.5 versus 18.0 IU/ml for anti-FHA, and 6.0 versus 9.0 IU/ml for anti-PRN). These findings support the concept of infant protection by maternal antibodies and the strategy of pertussis booster immunization in pregnant women (253). A case-control study in England and Wales between October 2012 and July 2013 evaluating infants <8 weeks of age at onset with pertussis infection found that the mothers of 10 infected infants (17%) and 39 controls (71%) had received pertussis vaccine in pregnancy, giving an unadjusted vaccine effectiveness of 91% and an adjusted effectiveness of 93% (260). In their study of 33 pregnant women who received Tdap between 30 and 32 weeks, Munoz et al. found no Tdap-associated serious adverse events in women or infants, and growth and development were similar in the treatment and placebo infant groups (249). Injection site and systemic reactogenicity rates in pregnant women were not significantly different from those observed among postpartum or non-pregnant women. In a large California retrospective observational cohort study of women with singleton pregnancies that ended in live birth, Tdap during pregnancy was not associated with increased risk of hypertensive disorders of pregnancy or preterm or small-for-gestational-age birth, although a small but statistically significant increased risk of chorioamnionitis was ob-

served (adjusted relative ratio, 1.19) (261). Another large single-center retrospective study comparing pregnancy outcomes between those who accepted or declined Tdap at 32 weeks of gestation found no increase in chorioamnionitis in vaccinated women (262). There was also no difference in stillbirths, major malformations, 5-min Apgar score, cord blood pH, or neonatal complications, including ventilation requirements, sepsis, intraventricular hemorrhage, or death. Morgan et al. also compared women who received Tdap vaccination during the current and a prior pregnancy in the past 5 years compared with multiparous women who received Tdap only in the current pregnancy, and no difference in neonatal outcomes was noted, pointing to the safety of repeated Tdap administration with subsequent pregnancies (262).

There is concern regarding maternal Tdap immunization and the blunting of the immune response of the infant to the primary immunization series. This was addressed in a recent study by Hardy-Fairbanks et al. (258). They reported that in the critical period of susceptibility from birth to 2 months of age, the pertussis antibody in infants of mothers vaccinated with Tdap during pregnancy remained higher than those of control infants (3.2- to 22.8-fold greater). Even though antibody to pertussis antigens was lower in the Tdap group after the primary series, there was not a notable difference before and after the booster DTaP at 12 to 18 months. Hence, maternal Tdap immunization offered infants protection during the most vulnerable period, when morbidity and mortality associated with infant pertussis is the greatest.

Another approach is to immunize infants at birth, followed by an accelerated schedule; this should provide some early protection and prevent deaths. However, there is also concern that immunization at birth blunts the subsequent immune response of the infant following the routine schedule at 2, 4, and 6 months (263–267). This approach has not been adopted. Tiwari et al. analyzed fatal and nonfatal pertussis cases in infants and found that the first pertussis vaccine dose and antibiotic treatment protect against death, hospitalization, and pneumonia (268). Compared with no vaccine doses, the receipt of a ≥1 pertussis vaccine doses was strongly protective against fatal pertussis (odds ratio, 0.17; 95% confidence interval, 0.08 to 0.6).

Over the years, pertussis vaccine recommendations have undergone many changes. In the United States, the most recent recommendations of the Committee on Infectious Diseases of the American Academy of Pediatrics and the ACIP generally should be followed (200, 269). Contraindications to pertussis vaccine include severe allergic reaction after a previous dose or to a vaccine component or encephalopathy not attributable to another cause within 7 days of vaccination. Precautions include moderate or severe illness with or without fever, Guillain-Barré syndrome within 6 weeks of a prior dose of vaccine, Arthus-type reaction, progressive or unstable neurologic disorder, uncontrolled seizures, or progressive encephalopathy until a treatment regimen has been established and the condition stabilized (270). Precautions specifically listed for either whole-cell DTP or DTaP include temperature of ≥105°F within 48 h not attributable to another identifiable cause, collapse, or shock-like state (hypotonic hyporesponsive episode) within 48 h, persistent crying lasting greater than or equal to 3 h occurring within 48 h, and convulsions with or without fever within 3 days (271).

WHY THE RESURGENCE OF PERTUSSIS?

There have been several possible reasons postulated for the resurgence of reported pertussis. These include molecular changes in the organism and increased awareness and diagnostic capabilities, as well as lessened vaccine efficacy and waning immunity (74, 272). Of these, evidence of waning immunity with current vaccines and schedules (273)

and targeted immunization to protect susceptible and fragile populations have been the main public health challenges.

There is evidence that the switch from whole-cell pertussis vaccines to acellular products has led to more rapidly waning immunity and, as a result, an upsurge in pertussis cases. A recent study after the 2012 Washington state pertussis epidemic looked at Tdap vaccine efficacy and duration of protection. It was a matched case-control study which included adolescents 11 to 19 years of age with suspected, probable, and confirmed pertussis. Among adolescents who received all-acellular vaccines, the investigators concluded that overall, Tdap vaccine effectiveness was 73% at 1 year and declined to 34% at 2 to 4 years (274). In Wisconsin's 2012 pertussis outbreak, a similar study was done also looking at vaccine effectiveness of Tdap for preventing pertussis among adolescents during a statewide outbreak of pertussis. The investigators found that Tdap effectiveness in preventing laboratory-confirmed pertussis during the 2012 statewide outbreak decreased rapidly with increasing time since Tdap receipt, with values of 75.3%, 68.2%, 34.5%, and 11.9% among those who received Tdap during 2012, 2011, 2010, and 2009/2008, respectively (275). Both studies revealed waning protection, indicating that it is likely is a major contributor to increasing pertussis incidence in this age group. A recent meta-analysis of studies that contained a measure of long-term immunity to pertussis after 3 or 5 doses of DTaP found evidence of waning immunity and estimated that the average duration of vaccine protection from DTaP is approximately 3 years, assuming 85% vaccine efficacy (276).

Factors thought to be most important relating to DTaP vaccine failure are the decay of antibody over time; a TH1/TH2 response (those who were primed by DTaP) versus a TH1, TH17 cellular response (those who were primed in infancy by infection or DTP); incomplete antigen package; incorrect balance of antigens in the vaccine;

linked-epitope suppression; and the occurrence of pertactin-deficient *Bordetella pertussis* strains (73, 76, 277–279).

To protect those at greatest risk from this disease, several strategies have been put into place. Cocooning by immunizing those around unimmunized babies was recommended. Teenagers were boosted with Tdap after the rise of teens as a source of pertussis was seen. Many adults (pregnant mothers and those who live with or care for young children) got a dose of Tdap. However, there are still no recommendations of repeat or booster vaccines for adults who recently got a Tdap vaccination, despite evidence that antibody wanes after 2 to 3 years. Natural infection also does not result in lasting immunity.

Since 2006, the ACIP has recommended targeted immunization of postpartum women and close contacts of infants (104). However, Tdap immunization of postpartum women alone was shown to not be sufficient to reduce pertussis illness in infants ≤6 months of age (242). Pertussis contacts are often siblings and other household members. With this in mind, various cocooning programs have been or are being established (240–247). However, successful comprehensive immunization is difficult to achieve. These programs include postpartum immunization of the mother, the father, grandparents, and siblings and immunization of mothers-to-be during the 2nd or 3rd trimester of pregnancy. A California study where Tdap vaccine was offered during visiting hours to contacts 7 years of age and older and to postpartum patients who had not received Tdap during pregnancy later estimated on the basis of retrospective phone interviews that 84.8% of all family members received Tdap and 76% of households reported a complete cocoon, while for the control group, only 52.2% and 29.3%, respectively, were immunized (280). However, cocooning strategies require significant financial and human resources and are difficult to implement; therefore, many programs have not reported such success (281).

A study in the greater Houston metropolitan area expanding access to free Tdap vaccine to contacts (aside from mothers) of young infants did not show reduced severe pertussis in infants (282). In fact, the investigators found that the age at diagnosis of pertussis actually decreased after maternal postpartum immunization and cocooning were introduced, and more infants were admitted to the intensive care unit, possibly reflecting the increased awareness about the need for close monitoring for pertussis complications. A Washington state study looking at the impact of the 2012 pertussis epidemic on infant vaccination did not find a difference in statewide up-to-date status between time points preepidemic, during the epidemic, or postepidemic (283). National pertussis immunization coverage for adults 19 to 64 years of age who reported living with an infant <1 year of age was 25.9% in 2012, despite widely known recommendations for household contact immunization (284).

In 2010, there were 10 infant deaths for the 9,120 cases of pertussis reported in the United States. In 2014, only 3 infant deaths were reported despite >10,000 notified cases of pertussis. This may be in part due to the ACIP recommendation in 2011, when Tdap during pregnancy was recommended in an effort to protect pregnant women and their infants (240, 285).

With now ample evidence of the safety and immunogenicity of Tdap during pregnancy, pertussis immunization rates during pregnancy are <20%, despite the strong recommendation by the ACIP for maternal immunization (286, 287). In a study by the CDC in 16 states and New York City participating in the Pregnancy Risk Assessment Monitoring System supplemental data collection, the median proportions of women with live births from September to December 2011 who reported receiving Tdap vaccination before pregnancy, during pregnancy, and after delivery were 13.9%, 9.8% and 30.9%, respectively (288). They also found that vaccination coverage was lower for non-Hispanic black women, those with Medicaid health care coverage for prenatal care, and those starting prenatal care after the first trimester of pregnancy. Implementing prenatal vaccination in the United States has been difficult due to financial concerns such as cost of vaccine, vaccine storage and maintenance, and inadequate reimbursement (286, 289). A study in Wisconsin showed that a health care provider recommendation and offer of vaccination are among the strongest predictors of whether a woman will be vaccinated during pregnancy. After the February 2013 ACIP recommendation, Tdap vaccination of pregnant women in Wisconsin steadily increased. The percentage of women who received Tdap during pregnancy increased from 13.8% of women delivering during January 2013 (63.1% of whom received Tdap 2 to 13 weeks before delivery) to 51.0% of women delivering during March 2014 (90.9% of whom received Tdap 2 to 13 weeks before delivery) (290). During the 2014 California epidemic, of 211 infants aged <4 months whose mothers' Tdap immunization histories were available, only 17% had mothers who reported receiving Tdap at 27 to 36 weeks' gestation during the most recent pregnancy (7).

Studies comparing the cost benefit of cocooning strategies versus immunization of pregnant women have been favorable towards immunizing pregnant women. This strategy is felt to prevent a larger number of pertussis cases, hospitalizations, and deaths in infants <1 year old while also being more cost-effective (291, 292). Neonatal vaccination against pertussis is under investigation as well (267).

CONCLUSIONS

Pertussis has been emerging in the United States and many other countries over the last decade. Thanks to ongoing research and public health efforts, there has been much progress in the awareness of pertussis by health care providers, greater availability of rapid and sensitive PCR diagnostic methods, and significantly improved understanding of the immune response to vaccines and natural illness. Our goal as health care providers is to continue these efforts in order to prevent devastating pertussis infections from taking the lives of our most fragile hosts, very young infants. Continued education efforts to immunize children and adults, in particular pregnant women, need to remain strong given that whooping cough is here to stay for the foreseeable future. Further research efforts should be concentrated on exploring the option of immunizing newborns and developing vaccines with long-lasting efficacy. In the meantime, educating ourselves on rapid recognition and appropriate treatment of *B. pertussis* infection continues to be crucial for better control of this disease.

ACKNOWLEDGMENTS

UH is a member of The Global Pertussis Initiative (GPI) which is supported by Sanofi Pasteur SA. The views and opinions expressed in this article are solely those of the author independent of the GPI or Sanofi Pasteur SA.

CITATION

Nieves DJ, Heininger U. 2016. *Bordetella pertussis*. Microbiol Spectrum 4(3):EI10-0008-2015.

REFERENCES

1. **Cherry JD.** 1984. The epidemiology of pertussis and pertussis immunization in the United Kingdom and the United States: a comparative study. *Curr Probl Pediatr* **14**(2):1–78.
2. **Mattoo S, Cherry JD.** 2005. Molecular pathogenesis, epidemiology, and clinical manifestations of respiratory infections due to *Bordetella pertussis* and other *Bordetella* subspecies. *Clin Microbiol Rev* **18**:326–382.
3. **Center for Disease Control and Prevention.** 2015. *Pertussis (whooping cough); surveillance and reporting.* Centers for Disease Control and

Prevention, Atlanta, GA. http://www.cdc.gov/pertussis/surv-reporting.html.

4. **World Health Organization.** 2015. *Pertussis.* World Health Organization, Geneva, Switzerland. http://www.who.int/immunization/monitoring_surveillance/burden/vpd/surveillance_type/passive/pertussis/en/. (Updated 4 August 2015.)

5. **Centers for Disease Contol and Prevention.** 2015. 2014 final pertussis surveillance report. *MMWR Morb Mortal Wkly Rep* **63**(53). http://www.cdc.gov/pertussis/downloads/pertussis-surv-report-2014.pdf.

6. **Murray EL, Nieves D, Bradley JS, Gargas J, Mason WH, Lehman D, Harriman K, Cherry JD.** 2013. Characteristics of severe *Bordetella pertussis* infection among infants ≤90 days of age admitted to pediatric intensive care units —Southern California, September 2009–June 2011. *J Pediatr Infect Dis* **2:**1–6.

7. **Winter K, Glaser C, Watt J, Harriman K, Centers for Disease Control and Prevention.** 2014. Pertussis epidemic—California, 2014. *MMWR Morb Mortal Wkly Rep* **63:**1129–1132.

8. **Gordon JE, Hood RI.** 1951. Whooping cough and its epidemiological anomalies. *Am J Med Sci* **222:**333–361.

9. **Heininger U, Stehr K, Schmitt-Grohe S, Lorenz C, Rost R, Christenson PD, Uberall M, Cherry JD.** 1994. Clinical characteristics of illness caused by *Bordetella parapertussis* compared with illness caused by *Bordetella pertussis. Pediatr Infect Dis* **13:**306–309.

10. **Cherry JD, Seaton BL.** 2012. Patterns of *Bordetella parapertussis* respiratory illnesses: 2008–2010. *Clin Infect Dis* **54:**534–537.

11. **Eldering G, Kendrick P.** 1938. *Bacillus parapertussis*: a species resembling both *Bacillus pertussis* and *Bacillus bronchisepticus* but identical with neither. *J Bacteriol* **35:**561–572.

12. **Porter JF, Connor K, Donachie W.** 1994. Isolation and characterization of *Bordetella parapertussis*-like bacteria from ovine lungs. *Microbiology* **140**(Part 2):**255–261.

13. **Stefanelli P, Mastrantonio P, Hausman SZ, Giuliano M, Burns DL.** 1997. Molecular characterization of two *Bordetella bronchiseptica* strains isolated from children with coughs. *J Clin Microbiol* **35:**1550–1555.

14. **Tamion F, Girault C, Chevron V, Pestel M, Bonmarchand G.** 1996. *Bordetella bronchoseptica* pneumonia with shock in an immunocompetent patient. *Scand J Infect Dis* **28:**197–198.

15. **Woolfrey BF, Moody JA.** 1991. Human infections associated with *Bordetella bronchiseptica. Clin Microbiol Rev* **4:**243–255.

16. **Bauwens JE, Spach DH, Schacker TW, Mustafa MM, Bowden RA.** 1992. *Bordetella bronchiseptica* pneumonia and bacteremia following bone marrow transplantation. *J Clin Microbiol* **30:**2474–2475.

17. **Gueirard P, Weber C, Le Coustumier A, Guiso N.** 1995. Human *Bordetella bronchiseptica* infection related to contact with infected animals: persistence of bacteria in host. *J Clin Microbiol* **33:**2002–2006.

18. **Kontor EJ, Wegrzyn RJ, Goodnow RA.** 1981. Canine infectious tracheobronchitis: effects of an intranasal live canine parainfluenza-*Bordetella bronchiseptica* vaccine on viral shedding and clinical tracheobronchitis (kennel cough). *Am J Vet Res* **42:**1694–1698.

19. **Magyar T, Chanter N, Lax AJ, Rutter JM, Hall GA.** 1988. The pathogenesis of turbinate atrophy in pigs caused by *Bordetella bronchiseptica. Vet Microbiol* **18:**135–146.

20. **Ner Z, Ross LA, Horn MV, Keens TG, MacLaughlin EF, Starnes VA, Woo MS.** 2003. *Bordetella bronchiseptica* infection in pediatric lung transplant recipients. *Pediatr Transplant* **7:**413–417.

21. **Yih WK, Silva EA, Ida J, Harrington N, Lett SM, George H.** 1999. *Bordetella holmesii*-like organisms isolated from Massachusetts patients with pertussis-like symptoms. *Emerg Infect Dis* **5:**441–443.

22. **Mazengia E, Silva EA, Peppe JA, Timperi R, George H.** 2000. Recovery of *Bordetella holmesii* from patients with pertussis-like symptoms: use of pulsed-field gel electrophoresis to characterize circulating strains. *J Clin Microbiol* **38:**2330–2333.

23. **Mink CM, O'Brien CH, Wassilak S, Deforest A, Meade BD.** 1994. Isotype and antigen specificity of pertussis agglutinins following whole-cell pertussis vaccination and infection with *Bordetella pertussis. Infect Immun* **62:**1118–1120.

24. **Mooi FR, van Loo IH, van Gent M, He Q, Bart MJ, Heuvelman KJ, de Greeff SC, Diavatopoulos D, Teunis P, Nagelkerke N, Mertsola J.** 2009. *Bordetella pertussis* strains with increased toxin production associated with pertussis resurgence. *Emerg Infect Dis* **15:**1206–1213.

25. **Robinson A, Irons LI, Seabrook RN, Pearce A, Matheson M, Funnell SGP.** 1990. Structure-function studies of *Bordetella pertussis* fimbriae, p 126–135. *In* Manclark CR (ed), *Proceedings of the Sixth International Symposium on Pertussis.* DHHS publication no (FDA) 90. Department of Health and Human Services, US Public Health Service, Bethesda, MD.

26. **Weiss AA, Hewlett EL.** 1986. Virulence factors of *Bordetella pertussis. Annu Rev Microbiol* **40:** 661–686.

27. **Cherry JD, Gornbein J, Heininger U, Stehr K.** 1998. A search for serologic correlates of immunity to *Bordetella pertussis* cough illnesses. *Vaccine* **16:**1901–1906.

28. **Storsaeter J, Hallander HO, Gustafsson L, Olin P.** 1998. Levels of anti-pertussis antibodies related to protection after household exposure to *Bordetella pertussis. Vaccine* **16:**1907–1916.

29. **Abramson T, Kedem H, Relman DA.** 2001. Proinflammatory and proapoptotic activities associated with *Bordetella pertussis* filamentous hemagglutinin. *Infect Immun* **69:**2650–2658.

30. **Leininger E, Roberts M, Kenimer JG, Charles IG, Fairweather N, Novotny P, Brennan MJ.** 1991. Pertactin, an Arg-Gly-Asp containing *Bordetella pertussis* surface protein that promotes adherence of mammalian cells. *Proc Natl Acad Sci* **88:**345–349.

31. **Cherry JD, Brunell PA, Golden GS, Karzon DT.** 1988. Report of the Task Force on Pertussis and Pertussis Immunization—1988. *Pediatrics* **81**(Suppl):939–984.

32. **Cotter PA, Miller JF.** 2001. *Bordetella*, p 619–674. *In* Groisman EA (ed), *Principles of Bacterial Pathogenesis*. Academic Press, San Diego, CA.

33. **Henderson MW, Inatsuka CS, Sheets AJ, Williams CL, Benaron DJ, Donato GM, Gray MC, Hewlett EL, Cotter PA.** 2012. Contribution of *Bordetella* filamentous hemagglutinin and adenylate cyclase toxin to suppression and evasion of interleukin-17-mediated inflammation. *Infect Immun* **80:**2061–2075.

34. **Kimura A, Mountzouros KT, Relman DA, Falkow S, Cowell JL.** 1990. *Bordetella pertussis* filamentous hemagglutinin: evaluation as a protective antigen and colonization factor in a mouse respiratory infection model. *Infect Immun* **58:**7–16.

35. **Makhov AM, Hannah JH, Brennan MJ, Trus BL, Kocsis E, Conway JF, Wingfield PT, Simon MN, Steven AC.** 1994. Filamentous hemagglutinin of *Bordetella pertussis*. A bacterial adhesin formed as a 50-nm monomeric rigid rod based on a 19-residue repeat motif rich in beta strands and turns. *J Mol Biol* **241:**110–124.

36. **Tuomanen E.** 1988. *Bordetella pertussis* adhesins, p 75–94. *In* Wardlaw AC, Parton R (ed), *Pathogenesis and Immunity in Pertussis*. John Wiley & Sons, New York, NY.

37. **Vidakovics MLA, Lamberti Y, van der Pol WL, Yantorno O, Rodriguez ME.** 2006. Adenylate cyclase influences filamentous haemagglutinin-medicated attachment of *Bordetella pertussis* to epithelial alveolar cells. *FEMS Immunol Med Microbiol* **48:**140–147.

38. **Sato H, Sato Y.** 1984. *Bordetella pertussis* infection in mice: correlation of specific antibodies against two antigens, pertussis toxin, and filamentous hemagglutinin with mouse protectivity in an intracerebral or aerosol challenge system. *Infect Immun* **46:**415–421.

39. **Shahin RD, Amsbaugh DF, Leef MF.** 1992. Mucosal immunization with filamentous hemagglutinin protects against *Bordetella pertussis* respiratory infection. *Infect Immun* **60:**1482–1488.

40. **Inatsuka CS, Xu Q, Vujkovic-Cvijin I, Wong S, Stibitz S, Miller JF, Cotter PA.** 2010. Pertactin is required for *Bordetella* species to resist neutrophil-mediated clearance. *Infect Immun* **78:**2901–2909.

41. **Leininger E, Kenimer JG, Brennan MJ.** 1990. Surface proteins of *Bordetella pertussis*: role in adherence, p 25–26. *In* Manclark CR (ed), *Proceedings of the Sixth International Symposium on Pertussis*. DHHS publication no (FDA) 90. Department of Health and Human Services, US Public Health Service, Bethesda, MD.

42. **Novotny P.** 1990. Pathogenesis in *Bordetella* species. *J Infect Dis* **161:**581–583.

43. **Novotny P, Chubb AP, Cownley K, Charles IG.** 1991. Biologic and protective properties of the 69-kDa outer membrane protein of *Bordetella pertussis*: a novel formulation for an acellular pertussis vaccine. *J Infect Dis* **164:**114–122.

44. **Hellwig SM, Rodriguez ME, Berbers GA, van de Winkel JG, Mooi FR.** 2003. Crucial role of antibodies to pertactin in *Bordetella pertussis* immunity. *J Infect Dis* **188:**738–742.

45. **Cherry JD.** 1997. Comparative efficacy of acellular pertussis vaccines: an analysis of recent trials. *Pediatr Infect Dis J* **16**(Suppl):90–96.

46. **Cherry JD, Olin P.** 1999. Commentaries: the science and fiction of pertussis vaccines. *Pediatrics* **104:**1381–1383.

47. **Gustafsson L, Hallander HO, Olin P, Reizenstein E, Storsaeter J.** 1996. A controlled trial of a two-component acellular, a five-component acellular, and a whole-cell pertussis vaccine. *N Engl J Med* **334:**349–355.

48. **Carbonetti NH.** 2010. Pertussis toxin and adenylate cyclase toxin: key virulence factors of *Bordetella pertussis* and cell biology tools. *Future Microbiol* **5:**455–469.

49. **Hewlett EL, Gordon VM.** 1988. Adenylate cyclase toxin of *Bordetella pertussis*, p 193–209. *In* Wardlaw AC, Parton R (ed), *Pathogenesis and Immunity in Pertussis*. John Wiley & Sons, New York, NY.

50. **Khelef N, Sakamoto H, Guiso N.** 1992. Both adenylate cyclase and hemolytic activities are required by *Bordetella pertussis* to initiate infection. *Microb Pathog* **12:**227–235.

51. **Weiss AA, Hewlett EL, Myers GA, Falkow S.** 1984. Pertussis toxin and extracytoplasmic

adenylate cyclase as virulence factors of *Bordetella pertussis*. *J Infect Dis* **150:**219–222.

52. **Cerny O, Kamanova J, Masin J, Bibova I, Skopova K, Sebo P.** 2015. *Bordetella pertussis* adenylate cyclase toxin blocks induction of bactericidal nitric oxide in macrophages through cAMP-dependent activation of the SHP-1 phosphatase. *J Immunol* **194:**4901–4913.

53. **Nakase Y, Endoh M.** 1988. Heat-labile toxin of *Bordetella pertussis*, p 217–229. *In* Wardlaw AC, Parton R (ed), *Pathogenesis and Immunity in Pertussis*. John Wiley & Sons, New York, NY.

54. **Cundell DR, Kanthakumar K, Taylor GW, Goldman WE, Flak T, Cole PJ, Wilson R.** 1994. Effect of tracheal cytotoxin from *Bordetella pertussis* on human neutrophil function in vitro. *Infect Immun* **62:**639–643.

55. **Goldman WE.** 1988. Tracheal cytotoxin of *Bordetella pertussis*, p 237–246. *In* Wardlaw AC, Parton R (ed), *Pathogenesis and Immunity in Pertussis*. John Wiley & Sons, New York, NY.

56. **Fennelly NK, Sisti F, Higgins SC, Ross PJ, van der Heide H, Mooi FR, Boyd A, Mills KHG.** 2008. *Bordetella pertussis* expresses a functional type III secretion system that subverts protective innate and adaptive immune responses. *Infect Immun* **76:**1257–1266.

57. **Linnemann CC, Jr, Ramundo N, Perlstein PH, Minton SD, Englender GS.** 1975. Use of pertussis vaccine in an epidemic involving hospital staff. *Lancet* **ii:**540–543.

58. **Chaby R, Caroff M.** 1988. Lipopolysaccharides of *Bordetella pertussis* endotoxin, p 247–272. *In* Wardlaw AC, Parton R (ed), *Pathogenesis and Immunity in Pertussis*. John Wiley & Sons, New York, NY.

59. **Cody CL, Baraff LJ, Cherry JD, Marcy SM, Manclark CR.** 1981. Nature and rates of adverse reactions associated with DTP and DT immunizations in infants and children. *Pediatrics* **68:**650–660.

60. **Mountzouros KT, Kimura A, Cowell JL.** 1992. A bactericidal monoclonal antibody specific for the lipooligosaccharide of *Bordetella pertussis* reduces colonization of the respiratory tract of mice after aerosol infection with *B. pertussis*. *Infect Immun* **60:**5316–5318.

61. **Murry E, Nieves D, Bradley JS, Mason WH, Lehman D, Harrison R, et al.** 2012. *Characteristics of severe pertussis infections among infants ≤ 90 days of age admitted to pediatric intensive care units—Southern California, September 2009-June 2011.* European Society for Paediatric Infectious Diseases, May 10, 2012, Thessaloniki, Greece.

62. **Paddock CD, Sanden GN, Cherry JD, Gal AA, Langston C, Tatti KM, Wu KH, Goldsmith CS, Greer PW, Montague JL, Eliason MT, Holman RC, Guarner J, Shieh WJ, Zaki SR.** 2008. Pathology and pathogenesis of fatal *Bordetella pertussis* infection in infants. *Clin Infect Dis* **47:**328–338.

63. **Winter K, Harriman K, Murray E, Gornbein J, Hammer SJ, Yeganeh N, Adachi K, Cherry JD.** 2015. Risk factors associated with infant death from pertussis: a case-control study. *Clin Infect Dis* **61:**1099–1106.

64. **Hewitt M, Canning BJ.** 2010. Coughing precipitated by *Bordetella pertussis* infection. *Lung* **188**(Suppl 1)**:**S73–S79.

65. **Hedenskog S, Bjorksten B, Blennow M, Granstrom G, Granstrom M.** 1989. Immunoglobulin E response to pertussis toxin in whooping cough and after immunization with a whole-cell and an acellular pertussis vaccine. *Int Arch Allergy Appl Immunol* **89:**156–161.

66. **Manclark CR, Meade BD, Burstyn DG.** 1986. Serological response to *Bordetella pertussis*, p 388–394. *In* Rose NR, Friedman H, Fahey JL (ed), *Manual of Clinical Laboratory Immunology*, 3rd ed. American Society for Microbiology, Washington, DC.

67. **Onorato IM, Wassilak SG.** 1987. Laboratory diagnosis of pertussis: the state of the art. *Pediatr Infect Dis J* **6:**145–151.

68. **Cherry JD.** 1996. Historical review of pertussis and the classical vaccine. *J Infect Dis* **174** (Suppl)**:**259–263.

69. **Cherry JD.** 1999. Pertussis in the preantibiotic and prevaccine era, with emphasis on adult pertussis. *Clin Infect Dis* **28**(Suppl 2)**:**107–111.

70. **Cherry JD, Beer T, Chartrand SA, DeVille J, Beer E, Olsen MA, Christenson PD, Moore CV, Stehr K.** 1995. Comparison of values of antibody to *Bordetella pertussis* antigens in young German and American men. *Clin Infect Dis* **20:**1271–1274.

71. **Schmitt-Grohe S, Cherry JD, Heininger U, Uberall MA, Pineda E, Stehr K.** 1995. Pertussis in German adults. *Clin Infect Dis* **21:**860–866.

72. **Centers for Disease Control and Prevention.** 2012. Pertussis epidemic—Washington, 2012. *MMWR Morb Mortal Wkly Rep* **61:**517–526.

73. **Cherry JD.** 2012. Why do pertussis vaccines fail? *Pediatrics* **129:**968–970.

74. **Cherry JD.** 2012. Epidemic pertussis in 2012—the resurgence of a vaccine-preventable disease. *N Engl J Med* **367:**785–787.

75. **Cherry JD.** 2013. Pertussis: challenges today and for the future. *PLoS Pathog* **9**(7)**:**e1003418.

76. **Cherry JD, Heininger U, Richards DM, Storsaeter J, Gustafsson L, Ljungman M, Hallander HO.** 2010. Antibody response patterns

to *Bordetella pertussis* antigens in vaccinated (primed) and unvaccinated (unprimed) young children with pertussis. *Clin Vaccine Immunol* **17**:741–747.

77. **Klein NP, Bartlett J, Rowhani-Rahbar A, Fireman B, Baxter R.** 2012. Waning protection after fifth dose of acellular pertussis vaccine in children. *N Engl J Med* **367**:1012–1019.

78. **Liko J, Robison SG, Cieslak PR.** 2013. Priming with whole-cell versus acellular pertussis vaccine. *N Engl J Med* **368**:581–582.

79. **Misegades LK, Winter K, Harriman K, Talarico J, Messonnier NE, Clark TA, Martin SW.** 2012. Association of childhood pertussis with receipt of 5 doses of pertussis vaccine by time since last vaccine dose, California, 2010. *JAMA* **308**:2126–2132.

80. **Sheridan SL, Ware RS, Grimwood K, Lambert SB.** 2012. Number and order of whole cell pertussis vaccines in infancy and disease protection. *JAMA* **308**:454–456.

81. **Skoff TH, Cohn AC, Clark TA, Messonnier NE, Martin SW.** 2012. Early Impact of the US Tdap vaccination program on pertussis trends. *Arch Pediatr Adolesc Med* **166**:344–349.

82. **Tartof SY, Lewis M, Kenyon C, White K, Osborn A, Liko J, Zell E, Martin S, Messonnier NE, Clark TA, Skoff TH.** 2013. Waning immunity to pertussis following 5 doses of DTaP. *Pediatrics* **131**(4):e1047–e1052.

83. **Witt MA, Arias L, Katz PH, Truong ET, Witt DJ.** 2013. Reduced risk of pertussis among persons ever vaccinated with whole cell pertussis vaccine compared to recipients of acellular pertussis vaccines in a large US cohort. *Clin Infect Dis* **56**:1248–1254.

84. **Deen JL, Mink CA, Cherry JD, Christenson PD, Pineda EF, Lewis K, Blumberg DA, Ross LA.** 1995. Household contact study of *Bordetella pertussis* infections. *Clin Infect Dis* **21**:1211–1219.

85. **Tondella ML, Carlone GM, Messonnier N, Quinn CP, Meade BD, Burns DL, Cherry JD, Guiso N, Hewlett EL, Edwards KM, Xing D, Giammanco A, Wirsing von König CH, Han L, Hueston L, Robbins JB, Powell M, Mink CM, Poolman JT, Hildreth SW, Lynn F, Morris A.** 2009. International *Bordetella pertussis* assay standardization and harmonization meeting report. Centers for Disease Control and Prevention, Atlanta, Georgia, United States, 19–20 July 2007. *Vaccine* **27**:803–814.

86. **Cherry JD, Harriman K.** 2012. Why do vaccine-preventable disease outbreaks occur in the United States? *Infect Dis Special Ed* **15**:53–57.

87. **Weiss AA, Patton AK, Millen SH, Chang SJ, Ward JI, Bernstein DI.** 2004. Acellular pertus-sis vaccines and complement killing of *Bordetella pertussis*. *Infect Immun* **72**:7346–7351.

88. **Olsen LC.** 1975. Pertussis. *Medicine* (Baltimore) **54**:427–469.

89. **Wiertz EJ, Loggen HG, Walvoort HC, Kreeftenberg JG.** 1989. In vitro induction of antigen specific antibody synthesis and proliferation of T lymphocytes with acellular pertussis vaccines, pertussis toxin and filamentous haemagglutinin in humans. *J Biol Stand* **17**:181–190.

90. **Mahon BP, Brady MT, Mills KH.** 2000. Protection against *Bordetella pertussis* in mice in the absence of detectable circulating antibody: implications for long-term immunity in children. *J Infect Dis* **181**:2087–2091.

91. **Cherry JD, Heininger U.** 2014. Pertussis and other *Bordetella* infections, p 1616–1639. *In* Cherry JD, Harrison GJ, Kaplan SL, Steinbach WJ, Hotez PJ (ed), *Feigin and Cherry's Textbook of Pediatric Infectious Diseases*, 7th ed. Elsevier Saunders, Philadelphia, PA.

92. **Cherry JD.** 1999. Epidemiological, clinical, and laboratory aspects of pertussis in adults. *Clin Infect Dis* **28**(Suppl 2):112–117.

93. **Cherry JD.** 2005. The epidemiology of pertussis: a comparison of the epidemiology of the disease pertussis with the epidemiology of *Bordetella pertussis* infection. *Pediatrics* **115**:1422–1427.

94. **Cherry JD.** 2010. The present and future control of pertussis. *Clin Infect Dis* **51**:663–667.

95. **Cherry JD, Baraff LJ, Hewlett E.** 1989. The past, present, and future of pertussis. The role of adults in epidemiology and future control. *West J Med* **150**:319–328.

96. **Cherry JD, Tan T, Wirsing von Konig CH, Forsyth KD, Thisyakorn U, Greenberg D, Johnson D, Marchant C, Plotkin S.** 2012. Clinical definitions of pertussis: summary of a Global Pertussis Initiative roundtable meeting, February 2011. *Clin Infect Dis* **54**:1756–1764.

97. **De Serres G, Shadmani R, Duval B, Boulianne N, Dery P, Douville Fradet M, Rochette L, Halperin SA.** 2000. Morbidity of pertussis in adolescents and adults. *J Infect Dis* **182**:174–179.

98. **Linnemann CC, Jr, Nasenbeny J.** 1977. Pertussis in the adult. *Annu Rev Med* **28**:179–185.

99. **Mink CM, Cherry JD, Christenson P, Lewis K, Pineda E, Shlian D, Dawson JA, Blumberg DA.** 1992. A search for *Bordetella pertussis* infection in university students. *Clin Infect Dis* **14**:464–471.

100. **Nennig ME, Shinefield HR, Edwards KM, Black SB, Fireman BH.** 1996. Prevalence and incidence of adult pertussis in an urban population. *JAMA* **275**:1672–1674.

101. **Birkebaek NH, Kristiansen M, Seefeldt T, Degn J, Moller A, Heron I, Lehm Andersen P, Möller JK, Østergård L.** 1999. *Bordetella pertussis* and chronic cough in adults. *Clin Infect Dis* **29:**1239–1242.

102. **Postels-Multani S, Schmitt HJ, Wirsing von Konig CH, Bock HL, Bogaerts H.** 1995. Symptoms and complications of pertussis in adults. *Infection* **23:**139–142.

103. **Wright SW, Edwards KM, Decker MD, Zeldin MH.** 1995. Pertussis infection in adults with persistent cough. *JAMA* **273:**1044–1046.

104. **Kretsinger K, Broder KR, Cortese MM, Joyce MP, Ortega-Sanchez I, Lee GM, Tiwari T, Cohn AC, Slade BA, Iskander JK, Mijalski CM, Brown KH, Murphy TV, Centers for Disease Control and Prevention, Advisory Committee on Immunization Practices, Healthcare Infection Control Practices Advisory Committee.** 2006. Preventing tetanus, diphtheria, and pertussis among adults: use of tetanus toxoid, reduced diphtheria toxoid and acellular pertussis vaccine recommendations of the Advisory Committee on Immunization Practices (ACIP) and recommendation of ACIP, supported by the Healthcare Infection Control Practices Advisory Committee (HICPAC), for use of Tdap among health-care personnel. *MMWR Recommend Rep* **55**(RR-17)**:**1–37.

105. **Nieves D, Heininger U, Cherry J.** 2016. *Bordetella pertussis* and other *Bordetella* spp. infections, p 598–616. *In* Wilson CB, Nizet V, Maldonado YA, Remington JS, Klein JO (ed), *Remington and Klein's Infectious Diseases of the Fetus and Newborn Infant*, 8th ed. Elsevier Saunders, Philadelphia, PA.

106. **Beiter A, Lewis K, Pineda EF, Cherry JD.** 1993. Unrecognized maternal peripartum pertussis with subsequent fatal neonatal pertussis. *Obstet Gynecol* **82**(4 Part 2 Suppl)**:**691–693.

107. **Christie CD, Baltimore RS.** 1989. Pertussis in neonates. *Am J Dis Child* **143:**1199–1202.

108. **Elliott E, McIntyre P, Ridley G, Morris A, Massie J, McEniery J, Knight G.** 2004. National study of infants hospitalized with pertussis in the acellular vaccine era. *Pediatr Infect Dis J* **23:**246–252.

109. **Heininger U, Stehr K, Cherry JD.** 1992. Serious pertussis overlooked in infants. *Eur J Pediatr* **151:**342–343.

110. **Kowalzik F, Barbosa AP, Fernandes VR, Carvalho PR, Avila-Aguero ML, Goh DY, Goh A, de Miguel JG, Moraga F, Roca J, Campins M, Huang M, Quian J, Riley N, Beck D, Verstraeten T.** 2007. Prospective multinational study of pertussis infection in hospitalized infants and their household contacts. *Pediatr Infect Dis J* **26:**238–242.

111. **McGregor J, Ogle JW, Curry-Kane G.** 1986. Perinatal pertussis. *Obstet Gynecol* **68:**582–586.

112. **Castagnini LA, Munoz FM.** 2010. Clinical characteristics and outcomes of neonatal pertussis: a comparative study. *J Pediatr* **156:**498–500.

113. **Crowcroft NS, Booy R, Harrison T, Spicer L, Britto J, Mok Q, Heath P, Murdoch I, Zambon M, George R, Miller E.** 2003. Severe and unrecognised: pertussis in UK infants. *Arch Dis Child* **88:**802–806.

114. **Goulin GD, Kaya KM, Bradley JS.** 1993. Severe pulmonary hypertension associated with shock and death in infants infected with *Bordetella pertussis*. *Crit Care Med* **21:**1791–1794.

115. **Haberling DL, Holman RC, Paddock CD, Murphy TV.** 2009. Infant and maternal risk factors for pertussis-related infant mortality in the United States, 1999 to 2004. *Pediatr Infect Dis J* **28:**194–198.

116. **Heininger U, Stehr K, Schmidt-Schlapfer G, Penning R, Vock R, Kleemann W, Cherry JD.** 1996. *Bordetella pertussis* infections and sudden unexpected deaths in children. *Eur J Pediatr* **155:**551–553.

117. **Mikelova LK, Halperin SA, Scheifele D, Smith B, Ford-Jones E, Vaudry W, Jadavji T, Law B, Moore D, Members of the Immunization Monitoring Program, Active (IMPACT).** 2003. Predictors of death in infants hospitalized with pertussis: a case-control study of 16 pertussis deaths in Canada. *J Pediatr* **143:**576–581.

118. **Nicoll A, Gardner A.** 1988. Whooping cough and unrecognised postperinatal mortality. *Arch Dis Child* **63:**41–47.

119. **Sawal M, Cohen M, Irazuzta JE, Kumar R, Kirton C, Brundler M-A, Evans CA, Wilson JA, Raffeeq P, Azaz A, Rotta AT, Vora A, Vohra A, Abboud P, Mirkin LD, Cooper M, Dishop MK, Graf JM, Petros A, Klonin H.** 2009. Fulminant pertussis: a multi-center study with new insights into the clinico-pathological mechanisms. *Pediatric Pulmonol* **44:**970–980.

120. **Smith C, Vyas H.** 2000. Early infantile pertussis; increasingly prevalent and potentially fatal. *Eur J Pediatr* **159:**898–900.

121. **Somerville RL, Grant CC, Grimwood K, Murdoch D, Graham D, Jackson P, Meates-Dennis M, Nicholson R, Purvis D.** 2007. Infants hospitalised with pertussis: estimating the true disease burden. *J Paediatr Child Health* **43:**617–622.

122. **Vitek CR, Pascual FB, Baughman AL, Murphy TV.** 2003. Increase in deaths from pertussis among young infants in the United States in the 1990s. *Pediatr Infect Dis J* **22:**628–634.

123. **Centers for Disease Control and Prevention.** 2002. Pertussis: United States, 1997–2000. *MMWR Morb Mortal Wkly Rep* **51**:73–76.

124. **Halperin SA, Wang EE, Law B, Mills E, Morris R, Dery P, Lebel M, MacDonald N, Jadavji T, Vaudry W, Scheifele D, Delage G, Duclos P.** 1999. Epidemiological features of pertussis in hospitalized patients in Canada, 1991–1997: report of the Immunization Monitoring Program—Active (IMPACT). *Clin Infect Dis* **28**:1238–1243.

125. **De Berry BB, Lynch JE, Chung DH, Zwischenberger JB.** 2005. Pertussis with severe pulmonary hypertension and leukocytosis treated with extracorporeal membrane oxygenation. *Pediatr Surg Int* **21**:692–694.

126. **Donoso A, Leon J, Ramirez M, Rojas G, Oberpaur B.** 2005. Pertussis and fatal pulmonary hypertension: a discouraged entity. *Scand J Infect Dis* **37**:145–148.

127. **Grzeszczak MJ, Churchwell KB, Edwards KM, Pietsch J.** 2006. Leukopheresis therapy for severe infantile pertussis with myocardial and pulmonary failure. *Pediatr Crit Care Med* **7**:580–582.

128. **Halasa NB, Barr FE, Johnson JE, Edwards KM.** 2003. Fatal pulmonary hypertension associated with pertussis in infants: does extracorporeal membrane oxygenation have a role? *Pediatrics* **112**(6 Part 1):1274–1278.

129. **Pierce C, Klein N, Peters M.** 2000. Is leukocytosis a predictor of mortality in severe pertussis infection? *Intensive Care Med* **26**:1512–1514.

130. **Sreenan CD, Osiovich H.** 2001. Neonatal pertussis requiring extracorporeal membrane oxygenation. *Pediatr Surg Int* **17**:201–203.

131. **Williams GD, Numa A, Sokol J, Tobias V, Duffy BJ.** 1998. ECLS in pertussis: does it have a role? *Intensive Care Med* **24**:1089–1092.

132. **Rocha G, Flor-de-Lima F, Soares P, Soares H, Pissarra S, Prioenca E, Fernandes P, Quintas C, Martins T, Silva A, Guimarães H.** 2013. Severe pertussis in newborns and young vulnerable infants. *Pediatr Infect Dis J* **32**:1152–1154. doi:10.1097/INF.0b013e31829f0b1a.

133. **Aoyama T, Ide Y, Watanabe J, Takeuchi Y, Imaizumi A.** 1996. Respiratory failure caused by dual infection with *Bordetella pertussis* and respiratory syncytial virus. *Acta Paediatr Jpn* **38**:282–285.

134. **Cosnes-Lambe C, Raymond J, Chalumeau M, Pons-Catalano C, Moulin F, de Suremain N, Reglier-Poupet H, Lebon P, Poyart C, Gendrel D.** 2008. Pertussis and respiratory syncytial virus infections. *Eur J Pediatr* **167**:1017–1019.

135. **Dagan R, Hall CB, Menegus MA.** 1985. Atypical bacterial infections explained by a concomitant virus infection. *Pediatrics* **76**:411–414.

136. **Korppi M, Hiltunen J.** 2007. Pertussis is common in nonvaccinated infants hospitalized for respiratory syncytial virus infection. *Pediatr Infect Dis J* **26**:316–318.

137. **Lewis K, Saubolle MA, Tenover FC, Rudinsky MF, Barbour SD, Cherry JD.** 1995. Pertussis caused by an erythromycin-resistant strain of *Bordetella pertussis*. *Pediatr Infect Dis J* **14**:388–391.

138. **Miron D, Srugo I, Kra-Oz Z, Keness Y, Wolf D, Amirav I, Kassis I.** 2010. Sole pathogen in acute bronchiolitis: is there a role for other organisms apart from respiratory syncytial virus? *Pediatr Infect Dis J* **29**(1):e7–e10.

139. **Nieves DJ, Singh J, Ashouri N, McGuire T, Adler-Shohet FC, Arrieta AC.** 2011. Clinical and laboratory features of pertussis in infants at the onset of a California epidemic. *J Pediatr* **159**:1044–1046.

140. **Heininger U, Burckhardt MA.** 2011. *Bordetella pertussis* and concomitant viral respiratory tract infections are rare in children with cough illness. *Pediatr Infect Dis J* **30**:640–644.

141. **Marshall H, Clarke M, Rasiah K, Richmond P, Buttery J, Reynolds G, Andrews R, Nissen M, Wood N, McIntyre P.** 2015. Predictors of disease severity in children hospitalized for pertussis during an epidemic. *Pediatr Infect Dis J* **34**:339–345.

142. **Zamir CS, Dahan DB, Shoob H.** 2015. Pertussis in infants under one year old: risk markers and vaccination status—a case-control study. *Vaccine* **33**:2073–2078.

143. **Shojaei J, Saffar M, Hashemi A, Ghorbani G, Rezai M, Shahmohammadi S.** 2014. Clinical and laboratory features of pertussis in hospitalized infants with confirmed versus probable pertussis cases. *Ann Med Health Sci Res* **4**:910–914.

144. **Heininger U, Cherry JD, Eckhardt T, Lorenz C, Christenson P, Stehr K.** 1993. Clinical and laboratory diagnosis of pertussis in the regions of a large vaccine efficacy trial in Germany. *Pediatr Infect Dis J* **12**:504–509.

145. **Berger JT, Carcillo JA, Shanley TP, Wessel DL, Clark A, Holubkov R, Meert KL, Newth CJ, Berg RA, Heidemann S, Harrison R, Pollack M, Dalton H, Harvill E, Karanikas A, Liu T, Burr JS, Doctor A, Dean JM, Jenkins TL, Nicholson CE, Eunice Kennedy Shriver National Institute of Child Health and Human Development (NICHD) Collaborative Pediatric Critical Care Research Network (CPCCRN).** 2013. Critical pertussis illness in children: a multicenter prospective cohort study. *Pediatr Crit Care Med* **14**:356–365.

146. **Heininger U, Kleemann WJ, Cherry JD.** 2004. A controlled study of the relationship between *Bordetella pertussis* infections and sudden unexpected deaths among German infants. *Pediatrics* **114**(1):e9–e15.

147. **Lindgren C, Milerad J, Lagercrantz H.** 1997. Sudden infant death and prevalence of whooping cough in the Swedish and Norwegian communities. *Eur J Pediatr* **156**:405–409.

148. **Cherry JD, Paddock CD, Greer PW, Heininger U.** 2011. The respiratory pathology in infants with sudden unexpected deaths in whom respiratory specimens were initially PCR-positive or PCR-negative for *Bordetella pertussis*. *Infection* **39**:545–548.

149. **Mastrantonio P, Stefanelli P, Giuliano M, Herrera Rojas Y, Ciofi degli Atti M, Anemona A, Tozzi AE.** 1998. *Bordetella parapertussis* infection in children: epidemiology, clinical symptoms, and molecular characteristics of isolates. *J Clin Microbiol* **36**:999–1002.

150. **Hoppe JE.** 1999. Update on respiratory infection caused by *Bordetella parapertussis*. *Pediatr Infect Dis J* **18**:375–381.

151. **Iwata S, Aoyama T, Goto A, Iwai H, Sato Y, Akita H, Murase Y, Oikawa T, Iwata T, Kusano S, Kawashima C, Sunakawa K.** 1991. Mixed outbreak of *Bordetella pertussis* and *Bordetella parapertussis* in an apartment house. *Dev Biol Stand* **73**:333–341.

152. **Mertsola J.** 1985. Mixed outbreak of *Bordetella pertussis* and *Bordetella parapertussis* infection in Finland. *Eur J Clin Microbiol* **4**:123–128.

153. **Amador C, Chiner E, Calpe JL, Ortiz de la Table V, Martinez C, Pasquau F.** 1991. Pneumonia due to *Bordetella bronchiseptica* in a patient with AIDS. *Rev Infect Dis* **13**:771–772.

154. **Dworkin MS, Sullivan PS, Buskin SE, Harrington RD, Olliffe J, MacArthur RD, Lopez CE.** 1999. *Bordetella bronchiseptica* infection in human immunodeficiency virus-infected patients. *Clin Infect Dis* **28**:1095–1099.

155. **Wernli D, Emonet S, Schrenzel J, Harbarth S.** 2010. Evaluation of eight cases of confirmed *Bordetella bronchiseptica* infection and colonization over a 15-year period. *Clin Microbiol Infect* **17**:201–203.

156. **Mooi FR, Bruisten S, Linde I, Reubsaet F, Heuvelman K, van der Lee S, King AJ.** 2012. Characterization of *Bordetella holmesii* isolates from patients with pertussis-like illness in The Netherlands. *FEMS Immunol Med Microbiol* **64**:289–291.

157. **Njamkepo E, Bonacorsi S, Debruyne M, Gibaud SA, Guillot S, Guiso N.** 2011. Significant finding of *Bordetella holmesii* DNA in nasopharyngeal samples from French patients with suspected pertussis. *J Clin Microbiol* **49**:4347–4348.

158. **Rodgers L, Martin SW, Cohn A, Budd J, Marcon M, Terranella A, Mandal S, Salamon D, Leber A, Tondella ML, Tatti K, Spicer K, Emanuel A, Koch E, McGlone L, Pawloski L, Lemaile-Williams M, Tucker N, Iyer R, Clark TA, Diorio M.** 2013. Epidemiologic and laboratory features of a large outbreak of pertussis-like illnesses associated with cocirculating *Bordetella holmesii* and *Bordetella pertussis*—Ohio, 2010-2011. *Clin Infect Dis* **56**:322–331.

159. **Anderson RM, May RM.** 1985. Vaccination and herd immunity to infectious diseases. *Nature* **318**:323–329.

160. **Fine PE.** 1993. Herd immunity: history, theory, practice. *Epidemiol Rev* **15**:265–302.

161. **Centers for Disease Control and Prevention.** 2012. Summary of notifiable diseases—United States, 2010. *MMWR Morb Mortal Wkly Rep* **59**:1–111.

162. **Fine PE, Clarkson JA.** 1982. The recurrence of whooping cough: possible implications for assessment of vaccine efficacy. *Lancet* **i**:666–669.

163. **Fine PEM.** 1988. Epidemiological considerations for whooping cough eradication, p 451–467. *In* Wardlaw AC, Parton R (ed), *Pathogenesis and Immunity in Pertussis*. John Wiley & Sons, New York, NY.

164. **Bordet J, Gengou O.** 1906. Le microbe de la coqueluche. *Ann Inst Pasteur (Paris)* **20**:48–68.

165. **Heininger U.** 2010. Update on pertussis in children. *Expert Rev Anti Infect Ther* **8**:163–173.

166. **Baron S, Njamkepo E, Grimprel E, Begue P, Desenclos JC, Drucker J, Guiso N.** 1998. Epidemiology of pertussis in French hospitals in 1993 and 1994: thirty years after a routine use of vaccination. *Pediatr Infect Dis J* **17**:412–418.

167. **Bisgard KM, Pascual FB, Ehresmann KR, Miller CA, Cianfrini C, Jennings CE, Rebmann CA, Gabel J, Schauer SL, Lett SM.** 2004. Infant pertussis: who was the source? *Pediatr Infect Dis J* **23**:985–989.

168. **Wendelboe AM, Njamkepo E, Bourillon A, Floret DD, Gaudelus J, Gerber M, Grimprel E, Greenberg D, Halperin S, Liese J, Muñoz-Rivas F, Teyssou R, Guiso N, Van Rie A; Infant Pertussis Study Group.** 2007. Transmission of *Bordetella pertussis* to young infants. *Pediatr Infect Dis J* **26**:293–299.

169. **Long SS, Lischner HW, Deforest A, Clark JL.** 1990. Serologic evidence of subclinical pertussis in immunized children. *Pediatr Infect Dis J* **9**:700–705.

170. **Long SS, Welkon CJ, Clark JL.** 1990. Widespread silent transmission of pertussis in

families: antibody correlates of infection and symptomatology. *J Infect Dis* **161**:480–486.

171. **Skoff TH, Kenyon C, Cocoros N, Liko J, Miller L, Kudish K, Baumbach J, Zansky S, Faulkner A, Martin SW.** 2015. Sources of infant pertussis infection in the United States. *Pediatrics* **136**:635–641.

172. **Strebel PM, Cochi SL, Farizo KM, Payne BJ, Hanauer SD, Baughman AL.** 1993. Pertussis in Missouri: evaluation of nasopharyngeal culture, direct fluorescent antibody testing, and clinical case definitions in the diagnosis of pertussis. *Clin Infect Dis* **16**:276–285.

173. **Andre P, Caro V, Njamkepo E, Wendelboe AM, Van Rie A, Guiso N.** 2008. Comparison of serological and real-time PCR assays to diagnose *Bordetella pertussis* infection in 2007. *J Clin Microbiol* **46**:1672–1677.

174. **Farrell DJ, McKeon M, Daggard G, Loeffelholz MJ, Thompson CJ, Mukkur TK.** 2000. Rapid-cycle PCR method to detect *Bordetella pertussis* that fulfills all consensus recommendations for use of PCR in diagnosis of pertussis. *J Clin Microbiol* **38**:4499–4502.

175. **Grimprel E, Begue P, Anjak I, Betsou F, Guiso N.** 1993. Comparison of polymerase chain reaction, culture, and Western immunoblot serology for diagnosis of *Bordetella pertussis* infection. *J Clin Microbiol* **31**:2745–2750.

176. **Guthrie JL, Robertson AV, Tang P, Jamieson F, Drews SJ.** 2010. Novel duplex real-time PCR assay detects *Bordetella holmesii* in specimens from patients with pertussis-like symptoms in Ontario, Canada. *J Clin Microbiol* **48**:1435–1437.

177. **Heininger U, Schmidt-Schlapfer G, Cherry JD, Stehr K.** 2000. Clinical validation of a polymerase chain reaction assay for the diagnosis of pertussis by comparison with serology, culture, and symptoms during a large pertussis vaccine efficacy trial. *Pediatrics* **105**(3):E31.

178. **Lichtinghagen R, Diedrich-Glaubitz R, von Horsten B.** 1994. Identification of *Bordetella pertussis* in nasopharyngeal swabs using the polymerase chain reaction: evaluation of detection methods. *Eur J Clin Chem Clin Biochem* **32**:161–167.

179. **Lind-Brandberg L, Welinder-Olsson C, Lagergard T, Taranger J, Trollfors B, Zackrisson G.** 1998. Evaluation of PCR for diagnosis of *Bordetella pertussis* and *Bordetella parapertussis* infections. *J Clin Microbiol* **36**:679–683.

180. **Loeffelholz M.** 2012. Towards improved accuracy of *Bordetella pertussis* nucleic acid amplification tests. *J Clin Microbiol* **50**:2186–2190.

181. **Mastrantonio P, Stefanelli P, Giuliano M.** 1996. Polymerase chain reaction for the detection of *Bordetella pertussis* in clinical nasopharyngeal aspirates. *J Med Microbiol* **44**:261–266.

182. **Meade BD, Bollen A.** 1994. Recommendations for use of the polymerase chain reaction in the diagnosis of *Bordetella pertussis* infections. *J Med Microbiol* **41**:51–55.

183. **Register KB, Sanden GN.** 2006. Prevalence and sequence variants of IS481 in *Bordetella bronchiseptica*: implications for IS481-based detection of *Bordetella pertussis*. *J Clin Microbiol* **44**:4577–4583.

184. **Reizenstein E, Johansson B, Mardin L, Abens J, Mollby R, Hallander HO.** 1993. Diagnostic evaluation of polymerase chain reaction discriminative for *Bordetella pertussis*, *B. parapertussis*, and *B. bronchiseptica*. *Diagn Microbiol Infect Dis* **17**:185–191.

185. **Roorda L, Buitenwerf J, Ossewaarde JM, van der Zee A.** 2011. A real-time PCR assay with improved specificity for detection and discrimination of all clinically relevant *Bordetella* species by the presence and distribution of three insertion sequence elements. *BMC Res Notes* **4**:11.

186. **Schlapfer G, Cherry JD, Heininger U, Uberall M, Schmitt-Grohe S, Laussucq S, Just M, Stehr K.** 1995. Polymerase chain reaction identification of Bordetella pertussis infections in vaccinees and family members in a pertussis vaccine efficacy trial in Germany. *Pediatr Infect Dis J* **14**:209–214.

187. **Schlapfer G, Senn HP, Berger R, Just M.** 1993. Use of the polymerase chain reaction to detect *Bordetella pertussis* in patients with mild or atypical symptoms of infection. *Eur J Clin Microbiol Infect Dis* **12**:459–463.

188. **Tatti KM, Sparks KN, Boney KO, Tondella ML.** 2011. Novel multitarget real-time PCR assay for rapid detection of *Bordetella* species in clinical specimens. *J Clin Microbiol* **49**:4059–4066.

189. **van der Zee A, Agterberg C, Peeters M, Mooi F, Schellekens J.** 1996. A clinical validation of *Bordetella pertussis* and *Bordetella parapertussis* polymerase chain reaction: comparison with culture and serology using samples from patients with suspected whooping cough from a highly immunized population. *J Infect Dis* **174**:89–96.

190. **van Kruijssen AM, Templeton KE, van der Plas RN, van Doorn HR, Claas EC, Sukhai RN, Kuijper EJ.** 2007. Detection of respiratory pathogens by real-time PCR in children with clinical suspicion of pertussis. *Eur J Pediatr* **166**:1189–1191.

191. **Aintablian N, Walpita P, Sawyer MH.** 1998. Detection of *Bordetella pertussis* and respiratory

synctial virus in air samples from hospital rooms. *Infect Control Hosp Epidemiol* **19**:918–923.

192. **Mandal S, Tatti KM, Woods-Stout D, Cassiday PK, Faulkner AE, Griffith MM, Jackson ML, Pawloski LC, Wagner B, Barnes M, Cohn AC, Gershman KA, Messonnier NE, Clark TA, Tondella ML, Martin SW.** 2012. Pertussis pseudo-outbreak linked to specimens contaminated by *Bordetella pertussis* DNA from clinic surfaces. *Pediatrics* **129**(2):e424–e430.

193. **Conway SP, Balfour AH, Ross H.** 1988. Serologic diagnosis of whooping cough by enzyme-linked immunosorbent assay. *Pediatr Infect Dis J* **7**:570–574.

194. **Halperin SA, Bortolussi R, MacLean D, Chisholm N.** 1989. Persistence of pertussis in an immunized population: results of the Nova Scotia Enhanced Pertussis Surveillance Program. *J Pediatr* **115**(5 Part 1):686–693.

195. **Mertsola J, Ruuskanen O, Kuronen T, Meurman O, Viljanen MK.** 1990. Serologic diagnosis of pertussis: evaluation of pertussis toxin and other antigens in enzyme-linked immunosorbent assay. *J Infect Dis* **161**:966–971.

196. **Stehr K, Cherry JD, Heininger U, Schmitt-Grohe S, uberall M, Laussucq S, Eckhardt T, Meyer M, Engelhardt R, Christenson P, Pertussis Vaccine Study Group.** 1998. A comparative efficacy trial in Germany in infants who received either the Lederle/Takeda acellular pertussis component DTP (DTaP) vaccine, the Lederle whole-cell component DTP vaccine, or DT vaccine. *Pediatrics* **101**(1 Part 1):1–11.

197. **Viljanen MK, Ruuskanen O, Granberg C, Salmi TT.** 1982. Serological diagnosis of pertussis: IgM, IgA and IgG antibodies against *Bordetella pertussis* measured by enzyme-linked immunosorbent assay (ELISA). *Scand J Infect Dis* **14**:117–122.

198. **Wirsing von Konig CH, Gounis D, Laukamp S, Bogaerts H, Schmitt HJ.** 1999. Evaluation of a single-sample serological technique for diagnosing pertussis in unvaccinated children. *Eur J Clin Microbiol Infect Dis* **18**:341–345.

199. **Granstrom M, Lindberg AA, Askelof P, Hederstedt B.** 1982. Detection of antibodies in human serum against the fimbrial haemagglutinin of *Bordetella pertussis* by enzyme-linked immunosorbent assay. *J Med Microbiol* **15**:85–96.

200. **American Academy of Pediatrics.** 2015. Pertussis (whooping cough), p 608–621. *In* Kimberlin D, Brady MT, Jackson MA, Long S (ed), *Red Book: 2015 Report of the Committee on Infectious Diseases*, 30th ed. American Academy of Pediatrics, Elk Grove Village, IL.

201. **Henry R, Dorman D, Skinner J, Mellis C.** 1981. Limitations of erythromycin in whooping cough. *Med J Aust* **2**:108–109.

202. **Bass JW.** 1986. Erythromycin for treatment and prevention of pertussis. *Pediatr Infect Dis* **5**:154–157.

203. **Bergquist SO, Bernander S, Dahnsjo H, Sundelof B.** 1987. Erythromycin in the treatment of pertussis: a study of bacteriologic and clinical effects. *Pediatr Infect Dis J* **6**:458–461.

204. **Hoppe JE.** 1998. State of art in antibacterial susceptibility of *Bordetella pertussis* and antibiotic treatment of pertussis. *Infection* **26**:242–246.

205. **Centers for Disease Control and Prevention.** 2005. Recommended antimicrobial agents for the treatment and postexposure prophylaxes of pertussis: 2005 CDC guidelines. *MMWR Morb Mortal Wkly Rep* **54**:1–16.

206. **Halperin SA, Bortolussi R, Langley JM, Miller B, Eastwood BJ.** 1997. Seven days of erythromycin estolate is as effective as fourteen days for the treatment of *Bordetella pertussis* infections. *Pediatrics* **100**:65–71.

207. **Honein MA, Paulozzi LJ, Himelright IM, Lee B, Cragan JD, Patterson L, Correa A, Hall S, Erickson JD.** 1999. Infantile hypertrophic pyloric stenosis after pertussis prophylaxis with erythromycin: a case review and cohort study. *Lancet* **354**:2101–2105.

208. **Morrison W.** 2007. Infantile hypertrophic pyloric stenosis in infants treated with azithromycin. *Pediatr Infect Dis J* **26**:186–188.

209. **Centers for Disease Control and Prevention.** 1999. Hypertrophic pyloric stenosis in infants following pertussis prophylaxis with erythromycin—Knoxville, Tennessee, 1999. *MMWR Morb Mortal Wkly Rep* **48**:1117–1120.

210. **Tiwari T, Murphy TV, Moran J, National Immunization Program, Centers for Disease Control and Prevention.** 2005. Recommended antimicrobial agents for the treatment and postexposure prophylaxis of pertussis: 2005 CDC guidelines. *MMWR Recommend Rep.* **54**(RR-14):1–16.

211. **Hoppe JE, Halm U, Hagedorn HJ, Kraminer-Hagedorn A.** 1989. Comparison of erythromycin ethylsuccinate and co-trimoxazole for treatment of pertussis. *Infection* **17**:227–231.

212. **Guillot S, Descours G, Gillet Y, Etienne J, Floret D, Guiso N.** 2012. Macrolide-resistant *Bordetella pertussis* infection in newborn girl, France. *Emerg Infect Dis* **18**:966–968.

213. **Korgenski EK, Daly JA.** 1997. Surveillance and detection of erythromycin resistance in *Bordetella pertussis* isolates recovered from a pediatric population in the Intermountain

West region of the United States. *J Clin Microbiol* **35:**2989–2991.

214. **Lee B.** 2000. Progressive respiratory distress in an infant treated for presumed pertussis. *Pediatr Infect Dis J* **19:**475, 492–493.

215. **Ohtsuka M, Kikuchi K, Shimizu K, Takahashi N, Ono Y, Sasaki T, Hiramatsu K.** 2009. Emergence of quinolone-resistant *Bordetella pertussis* in Japan. *Antimicrob Agents Chemother* **53:**3147–3149.

216. **Donoso AF, Cruces PI, Camacho JF, Leon JA, Kong JA.** 2006. Exchange transfusion to reverse severe pertussis-induced cardiogenic shock. *Pediatr Infect Dis J* **25:**846–848.

217. **Romano MJ, Weber MD, Weisse ME, Siu BL.** 2004. Pertussis pneumonia, hypoxemia, hyperleukocytosis, and pulmonary hypertension: improvement in oxygenation after a double volume exchange transfusion. *Pediatrics* **114**(2):e264–e266.

218. **Nieves D, Bradley JS, Gargas J, Mason WH, Lehman D, Lehman SM, Murray EL, Harriman K, Cherry JD.** 2013. Exchange blood transfusion in the management of severe pertussis in young infants. *Pediatr Infect Dis J* **32:**698–699.

219. **Taffarel P, Bonetto G, Haimovich A.** 2012. Severe pertussis, progression and exchange transfusion as an alternative treatment. Case reports. *Arch Argent Pediatr* **110:**327–330. (In Spanish.)

220. **Bettiol S, Thompson MJ, Roberts NW, Perera R, Heneghan CJ, Harnden A.** 2010. Symptomatic treatment of the cough in whooping cough. *Cochrane Database Syst Rev* **2010**(1):CD003257.

221. **Zoumboulakis D, Anagnostakis D, Albanis V, Matsaniotis N.** 1973. Steroids in treatment of pertussis. A controlled clinical trial. *Arch Dis Child* **48:**51–54.

222. **Iida T, Kunitani A, Komase Y, Yamamoto A.** 1983. Studies on experimental infection with *Bordetella pertussis*: effect of cortisone on the infection and immunity in mice. *Jpn J Exp Med* **33:**283–295.

223. **Roberts I, Gavin R, Lennon D.** 1992. Randomized controlled trial of steroids in pertussis. *Pediatr Infect Dis J* **11:**982–983.

224. **Broomhall J, Herxheimer A.** 1984. Treatment of whooping cough: the facts. *Arch Dis Child* **59:**185–187.

225. **Pillay V, Swingler G.** 2003. Symptomatic treatment of the cough in whooping cough. *Cochrane Database Syst Rev* **2003**(4):CD003257.

226. **Cherry JD.** 1990. 'Pertussis vaccine encephalopathy': it is time to recognize it as the myth that it is. *JAMA* **263:**1679–1680.

227. **Hewlett EL, Cherry JD.** 1990. New and improved vaccines against pertussis, p 231–250. *In* Woodrow GC, Levine MM (ed), *New Generation Vaccines*. Marcel Dekker, New York, NY.

228. **Sato Y, Kimura M, Fukumi H.** 1984. Development of a pertussis component vaccine in Japan. *Lancet* **i:**122–126.

229. **Cherry JD, Mortimer EA Jr.** 1987. Acellular and whole-cell pertussis vaccines in Japan: report of a visit by US scientists. *JAMA* **257:**1375–1376.

230. **Kimura M, Kuno-Sakai H.** 1988. Pertussis vaccines in Japan. *Acta Paediatr Jpn* **30:**143–153.

231. **Noble GR, Bernier RH, Esber EC, Hardegree MC, Hinman AR, Klein D, Saah AJ.** 1987. Acellular and whole-cell pertussis vaccines in Japan. Report of a visit by US scientists. *JAMA* **257:**1351–1356.

232. **Edwards K, Decker MD.** 2013. Pertussis vaccines, p 447–492. *In* Plotkin S, Orenstein WA, Offit PA (ed), *Vaccines*, 5th ed. Saunders, Philadelphia.

233. **Le Saux N, Barrowman NJ, Moore DL, Whiting S, Scheifele D, Halperin S.** 2003. Decrease in hospital admissions for febrile seizures and reports of hypotonic-hyporesponsive episodes presenting to hospital emergency departments since switching to acellular pertussis vaccine in Canada: a report from IMPACT. *Pediatrics* **112:**348–353.

234. **Centers for Disease Control and Prevention.** 2006. Preventing tetanus, diphtheria, and pertussis among adults: use of tetanus toxoid, reduced diphtheria toxoid and acellular pertussis vaccine. *MMWR Morb Mortal Wkly Rep* **55**(RR-17):1–37.

235. **Centers for Disease Control and Prevention.** 2006. Preventing tetanus, diphtheria, and pertussis among adolescents: use of tetanus toxoid, reduced diphetheria toxoid and acellular pertussis vaccines. *MMWR Morb Mortal Wkly Rep* **55**(RR-3):1–34.

236. **Cherry JD.** 2005. Pertussis vaccines for adolescents and adults. *Pediatrics* **116:**755–756.

237. **Food and Drug Administration.** 2005. Product approval information-licensing action, package insert: BOOSTRIX. Tetanus toxoid, reduced diphtheria toxoid and acellular pertussis vaccine, adsorbed. *GlaxoSmithKline Biologicals*. US Department of Health and Human Services, Food and Drug Administration, Center for Biologics Evaluation and Research, Rockville, MD. http://www.fda.gov/cber/label/tdapgla122905LB.pdf.

238. **Food and Drug Administration.** 2006. Product approval information-licensing action, package insert: tetanus toxoid, reduced diphtheria toxoid and acellular pertussis vaccine adsorbed

ADACEL. *Sanofi Pasteur*. US Department of Health and Human Services, Food and Drug Administration, Center for Biologics Evaluation and Research, Rockville, MD. http://www.fda. gov/cber/label/tdapave012306LB.pdf.

239. **Heininger U, Cherry JD.** 2006. Pertussis immunization in adolescents and adults: *Bordetella pertussis* epidemiology should guide vaccination recommendations. *Expert Opin Biol Ther* **6:**1–13.

240. **Centers for Disease Control and Prevention.** 2011. Updated recommendations for use of tetanus toxoid, reduced diphtheria toxoid and acellular pertussis vaccine (Tdap) in pregnant women and persons who have or anticipate having close contact with an infant aged <12 months—Advisory Committee on Immunization Practices (ACIP), 2011. *MMWR Morb Mortal Wkly Rep* **60:**1424–1426.

241. **Grizas AP, Camenga D, Vazquez M.** 2012. Cocooning: a concept to protect young children from infectious diseases. *Curr Opin Pediatr* **24:**92–97.

242. **Castagnini LA, Healy CM, Rench MA, Wootton SH, Munoz FM, Baker CJ.** 2012. Impact of maternal postpartum tetanus and diphtheria toxoids and acellular pertussis immunization on infant pertussis infection. *Clin Infect Dis* **54:**78–84.

243. **Healy CM, Rench MA, Castagnini LA, Baker CJ.** 2009. Pertussis immunization in a high-risk postpartum population. *Vaccine* **27:**5599–5602.

244. **Libster R, Edwards KM.** 2012. How can we best prevent pertussis in infants? *Clin Infect Dis* **54:**85–87.

245. **Prato R, Martinelli D, Marchetti F, Fortunato F, Tafuri S, Germinario CA.** 2012. Feasibility of a cocoon strategy for the prevention of pertussis in Italy: a survey of prevention department healthcare providers. *Pediatr Infect Dis J* **31:**1304–1307.

246. **Walter EB, Allred N, Rowe-West B, Chmielewski K, Kretsinger K, Dolor RJ.** 2009. Cocooning infants: Tdap immunization for new parents in the pediatric office. *Acad Pediatr* **9:**344–347.

247. **Wiley KE, Zuo Y, Macartney KK, McIntyre PB.** 2013. Sources of pertussis infection in young infants: a review of key evidence informing targeting of the cocoon strategy. *Vaccine* **31:**618–625.

248. **California Department of Public Health Immunization Branch.** 2010. *Pertussis vaccination recommendations 2010.* California Department of Health Immunization Branch, Sacramento, CA. http://www.cdph.ca.gov/programs/imm unize/Documents/CDPHPertussisImmuni zationPolicy201007.pdf.

249. **Munoz FM, Bond NH, Maccato M, Pinell P, Hammill HA, Swamy GK, Walter EB, Jackson LA, Englund JA, Edwards MS, Healy CM, Petrie CR, Ferreira J, Goll JB, Baker CJ.** 2014. Safety and immunogenicity of tetanus diphtheria and acellular pertussis (Tdap) immunization during pregnancy in mothers and infants: a randomized clinical trial. *JAMA* **311:**1760–1769.

250. **Cherry JD.** 2015. Tetanus-diphtheria-pertussis immunization in pregnant women and the prevention of pertussis in young infants. *Clin Infect Dis* **60:**338–340.

251. **Centers for Disease Control and Prevention.** 2015. *Tdap for pregnant women: information for providers.* Centers for Disease Control and Prevention, Atlanta, GA. http://www.cdc.gov/ pertussis/pregnant/index.html.

252. **Gall SA, Myers J, Pichichero M.** 2011. Maternal immunization with tetanus-diphtheria-pertussis vaccine: effect on maternal and neonatal serum antibody levels. *Am J Obstet Gynecol* **204**(4):334e1–334e5.

253. **Heininger U, Riffelmann M, Bar G, Rudin C, von Konig CH.** 2013. The protective role of maternally derived antibodies against *Bordetella pertussis* in young infants. *Pediatr Infect Dis J* **32:**695–698.

254. **Heininger U, Riffelmann M, Leineweber B, Wirsing von Koenig CH.** 2009. Maternally derived antibodies against *Bordetella pertussis* antigens pertussis toxin and filamentous hemagglutinin in preterm and full term newborns. *Pediatr Infect Dis J* **28:**443–445.

255. **Halperin BA, Morris A, Mackinnon-Cameron D, Mutch J, Langley JM, McNeil SA, Macdougall D, Halperin SA.** 2011. Kinetics of the antibody response to tetanus-diphtheria-acellular pertussis vaccine in women of childbearing age and postpartum women. *Clin Infect Dis* **53:**885–892.

256. **Mooi FR, de Greeff SC.** 2007. The case for maternal vaccination against pertussis. *Lancet Infect Dis* **7:**614–624.

257. **Healy CM, Rench MA, Baker CJ.** 2013. Importance of timing of maternal combined tetanus, diphtheria, and acellular pertussis (Tdap) immunization and protection of young infants. *Clin Infect Dis* **56:**539–544.

258. **Hardy-Fairbanks AJ, Pan SJ, Decker MD, Johnson DR, Greenberg DP, Kirkland KB, Talbot EA, Bernstein HH.** 2013. Immune responses in infants whose mothers received Tdap vaccine during pregnancy. *Pediatr Infect Dis J* **32:**1257–1260.

259. **Donegan K, King B, Bryan P.** 2014. Safety of pertussis vaccination in pregnant women in UK: observational study. *BMJ* **349:**g4219.

260. **Dabrera G, Amirthalingam G, Andrews N, Campbell H, Ribeiro S, Kara E, Fry NK, Ramsay M.** 2015. A case-control study to estimate the effectiveness of maternal pertussis vaccination in protecting newborn infants in England and Wales, 2012-2013. *Clin Infect Dis* **60:**333–337.

261. **Kharbanda EO, Vazquez-Benitez G, Lipkind HS, Klein NP, Cheetham TC, Naleway A, Omer SB, Hambidge SJ, Lee GM, Jackson ML, McCarthy NL, DeStefano F, Nordin JD.** 2014. Evaluation of the association of maternal pertussis vaccination with obstetric events and birth outcomes. *JAMA* **312:**1897–1904.

262. **Morgan JL, Baggari SR, McIntire DD, Sheffield JS.** 2015. Pregnancy outcomes after antepartum tetanus, diphtheria, and acellular pertussis vaccination. *Obstet Gynecol* **125:**1433–1438.

263. **Baraff LJ, Leake RD, Burstyn DG, Payne T, Cody CL, Manclark CR, St Geme JW Jr.** 1984. Immunologic response to early and routine DTP immunization in infants. *Pediatrics* **73:**37–42.

264. **Burstyn DG, Baraff LJ, Peppler MS, Leake RD, St Geme J Jr, Manclark CR.** 1983. Serological response to filamentous hemagglutinin and lymphocytosis-promoting toxin of *Bordetella pertussis. Infect Immun* **41:**1150–1156.

265. **Knuf M, Schmitt HJ, Wolter J, Schuerman L, Jacquet JM, Kieninger D, Siegrist CA, Zepp F.** 2008. Neonatal vaccination with an acellular pertussis vaccine accelerates the acquisition of pertussis antibodies in infants. *J Pediatr* **152:**655–660, 60e1.

266. **Ulloa-Gutierrez R.** 2009. Pertussis vaccination in newborns. *Expert Rev Vaccines* **8:**153–157.

267. **Wood N, McIntyre P, Marshall H, Roberton D.** 2010. Acellular pertussis vaccine at birth and one month induces antibody responses by two months of age. *Pediatr Infect Dis J* **29:**209–215.

268. **Tiwari TS, Baughman AL, Clark TA.** 2015. First pertussis vaccine dose and prevention of infant mortality. *Pediatrics* **135:**990–999.

269. **Centers for Disease Control and Prevention.** 2013. Updated recommendations for use of tetanus toxoid, reduced diphtheria toxoid, and acellular pertussis vaccine (Tdap) in pregnant women—Advisory Committee on Immunization Practices (ACIP), 2012. *MMWR Morb Mortal Wkly Rep* **62:**131–135.

270. **National Center for Immunization and Respiratory Diseases.** 2011. General recommendations on immunization—recommendations of the Advisory Committee on Immunization Practices (ACIP). *MMWR Recommend Rep* **60:**1–64.

271. **Centers for Disease Control and Prevention.** 1997. Pertussis vaccination: use of acellular pertussis vaccines among infants and young children. Recommendations of the Advisory Committee on Immunization Practices (ACIP). *MMWR Recommend Rep* **46**(RR-7)**:**1–25.

272. **Skoff TH, Baumbach J, Cieslak PR.** 2015. Tracking pertussis and evaluating control measures through Enhanced Pertussis Surveillance, Emerging Infections Program, United States. *Emerg Infect Dis* **21:**1568–1573.

273. **Haller S, Dehnert M, Karagiannis I, Rieck T, Siffczyk C, Wichmann O, Poethko-Mueller C, Hellenbrand W.** 2015. Effectiveness of routine and booster pertussis vaccination in children and adolescents, federal state of Brandenburg, Germany, 2002–2012. *Pediatr Infect Dis J* **34:**513–519.

274. **Acosta AM, DeBolt C, Tasslimi A, Lewis M, Stewart LK, Misegades LK, Messonnier NE, Clark TA, Martin SW, Patel M.** 2015. Tdap vaccine effectiveness in adolescents during the 2012 Washington State pertussis epidemic. *Pediatrics* **135:**981–989.

275. **Koepke R, Eickhoff JC, Ayele RA, Petit AB, Schauer SL, Hopfensperger DJ, Conway JH, Davis JP.** 2014. Estimating the effectiveness of tetanus-diphtheria-acellular pertussis vaccine (Tdap) for preventing pertussis: evidence of rapidly waning immunity and difference in effectiveness by Tdap brand. *J Infect Dis* **210:**942–953.

276. **McGirr A, Fisman DN.** 2015. Duration of pertussis immunity after DTaP immunization: a meta-analysis. *Pediatrics* **135:**331–343.

277. **Cherry JD.** 2015. Epidemic pertussis and acellular pertussis vaccine failure in the 21st century. *Pediatrics* **135:**1130–1132.

278. **Warfel JM, Merkel TJ.** 2013. *Bordetella pertussis* infection induces a mucosal IL-17 response and long-lived Th17 and Th1 immune memory cells in nonhuman primates. *Mucosal Immunol* **6:**787–796.

279. **Pawloski LC, Queenan AM, Cassiday PK, Lynch AS, Harrison MJ, Shang W, Williams MM, Bowden KE, Burgos-Rivera B, Qin X, Messonnier N, Tondella ML.** 2014. Prevalence and molecular characterization of pertactin-deficient *Bordetella pertussis* in the United States. *Clin Vaccine Immunol* **21:**119–125.

280. **Rosenblum E, McBane S, Wang W, Sawyer M.** 2014. Protecting newborns by immunizing family members in a hospital-based vaccine clinic: a successful Tdap cocooning program

during the 2010 California pertussis epidemic. *Public Health Rep* **129:**245–251.

281. **Urwyler P, Heininger U.** 2014. Protecting newborns from pertussis—the challenge of complete cocooning. *BMC Infect Dis* **14:**397.

282. **Healy CM, Rench MA, Wootton SH, Castagnini LA.** 2015. Evaluation of the impact of a pertussis cocooning program on infant pertussis infection. *Pediatr Infect Dis J* **34:**22–26.

283. **Wolf ER, Opel D, DeHart MP, Warren J, Rowhani-Rahbar A.** 2014. Impact of a pertussis epidemic on infant vaccination in Washington state. *Pediatrics* **134:**456–464.

284. **Williams WW, Lu PJ, O'Halloran A, Bridges CB, Pilishvili T, Hales CM, Markowitz LE.** 2014. Noninfluenza vaccination coverage among adults—United States, 2012. *MMWR Morb Mortal Wkly Rep* **63:**95–102.

285. **Sawyer MH, Long SS.** 2015. Tdap in every pregnancy: circling the wagons around the newborn. *Pediatrics* **135:**e1483–e1484.

286. **Housey M, Zhang F, Miller C, Lyon-Callo S, McFadden J, Garcia E, Potter R, Centers for Disease Control and Prevention.** 2014. Vaccination with tetanus, diphtheria, and acellular pertussis vaccine of pregnant women enrolled in Medicaid—Michigan, 2011–2013. *MMWR Morb Mortal Wkly Rep* **63:**839–842.

287. **Kharbanda EO, Vazquez-Benitez G, Lipkind H, Naleway AL, Klein NP, Cheetham TC, Hambidge SJ, Vellozzi C, Nordin JD.** 2014. Receipt of pertussis vaccine during pregnancy across 7 Vaccine Safety Datalink sites. *Prev Med* **67:**316–319.

288. **Ahluwalia IB, Ding H, D'Angelo D, Shealy KH, Singleton JA, Liang J, Rosenberg KD, Centers for Disease Control and Prevention.** 2015. Tetanus, diphtheria, pertussis vaccination coverage before, during, and after pregnancy—16 states and New York City, 2011. *MMWR Morb Mortal Wkly Rep* **64:**522–526.

289. **Harriman K, Winter K.** 2014. Pertussis vaccine uptake during pregnancy: we need to do better in the U.S. *Prev Med* **67:**320–321.

290. **Koepke R, Kahn D, Petit AB, Schauer SL, Hopfensperger DJ, Conway JH, Davis JP, Centers for Disease Control and Prevention.** 2015. Pertussis and influenza vaccination among insured pregnant women—Wisconsin, 2013-2014. *MMWR Morb Mortal Wkly Rep* **64:**746–750.

291. **Fernandez-Cano MI, Armadans Gil L, Campins Marti M.** 2015. Cost-benefit of the introduction of new strategies for vaccination against pertussis in Spain: cocooning and pregnant vaccination strategies. *Vaccine* **33:**2213–2220.

292. **Terranella A, Asay GR, Messonnier ML, Clark TA, Liang JL.** 2013. Pregnancy dose Tdap and postpartum cocooning to prevent infant pertussis: a decision analysis. *Pediatrics* **131**(6):e1748–e1756.

Invasive Infections with Nontyphoidal *Salmonella* in Sub-Saharan Africa

18

BARBARA E. MAHON[1] and PATRICIA I. FIELDS[1]

INTRODUCTION AND DISEASE BURDEN

Worldwide, *Salmonella* infection typically causes gastroenteritis and rarely causes invasive infections of normally sterile sites. A well-known exception is enteric fever (invasive infection caused by *Salmonella enterica* serotypes Typhi, Paratyphi A, Paratyphi B, or Paratyphi C), a syndrome of acute febrile illness, often with abdominal pain, headache, and other manifestations. However, nontyphoidal *Salmonella* (NTS) serotypes can also cause invasive infections, which often present as sepsis rather than as typical enteric fever (1). Vulnerable populations, such as infants, young children, and immunocompromised people of any age, are at risk. Invasive NTS infections in Africa cause an enormous burden of illness—Africa is estimated to account for more than half of the 3.4 million invasive NTS infections (2)—and these infections are often devastating, with a mortality rate estimated at 20% in African settings (3), even with appropriate antimicrobial therapy. Although invasive NTS infection has been recognized for decades as an important cause of invasive bacterial infection in sub-Saharan Africa, until recently it received relatively little attention (4, 5). However, this is changing, with increasing attention from the scientific community and from both governmental and

[1]Division of Foodborne, Waterborne, and Environmental Diseases, National Center for Emerging and Zoonotic Infectious Diseases, Centers for Disease Control and Prevention, Atlanta, GA 30329.
Emerging Infections 10
Edited by W. Michael Scheld, James M. Hughes and Richard J. Whitley
© 2016 American Society for Microbiology, Washington, DC
doi:10.1128/microbiolspec.EI10-0015-2016

nongovernmental organizations focused on understanding the sources of these infections and developing effective tools for prevention (4, 6).

The diagnosis of NTS infection relies on microbiological testing, typically culture of stool, blood, or other clinical specimens. The capacity to conduct such testing is unavailable in much of Africa (7, 8). Consequently, population-based surveillance information on the incidence of invasive NTS infections is also limited. Much of what is known comes from studies conducted in health care facilities or relatively small geographic areas that have enhanced microbiologic capacity, often developed to support research studies on other topics. For example, important information about invasive NTS infections has emerged from research programs on vaccine-preventable diseases, HIV infection, malaria, and other infectious diseases.

In many areas of sub-Saharan Africa, NTS is now recognized as the most common cause of community-acquired invasive bacterial infection, with an estimated overall incidence of 227 cases per 100,000 population annually (3). To some extent, this reflects the successful implementation of childhood vaccination for *Streptococcus pneumoniae* and *Haemophilus influenzae* in many countries, with great reductions in the burden of childhood invasive infections caused by these pathogens (4). However, the prominence of invasive NTS infection is not simply due to control of other infections. Early in the HIV epidemic, it became clear that invasive NTS infection was a common opportunistic infection in immunocompromised HIV-infected people throughout the world; the high prevalence of HIV in sub-Saharan Africa has contributed greatly to the high incidence of invasive NTS disease in the region. However, the incidence of invasive NTS disease varies substantially from place to place and time to time. For example, incidence rates exceeding 2,000 per 100,000 children under 5 years old per year have recently been reported in rural Kenya (9, 10), whereas in Mozambique in the

same time frame, incidence was an order of magnitude lower, at just over 200 cases per 100,000 infants (11).

Salmonella is well known as a cause of outbreaks, some of which can extend over months or years. Because much of the information from Africa comes from point-in-time studies, rather than from ongoing disease surveillance, and because outbreak detection and investigation is limited, it is not clear what proportion of NTS infections are outbreak-associated, as opposed to sporadic. However, there are suggestions that outbreak-type dynamics may be driving the epidemiology of invasive NTS disease, at least to some extent. It is certainly clear that large, sustained outbreaks have occurred, because investigators in Malawi have documented serial outbreaks of invasive NTS disease caused by NTS of different serotypes and antimicrobial resistance patterns (12, 13), and investigators in Mali have documented a large, sustained outbreak caused by *Salmonella* Enteritidis (14). Similarly, in areas of Kenya that previously experienced the highest rates of invasive NTS disease ever reported (9), a recent report shows decreasing—although still very high—incidence from 2009 to 2014 (15). Progressive declines in annual incidence have also been reported in children in Mozambique and Malawi (11, 16). In the absence of other interventions or events that would have led to decreasing incidence, these observations suggest that large outbreaks or even a continent-wide epidemic may be or may have been responsible for a substantial part of the large burden of invasive NTS disease.

This chapter reviews the current state of knowledge on invasive NTS infections in Africa, focusing on epidemiologic aspects of these infections and opportunities for prevention while also addressing microbiologic aspects. Much is not known regarding the sources and transmission of these infections, and thus the ability to prevent them is hampered. However, prevention is much needed, because these infections are not only common and serious, but emerging antimicrobial resistance makes them increasingly difficult to treat.

CLINICAL FEATURES AND RISK FACTORS

Like most infectious diseases, invasive NTS infections can range from mild to severe. Because most studies have been conducted among inpatients, the published descriptions of clinical features lean toward the more severe end of the clinical spectrum. However, all indications are that, as in other settings, two major groups—young children and HIV-infected adults—suffer the great majority of these infections. It is also clear that mortality is substantial, typically around 20% in populations with standard access to medical services (12). In studies focused only on inpatients, mortality can exceed 50%, but even in community-based studies that include less severe illnesses that might not otherwise come to medical attention, mortality is in the 2 to 5% range (9).

Invasive NTS Infection in Children

In children, invasive NTS infections often present with a nonspecific febrile or toxic picture. Estimates of the proportion of patients with a history of antecedent diarrhea vary from about a quarter to a half (11, 17–19). In children for whom diarrhea is not reported, it is not clear whether relatively mild diarrhea might have occurred, but it is clear that many children do not present with the prominent bloody diarrhea often associated with severe enteric *Salmonella* infection. Indeed, many children present with respiratory symptoms that may even meet criteria for acute lower respiratory tract infection (17, 19–21). Most children have a septic picture, with positive blood cultures, but a small proportion have invasive focal infections, including meningitis, abscesses, osteomyelitis, septic arthritis, thoracic empyema, and even panophthalmitis (17, 22). Reported mor-

tality has ranged widely, from about 3 to 20%, likely reflecting both variation in study methods, as discussed above, and the availability of effective antibiotics and other care.

Regardless of the overall case fatality ratio, however, multiple studies have shown that infants are more likely to die than older children (12, 23–25). Children who survive occasionally experience recrudescent disease, but this occurs less frequently in children than in adults. Aside from any other immunocompromising factors, and consistent with patterns seen in other countries (26), young age is itself an important risk factor for invasive NTS infection. Rates of infection in children under 5 years old are many-fold higher than in older children (10), and the highest rates of all are in the first year of life (27). However, infection is relatively uncommon in the first several months of life, peaking at around six months of age. This peak is a few months later than in developed countries, perhaps reflecting the waning of protection from maternal antibodies and from breastfeeding; as in other areas of the world, breastfeeding appears to be protective (22). It may also reflect rates of exposure to NTS from food, water, or environmental sources, though the sources of NTS infection in infants are not clearly known. Young age—less than a year old in a Kenyan study—is also a risk factor for greater disease severity (28).

Much research on invasive NTS infections in young children has focused on the role of malaria. Malaria—either concurrent or recent—is strongly associated at both the individual and population levels with invasive NTS infection (18, 27, 29, 30). Severe malaria is particularly strongly associated (25, 31). The reasons for this association are not fully understood but may involve effects on free iron availability (32), neutrophil function (33) and facilitation of NTS invasion of the bloodstream due to damage to the gut intestinal barrier (34, 35). The effect of malaria seems to be specific to NTS; whereas invasive NTS disease is strongly associated with malaria, other pathogens that cause bacteremia are not (10, 27, 36). Regardless of the reason, several studies conducted in various countries have shown marked reductions in invasive NTS infections with declining prevalence of malaria (16, 29, 37, 38). This gives hope that an effective malaria vaccine might indirectly lower risk of invasive NTS infection, at least to some extent.

Other well-documented risk factors for invasive NTS infection in children include malnutrition (18, 19, 23, 27), HIV infection (5, 18, 20, 30), anemia (27), concurrent schistosomiasis (39), and sickle cell disease. Although child malnutrition is common in the general population in much of sub-Saharan Africa, it is even more common in these children with invasive NTS infection. For example, in a multivariate analysis of data from Tanzania on children admitted to hospital with acute febrile illness, children with invasive NTS disease were twice as likely to have severe acute malnutrition as children with other diagnoses (27). In addition to its direct effects on the immune system, malnutrition can impair the intestinal endothelial barrier, which may predispose to invasion of NTS that might only have caused enteric infection otherwise. HIV infection is not as common in children as in adults with invasive NTS infection. Nonetheless, it is an important risk factor, especially in children who are not receiving antiretroviral therapy. Mortality in NTS infection exceeds 20% in children with HIV infection (19, 23, 30). In schistosomiasis, adult worms attach to the portal and mesenteric blood vessels. They are thought to provide a sanctuary for salmonellae to multiply and seed the bloodstream (39). Invasive NTS infection is also common in children with sickle cell anemia and other hemoglobinopathies. In coastal Kenya, about 5 to 10% of children hospitalized with invasive NTS disease had sickle cell disease (18). Few other studies of invasive NTS disease in Africa have documented sickle cell status, but it is known to be common throughout Africa and likely contributes to the overall burden of invasive NTS disease.

Sickle cell disease, malaria, and malnutrition may all play a role in the observed association of invasive NTS disease with anemia. Not surprisingly, these risk factors appear to interact, with even higher risk of invasive NTS infection in children with two or more of the risk factors discussed above (16, 40).

Invasive NTS Infection in Adults

Early in the HIV epidemic, invasive NTS infection was recognized as a common presentation in severely immunocompromised patients (41). In Africa, the majority of invasive NTS infection in adults occurs in patients with HIV infection (18, 42, 43), usually untreated. Like children, adults often present without a history of antecedent diarrhea, though diarrhea is more common in adults with invasive NTS disease than those who are admitted for other reasons (18). The presentation is commonly described as being consistent with enteric fever (44), although a septic picture is also common. Mortality is high, especially in patients with advanced HIV disease, in whom it can exceed 50% (42). However, even in HIV-negative patients, mortality of 32% was reported in Malawi (42). For survivors, recrudescent or recurrent invasive NTS infection occurs in a substantial proportion. HIV infection is a strong risk factor; recurrence has been reported to occur in more than 40% of HIV-infected patients with invasive NTS disease (45, 46).

MICROBIOLOGY

Although many *Salmonella* serotypes have been described, just a few are responsible for most invasive infections. In sub-Saharan Africa, the NTS serotypes that cause most invasive disease are Typhimurium and Enteritidis (8, 12, 14, 19, 24, 28, 42, 44, 47–50), which are also among the most common serotypes causing both gastrointestinal and invasive *Salmonella* infections globally. Although serotypes Typhimurium and Enter-itidis appear to be frequent causes of invasive infection continent-wide, other serotypes have been reported in invasive infections, with specific serotypes appearing relatively frequently in specific geographic areas. Serotype Concord is a frequent cause of invasive infection in Ethiopia (51); serotype Isangi in South Africa (52); and serotypes Newport, Virchow, Derby, and Braenderup in Kenya (28, 53). Many other serotypes have been reported, though rarely.

Very limited information on the propor-tion of NTS infections that are invasive is available from Africa, in large part because microbiologic evaluation of diarrheal ill-nesses is quite rare, even in settings where blood and CSF cultures can be performed. Much of the information regarding the relative propensity of nontyphoidal serotypes to cause invasive disease comes from Kenya. This information reveals two patterns. First, a broader range of serotypes is isolated from stool than from blood. Second, however, the serotypes commonly isolated from blood are also commonly isolated from stool, though relatively less commonly than from blood. For example, in reports from the mid-1990s through the late 2000s from a hospital serving a rural population on the coast, *Salmonella* Typhimurium and Enteritidis accounted for 85 to 95% of *Salmonella* iso-lated from invasive infections in children but only 33 to 68% of *Salmonella* isolated from stool. By contrast, other serotypes accounted for up to 67% of *Salmonella* isolated from stool but less than 15% of invasive infections (24, 28, 54). Similarly, in a report from two other settings in Kenya covering 2006 through 2009, *Salmonella* Typhimurium accounted for 84% and 53% of *Salmonella* isolated from blood and stool, respectively (10). Given that the populations in which most invasive NTS disease occurs—young, often malnourished, children and HIV-infected adults—have com-promised immunity, these data imply that *Salmonella* Typhimurium and Enteritidis are more prone than other serotypes to causing

invasive disease in these immunocompro-mised populations. A similar observation was made early in the HIV epidemic in the United States, where surveillance data showed that *Salmonella* Typhimurium and Enteritidis, but not Heidelberg, were disproportionately asso-ciated with invasive infections in regions and age groups with a high prevalence of HIV infection (41).

Salmonella Typhimurium is particularly common in invasive infections in Africa, accounting for more than 90% of isolates in some series (44). In recent years, a specific strain of *Salmonella* Typhimurium, multi-locus sequence type 313, or ST313, has caused epidemics of invasive disease (12). This strain was first recognized during the HIV epidem-ic that has been so prominent in Africa (55). Although ST313 does appear to be very prone to causing invasive infections in compro-mised hosts, apparently it also causes more typical gastrointestinal infections; a South African report notes that ST313 is commonly isolated from stool in diarrheal illness in otherwise healthy people (56). To the same point, six of nine ceftriaxone-resistant *Sal-monella* Typhimurium isolates from people with severe illness in 2009 to 2011 charac-terized by whole-genome sequencing were from stool isolates. Although the multilocus sequence type was not reported, these iso-lates were genotypically closely related and were likely ST313 (57).

In the last several years, many studies have used phenotypic and genetic methods to characterize ST313 strains. These strains initially fell into two (55, 58) and then three (59) distinct clusters based on genome se-quencing comparisons. All three lineages are resistant to multiple antimicrobial agents, which likely contributed to their rapid clonal expansion in a population of suscep-tible NTS. Comparisons to other *Salmonella* Typhimurium strains indicated that eight ST19 strains that were associated with in-vasive disease in Africa were scattered throughout the phylogenetic tree (55). This observation indicates that while other types may not be as common as ST313, they can also cause invasive disease in susceptible people in Africa. ST313 strains possess multiple pseudogenes, a characteristic which has been noted to be a marker for host adaptation. Different lineages possess somewhat different pseudogene repertoires (60, 61). Roles for some of the pseudogenes in virulence for humans have been suggested (55, 60–62). Phage type DT2 strains, which are known to be host-adapted to birds, were also noted to have multiple pseudogenes (63). In a whole-genome sequence comparison, ST313 strains appeared to be more closely related to the DT2 strains than to representative ST19 strains (63); a comparison of pseudogene profile between ST313 and DT2 was not made.

Experiments using *in vitro* models of infection to investigate potential virulence differences between ST313 and other *S.* Typhimurium strains have not provided a clear picture of the virulence properties of ST313. Using a mouse oral infection model, one study showed that an ST313 strain has a 50% lethal dose similar to an ST19 strain (64), while another showed similar levels of systemic colonization for ST313 and ST19 but a lower inflammatory response for ST313 (61). A study using cell culture models showed that an ST313 strain produced less inflammatory response than an ST19 strain (65). In a chicken oral challenge model, both ST313 and ST19 strains caused invasive infections, with invasion occurring somewhat more slowly with the ST19 strain (66). A variety of macrophage models suggested that ST313 strains had a survival phenotype intermediate between ST19 strains, which were killed by human macrophages, and *S. enterica* serotypes Typhi and Paratyphi A, which are known to be highly invasive in humans and which survived and grew in human macrophages (67). The genetic diversity of *Salmonella* Typhimurium may be an explanation for the variable results in the *in vitro* models; results may depend on the model system used and the strains that are being compared.

Diversity in host range and ability to infect humans has been suggested for *Salmonella* Typhimurium (68). For example, phage type D2 has been noted to be adapted to birds and not commonly associated with human infections (68). Given the existence of *Salmonella* Typhimurium strains that are host-restricted to birds, it may be appropriate to consider the hypothesis that the apparent relative rarity of gastrointestinal infections due to ST313 in Africa is a reflection of low pathogenicity in healthy humans. Alternatively, it has been suggested that the *spv* genes found in some *Salmonella* serotypes including *Salmonella* Typhimurium and Enteritidis may contribute to more severe infections in immunocompromised individuals (69). Further understanding of the biological and epidemiological implications of the unique characteristics of ST313 could be valuable, particularly if it leads to a better understanding of sources of exposure, events leading to severe disease, and interventions that could decrease disease burden.

SOURCES AND TRANSMISSION

Known important routes of transmission for *Salmonella* worldwide include food-borne, waterborne, direct animal contact, and person-to-person routes. In the United States and other developed countries, food-borne transmission predominates (70). As summarized above, much is known about host risk factors for invasive NTS disease, such as HIV infection, malnutrition, malaria, and other host-compromising conditions. These host risk factors increase the risk of invasive disease occurring after exposure to NTS. They also confer greater risk for severe disease and death in those who become ill. Little is known, however, about risk factors for exposure to NTS in sub-Saharan Africa in the first place, and this lack of knowledge makes it difficult to design rational interventions to decrease exposure. By contrast, many studies have shown that risk factors for typhoid fever include crowding, poor sanitation, and lack of access to safe food and water (1). These factors relate to the risk of exposure to *Salmonella* Typhi itself and point directly toward interventions that can decrease the risk of disease. More information about the sources of exposure to NTS, especially *Salmonella* Typhimurium and Enteritidis, is urgently needed to inform disease control efforts.

Globally, much of what is known about routes of NTS transmission to humans comes from outbreak investigations that reveal sources and routes of exposure for a group of ill people with a source in common; reservoirs and sources vary by serotype (71). In sub-Saharan Africa, outbreak detection and investigation are less well developed, with no information on the sources of NTS outbreaks available from most countries. The few published outbreak investigations tend to be of outbreaks associated with institutions, especially hospitals (52, 72–74). Since hospitalized populations are likely to include many people with host risk factors for invasive NTS disease, the occurrence of an outbreak associated with a hospital could be consistent with almost any route of transmission, especially food-borne, waterborne, and person-to-person. For instance, a primarily nosocomial outbreak of noninvasive *Salmonella* Typhimurium infections was reported on a children's ward in South Africa in 2012, but the investigation did not reveal a source or mode of transmission (73). By contrast, the investigation of a 2000–2001 nosocomial *Salmonella* Isangi outbreak from another South African hospital showed spread to patients in beds and cubicles contiguous to that of the index case, suggesting a role for either direct or indirect transmission from person to person (52).

Another approach to identifying sources of NTS has been to seek matching strains in household members, animals, and environments of patients. The most comprehensive of these studies, which was conducted in Nairobi slums, identified young children with invasive NTS disease and then did compre-

hensive culturing of family members, household and neighborhood animals, water sources, food, and local vendors. In all, NTS was isolated from 7% of family members, and the serotype matched in 65% of them (28). This observation does not elucidate whether the family members were simply exposed to the same source as the case or whether person-to-person transmission occurred. In this study, NTS was isolated from few nonhuman sources, but four isolates from water or soil matched the serotype and pulsed-field gel electrophoresis pattern of the isolate from the ill child (28). Again, though, detecting the same strain in the environment offers little insight into whether the patient was exposed through an environmental source, whether the patient contaminated the environment during the illness, or whether the NTS found in both the patient and the environment originated from another source, such as an animal.

Several studies have cultured livestock, poultry, and retail meats and have found NTS, often with a different distribution of serotypes than are found in humans (75–78). However, this pattern of differing serotype distributions is seen in settings where food-borne transmission is known to be common (79), so again it offers little clue as to sources. There are hints that poultry might be an important source of NTS in sub-Saharan Africa, as it is in the rest of the world. In Kenya, in the context of increasing incidence of human Enteritidis infections, a serotype strongly linked to eggs, investigators noted that rearing chickens for eggs had become increasingly common in the population (80). Finally, an intriguing study in South Africa compared pulsed-field gel electrophoresis patterns of NTS isolates from noninvasive human infections and captive wild animals, showing marked similarities in strains. This may imply a common source of exposure. The authors speculate that chicken, a common source of NTS globally, could be a source, since it is frequently part of the diet fed to captive wild animals (81).

In the absence of more definitive information on sources and routes of transmission, we are left to try to extrapolate from other information. The pronounced seasonality of invasive NTS disease, with increased incidence during and after the rainy season in Malawi (12), Kenya (28), and other countries has led some investigators to wonder whether this pattern implies an important role for waterborne transmission or whether general environmental contamination or person-to-person transmission might increase during the rainy season. Comparisons between NTS and *Salmonella* Typhi, which has a human reservoir, may offer other clues. In a 4-year study comparing the incidence of invasive NTS disease to typhoid fever in a rural and an urban setting in Kenya, NTS greatly predominated in the rural setting, whereas Typhi predominated in the urban setting (10). In Tanzania, a similar dichotomy was reported among children, with an NTS: Typhi ratio of 15:1 in the rural area and 1:6 in the urban area. It is tempting to speculate that this pattern might reflect sources of infection, with Typhi (human to human) being more common in the urban setting and NTS (animal to human) being more common in the rural setting. In summary, though, knowledge of the sources and routes of transmission of NTS in sub-Saharan Africa remains unclear at best, and this limits the ability to target interventions. In particular, if person-to-person transmission accounts for a large proportion of cases, then different interventions would be indicated than if, as in the rest of the world, contaminated food and water and contact with infected animals and environments are the major issues.

ANTIMICROBIAL RESISTANCE

Although antimicrobial therapy is not recommended for most uncomplicated gastrointestinal NTS infections, it is critically important for treatment of invasive infections. This was documented dramatically in an early paper on invasive NTS disease in Rwandan children, in whom mortality was 10% in those treated with an effective antibiotic (cefotaxime in this setting) but close to 80% in those who did not receive such treatment (22). Thus, the emergence and spread of resistance to antimicrobial agents commonly used for treatment of invasive NTS infections in Africa is an ominous development. This is especially true because the widespread limitations in microbiologic diagnostic capacity in much of Africa means that infections are often treated empirically. When resistance to empiric regimens emerges, it may not be identified promptly, and large numbers of patients may not be treated with appropriate alternative agents, if alternatives are even available. Moreover, because children with invasive NTS infection may meet clinical criteria for pneumonia, which is usually caused by pathogens other than NTS, selection of antimicrobial agents poses a conundrum; agents that are recommended for empiric treatment of pneumonia, e.g., penicillin and chloramphenicol, are often ineffective in invasive NTS infection, and many agents effective against NTS are not ideal choices for the pathogens that cause pneumonia.

Beginning in the 1980s and accelerating since then, waves of antimicrobial resistance have greatly complicated the treatment of invasive NTS infections in Africa. The initial challenge was from resistance to several agents classically used for treatment of NTS infections, including chloramphenicol, ampicillin, and co-trimoxazole, as well as other agents. In Rwanda, invasive infections with such resistant isolates, as well as successful treatment with the third-generation cephalosporin cefotaxime, were described in children in the 1980s (17, 22). In Kenya in the mid-to-late 1990s, about half of invasive infections in children in a rural community were caused by NTS resistant to these agents (54), though resistance to chloramphenicol was somewhat less common. At that time, resistance to third-generation cephalosporins and fluoroquinolones was not seen

(82). Similarly, in invasive NTS infections in adults in Kenya, the proportion resistant to these three agents was about 40% by 2003 (80). In Malawi in the late 1990s and early 2000s, successive epidemics of invasive infections resistant to these agents were caused by multi-drug resistant (MDR) Enteritidis and subsequently by MDR Typhimurium. In this primarily urban setting, resistance to all three agents increased rapidly over a period of several months to a year and a half from zero to about 80% of isolates (12). Whenever molecular characterization of resistance has been conducted, the resistance determinants have been shown to be plasmid-borne, implying that horizontal transfer between bacteria can readily occur. In sum, the emergence and spread of resistance to these inexpensive and widely available agents has essentially spelled the end of their usefulness of for treatment of invasive NTS infections in many areas. Clinicians have had to turn to more expensive agents, such as third-generation cephalosporins (e.g., ceftriaxone) and fluoroquinolones (e.g., ciprofloxacin), when these agents were available.

Recently, NTS isolates with resistance to third-generation cephalosporins, and in some cases to fluoroquinolones as well, have become increasingly common. In 2000, a nosocomial outbreak of Isangi infections that produced an extended-spectrum beta lactamase (ESBL) and thus were resistant to ceftriaxone was reported from South Africa (52). Since then, Typhimurium resistant to third-generation cephalosporin has been reported from Malawi (83), Kenya (9, 57, 84), South Africa (3), and the Democratic Republic of the Congo (85). The Malawi report illustrates how quickly resistance can be acquired; the patient was a woman with HIV infection who had an initial NTS infection that was MDR but susceptible to ceftriaxone and ciprofloxacin. She was treated as an inpatient with ceftriaxone and discharged on oral ciprofloxacin and was readmitted a month later with recrudescent disease; the isolate was MDR and also

resistant to both ciprofloxacin and ceftriaxone (83). Genomic analysis suggested that this episode did not reflect reinfection with a new strain but rather acquisition of additional resistance determinants by the initial strain. Similarly, ceftriaxone resistance, along with resistance to multiple other agents, increased from less than 10% to more than 50% over about 2 years in NTS isolated in invasive Typhimurium infections in young children (9). An IncHI2 plasmid bearing CTX-M extended-spectrum beta-lactamase (ESBL) genes as well as genes conferring resistance to multiple other antimicrobial agents was identified in isolates from both Malawi and Kenya (57, 83), and beta lactamase genes of the TEM and CMY classes were reported from South Africa (3, 52). Fluoroquinolone resistance in isolates that do not produce ESBLs have also been reported (86). To our knowledge, NTS isolates resistant to carbapenems (e.g., imipenem, meropenem) have not been reported, but carbapenems are unavailable in most health care settings in Africa.

Antimicrobial resistance is complex, and although a pattern of increasing resistance has been seen in almost all studies, some exceptions exist. In a rural area of Kenya, a marked decrease in resistance to amoxicillin and co-trimoxazole in NTS isolated from children with invasive disease, from just under 70% to both agents in 1994–1997 to just over 10% in 2002–2005 was documented (53). While this offers hope that high rates of resistance might be reversible, information on antimicrobial usage trends in this area was not available, so it is not clear whether selective pressure was decreased or whether other factors, such as changes in medical care or in the distribution of NTS serotypes causing invasive disease, may have contributed to the decrease in resistance rates.

In summary, antimicrobial resistance poses a serious threat to our ability to treat invasive NTS infections in Africa. Effective antimicrobial stewardship—both for agents used in human medicine and for those used in animal agriculture—is critical to preserve the effectiveness of these agents. Antimicrobial agents are widely available without a prescription in most areas. Surveillance for antimicrobial resistance in NTS is needed to detect emerging resistance as early as possible. Protocols for empiric treatment need to reflect the prevailing resistance patterns while also acknowledging the limited availability and affordability of agents such as carbapenems and even third-generation cephalosporins (87)—a challenging task, indeed (87). That so many NTS isolates from invasive infections display resistance that makes them effectively untreatable, given the local availability of extended-spectrum agents, emphasizes the importance of primary prevention of invasive NTS infections.

INTERVENTIONS

Public health, environmental, and medical interventions to address the toll of invasive NTS disease in sub-Saharan Africa can be considered in three major categories—interventions to prevent exposure to NTS, interventions to prevent the occurrence of disease if exposure does occur, and interventions to prevent severe disease and death in those who become ill. All are important.

Although, as discussed above, the routes of exposure to NTS in sub-Saharan Africa are not well understood, improvements in sanitation and hygiene in general are likely to decrease exposure to NTS by any route. Most enteric pathogens have transmission pathways in common, and it has been observed in other settings—for instance, when improvements in sanitation and hygiene undertaken in Mexico to control cholera were associated with marked decreases in all-cause diarrheal mortality in young children (88)—that such improvements have protean benefits. Nonetheless, better information about sources of NTS infection might help with the design of interventions that would be particularly appropriate for sub-Saharan Africa. En-

hanced capacity for outbreak detection and investigation would be particularly valuable. Whole-genome sequencing also has promise as part of efforts to link human infections with their sources (56, 89).

Interventions to decrease the risk of progression to invasive infection after exposure to NTS are also critical. Several of the important risk factors for invasive NTS disease are themselves targets of concerted public health action. Great efforts have been and are being made to prevent HIV infection and to provide treatment when it occurs (90). Economic development as well as targeted programs can help to prevent childhood malnutrition. Malaria is also an enormously important public health problem (91), and efforts to control it through such measures as insecticide-treated bed nets appear to have had a major impact on invasive NTS disease as well as on malaria itself. The possibility that an effective malaria vaccine would have indirect impact in preventing invasive NTS disease is exciting and important. A recent study from Malawi modeling the impact of HIV infection, acute malnutrition, malaria, and other factors on invasive NTS disease validated the notion that public health interventions to reduce them have likely had both individual and synergistic impact on rates of invasive NTS disease in children (16).

Effective NTS vaccines are an attractive idea. Studies in Malawi have demonstrated that most children developed anti-NTS antibodies by two years of age, as well as cell-mediated immunity, and that this antibody enabled NTS killing *in vitro*, suggesting that a vaccine that stimulates production of such antibodies might be possible (92, 93). Several candidate live attenuated vaccines and glycoconjugate vaccines targeted at serogroup-specific surface antigens have been developed and are in early development (14, 94–99). Although these vaccines are promising, it is difficult to predict whether any of them would be safe and effective. It is unlikely that an NTS vaccine could be licensed and available in less than 5 to

10 years, so other actions to control invasive NTS disease should not be postponed in anticipation of a vaccine.

Finally, prevention of severe infection and death will rely not only on general development of the medical system, including primary prevention through infection prevention and control within health care facilities, but also on the availability of effective antimicrobial agents to treat these infections. The emergence and spread of antimicrobial resistance has rightly been described as a public health crisis that threatens the ability to treat many infections, invasive NTS disease among them (100). Global, regional, and local action to preserve the effectiveness of antimicrobial agents involves surveillance for the emergence and prevalence of resistance and stewardship of antimicrobial agents used for humans and for animals. Already, many invasive NTS infections are essentially untreatable in many health care facilities in sub-Saharan Africa, and prevention of further development and spread of resistance is urgently needed.

CONCLUSION

Invasive nontyphoidal *Salmonella* (NTS) infections in Africa cause an enormous burden of illness and high mortality and, in some areas, NTS is the most common cause of invasive bacterial infection. Populations with compromised immunity—young children, especially those with malnutrition or malaria, and HIV-infected adults—are at the highest risk. As in the rest of the world, Typhimurium and Enteritidis are the most common serotypes causing invasive NTS infections in Africa. A specific strain of Typhimurium, multilocus sequence type 313, has recently caused epidemics of invasive disease. Antimicrobial therapy is critically important for treatment of invasive NTS infections. Waves of antimicrobial resistance, recently including third-generation cephalosporins, have emerged and spread across the continent, threatening the ability to treat these infec-

tions. Improvements in antimicrobial stewardship are important in Africa, as in the rest of the world. Several NTS vaccines are in early development and, if shown to be safe and effective, could be promising, but vaccines will not be widely available for years, so other control strategies must also be pursued. Because of the strong association of invasive NTS disease in children with malaria, effective malaria control programs may also help reduce invasive NTS disease to some extent. Little is known about the sources of exposure to NTS in Africa or about the relative importance of foodborne or waterborne transmission or direct contact with infected animals or people, making the rational design of interventions to prevent exposure difficult. However, improved sanitation and access to safe water and food would likely have an important impact on exposure to NTS in Africa.

ACKNOWLEDGMENTS

We gratefully acknowledge Anya Rosen-Gooding for assistance with the literature review.

The findings and conclusions in this report are those of the authors and do not necessarily represent the official position of the Centers for Disease Control and Prevention.

CITATION

Mahon BE, Fields PI. 2016. Invasive infections with nontyphoidal *Salmonella* in sub-Saharan Africa. Microbiol Spectrum 4(3): EI10-0015-2016.

REFERENCES

1. **Crump JA, Sjolund-Karlsson M, Gordon MA, Parry CM.** 2015. Epidemiology, clinical presentation, laboratory diagnosis, antimicrobial resistance, and antimicrobial management of invasive *Salmonella* infections. *Clin Microbiol Rev* **28:**901–937.
2. **Ao TT, Feasey NA, Gordon MA, Keddy KH, Angulo FJ, Crump JA.** 2015. Global burden of

invasive nontyphoidal *Salmonella* disease, 2010. *Emerg Infect Dis* **21:**941–949.

3. **Kruger T, Szabo D, Keddy KH, Deeley K, Marsh JW, Hujer AM, Bonomo RA, Paterson DL.** 2004. Infections with nontyphoidal *Salmonella* species producing TEM-63 or a novel TEM enzyme, TEM-131, in South Africa. *Antimicrob Agents Chemother* **48:**4263–4270.

4. **Crump JA, Heyderman RS.** 2014. Invasive *Salmonella* infections in Africa. *Trans R Soc Trop Med Hyg* **108:**673–675.

5. **Feasey NA, Dougan G, Kingsley RA, Heyderman RS, Gordon MA.** 2012. Invasive non-typhoidal *Salmonella* disease: an emerging and neglected tropical disease in Africa. *Lancet* **379:**2489–2499.

6. **Imran Khan M, Freeman AJ, Gessner BD, Sahastrabuddhe S.** 2015. The need for an information communication and advocacy strategy to guide a research agenda to address burden of invasive nontyphoidal *Salmonella* infections in Africa. *Clin Infect Dis* **61:**S380–S385.

7. **Archibald LK, Reller LB.** 2001. Clinical microbiology in developing countries. *Emerg Infect Dis* **7:**302–305.

8. **Reddy EA, Shaw AV, Crump JA.** 2010. Community-acquired bloodstream infections in Africa: a systematic review and meta-analysis. *Lancet Infect Dis* **10:**417–432.

9. **Oneko M, Kariuki S, Muturi-Kioi V, Otieno K, Otieno VO, Williamson JM, Folster J, Parsons MB, Slutsker L, Mahon BE, Hamel MJ.** 2015. Emergence of community-acquired, multidrug-resistant invasive nontyphoidal *Salmonella* disease in rural western Kenya, 2009–2013. *Clin Infect Dis* **61:**S310–S316.

10. **Tabu C, Breiman RF, Ochieng B, Aura B, Cosmas L, Audi A, Olack B, Bigogo G, Ongus JR, Fields P, Mintz E, Burton D, Oundo J, Feikin DR.** 2012. Differing burden and epidemiology of non-Typhi *Salmonella* bacteremia in rural and urban Kenya, 2006-2009. *PLoS One* **7:**e31237. doi:10.1371/journal.pone.0031237.

11. **Mandomando I, Bassat Q, Sigaúque B, Massora S, Quintó L, Acacio S, Nhampossa T, Vubil D, Garrine M, Macete E, Aide P, Sacoor C, Herrera-León S, Ruiz J, Tennant SM, Menéndez C, Alonso PL.** 2015. Invasive *Salmonella* infections among children from rural Mozambique, 2001–2014. *Clin Infect Dis* **61:**S339–S345.

12. **Gordon MA, Graham SM, Walsh AL, Wilson L, Phiri A, Molyneux E, Zijlstra EE, Heyderman RS, Hart CA, Molyneux ME.** 2008. Epidemics of invasive *Salmonella enterica* serovar Enteritidis and *S. enterica* serovar Typhimurium infection associated with multidrug resistance among adults and children in Malawi. *Clin Infect Dis* **46:**963–969.

13. **Feasey NA, Masesa C, Jassi C, Faragher EB, Mallewa J, Mallewa M, MacLennan CA, Msefula C, Heyderman RS, Gordon MA.** 2015. Three epidemics of invasive multidrug-resistant *Salmonella* bloodstream infection in Blantyre, Malawi, 1998–2014. *Clin Infect Dis* **61:**S363–S371.

14. **Tapia MD, Tennant SM, Bornstein K, Onwuchekwa U, Tamboura B, Maiga A, Sylla MB, Sissoko S, Kourouma N, Toure A, Malle D, Livio S, Sow SO, Levine MM.** 2015. Invasive nontyphoidal *Salmonella* infections among children in Mali, 2002-2014: microbiological and epidemiologic features guide vaccine development. *Clin Infect Dis* **61:**S332–338.

15. **Verani JR, Toroitich S, Auko J, Kiplang'at S, Cosmas L, Audi A, Mogeni OD, Aol G, Oketch D, Odiembo H, Katieno J, Wamola N, Onyango CO, Juma BW, Fields BS, Bigogo G, Montgomery JM.** 2015. Burden of invasive nontyphoidal *Salmonella* disease in a rural and urban site in Kenya, 2009–2014. *Clin Infect Dis* **61:**S302–S309.

16. **Feasey NA, Everett D, Faragher EB, Roca-Feltrer A, Kang'ombe A, Denis B, Kerac M, Molyneux E, Molyneux M, Jahn A, Gordon MA, Heyderman RS.** 2015. Modelling the contributions of malaria, HIV, malnutrition and rainfall to the decline in paediatric invasive non-typhoidal *Salmonella* disease in Malawi. *PLoS Negl Trop Dis* **9:**e0003979. doi:10.1371/journal.pntd.0003979.

17. **Lepage P, Bogaerts J, Van Goethem C, Hitimana DG, Nsengumuremyi F.** 1990. Multiresistant *Salmonella typhimurium* systemic infection in Rwanda. Clinical features and treatment with cefotaxime. *J Antimicrob Chemother* **26**(Suppl A):53–57.

18. **Muthumbi E, Morpeth SC, Ooko M, Mwanzu A, Mwarumba S, Mturi N, Etyang AO, Berkley JA, Williams TN, Kariuki S, Scott JAG.** 2015. Invasive salmonellosis in Kilifi, Kenya. *Clin Infect Dis* **61:**S290–S301.

19. **Brent AJ, Oundo JO, Mwangi I, Ochola L, Lowe B, Berkley JA.** 2006. *Salmonella* bacteremia in Kenyan children. *Pediatr Infect Dis J* **25:**230–236.

20. **Berkley JA, Lowe BS, Mwangi I, Williams T, Bauni E, Mwarumba S, Ngetsa C, Slack MP, Njenga S, Hart CA, Maitland K, English M, Marsh K, Scott JA.** 2005. Bacteremia among children admitted to a rural hospital in Kenya. *N Engl J Med* **352:**39–47.

21. **Cheesbrough JS, Taxman BC, Green SD, Mewa FI, Numbi A.** 1997. Clinical definition

for invasive *Salmonella* infection in African children. *Pediatr Infect Dis J* **16**:277–283.

22. **Lepage P, Bogaerts J, Nsengumuremyi F, Hitimana DG, Van Goethem C, Vandepitte J, Butzler JP.** 1984. Severe multiresistant *Salmonella typhimurium* systemic infections in Central Africa: clinical features and treatment in a paediatric department. *J Antimicrob Chemother* **14**(Suppl B):153–159.

23. **Graham SM, Molyneux EM, Walsh AL, Cheesbrough JS, Molyneux ME, Hart CA.** 2000. Nontyphoidal *Salmonella* infections of children in tropical Africa. *Pediatr Infect Dis J* **19**:1189–1196.

24. **Kariuki S, Revathi G, Kariuki N, Kiiru J, Mwituria J, Hart CA.** 2006. Characterisation of community acquired non-typhoidal *Salmonella* from bacteraemia and diarrhoeal infections in children admitted to hospital in Nairobi, Kenya. *BMC Microbiol* **6**:101.

25. **Oundo JO, Muli F, Kariuki S, Waiyaki PG, Iijima Y, Berkley J, Kokwaro GO, Ngetsa CJ, Mwarumba S, Torto R, Lowe B.** 2002. Non-Typhi salmonella in children with severe malaria. *East Afr Med J* **79**:633–639.

26. **Cheng LH, Crim SM, Cole CR, Shane AL, Henao OL, Mahon BE.** 2013. Epidemiology of infant salmonellosis in the United States, 1996-2008: a Foodborne Diseases Active Surveillance Network study. *J Pediatr Infect Dis* **2**:232–239.

27. **Biggs HM, Lester R, Nadjm B, Mtove G, Todd JE, Kinabo GD, Philemon R, Amos B, Morrissey AB, Reyburn H, Crump JA.** 2014. Invasive *Salmonella* infections in areas of high and low malaria transmission intensity in Tanzania. *Clin Infect Dis* **58**:638–647.

28. **Kariuki S, Revathi G, Kariuki N, Kiiru J, Mwituria J, Muyodi J, Githinji JW, Kagendo D, Munyalo A, Hart CA.** 2006. Invasive multidrug-resistant non-typhoidal *Salmonella* infections in Africa: zoonotic or anthroponotic transmission? *J Med Microbiol* **55**:585–591.

29. **Scott JA, Berkley JA, Mwangi I, Ochola L, Uyoga S, Macharia A, Ndila C, Lowe BS, Mwarumba S, Bauni E, Marsh K, Williams TN.** 2011. Relation between falciparum malaria and bacteraemia in Kenyan children: a population-based, case-control study and a longitudinal study. *Lancet* **378**:1316–1323.

30. **Graham SM, Walsh AL, Molyneux EM, Phiri AJ, Molyneux ME.** 2000. Clinical presentation of non-typhoidal *Salmonella* bacteraemia in Malawian children. *Trans R Soc Trop Med Hyg* **94**:310–314.

31. **Mtove G, Amos B, von Seidlein L, Hendriksen I, Mwambuli A, Kimera J, Mallahiyo R, Kim**

DR, Ochiai RL, Clemens JD, Reyburn H, Magesa S, Deen JL. 2010. Invasive salmonellosis among children admitted to a rural Tanzanian hospital and a comparison with previous studies. *PLoS One* **5**:e9244. doi:10.1371/journal.pone.0009244.

32. **Morpeth SC, Ramadhani HO, Crump JA.** 2009. Invasive non-Typhi *Salmonella* disease in Africa. *Clin Infect Dis* **49**:606–611.

33. **Cunnington AJ, de Souza JB, Walther M, Riley EM.** 2012. Malaria impairs resistance to *Salmonella* through heme- and heme oxygenase-dependent dysfunctional granulocyte mobilization. *Nat Med* **18**:120–127.

34. **Davis TM, Pongponratan E, Supanaranond W, Pukrittayakamee S, Helliwell T, Holloway P, White NJ.** 1999. Skeletal muscle involvement in falciparum malaria: biochemical and ultrastructural study. *Clin Infect Dis* **29**:831–835.

35. **Seydel KB, Milner DA Jr, Kamiza SB, Molyneux ME, Taylor TE.** 2006. The distribution and intensity of parasite sequestration in comatose Malawian children. *J Infect Dis* **194**:208–205.

36. **Walsh AL, Molyneux EM, Kabudula M, Phiri AJ, Molyneux ME, Graham SM.** 2002. Bacteraemia following blood transfusion in Malawian children: predominance of *Salmonella*. *Trans R Soc Trop Med Hyg* **96**:276–277.

37. **Mackenzie G, Ceesay SJ, Hill PC, Walther M, Bojang KA, Satoguina J, Enwere G, D'Alessandro U, Saha D, Ikumapayi UN, O'Dempsey T, Mabey DC, Corrah T, Conway DJ, Adegbola RA, Greenwood BM.** 2010. A decline in the incidence of invasive non-typhoidal *Salmonella* infection in The Gambia temporally associated with a decline in malaria infection. *PLoS One* **5**:e10568. doi:10.1371/journal.pone.0010568.

38. **Mtove G, Amos B, Nadjm B, Hendriksen IC, Dondorp AM, Mwambuli A, Kim DR, Ochiai RL, Clemens JD, von Seidlein L, Reyburn H, Deen J.** 2011. Decreasing incidence of severe malaria and community-acquired bacteraemia among hospitalized children in Muheza, north-eastern Tanzania, 2006-2010. *Malar J* **10**:320.

39. **Gendrel D, Kombila M, Beaudoin-Leblevec G, Richard-Lenoble D.** 1994. Nontyphoidal salmonellal septicemia in Gabonese children infected with *Schistosoma intercalatum*. *Clin Infect Dis* **18**:103–105.

40. **Bronzan RN, Taylor TE, Mwenechanya J, Tembo M, Kayira K, Bwanaisa L, Njobvu A, Kondowe W, Chalira C, Walsh AL, Phiri A, Wilson LK, Molyneux ME, Graham SM.** 2007. Bacteremia in Malawian children with severe malaria: prevalence, etiology, HIV

coinfection, and outcome. *J Infect Dis* **195**:895–904.

41. **Levine WC, Buehler JW, Bean NH, Tauxe RV.** 1991. Epidemiology of nontyphoidal *Salmonella* bacteremia during the human immunodeficiency virus epidemic. *J Infect Dis* **164**:81–87.

42. **Gordon MA, Walsh AL, Chaponda M, Soko D, Mbvwinji M, Molyneux ME, Gordon SB.** 2001. Bacteraemia and mortality among adult medical admissions in Malawi: predominance of non-Typhi salmonellae and *Streptococcus pneumoniae. J Infect* **42**:44–49.

43. **Gilks CF, Brindle RJ, Otieno LS, Simani PM, Newnham RS, Bhatt SM, Lule GN, Okelo GB, Watkins WM, Waiyaki PG, Were JBO, Otieno LS, Simani PM, Bhatt SM, Lule GN, Okelo GBA, Brindle RJ, Newnham RS, Gilks CF, Warrell DA.** 1990. Life-threatening bacteraemia in HIV-1 seropositive adults admitted to hospital in Nairobi, Kenya. *Lancet* **336**:545–549.

44. **Arthur G, Nduba VN, Kariuki SM, Kimari J, Bhatt SM, Gilks CF.** 2001. Trends in bloodstream infections among human immunodeficiency virus-infected adults admitted to a hospital in Nairobi, Kenya, during the last decade. *Clin Infect Dis* **33**:248–256.

45. **Gordon MA, Banda HT, Gondwe M, Gordon SB, Boeree MJ, Walsh AL, Corkill JE, Hart CA, Gilks CF, Molyneux ME.** 2002. Nontyphoidal *Salmonella* bacteraemia among HIV-infected Malawian adults: high mortality and frequent recrudescence. *AIDS* **16**:1633–1641.

46. **Okoro CK, Kingsley RA, Quail MA, Kankwatira AM, Feasey NA, Parkhill J, Dougan G, Gordon MA.** 2012. High-resolution single nucleotide polymorphism analysis distinguishes recrudescence and reinfection in recurrent invasive nontyphoidal *Salmonella* Typhimurium disease. *Clin Infect Dis* **54**:955–963.

47. **Gordon MA.** 2011. Invasive nontyphoidal *Salmonella* disease: epidemiology, pathogenesis and diagnosis. *Curr Opin Infect Dis* **24**:484–489.

48. **Kurtz JR, Petersen HE, Frederick DR, Morici LA, McLachlan JB.** 2014. Vaccination with a single CD4 T cell peptide epitope from a *Salmonella* type III-secreted effector protein provides protection against lethal infection. *Infect Immun* **82**:2424–2433.

49. **Obaro SK, Hassan-Hanga F, Olateju EK, Umoru D, Lawson L, Olanipekun G, Ibrahim S, Munir H, Ihesiolor G, Maduekwe A, Ohiaeri C, Adetola A, Shetima D, Jibir BW, Nakaura H, Kocmich N, Ajose T, Idiong D, Masokano K, Ifabiyi A, Ihebuzor N, Chen B, Meza J,** Akindele A, Rezac-Elgohary A, Olaosebikan R, Suwaid S, Gambo M, Alter R, Davies HD, Fey PD. 2015. *Salmonella* bacteremia among children in central and northwest Nigeria, 2008–2015. *Clin Infect Dis* **61**:S325–S331.

50. **Kwambana-Adams B, Darboe S, Nabwera H, Foster-Nyarko E, Ikumapayi UN, Secka O, Betts M, Bradbury R, Wegmüller R, Lawal B, Saha D, Hossain MJ, Prentice AM, Kampmann B, Anderson S, Dalessandro U, Antonio M.** 2015. *Salmonella* infections in The Gambia, 2005–2015. *Clin Infect Dis* **61**:S354–S362.

51. **Beyene G, Nair S, Asrat D, Mengistu Y, Engers H, Wain J.** 2011. Multidrug resistant *Salmonella* Concord is a major cause of salmonellosis in children in Ethiopia. *J Infect Dev Ctries* **5**:23–33.

52. **Wadula J, von Gottberg A, Kilner D, de Jong G, Cohen C, Khoosal M, Keddy K, Crewe-Brown H.** 2006. Nosocomial outbreak of extended-spectrum beta-lactamase-producing *Salmonella* Isangi in pediatric wards. *Pediatr Infect Dis J* **25**:843–844.

53. **Kariuki S, Revathi G, Kiiru J, Lowe B, Berkley JA, Hart CA.** 2006. Decreasing prevalence of antimicrobial resistance in nontyphoidal *Salmonella* isolated from children with bacteraemia in a rural district hospital, Kenya. *Int J Antimicrob Agents* **28**:166–171.

54. **Oundo JO, Kariuki S, Maghenda JK, Lowe BS.** 2000. Antibiotic susceptibility and genotypes of non-typhi *Salmonella* isolates from children in Kilifi on the Kenya coast. *Trans R Soc Trop Med Hyg* **94**:212–215.

55. **Okoro CK, Kingsley RA, Connor TR, Harris SR, Parry CM, Al-Mashhadani MN, Kariuki S, Msefula CL, Gordon MA, de Pinna E, Wain J, Heyderman RS, Obaro S, Alonso PL, Mandomando I, MacLennan CA, Tapia MD, Levine MM, Tennant SM, Parkhill J, Dougan G.** 2012. Intracontinental spread of human invasive *Salmonella* Typhimurium pathovariants in sub-Saharan Africa. *Nat Genet* **44**:1215–1221.

56. **Wain J, Keddy KH, Hendriksen RS, Rubino S.** 2013. Using next generation sequencing to tackle non-typhoidal *Salmonella* infections. *J Infect Dev Ctries* **7**:1–5.

57. **Kariuki S, Okoro C, Kiiru J, Njoroge S, Omuse G, Langridge G, Kingsley RA, Dougan G, Revathi G.** 2015. Ceftriaxone-resistant *Salmonella enterica* serotype Typhimurium sequence type 313 from Kenyan patients is associated with the $bla_{CTX-M-15}$ gene on a novel IncHI2 plasmid. *Antimicrob Agents Chemother* **59**:3133–3139.

58. **Msefula CL, Kingsley RA, Gordon MA, Molyneux E, Molyneux ME, MacLennan**

CA, Dougan G, Heyderman RS. 2012. Genotypic homogeneity of multidrug resistant *S.* Typhimurium infecting distinct adult and childhood susceptibility groups in Blantyre, Malawi. *PLoS One* **7:**e42085. doi:10.1371/journal.pone.0042085.

59. Leekitcharoenphon P, Friis C, Zankari E, Svendsen CA, Price LB, Rahmani M, Herrero-Fresno A, Fashae K, Vandenberg O, Aarestrup FM, Hendriksen RS. 2013. Genomics of an emerging clone of *Salmonella* serovar Typhimurium ST313 from Nigeria and the Democratic Republic of Congo. *J Infect Dev Ctries* **7:**696–706.

60. Okoro CK, Barquist L, Connor TR, Harris SR, Clare S, Stevens MP, Arends MJ, Hale C, Kane L, Pickard DJ, Hill J, Harcourt K, Parkhill J, Dougan G, Kingsley RA. 2015. Correction: signatures of adaptation in human invasive *Salmonella* Typhimurium ST313 populations from sub-Saharan Africa. *PLoS Negl Trop Dis* **9:**e0003848. doi:10.1371/journal.pntd.0003848.

61. Okoro CK, Barquist L, Connor TR, Harris SR, Clare S, Stevens MP, Arends MJ, Hale C, Kane L, Pickard DJ, Hill J, Harcourt K, Parkhill J, Dougan G, Kingsley RA. 2015. Signatures of adaptation in human invasive *Salmonella* Typhimurium ST313 populations from sub-Saharan Africa. *PLoS Negl Trop Dis* **9:**e0003611. doi:10.1371/journal.pntd.0003848.

62. Kingsley RA, Msefula CL, Thomson NR, Kariuki S, Holt KE, Gordon MA, Harris D, Clarke L, Whitehead S, Sangal V, Marsh K, Achtman M, Molyneux ME, Cormican M, Parkhill J, MacLennan CA, Heyderman RS, Dougan G. 2009. Epidemic multiple drug resistant *Salmonella* Typhimurium causing invasive disease in sub-Saharan Africa have a distinct genotype. *Genome Res* **19:**2279–2287.

63. Kingsley RA, Kay S, Connor T, Barquist L, Sait L, Holt KE, Sivaraman K, Wileman T, Goulding D, Clare S, Hale C, Seshasayee A, Harris S, Thomson NR, Gardner P, Rabsch W, Wigley P, Humphrey T, Parkhill J, Dougan G. 2013. Genome and transcriptome adaptation accompanying emergence of the definitive type 2 host-restricted *Salmonella enterica* serovar Typhimurium pathovar. *MBio* **4:**e00565-13. doi:10.1128/mBio.00565-13.

64. Yang J, Barrila J, Roland KL, Kilbourne J, Ott CM, Forsyth RJ, Nickerson CA. 2015. Characterization of the invasive, multidrug resistant non-typhoidal *Salmonella* strain D23580 in a murine model of infection. *PLoS Negl Trop Dis* **9:**e0003839. doi:10.1371/journal.pntd.0003839.

65. Carden S, Okoro C, Dougan G, Monack D. 2015. Non-typhoidal *Salmonella* Typhimurium ST313 isolates that cause bacteremia in humans stimulate less inflammasome activation than ST19 isolates associated with gastroenteritis. *Pathog Dis* **73:**ftu023.

66. Parsons BN, Humphrey S, Salisbury AM, Mikoleit J, Hinton JC, Gordon MA, Wigley P. 2013. Invasive non-typhoidal *Salmonella* Typhimurium ST313 are not host-restricted and have an invasive phenotype in experimentally infected chickens. *PLoS Negl Trop Dis* **7:** e2487. doi:10.1371/journal.pntd.0002487.

67. Ramachandran G, Perkins DJ, Schmidlein PJ, Tulapurkar ME, Tennant SM. 2015. Invasive *Salmonella* Typhimurium ST313 with naturally attenuated flagellin elicits reduced inflammation and replicates within macrophages. *PLoS Negl Trop Dis* **9:**e3394. doi:10.1371/journal.pntd.0003394.

68. Rabsch W, Andrews HL, Kingsley RA, Prager R, Tschape H, Adams LG, Baumler AJ. 2002. *Salmonella enterica* serotype Typhimurium and its host-adapted variants. *Infect Immun* **70:**2249–2255.

69. Guiney DG, Fierer J. 2011. The Role of the *spv* genes in *Salmonella* pathogenesis. *Front Microbiol* **2:**129.

70. Scallan E, Hoekstra RM, Angulo FJ, Tauxe RV, Widdowson MA, Roy SL, Jones JL, Griffin PM. 2011. Foodborne illness acquired in the United States: major pathogens. *Emerg Infect Dis* **17:**7–15.

71. Jackson BR, Griffin PM, Cole D, Walsh KA, Chai SJ. 2013. Outbreak-associated *Salmonella enterica* serotypes and food commodities, United States, 1998-2008. *Emerg Infect Dis* **19:**1239–1244.

72. Niehaus AJ, Apalata T, Coovadia YM, Smith AM, Moodley P. 2011. An outbreak of foodborne salmonellosis in rural KwaZulu-Natal, South Africa. *Foodborne Pathog Dis* **8:**693–697.

73. Smith AM, Mthanti MA, Haumann C, Tyalisi N, Boon GP, Sooka A, Keddy KH, GERMS-SA Surveillance Network. 2014. Nosocomial outbreak of *Salmonella enterica* serovar Typhimurium primarily affecting a pediatric ward in South Africa in 2012. *J Clin Microbiol* **52:**627–631.

74. Hadfield TL, Monson MH, Wachsmuth IK. 1985. An outbreak of antibiotic-resistant *Salmonella enteritidis* in Liberia, West Africa. *J Infect Dis* **151:**790–795.

75. Kagambega A, Lienemann T, Aulu L, Traore AS, Barro N, Siitonen A, Haukka K. 2013. Prevalence and characterization of *Salmonella*

enterica from the feces of cattle, poultry, swine and hedgehogs in Burkina Faso and their comparison to human *Salmonella* isolates. *BMC Microbiol* **13**:253.

76. **Magwedere K, Rauff D, De Klerk G, Keddy KH, Dziva F.** 2015. Incidence of nontyphoidal *Salmonella* in food-producing animals, animal feed, and the associated environment in South Africa, 2012–2014. *Clin Infect Dis* **61**:S283–S289.

77. **Kidanemariam A, Engelbrecht M, Picard J.** 2010. Retrospective study on the incidence of *Salmonella* isolations in animals in South Africa, 1996 to 2006. *J S Afr Vet Assoc* **81**:37–44.

78. **Dione MM, Ikumapayi UN, Saha D, Mohammed NI, Geerts S, Ieven M, Adegbola RA, Antonio M.** 2011. Clonal differences between non-typhoidal *Salmonella* (NTS) recovered from children and animals living in close contact in the Gambia. *PLoS Negl Trop Dis* **5**:e1148. doi:10.1371/journal.pntd.0001148.

79. **National Antimicrobial Resistance Monitoring System.** 2015. *NARMS Integrated Report: 2012-2013*. U.S. FDA, Silver Spring, MD.

80. **Kariuki S, Revathi G, Kariuki N, Muyodi J, Mwituria J, Munyalo A, Kagendo D, Murungi L, Anthony Hart C.** 2005. Increasing prevalence of multidrug-resistant nontyphoidal salmonellae, Kenya, 1994-2003. *Int J Antimicrob Agents* **25**:38–43.

81. **Smith AM, Ismail H, Henton MM, Keddy KH, GERMS-SA Surveillance Network.** 2014. Similarities between *Salmonella* Enteritidis isolated from humans and captive wild animals in South Africa. *J Infect Dev Ctries* **8**:1615–1619.

82. **Bejon P, Mwangi I, Ngetsa C, Mwarumba S, Berkley JA, Lowe BS, Maitland K, Marsh K, English M, Scott JA.** 2005. Invasive Gram-negative bacilli are frequently resistant to standard antibiotics for children admitted to hospital in Kilifi, Kenya. *J Antimicrob Chemother* **56**:232–235.

83. **Feasey NA, Cain AK, Msefula CL, Pickard D, Alaerts M, Aslett M, Everett DB, Allain TJ, Dougan G, Gordon MA, Heyderman RS, Kingsley RA.** 2014. Drug resistance in *Salmonella enterica* ser. Typhimurium bloodstream infection, Malawi. *Emerg Infect Dis* **20**:1957–1959.

84. **Kariuki S, Onsare RS.** 2015. Epidemiology and genomics of invasive nontyphoidal *Salmonella* infections in Kenya. *Clin Infect Dis* **61**:S317–S324.

85. **Kalonji LM, Post A, Phoba M-F, Falay D, Ngbonda D, Muyembe J-J, Bertrand S,** Ceyssens P-J, Mattheus W, Verhaegen J, Barbé B, Kuijpers L, Van Geet C, Lunguya O, Jacobs J. 2015. Invasive *Salmonella* infections at multiple surveillance sites in the Democratic Republic of the Congo, 2011–2014. *Clin Infect Dis* **61**:S346–S353.

86. **Govender N, Smith AM, Karstaedt AS, Keddy KH, Group for Enteric, Respiratory, and Meningeal Disease Surveillance in South Africa (GERMS-SA).** 2009. Plasmid-mediated quinolone resistance in *Salmonella* from South Africa. *J Med Microbiol* **58**:1393–1394.

87. **Kariuki S, Gordon MA, Feasey N, Parry CM.** 2015. Antimicrobial resistance and management of invasive *Salmonella* disease. *Vaccine* **33**(Suppl 3):C21–C29.

88. **Sepulveda J, Valdespino JL, Garcia-Garcia L.** 2006. Cholera in Mexico: the paradoxical benefits of the last pandemic. *Int J Infect Dis* **10**:4–13.

89. **Mather AE, Vaughan TG, French NP.** 2015. Molecular approaches to understanding transmission and source attribution in nontyphoidal *Salmonella* and their application in Africa. *Clin Infect Dis* **61**:S259–S265.

90. **World Health Organization.** 2015. *Global Health Sector Response to HIV, 2000-2015: Focus on Innovations in Africa: Progress Report*. http://apps.who.int/iris/bitstream/10665/198065/1/9789241509824_eng.pdf. WHO, Geneva, Switzerland.

91. **World Health Organization.** 2015. *Achieving the Malaria MDG Target: Reversing the Incidence of Malaria 2000-2015*. http://apps.who.int/iris/bitstream/10665/184521/1/9789241509442_eng.pdf. WHO, Geneva, Switzerland.

92. **MacLennan CA, Gondwe EN, Msefula CL, Kingsley RA, Thomson NR, White SA, Goodall M, Pickard DJ, Graham SM, Dougan G, Hart CA, Molyneux ME, Drayson MT.** 2008. The neglected role of antibody in protection against bacteremia caused by nontyphoidal strains of *Salmonella* in African children. *J Clin Invest* **118**:1553–1562.

93. **Nyirenda TS, Gilchrist JJ, Feasey NA, Glennie SJ, Bar-Zeev N, Gordon MA, MacLennan CA, Mandala WL, Heyderman RS.** 2014. Sequential acquisition of T cells and antibodies to nontyphoidal *Salmonella* in Malawian children. *J Infect Dis* **210**:56–64.

94. **Rondini S, Micoli F, Lanzilao L, Gavini M, Alfini R, Brandt C, Clare S, Mastroeni P, Saul A, MacLennan CA.** 2015. Design of glycoconjugate vaccines against invasive African *Salmonella enterica* serovar Typhimurium. *Infect Immun* **83**:996–1007.

95. **Goh YS, MacLennan CA.** 2013. Invasive African nontyphoidal *Salmonella* requires high levels of complement for cell-free antibody-dependent killing. *J Immunol Methods* **387:**121–129.

96. **Simon R, Levine MM.** 2012. Glycoconjugate vaccine strategies for protection against invasive *Salmonella* infections. *Human Vaccin Immunother* **8:**494–498.

97. **Simon R, Tennant SM, Wang JY, Schmidlein PJ, Lees A, Ernst RK, Pasetti MF, Galen JE, Levine MM.** 2011. *Salmonella enterica* serovar Enteritidis core O polysaccharide conjugated to H:g,m flagellin as a candidate vaccine for protection against invasive infection with *S.* Enteritidis. *Infect Immun* **79:**4240–4249.

98. **Simon R, Wang JY, Boyd MA, Tulapurkar ME, Ramachandran G, Tennant SM, Pasetti M, Galen JE, Levine MM.** 2013. Sustained protection in mice immunized with fractional doses of *Salmonella* Enteritidis core and O polysaccharide-flagellin glycoconjugates. *PLoS One* **8:**e64680. doi:10.1371/journal.pone.0064680.

99. **Tennant SM, Levine MM.** 2015. Live attenuated vaccines for invasive *Salmonella* infections. *Vaccine* **33**(Suppl 3)**:**C36–C41.

100. **World Health Organization.** 2015. *Global Action Plan on Antimicrobial Resistance.* http://apps.who.int/iris/bitstream/10665/193736/1/9789241509763_eng.pdf. WHO, Geneva, Switzerland.

19

Fungal Infections Associated with Contaminated Steroid Injections

CAROL A. KAUFFMAN[1,3] and ANURAG N. MALANI[2,3]

INTRODUCTION

By late September 2012, several cases of fungal meningitis were reported from different states. Investigation by the Centers for Disease Control and Prevention (CDC) quickly led to the discovery that the causative organism was a rare, usually nonpathogenic brown-black mold, *Exserohilum rostratum*, and that infection was associated with epidural injection of methylprednisolone acetate that had been contaminated at the compounding center at which it was produced. Although the contaminated lots of methylprednisolone were recalled as soon as the link was discovered, a total of 17,675 vials of potentially contaminated methylprednisolone acetate had been shipped to 76 facilities in 23 states (1). It is estimated that as many as 13,534 patients had been exposed to this product before the recall went into effect.

As the outbreak progressed, it became clear that a disproportionate number of cases were occurring in Michigan. When the CDC issued their last update on this outbreak in October 2013, there were a total of 751 cases, and 264 (35%) were reported from Michigan (2). Most patients were cared for at one hospital, St. Joseph Mercy Hospital (SJMH), in Ann Arbor, MI. We review the

Division of Infectious Diseases, Department of Internal Medicine; [1]Veterans Affairs Ann Arbor Healthcare System; [2]St. Joseph Mercy Hospital; [3]University of Michigan Medical School, Ann Arbor, MI 48105.
Emerging Infections 10
Edited by W. Michael Scheld, James M. Hughes and Richard J. Whitley
© 2016 American Society for Microbiology, Washington, DC
doi:10.1128/microbiolspec.EI10-0005-2015

epidemiology of the outbreak and discuss our own experiences with the clinical manifestations of *E. rostratum* infection, which varied from life-threatening stroke to localized epidural abscesses to unremitting arachnoiditis. Treatment with antifungal agents was usually, but not always, successful but was accompanied by many adverse effects, some of which had not been reported previously. The legal and political ramifications of this outbreak, which became the largest healthcare-associated outbreak ever reported in the United States, are ongoing.

EPIDEMIOLOGY

The Beginning of the Outbreak

The inception of this outbreak occurred on 18 September 2012, when the Tennessee Department of Health was alerted by an astute physician that a patient in Nashville had died of culture-confirmed *Aspergillus fumigatus* meningitis and that this patient had received an epidural steroid injection 46 days earlier (3). By 25 September, 7 additional patients who had received epidural steroid injections at the same clinic were identified as having neutrophilic nonbacterial meningitis, and soon after, a similar case was reported from North Carolina (1). In-

vestigation by the CDC determined that all affected patients had received an injection of preservative-free methylprednisolone acetate compounded at the New England Compounding Center (NECC) in Framingham, MA. The company was immediately notified that their product was implicated (4). Three lots, designated by their date of release as 05212012@68, 06292012@26, and 08102012@51, were contaminated (5). All patients who had received an injection from one of these 3 lots were contacted through state and local health departments, and all clinics that had purchased one of these 3 lots were told to immediately stop giving injections of this material.

By 1 October 2012, the CDC had convened an expert panel to consult on case definitions and treatment regimens for fungal meningitis. Case definitions were established (Table 1). On 4 October 2012, the first health advisory notice was posted regarding this outbreak of fungal meningitis, and the Food and Drug Administration (FDA) reported that fungi were found in unopened vials of methylprednisolone acetate from the implicated lots (6). Both specimens from patients and material from the unopened vials revealed the rarely pathogenic dematiaceous mold *Exserohilum rostratum* (7).

As soon as a dematiaceous mold was identified as the likely pathogen, analogy was

TABLE 1 CDC case definitions of probable and confirmed fungal infections associated with contaminated methylprednisolone injection[a]

Type of infection	Probable infection[b] in a person who had received an injection after 21 May 2012 from 1 of 3 implicated MPA lots[c]
Meningitis	Signs and symptoms of meningitis (headache, fever, meningismus, or photophobia); unknown etiology; epidural or paraspinal injection; CSF pleocytosis (≥5 WBCs/μl adjusted for RBC)
Posterior circulation stroke	Signs and symptoms of stroke; epidural or paraspinal injection; no cardioembolic source; lumbar puncture not performed or CSF pleocytosis if performed
Spinal or paraspinal infections	Osteomyelitis, abscess, phlegmon, or soft tissue infection; unknown etiology; epidural or paraspinal injection
Peripheral osteoarticular infections	Osteomyelitis or worsening inflammatory arthritis; unknown etiology; injection of an osteoarticular structure

[a]MPA, methylprednisolone acetate; CSF, cerebrospinal fluid; WBCs, white blood cells; RBC, red blood cell.
[b]A confirmed case met the definitions for probable infection and had evidence of fungal infection by culture, histopathology, or molecular assay.
[c]Three implicated lots produced by the NECC were 05212012@68, 06292012@26, and 08102012@51.

made to an almost identical outbreak that had occurred a decade before (8). In 2002, four patients, one of whom died, developed meningitis after receiving an epidural injection with methylprednisolone acetate that was contaminated with *Exophiala dermatitidis*. A compounding center in South Carolina had manufactured the product, and unopened vials at that center were found to contain *E. dermatitidis*. What was dramatically different about the NECC outbreak was that the contaminated product had been shipped widely throughout the United States and more than 13,000 patients had been exposed.

The investigation traced back those patients who had received injections soon after the release of the first contaminated lot on 21 May 2012. The first infection that was documented was a spinal or paraspinal infection on 7 July 2012, and the first case of meningitis had symptoms beginning on 16 July 2012 (5) (Fig. 1). Further studies revealed that the lot released on 29 June 2012 (06292012@26) was associated with a higher attack rate than the other two contaminated lots (9).

Evolution of the Outbreak

At the outset, most patients were diagnosed with meningitis, and a small number experienced a stroke (10, 11). By mid-October 2012, spinal and paraspinal infections became the predominant types of infection (12, 13). It was not unusual for a patient who was doing well on voriconazole for treatment of meningitis to return to the hospital with increasing back pain at the site of the injection and then to be found by magnetic resonance imaging (MRI) study to have localized spinal or paraspinal infection and/or arachnoiditis. Other patients

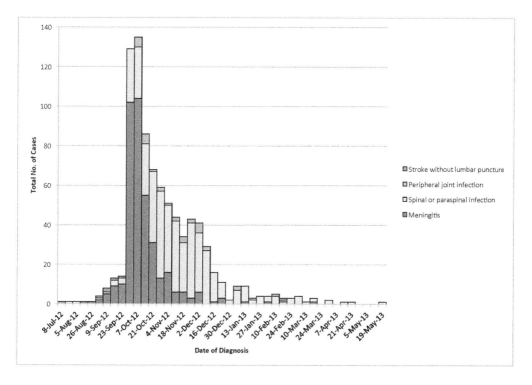

FIGURE 1 **Epidemiological curve of fungal infections associated with injection of contaminated methylprednisolone acetate manufactured by the NECC. Reproduced from reference 5 with permission.**

never had meningitis but presented with only spinal or paraspinal infection. Soon the number of cases of spinal or paraspinal infection surpassed the number of meningitis cases, and by October 2013, 476 patients (63%) had either isolated spinal or paraspinal infection or both spinal or paraspinal infection and meningitis (2).

The median incubation period was 47 days (range, 0 to 249 days); this was shorter for patients who experienced a stroke without documented meningitis (median, 24 days, and range, 3 to 157 days) and patients who had meningitis (median, 35 days, and range, 1 to 200 days) and longer for those who had spinal or paraspinal infection (median, 58 days, and range, 10 to 249 days) and osteoarticular infection (median, 65 days, and range, 22 to 190 days) (5). One theory for why spinal and paraspinal infections presented late in the outbreak is that the steroid injection may have masked early signs and symptoms of local inflammation and led to delayed clinical presentation. Additionally, the incubation period for a localized *Exserohilum* infection to become clinically evident may be prolonged, as noted with other central nervous system (CNS) brown-black mold infections (8, 14).

In Michigan, 4 facilities received 2,225 vials of contaminated methylprednisolone acetate, and 1,791 residents of Michigan received a total of 2,537 injections in tissues other than peripheral joints (mostly epidural injections) (12). In a pain facility near Ann Arbor, approximately 544 persons received 1 or more epidural injections of contaminated methylprednisolone acetate—all from the most contaminated lot, 06292012@26. Most patients who developed symptoms were cared for at SJMH. A striking finding was that a disproportionate number of cases of spinal or paraspinal infection were reported from Michigan. Of the 264 cases seen in Michigan, 166 (63%) involved only spinal or paraspinal infections and an additional 46 (17%) included both a spinal or paraspinal infection and meningitis (12, 13, 15).

MYCOLOGICAL ASPECTS

Exserohilum rostratum is a dematiaceous (brown-black) fungus that is found in soil and on plants throughout the world but most frequently in tropical and subtropical climates. The cell wall contains melanin, and colonies on Sabouraud's dextrose agar are brown-black. The conidia are large, septate, darkly pigmented structures. The organisms are primarily plant pathogens and rarely infect humans; only 3 species, *E. rostratum, E. longirostratum*, and *E. mcginnisii*, have been reported to cause disease in humans (16). Those cases that have been reported prior to this outbreak were either localized infections related to traumatic inoculation of the conidia or disseminated infection in immunosuppressed hosts (16–20). A review of the preoutbreak literature, from 1975 through 2012, found 48 cases of infection with *Exserohilum* species, of which only 29 were identified as *E. rostratum* (16). Only one patient had CNS infection as one manifestation of disseminated disease (17). Most reported infections were sinusitis, localized cutaneous lesions, or keratitis.

In vitro antifungal susceptibility studies for 34 *Exserohilum* isolates found that the organisms generally were susceptible to amphotericin B, itraconazole, voriconazole, and posaconazole. Echinocandin susceptibility was variable, and the organisms were resistant to fluconazole and flucytosine (21). Subsequent studies on outbreak strains confirmed these findings (22). It should be noted that the MIC_{90} consistently is slightly higher for voriconazole (0.2 to 2 µg/ml) than for itraconazole (0.03 to 1 µg/ml) and posaconazole (0.03 to 1 µg/ml) (21, 22).

Whole-genome sequencing of strains from patients and from unopened vials of methylprednisolone acetate from 2 of the 3 implicated lots produced at the NECC revealed almost identical genomes, with no more than 2 single nucleotide polymorphisms noted between strains (23). Randomly selected environmental strains differed greatly from the outbreak strains.

CLINICAL ASPECTS

By October 2013, there were 751 cases of fungal infection reported in the multistate fungal outbreak, with 64 deaths (8.5%) (2). Among the 751 identified patients who had fungal infections, 325 had spinal or paraspinal infections, 233 had meningitis, 151 had both spinal or paraspinal infections and meningitis, and 7 had strokes without documented meningitis (a lumbar puncture was not performed in these 7 patients). Additionally, there were 33 patients who had a peripheral osteoarticular infection and 2 who had both a spinal or paraspinal infection and a peripheral osteoarticular infection (2). Among 728 patients for whom data were available, the median age was 64 years (range, 15 to 97), and 432 (59%) were women. Underlying immunosuppression was present in only 60 patients (8%) (5).

Meningitis

Approximately 90% of patients presenting with meningitis reported a headache, and about half experienced neck pain or stiffness (5). Less common symptoms at presentation were fever, photophobia, and neurological symptoms (15). About one-quarter of patients reported back pain (5).

For the patients with meningitis, the first cerebrospinal fluid (CSF) sample showed a median white blood cell (WBC) count of 83 cells/µl (range, 6 to 15,400 cells/µl); the median glucose concentration was 53 mg/dl (range, 3 to 249 mg/dl), and the median protein level was 84 mg/dl (range, 13 to 2,830 mg/dl) (15).

The occurrence of a stroke was reported for 40 patients (5%). In 33 patients, the stroke occurred in addition to documented meningitis. In the remaining 7 patients, who did not have a lumber puncture performed, stroke was presumed to be associated with fungal infection. The type of stroke was reported for 34 patients: 24 were ischemic, 6 were hemorrhagic, and 4 were both. Almost all strokes (96%) involved the posterior circulation, and over half of the patients who suffered a stroke died (5). The CSF showed a higher WBC count, a lower glucose level, and a higher protein level for those who had a stroke than for patients who had only meningitis (15).

Of the approximately 384 patients with fungal meningitis, 151 (39%) developed concomitant localized spinal or paraspinal infection (epidural abscess, phlegmon, diskitis, vertebral osteomyelitis, or arachnoiditis) (2, 5). Arachnoiditis (characterized by nodular or linear enhancement of the nerve roots

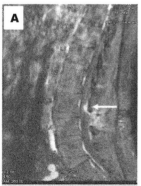
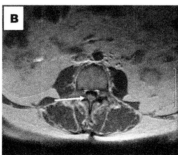
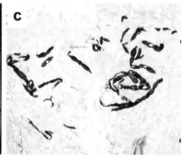

FIGURE 2 **(A) Sagittal T1 fat-saturated, postcontrast image of the lumbar spine shows dorsal intradural enhancement (arrow). (B) Axial T1 postcontrast image shows intradural enhancement and clumping (arrow) in the thecal sac, consistent with arachnoiditis. (C) Operative pathology from the intradural abscess shows fungal hyphae by Gomori methenamine silver staining.**

of the cauda equina on MRI) was commonly found among patients who had meningitis (Fig. 2). In a review of 63 cases of arachnoiditis from the 6 states (Michigan, Tennessee, Indiana, New Jersey, Florida, and Virginia) with the most reported cases, lumbar puncture was performed in 58 (92%); 52 of the 58 (90%) patients had CSF pleocytosis. The median WBC count in CSF was increased 10-fold among those patients who had arachnoiditis compared with those who had meningitis alone (539 versus 47 cells/μl). Most patients with arachnoiditis (78%) had both headache and back pain (15).

A multivariable logistic-regression model evaluating risk factors for CNS disease (meningitis, stroke, arachnoiditis, and intradural abscess) in comparison with non-CNS disease (spinal or paraspinal infection) in patients in Michigan showed that the presence of hypertension (odds ratio, 4.28; 95% confidence interval, 1.47 to 12.48) and receipt of a translaminar epidural injection (odds ratio, 3.83; 95% confidence interval, 1.60 to 9.20) were independently associated with CNS disease (15). Earlier work from Tennessee showed that patients who received an injection of methylprednisolone by a translaminar approach had a higher rate of developing infection than those who received an injection by the transforaminal route; most of the patients in that series had meningitis and not spinal or paraspinal infection (9).

Spinal and Paraspinal Infections

As the outbreak evolved, there was a predominance of patients who manifested symptoms and signs of spinal or paraspinal infections at the injection site (Fig. 3). This phenomenon was most evident in Michigan (1, 13, 24). In a review of 153 spinal and paraspinal infections from SJMH, it was found that the median time from the last epidural or paraspinal injection to diagnosis was 52 days (range, 21 to 232 days). Within this group, the median time from the last injection to diagnosis was 56 days (range, 23 to 232 days) for the 112 patients who presented with spinal or paraspinal infection alone, compared with a median time from injection to diagnosis of 44 days (range, 21 to 75 days) for the 41 patients who had both meningitis and spinal or paraspinal infection (13).

The symptoms reported most commonly among patients with spinal or paraspinal

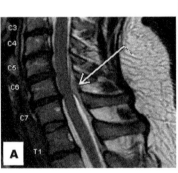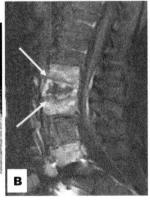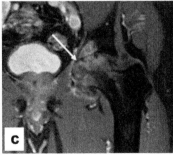

FIGURE 3 **(A) Sagittal T2-weighted image of the cervical spine shows a dorsal epidural fluid collection consistent with a phlegmon or abscess. Tissue obtained at surgery showed fungal hyphae. (B) Linear endplate enhancement consistent with diskitis or osteomyelitis of the lumbar spine. (C) Coronal T1 fat-saturated, postcontrast image shows edema and enhancement in the left femoral head and acetabulum consistent with septic arthritis or osteomyelitis.**

infections were back pain (63%) and headache (36%) (5, 12, 13). However, some patients experienced little to no change in chronic back or neck pain yet were found to have spinal or paraspinal infection (24). Given the insidious onset of spinal or paraspinal infection at the injection site and the often subtle clinical findings, contrast-enhanced MRI screening was initiated at SJMH. In a cohort of 172 patients who underwent screening MRI, 36 (21%) were found to have an abnormal MRI, with findings that included epidural or paraspinal abscess or phlegmon, arachnoiditis, spinal osteomyelitis and/or diskitis, and moderate to severe epidural, paraspinal, or intradural enhancement. Thirty-five of the 36 patients with abnormal MRIs were found to have spinal or paraspinal infection, including 13 (37%) patients who had no change in back or neck pain, no lower-extremity weakness, and no evidence of radiculopathy (24). A single MRI was not always sufficient to detect infection. Some patients for whom the initial MRI showed no evidence of infection were later found to have spinal or paraspinal infection when an MRI was repeated (13).

Evolving guidance from the CDC called for clinicians to remain vigilant when following up patients who had received spinal or paraspinal injections of contaminated methylprednisolone and recommended a contrast-enhanced MRI for anyone who had new or worsening symptoms at the injection site. The CDC also added that consideration should be given to obtaining a contrast-enhanced MRI for patients with persistent pain that was similar to their baseline symptoms (25).

Surgical intervention, usually a total laminectomy or hemi-laminectomy, was often required to decompress neural elements, remove infectious material, and obtain tissue for diagnostic purposes. At SJMH, surgical intervention was performed in 116 (76%) of 153 patients with spinal or paraspinal infection. Epidural phlegmon and abscess were the most common intraoperative findings (13).

It remains unexplained why Michigan had a disproportionate number of spinal or paraspinal infections. Only 13% of potentially contaminated vials were shipped to the state, yet over 50% of spinal and paraspinal infections were reported from Michigan (12). Possible explanations include state-specific variation in injection approach or possibly higher levels of contamination with *Exserohilum* in the vials shipped to Michigan. It is also possible that the use of MRI to screen for localized infection, regardless of symptoms, led to enhanced diagnosis.

Peripheral Osteoarticular Infections

Of the 13,534 patients that been potentially exposed to methylprednisolone acetate from one of the three lots, 12,068 (89%) had been exposed by epidural, spinal, or paraspinal injections and 1,648 (12%) had been exposed by injections into peripheral joints or adjacent structures. The attack rate was higher for meningitis and spinal or paraspinal infections than for peripheral osteoarticular infections (5). Patients with peripheral osteoarticular infections were exposed to contaminated methylprednisolone through injection into shoulder, hip, knee, ankle, and tendon insertion sites as well as various bursae (Fig. 3). Joint aspiration yielded a median WBC count of 515 cells/μl (range, 6 to 24,000 cells/μl) (5). The most common symptom among these patients was joint pain (84%). Surgical intervention, including incision and drainage, washout, bursectomy, or total arthroplasty, was often required to treat these infections.

Long-Term Outcomes

Recent data from a long-term follow-up study being conducted by the Mycoses Study Group Education and Research Consortium reveal that most patients with fungal infections associated with contaminated methylprednisolone acetate have done well following treatment (26). Of the approximately 450 patients in the long-term follow-up study, most patients received antifungal treatment for approximately 6 months; a small subset continues to require antifungal treatment. Only 8 (1%) of 751 patients have experienced a relapse (27). Among the six relapsed cases with known time from initial completion of antifungal therapy to relapse, the median time to relapse was 90 days (range, 20 to 662 days). Two additional cases have been recently identified, for a total of 753 cases to date (27).

DIAGNOSIS

A patient who met the case definition was confirmed as having a proven case if a fungal infection was established by culture, histopathology, or molecular assay (Table 1).

Culture

Growth of *E. rostratum* in culture was an insensitive diagnostic tool in this outbreak. An interim analysis of 268 patients who had samples sent to the CDC showed that only 96 had definite evidence of *E. rostratum*. Of the 96, only 30 had *E. rostratum* isolated in culture; 15 of these 30 also had a positive PCR. An additional 66 patients had only a positive PCR assay for *E. rostratum* (15). Very quickly, PCR became the preferred tool to establish the diagnosis of *E. rostratum* infection (22). There are no data on the overall rate of culture positivity among patients in the outbreak. The difficulty of growing fungi from the CSF in this outbreak is unexplained but is well known for several other fungal infections, such as coccidioidomycosis and histoplasmosis (28).

Polymerase Chain Reaction

Early in the outbreak investigation, the CDC developed a novel real-time PCR detection test with broad-range fungal primers, including an *Exserohilum*-specific primer (29).

Among 139 patients who had both real-time PCR and culture results obtained for the same specimen, PCR was found to be more sensitive than culture for detecting fungus, 47% versus 14%.

A total of 751 clinical specimens (547 CSF samples, 120 fresh-frozen tissue samples, 27 formalin-fixed paraffin-embedded tissue samples, and 38 other body fluid samples, including synovial and epidural fluid) from probable and proven cases of fungal infection were tested at the CDC (22). *E. rostratum* DNA was detected in 90 CSF samples from 82 patients (23% of all patients from whom CSF was submitted). CSF samples from which *E. rostratum* was identified by culture or PCR had significantly more WBCs (970/µl versus 25/µl [$P < 0.001$]) than samples from which fungi could not be detected or isolated. All CSF samples from 136 patients initially suspected to have fungal meningitis but shown to have no WBCs in their CSF were negative by PCR testing (22).

Histopathology

Histopathology was described for 40 patients whose samples were sent to the CDC (30). The histopathological features of fatal *Exserohilum* cases included necrosuppurative to granulomatous meningitis and vasculitis with thrombi and abundant angioinvasive fungi and extensive involvement of the basilar arterial circulation of the brain. A hypothesis for pathogenesis of *E. rostratum* migration to the brain was suggested to involve fungal penetration into the CSF at the injection site, with transport through CSF to the basal cisterns and subsequent invasion of the basilar arteries, rather than migration through the vasculature.

Identifications of hyphae were similar for the Gomori methenamine silver stain and polyfungal immunohistochemistry. However, immunohistochemistry proved to be more sensitive because it labeled remnants of degraded fungi in areas of inflammation that lacked intact hyphae. Immunohistochemistry also was more sensitive than PCR for detecting *Exserohilum* in formalin-fixed paraffin-embedded tissues. The lower sensitivity of PCR may be due to few intact fungi in tissues and difficulty with breaking down fungal cell walls during the DNA extraction process (30).

CSF (1,3) beta-D-glucan

The (1,3) beta-D-glucan assay detects this cell wall constituent, which is present in many different fungi. In this outbreak, this assay performed on CSF proved to be both sensitive and specific for fungal meningitis (31–33). The largest study tested CSF specimens from 233 patients from Michigan and Tennessee. Forty-five patients had meningitis (28 proven), 53 had spinal or paraspinal infection (19 proven), and 135 did not develop disease (33). Using the manufacturer's cutoff (≥80 pg/ml), the sensitivity and specificity were 96% and 95% for proven meningitis and 84% and 95% for probable or proven meningitis. The optimal cutoff for proven meningitis was found to be 66 pg/ml (sensitivity, 100%, and specificity, 94%); for probable or proven meningitis, it also was 66 pg/ml (sensitivity, 91%, and specificity, 92%). A second study included specimens from 41 proven cases of fungal meningitis and 66 controls; the optimal cutoff was found to be 138 pg/ml, which provided 100% sensitivity and 98% specificity for the diagnosis of fungal meningitis that was confirmed microbiologically (32). Testing samples obtained serially from a small number of patients showed that beta-D-glucan levels that decline with therapy may predict therapeutic response.

TREATMENT

Initial Treatment Regimens

Because fungal CNS infections caused by molds are uncommon, the CDC sought advice from a panel of physicians who had expertise in treating fungal infections. The initial treatment regimen that was suggested was liposomal amphotericin B, 7.5 mg/kg intravenously (i.v.) daily, combined with voriconazole, 6 mg/kg i.v. twice daily. This recommendation was based on the presumption that the pathogen was likely *A. fumigatus*, because the index case had this organism isolated from CSF (3). When it became apparent that further cases were caused not by *A. fumigatus* but rather by *E. rostratum*, recommendations for treatment were changed (10). Treatment recommendations also were modified because many patients, especially those who were elderly, did not tolerate high doses of liposomal amphotericin B and voriconazole, and because it became apparent that antifungal therapy would have to be safe enough to be given for months.

The recommended dosage of liposomal amphotericin B was decreased to 5 to 6 mg/kg i.v. daily, and it was recommended that combination therapy with liposomal amphotericin B and voriconazole be reserved for patients who had severe or refractory disease (34). For patients with mild to moderate meningitis and localized spinal or paraspinal infections, the recommendation was to treat with voriconazole alone, starting at a dosage of 6 mg/kg twice daily (34).

The standard practice for administering voriconazole is to modify the daily dose based on the serum concentration, aiming to achieve a level between 1 µg/ml and 5 µg/ml (35, 36). For patients in this outbreak who had CNS mold infections, the aim was to achieve a serum concentration of 2 to 5 µg/ml to better ensure adequate voriconazole concentrations in the CSF (37, 38). In some patients, this led to a dose reduction from that given initially, but in many, a higher daily dose of voriconazole was required to achieve these concentrations.

For patients who had osteoarticular infections, voriconazole monotherapy was recommended using a loading dose of 6 mg/kg for two doses, followed by 4 mg/kg twice daily.

These patients were less ill, and the penetration of voriconazole into the joint space is excellent. It was thought that there was no compelling reason to add amphotericin B to treat these infections. Surgical debridement was recommended when feasible (39).

Amphotericin B

The recommendation to use liposomal amphotericin B for patients in this outbreak was based on past experience with treatment of other CNS dematiaceous mold infections (14, 40). Liposomal amphotericin B was recommended because of animal data suggesting that higher CSF and brain concentrations could be achieved with this formulation than with amphotericin B lipid complex or amphotericin B deoxycholate (41). Most patients who were treated with amphotericin B as initial therapy received this agent for several days to weeks. However, some patients who failed to respond to voriconazole monotherapy or who had recalcitrant arachnoiditis were treated with liposomal amphotericin B for months. Excluding the few patients who were treated for months for severe arachnoiditis, the median time liposomal amphotericin B was given to 115 patients who had spinal or paraspinal infections at SJMH was 13 days.

Adverse effects

The adverse effects of amphotericin B are well known and occurred in most patients who were treated with this agent in the outbreak. The extent of electrolyte disturbance, specifically tubular loss of potassium and magnesium, was dramatic in some patients and required aggressive i.v. replacement therapy in the hospital to correct the deficits. Nephrotoxicity, not unexpectedly, was more severe in older adults and those with preexisting chronic kidney disease. Infusion reactions were generally not severe, but routine pretreatment with hydrocortisone, diphenhydramine, and acetaminophen was given to many patients.

Voriconazole

Voriconazole was selected over posaconazole and itraconazole for several reasons. First and foremost, there was experience in the use of voriconazole for various invasive mold infections (42, 43). Second, there were some data, later confirmed for the isolates from this outbreak, that showed *in vitro* activity of voriconazole against *Exserohilum* species (21, 22). Third, both i.v. and oral formulations were available, and oral administration on an empty stomach produced serum levels similar to those achieved by i.v. administration. Fourth, concentrations of voriconazole in CSF are approximately 50% of serum levels, and levels in both CSF and serum are above the MIC for many dematiaceous molds (21, 38). By comparison, posaconazole and itraconazole, although slightly more active *in vitro* against dematiaceous molds, at the time were not available in an i.v. formulation, neither achieved substantial levels in CSF, and absorption of the oral formulations was often erratic.

Adverse effects

Adverse effects associated with the use of voriconazole are well described. Most commonly these include hepatotoxicity, transient photopsia (seeing bright spots and flashing lights), visual hallucinations, and rash (44). Because this agent was used at relatively high doses for prolonged periods in patients who did not have a hematological malignancy, had not received a transplant, and had not been given immunosuppressive drugs, adverse effects came to the fore that had been documented only rarely or had been masked by these serious underlying illnesses.

The most obvious was alopecia, which was dramatic in these patients who had no other reason to lose their hair. At SJMH, a cross-sectional survey of 152 patients who were treated with voriconazole for at least a month found that 82% had developed alopecia, mostly involving the scalp but also involving the extremities, eyebrows, and eyelashes

(45). The loss of scalp hair was profound enough in 19 patients that they wore a wig or a head covering to hide the loss. The mean time to onset of alopecia was 75 days after beginning voriconazole. Alopecia was reversible, with 69% of patients reporting regrowth of hair within 3 months of stopping voriconazole. The reversal of alopecia also occurred among patients who switched from voriconazole to other azoles (itraconazole or posaconazole), suggesting that alopecia is not a class effect of azoles. Most of those who had alopecia also noticed brittle or split nails, and a few patients lost nails. Alopecia and nail changes did not appear to be related to the daily dose of voriconazole or serum concentrations of voriconazole.

Although CNS effects due to voriconazole are well known, the extent of dysfunction while on voriconazole was striking. Patients routinely complained of feeling "foggy" and being unable to concentrate on day-to-day tasks. Family members noted that patients were increasingly forgetful and at times were confused. These adverse CNS effects were not associated with high serum concentrations of voriconazole. They disappeared when voriconazole was stopped or when another azole was substituted for voriconazole. In contrast, hallucinations definitely were dose related and were seen predominantly when patients received high doses of voriconazole i.v. and had serum voriconazole levels of >5 μg/ml, as noted previously (35). Decreasing the dose or changing the route of administration of voriconazole often led to resolution of hallucinations.

Periostitis is a rarely described side effect of voriconazole (46–48). Periostitis was seen in this outbreak, most likely because voriconazole was given at high doses for a prolonged period (49). The prominent manifestation of this uncommon side effect is bone pain, and the bones most commonly involved are the ribs and wrist bones (49). Radiographic diagnosis can be made by finding abnormal uptake on a whole-body bone scan (Fig. 4).

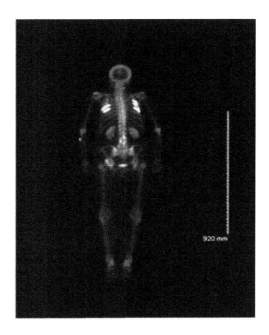

FIGURE 4 **Whole-body bone scan of a woman who had been on voriconazole for 4 months for meningitis and arachnoiditis shows uptake in the left and right ribs posteriorly consistent with periostitis.**

The pathogenesis of voriconazole-associated periostitis is related to fluoride toxicity, which has been documented by elevated serum fluoride concentrations 4- to 7-fold above normal in all patients with this adverse effect (46, 48, 49). The excess fluoride molecules replace calcium molecules in bone and cause bone pain and osteomalacia. The structure of voriconazole contains 3 fluorine molecules, more than in any other azole antifungal agent. The development of periostitis has been correlated with the daily and the cumulative dosage of voriconazole; thus, the amount of fluoride consumed, and not serum voriconazole concentrations, predicts the development of periostitis. All symptoms resolve when the dose of voriconazole is decreased or the drug is discontinued.

Voriconazole, as well as other azoles, has been known to cause rashes, chapped lips, and dry skin. However, voriconazole is unique in its propensity to cause photosensitivity rashes. The photosensitivity is severe in some patients, and with continued administration of voriconazole, actinic changes and ultimately multicentric squamous cell skin cancers can arise in sun-damaged areas (50, 51). Melanomas also have been reported for patients on long-term therapy with voriconazole (52).

Voriconazole has many drug-drug interactions because it is metabolized by 3 different cytochrome P-450 enzyme systems (44). Drugs, such as rifampin and carbamazepine, that induce cytochrome P-450 activity greatly decrease voriconazole levels. Voriconazole interferes with the metabolism of many drugs, and interactions with cyclosporine, tacrolimus, sirolimus, and warfarin can result in toxic levels of these drugs. The coadministration of voriconazole and other agents, such as statins, benzodiazepines, and calcium channel blockers, should be avoided or done with careful attention paid to decreasing the doses of these agents. Because of its propensity to prolong the QTc interval, voriconazole must be used with caution with drugs, such as amiodarone, quetiapine, citalopram, and fluoroquinolones, that also prolong the QTc. Frequent monitoring of electrocardiograms is required when voriconazole is used concomitantly with medications that prolong the QTc interval.

Other Azoles

As treatment with voriconazole continued for months among patients who had meningitis and/or localized spinal or paraspinal infections, many of the side effects of voriconazole became limiting. The CNS effects were especially bothersome, and the adverse effects seen after long-term therapy, such as alopecia and periostitis, led clinicians and patients to change therapy to itraconazole or posaconazole. These two agents have activity against *E. rostratum* (21) but were not recommended initially because the levels attained in the CNS were low and absorption of the oral formulations was not reliable (34). However, for patients who had responded to initial antifungal therapy and were doing well and for those who had not meningitis but rather paraspinal or osteoarticular infections, these agents became more attractive as the side effects of voriconazole became more problematic. Most patients at SJMH who required antifungal therapy for more than 6 months had their therapy changed to itraconazole. A few had adverse effects, primarily nausea, vomiting, and abdominal discomfort, with this agent, and they were then treated with posaconazole. For both drugs, measurement of serum drug concentrations was essential for successful management. Currently, long-term follow-up data are not available regarding how many patients were changed to oral itraconazole or posaconazole and how they responded.

CAN THIS HAPPEN AGAIN?

This large outbreak served as a dramatic wake-up call regarding the risks of compounded drugs. This was not the first time that medications produced by a compounding center had been found to be contaminated and to cause life-threatening or sight-threatening disease. This outbreak, except for its size and the involvement of a different dematiaceous mold, was almost an exact replica of an outbreak a decade earlier (8). Earlier in 2012, two outbreaks involving one compounding center led to visual loss in 39 of 40 patients (98%). That compounding center, Franck's Compounding Lab, sold brilliant blue G dye (used during retinal surgery) that was contaminated with *Fusarium* species and triamcinolone acetonide for intraocular injection that was contaminated with the dematiaceous mold *Bipolaris hawaiiensis* (53).

Compounded drugs are prepared for individual patients in formulations and dosages that are not available from pharmaceutical firms; this includes chemotherapeutic agents, preservative-free and dye-free preparations, medications with different flavorings for children, and other products (54). Clearly, there is an important role for compounding pharmacies in providing specific medications for specific patients.

The regulation of compounding pharmacies differs greatly from that of pharmaceutical firms in that they are not regulated by the FDA but instead are under the purview of individual state boards of pharmacy. The FDA was specifically blocked from exerting authority over compounding pharmacies by a series of legal decisions and congressional acts that occurred in the 1990s (55, 56). The FDA does have authority to enter a compounding pharmacy and inspect conditions at that firm if a problem has been identified, but the inspection can be delayed through various legal maneuvers by the company.

The basic tenet of a compounding pharmacy was ignored when the NECC did not produce drugs in response to prescriptions for individual patients but instead shipped large amounts of their product to many different states, resulting in hundreds of patients becoming infected. In this respect, they acted as if they were a pharmaceutical firm but without regulatory oversight by the FDA. When the FDA did inspect the NECC facility after the first cases were reported, multiple vials from one of the contaminated lots were found to contain particulate material, the cleanliness of the environment and the equipment did not meet expected standards, and it was noted that nonsterile products were used to prepare preservative-free drugs, such as methylprednisolone acetate.

As a result of this large outbreak that endangered many lives, Congress passed the Drug Quality and Security Act in November 2013. This law created a new class of compounding pharmacies that are able to produce medications in bulk and distribute them to many states. The law states that these compounding pharmacies will be designated as "outsourcing facilities" and will be regulated by the FDA. However, registering as an outsourcing facility is voluntary. Whether market pressure will force compounding pharmacies to enter this program if they wish to produce medications for more than single-patient use or whether it will be business as usual remains to be seen.

CONCLUSIONS

Injection of methylprednisolone acetate that had been manufactured by the New England Compounding Center and that was discovered to be contaminated with the brown-black mold, *Exserohilum rostratum*, caused infection in 751 patients in the fall of 2012. Of the 751 patients, 233 had meningitis, 7 had a stroke, 325 had spinal or paraspinal infection, 151 had both meningitis and spinal or paraspinal infection, and 35 had osteoarticular infection. Sixty-four patients died, mostly from meningitis or stroke. Treatment with a combination of liposomal amphotericin B and voriconazole for meningitis and voriconazole, with or without liposomal amphotericin B, plus surgical debridement for spinal or paraspinal infection appeared to be successful for many, but not all, patients. Congress enacted legislation increasing the oversight of compounding pharmacies by the Food and Drug Administration after this outbreak in hopes of averting similar devastating events in the future.

ACKNOWLEDGMENTS

Doctor Malani is a shareholder of Pfizer pharmaceuticals.

CITATION

Kauffman CA, Malani AN. 2016. Fungal infections associated with contaminated steroid injections. Microbiol Spectrum 4(3):EI10-0005-2015.

REFERENCES

1. **Pettit AC, Malani AN.** 2015. Outbreak of fungal infections associated with contaminated

methylprednisolone acetate: an update. *Curr Infect Dis Rep* **17:**441–448.

2. **Centers for Disease Control and Prevention.** *Multi-state fungal meningitis outbreak—current case count.* Centers for Disease Control and Prevention, Atlanta, GA. http://www.cdc.gov/hai/outbreaks/meningitis-map-large.html. Accessed 5 August 2015.

3. **Pettit AC, Kropski JA, Castilho JL, Schmitz JKE, Rauch CA, Mobley BC, Wang XJ, Spires SS, Pugh ME.** 2012. The index case for the fungal meningitis outbreak in the United States. *N Engl J Med* **367:**2119–2125.

4. **Smith R, Derado G, Wise M, Harris J, Chiller T, Meltzer M, Park B.** 2015. Estimated deaths and illnesses averted during fungal meningitis outbreak associated with contaminated steroid injections, United States, 2012-2013. *Emerg Infect Dis* **21:**933–940.

5. **Smith RM, Schaefer MK, Kainer MA, Wise M, Finks J, Duwve J, Fontaine E, Chu A, Carothers B, Reilly A, Fiedler J, Wiese AD, Feaster C, Gibson L, Griese S, Purfield A, Cleveland AA, Benedict K, Harris JR, Brandt ME, Blau D, Jernigan J, Weber JT, Park BJ, the Multistate Fungal Infection Outbreak Response Team.** 2013. Fungal infections associated with contaminated methylprednisolone injections. *N Engl J Med* **369:**1598–1609.

6. **Centers for Disease Control and Prevention Health Alert Network.** 2012. *Meningitis and stroke associated with potentially contaminated product.* Centers for Disease Control and Prevention, Atlanta, GA. http://emergency.cdc.gov/HAN/han00327.asp. Accessed 5 August 2015.

7. **Centers for Disease Control and Prevention.** 2012. Multistate outbreak of fungal infection associated with injection of methylprednisolone acetate solution from a single compounding pharmacy—United States, 2012. *MMWR Morb Mortal Wkly Rep* **61:**839–842.

8. **Centers for Disease Control and Prevention.** 2002. *Exophiala* infection from contaminated injectable steroids prepared by a compounding pharmacy—United States, July–November 2002. *MMWR Morb Mortal Wkly Rep* **51:**1109–1112.

9. **Kainer MA, Reagan DR, Nguyen DB, Wiese AD, Wise ME, Ward J, Park BJ, Kanago ML, Baumblatt J, Schaefer MK, Berger BE, Marder EP, Min JY, Dunn JR, Smith RM, Dreyzehner J, Jones TF, Tennessee Fungal Meningitis Investigation Team.** 2012. Fungal infections associated with contaminated methylprednisolone in Tennessee. *N Engl J Med* **367:**2194–2203.

10. **Kauffman CA, Pappas PG, Patterson TF.** 2013. Fungal infections associated with contaminated

methylprednisolone injections. *N Engl J Med* **368:**2495–2500.

11. **Kerkering TM, Grifasi ML, Baffoe-Bonnie AW, Bansal E, Garner DC, Smith JA, Demicco DD, Schleupner CJ, Aldoghaither RA, Savaliya VA.** 2013. Early clinical observations in prospectively followed patients with fungal meningitis related to contaminated epidural steroid injections. *Ann Intern Med* **158:**154–161.

12. **Centers for Disease Control and Prevention.** 2013. Spinal and paraspinal infections associated with contaminated methylprednisolone acetate injections—Michigan, 2012-2013. *MMWR Morb Mortal Wkly Rep* **62:**377–381.

13. **Moudgal V, Singal B, Kauffman CA, Brodkey JA, Malani AN, Olmstead RN, Kasotakis M, Koch S, Kaakaji R, Nyaku M, Neelakanta A, Valenstein P, Winter S, Otto MH, Jagarlamudi R, Kerr L, Czerwinski J, Vandenberg DM, Sutton SR, Murphy H, Halasyamani L.** 2014. Spinal and paraspinal fungal infections associated with contaminated methyloprednisolone injections. *Open Forum Infect Dis* doi:10.1093/ofid/ofu022.

14. **Revankar SG, Sutton DA, Rinaldi MG.** 2004. Primary central nervous system phaeohyphomycosis: a review of 101 cases. *Clin Infect Dis* **38:**206–216.

15. **Chiller TM, Roy M, Nguyen D, Guh A, Malani AN, Latham R, Peglow S, Kerkering T, Kaufman D, McFadden J, Collins J, Kainer M, Duwve J, Trump D, Blackmore C, Tan C, Cleveland AA, MacCannell T, Muehlenbachs A, Zaki SR, Brandt ME, Jernigan JA, Multistate Fungal Infection Clinical Investigation Team.** 2013. Clinical findings for fungal infections caused by methylprednisolone injections. *N Engl J Med* **369:**1610–1619.

16. **Katragou A, Pana Z-D, Perlin DS, Kontoyiannis DP, Walsh TJ, Roilides E.** 2014. *Exserohilum* infections: review of 48 cases before the 2012 United States outbreak. *Med Mycol* **52:**376–386.

17. **Adler A, Yaniv I, Samra Z, Yacobovich J, Fisher S, Avrahami G, Levy I.** 2006. *Exserohilum*: an emerging human pathogen. *Eur J Clin Microbiol Infect Dis* **25:**247–253.

18. **Acquino VM, Norvell JM, Krisher K, Mustafa MM.** 1995. Fatal disseminated infection due to *Exserohilum rostratum* in a patient with aplastic anemia: case report and review. *Clin Infect Dis* **20:**176–178.

19. **Lasala PR, Smith MB, McGinnis MR, Sackey K, Patel JA, Qiu S.** 2005. Invasive *Exserohilum* sinusitis in a patient with aplastic anemia. *Pediatr Infect Dis J* **24:**939–941.

20. Saint-Jean M, St-Germain G, Laferruere C, Tapiero B. 2007. Hospital-acquired phaeohyphomycosis due to *Exserohilum rostratum* in a child with leukemia. *Can J Infect Dis Med Microbiol* 18:200–202.

21. da Cunha KC, Sutton DA, Gene J, Capilla J, Cano J, Guarro J. 2012. Molecular identification and in vitro response to antifungal drugs of clinical isolates of *Exserohilum*. *Antimicrob Agents Chemother* 56:4951–4954.

22. Lockhart SR, Pham CD, Gade L, Iqbal N, Scheel CM, Cleveland AA, Whitney AM, Noble-Wang J, Chiller TM, Park BJ, Litvintseva AP, Brandt ME. 2013. Preliminary laboratory report of fungal infections associated with contaminated methylprednisolone injections. *J Clin Microbiol* 51:2654–2661.

23. Litvintseva AP, Hurst S, Gade L, Frace MA, Hilsabeck R, Schupp JM, Gillece JD, Roe C, Smith D, Keim P, Lockhart SR, Changayil S, Weil MR, MacCannell CDR, Brandt ME, Engelthaler DM. 2014. Whole-genome analysis of *Exserohilum rostratum* from an outbreak of fungal meningitis and other infections. *J Clin Microbiol* 52:3216–3222.

24. Malani AN, Vandenberg DM, Singal B, Kasotakis M, Koch S, Moudgal V, Jagarlamudi R, Neelakanta A, Otto MH, Halasyamani L, Kaakaji R, Kauffman CA. 2013. Magnetic resonance imaging screening to identify spinal and paraspinal infections associated with injections of contaminated methylprednisolone acetate. *JAMA* 309:2465–2472.

25. Centers for Disease Control and Prevention Health Alert Network. 2012. *Update: multistate outbreak of fungal infections among persons who received injections with contaminated medication.* Centers for Disease Control and Prevention, Atlanta, GA. http://emergency.cdc.gov/HAN/han00338.asp. Accessed 5 August 2015.

26. McCotter OZ, Smith RM, Westercamp M, Kerkering TM, Malani AN, Latham R, Peglow SL, Mody R, Pappas PG, Chiller TM. 2015. Notes from the field: update on multistate outbreak of fungal infections associated with contaminated methylprednisolone injections, 2012–2014. *MMWR Morb Mortal Wkly Rep* 64:1200–1201.

27. Smith RM, Tipple M, Chaudry MN, Schaefer MK, Park BJ. 2013. Relapse of fungal meningitis associated with contaminated methylprednisolone. *N Engl J Med* 368:2535–2536.

28. Ampel NM. 2011. Coccidioidomycosis, p 349–366. *In* Kauffman CA, Pappas PG, Sobel JD, Dismukes WE (ed), *Essentials of Clinical Mycology*, 2nd ed. Springer, New York, NY.

29. Gade L, Scheel CM, Pham CD, Lindsley MD, Iqbal N, Cleveland AA, Whitney AM, Lockhart SR, Brandt ME, Litvintseva AP. 2013. Detection of fungal DNA in human body fluids and tissues during a multistate outbreak of fungal meningitis and other infections. *Eukaryot Cell* 12:677–683.

30. Ritter JM, Muehlenbachs A, Blau DM, Paddock CD, Shieh WJ, Drew CP, Batten BC, Bartlett JH, Metcalfe MG, Pham CD, Locjhart SR, Patel M, Liu L, Jones TL, Greer PW, Montague JL, White E, Rollin DC, Seales C, Stewart D, Deming MV, Brandt ME, Zaki SR, Exserohilum Infections Working Group. 2013. *Exserohilum* infections associated with contaminated steroid injections: a clinicopathologic review of 40 cases. *Am J Pathol* 183:881–892.

31. Lyons JL, Roos KL, Marr KA, Neumann H, Trivedi JB, Kimbrough DJ, Steiner L, Thakur KT, Harrison DM, Zhang SX. 2013. Cerebrospinal fluid (1,3)-beta-D-glucan detection as an aid for diagnosis of iatrogenic fungal meningitis. *J Clin Microbiol* 51:1285–1287.

32. Litvintseva AP, Lindsley MD, Gade L, Smith R, Chiller T, Lyons JL, Thakur KT, Zhang SX, Grgurich DE, Kerkering TM, Brandt ME, Park BJ. 2014. Utility of (1-3)-beta-D-glucan testing for diagnostics and monitoring response to treatment during the multistate outbreak of fungal meningitis and other infections. *Clin Infect Dis* 58:622–630.

33. Malani AN, Singal B, Wheat LJ, Al Sous O, Summons TA, Durkin MM, Pettit AC. 2015. (1,3)-β-D-Glucan in cerebrospinal fluid for diagnosis of fungal meningitis associated with contaminated methylprednisolone injections. *J Clin Microbiol* 53:799–803.

34. Centers for Disease Control and Prevention. 2012. *Interim treatment guidance for central nervous system and parameningeal infections associated with injection of contaminated steroid products.* Centers for Disease Control and Prevention, Atlanta, GA. http://www.cdc.gov/hai/outbreaks/clinicians/index.html. Accessed 5 August 2015.

35. Pascual A, Calandra T, Bolay S, Buclin T, Bille J, Marchetti O. 2008. Voriconazole therapeutic drug monitoring in patients with invasive mycoses improves efficacy and safety outcomes. *Clin Infect Dis* 46:201–211.

36. Park WB, Kim N-H, Lee SH, Nam W-S, Yoon SH, Song K-H, Choe PG, Kim NJ, Jang I-J, Oh M-D, Yu K-S. 2012. The effect of therapeutic drug monitoring on safety and efficacy of voriconazole in invasive fungal infections: a randomized controlled trial. *Clin Infect Dis* 55:1080–1087.

37. Pascual A, Csajka C, Buclin T, Bolay S, Bile J, Calandra T, Marchetti O. 2012. Challenging recommended oral and intravenous voriconazole doses for improved efficacy and safety: population pharmacokinetics-based analysis of adult patients with invasive fungal infections. *Clin Infect Dis* **55:**381–390.

38. Lutsar I, Roffey S, Troke P. 2003. Voriconazole concentrations in the cerebrospinal fluid and brain tissue of guinea pigs and immunocompromised patients. *Clin Infect Dis* **37:**728–732.

39. Centers for Disease Control and Prevention. 2012. *Interim treatment guidance for osteoarticular infections associated with injection of contaminated steroid products.* Centers for Disease Control and Prevention, Atlanta, GA. http://www.cdc.gov/hai/outbreaks/clinicians/index.html. Accessed 5 August 2015.

40. Li DM, de Hoog GS. 2009. Cerebral phaeohyphomycosis—a cure at what lengths? *Lancet Infect Dis* **9:**376–383.

41. Groll AH, Giri N, Petraitis V, Petraitiene R, Candelario M, Bacher JS, Piscitelli SC, Walsh TJ. 2000. Comparative efficacy and distribution of lipid formulations of amphotericin B in experimental *Candida albicans* infection of the central nervous system. *J Infect Dis* **182:**274–282.

42. Schwartz S, Ruhnke M, Ribaud P, Corey L, Driscoll T, Cornely OA, Schuler U, Lutsar I, Troke P, Thiel E. 2005. Improved outcome in central nervous system aspergillosis using voriconazole treatment. *Blood* **106:**2641–2645.

43. Troke P, Aguirrebengoa K, Arteaga C, Ellis D, Heath CH, Lutsar I, Rovira M, Nguyen Q, Slavin M, Chen SCA, Global Scedosporium Study Group. 2008. Treatment of scedosporiosis with voriconazole: clinical experience with 107 patients. *Antimicrob Agents Chemother* **52:**1743–1750.

44. Malani AN, Kerr L, Kauffman CA. 2015. Voriconazole—how to use this antifungal agent and what to expect. *Semin Crit Care Respir Med* **36:**795–804.

45. Malani AN, Kerr L, Obear J, Singal B, Kauffman CA. 2014. Alopecia and nail changes associated with voriconazole therapy. *Clin Infect Dis* **59:**e61–e65.

46. Gerber B, Guggenberger R, Fasler D, Nair G, Manz MG, Stussi G, Schanz U. 2012. Reversible skeletal disease and high fluoride serum levels in hematologic patients receiving voriconazole. *Blood* **120:**2390–2394.

47. Wang TF, Wang T, Altman R, Eshaghian P, Lynch JP III, Ross JA, Belperio JA, Weigt SS, Saggar R, Gregson A, Kubak B, Saggar R. 2009. Periostitis secondary to prolonged voriconazole therapy in lung transplant recipients. *Am J Transpl* **9:**2845–2850.

48. Wermers RA, Cooper K, Razonable RR, Deziel PJ, Whitford GM, Kremers WK, Moyer TP. 2011. Fluoride excess and periostitis in transplant patients receiving long-term voriconazole therapy. *Clin Infect Dis* **52:**604–611.

49. Moon WJ, Scheller EL, Suneja A, Livermore JA, Malani AN, Moudgal V, Kerr LE, Ferguson E, Vandenberg DM. 2014. Plasma fluoride level as a predictor of voriconazole induced periostitis in patients with skeletal pain. *Clin Infect Dis* **59:**604–611.

50. Epaulard O, Villier C, Ravaud P, Chosidow O, Blanche S, Mamzer-Bruneel M-F, Thiebaut A, Leccia M-T, Lortholary O. 2013. A multistep voriconazole-related phototoxic pathway may lead to skin carcinoma: results from a French nationwide study. *Clin Infect Dis* **57:**e182–e188.

51. Williams K, Mansh M, Chin-Hong P, Singer J, Arron ST. 2014. Voriconazole-associated cutaneous malignancy: a literature review on photocarcinogenesis in organ transplant recipients. *Clin Infect Dis* **58:**997–1002.

52. Miller DD, Cowen EW, Nguyen JC, McCalmont TH, Fox LP. 2010. Melanoma associated with long-term voriconazole therapy. A new manifestation of chronic photosensitivity. *Arch Dermatol* **146:**300–304.

53. Mikosz CA, Smith RM, Kim M, Tyson C, Lee EH, Adams E, Straif-Bourgeois S, Sowadsky R, Arroyo S, Grant-Greene Y, Duran J, Vasquez Y, Robinson BF, Harris JR, Lockhart SR, Torok TJ, Mascola L, Park BJ, Fungal Endophthalmitis Outbreak Response Team. 2014. Fungal endophthalmitis associated with compounded products. *Emerg Infect Dis* **20:**248–256.

54. Drazen JM, Curfman GD, Baden LR, Morrissey S. 2012. Compounding errors. *N Engl J Med* **367:**2436–2437.

55. Outterson K. 2012. Regulating compounding pharmacies after NECC. *N Engl J Med* **367:**1969–1972.

56. Weissfeld AS. 2013. Straight from the headlines: what is going on in compounding pharmacies, and how can clinical microbiologists help? *J Clin Microbiol* **51:**3168–3171.

Emerging Fungal Infections in the Pacific Northwest: The Unrecognized Burden and Geographic Range of *Cryptococcus gattii* and *Coccidioides immitis*

20

SHAWN R. LOCKHART,[1] ORION Z. McCOTTER,[1] and TOM M. CHILLER[1]

INTRODUCTION

Fungal infections present a real challenge to public health, as they are ubiquitous in the environment and are not passed from human to human or generally transmitted by a vector, making exposure impossible to completely prevent. New opportunistic fungal pathogens are emerging in highly immunosuppressed (transplant) patients. These patient groups are highly susceptible to infections, and it is not unexpected that we find newly emerging infections. However, there are fungi that are known to be specific to certain geographic regions (often referred to as endemic) which are themselves emerging in new geographic areas and are not associated with immunosuppressed patients. Two of these such fungi are *Coccidioides immitis/ posadasii* in the Southwest United States and *Cryptococcus gattii*, with most cases being recognized in Southern California. When regional or endemic diseases are encountered outside of their traditional geographic boundaries, especially in nontravelers, diagnosis can be delayed, leading to significant morbidity and mortality. These two fungi have recently emerged in the Pacific Northwest (PNW) of the United States.

[1]Mycotic Diseases Branch, Centers for Disease Control and Prevention, Atlanta, GA 30333.

Emerging Infections 10
Edited by W. Michael Scheld, James M. Hughes and Richard J. Whitley
© 2016 American Society for Microbiology, Washington, DC
doi:10.1128/microbiolspec.EI10-0016-2016

EMERGENCE OF *CRYPTOCOCCUS GATTII* IN NORTH AMERICA

Cryptococcus species are saprophytic basid-iomycete fungi capable of causing invasive infection in humans, particularly in immu-nocompromised persons. There are two major human pathogens within the genus *Cryptococcus*, *Cryptococcus neoformans* and *Cryptococcus gattii* (1). *C. neoformans* and *C. gattii* differ significantly with regard to their geographic distributions, their ecologi-cal niches, and the clinical aspects of dis-eases they cause in humans. *C. neoformans* is found worldwide and has been isolated frequently in association with pigeon guano and certain types of trees, and it is most frequently seen in the context of meningo-encephalitis in immunocompromised pa-tients. Until recently, *C. gattii* was thought to be largely confined to tropical and sub-tropical regions, where it had been found primarily in association with *Eucalyptus* trees (2). It was believed that in the United States, *C. gattii* was largely confined to Southern California (3, 4). Although *C. gattii* can be a primary pathogen of healthy hosts, in a sur-vey of HIV⁺ patients in Southern California, a substantial number of the *Cryptococcus* isolates causing meningoencephalitis were *C. gattii* (5).

Although *C. gattii* was occasionally isolat-ed throughout the United States (6–8), the vast majority of North American cases prior to 2008 were seen in Southern California, which fit the narrative of confinement to a subtropical region (3, 4). With cases outside of California being exceedingly rare, it was a surprise to the clinical community when *C. gattii* cases were reported among ani-mals and people living in or traveling from Vancouver Island (VI), British Columbia, Canada, starting in 1999 (9–11). At the time of this outbreak, it was believed to be an anomaly, as *C. gattii* was not believed to be an organism found in temperate environments such as the PNW. The number of cases in-creased each year after 1999, and *C. gattii*

was isolated from multiple environmental sources, including coastal Douglas fir trees, a staple of the PNW forest and a tree species unrelated to the *Eucalyptus* trees that were thought to be the primary source of *C. gattii* (12–16). More puzzling was the fact that the VGII molecular types of *C. gattii* isolates from the PNW (designated VGIIa for the predominant molecular type comprising over 90% of the isolates and VGIIb for the minority molecular type comprising about 5 to 8% of the isolates) were different from the molecular type VGIII typically seen further south along the Pacific coast in Southern California (17–19). Of note, these two molec-ular types have recently been described as separate species within the *C. gattii* species complex, with molecular type VGII being named *C. deuterogattii* and molecular type VGIII as *C. basillisporus* (20).

The coastal Douglas fir biogeoclimatic zone characterizing the part of British Co-lumbia where most *C. gattii* cases originated extends down the Pacific coast into the United States, specifically west of the Cas-cade Mountains in Washington State and the Willamette Valley of Oregon (13, 21), so it was reasonable to conclude that the emer-gence might stretch into the United States. In 2004, a patient from the Orcas Islands in the Puget Sound had the first recorded case of *C. gattii* molecular type VGIIa in the United States (22), and shortly thereafter, in 2005, *C. gattii*-positive environmental samples from Washington State were de-scribed (14).

Between 2005 and 2011 the number of cases of *C. gattii* in humans and animals in the PNW of the United States increased (23–26). The majority of the isolates were VGIIa and VGIIb, as seen in the VI emergence, but there were also VGIII isolates similar to those seen in Southern California, especially among cats (24). In 2008, a new genotype, designated VGIIc, emerged in Oregon (25). This genotype was similar but not identical to the VGIIa and VGIIb genotypes seen previously. Retrospective analysis showed that the first case of cryptococcosis due to *C. gattii* VGIIc was recorded in Oregon in 2005.

As mentioned above, the majority of isolates from British Columbia and the PNW United States were of the genotype VGIIa, which is similar but not identical to isolates found in both Australia and Brazil (17, 18, 27, 28). A minority of cases were caused by genotype VGIIb, a genotype that had been isolated from Malaysia, Thailand, Australia, and Brazil (29). Whole-genome sequencing has been used to show that both the VGIIa and VGIIb clades are highly clonal, with approximately 21 single nucleotide polymorphisms over 18.4 million base pairs detected between any two isolates of VGIIa and just slightly higher than that between any two VGIIb isolates (27). The Oregon VGIIc genotype was also highly clonal, with an average of only 10 single nucleotide polymorphisms between any two isolates. When they were compared to other isolates of molecular type VGII from throughout the world, it was apparent that the VGIIa, VGIIb, and VGIIc isolates likely originated in South America and spread from there, although it is not clear if they arrived in North America first or detoured through Australia (27, 30, 31). Based on whole-genome analysis, it is apparent that *C. gattii* was introduced to the PNW at least four times, with VGIIa and VGIIc each introduced once and lineages of VGIIb introduced at least twice (27). Whole-genome sequencing of an isolate of VGIIb from a patient in Florida indicates that VGIIb may have been introduced to North America a third time as well (27, 32). While the genotypic diversity of the PNW isolates clearly indicates that there were multiple introductions, it is not yet clear when these introductions took place or why these particular genotypes were able to occupy this new niche, which was seemingly outside of the normal biogeoclimatic zone of *C. gattii*. There is no evidence of how these *C. gattii* lineages were introduced, but given their association with trees and plant material, it

could be speculated that they were introduced through agricultural products.

It is important to note that a single VGIIa clinical isolate was obtained from a patient in Seattle, WA, in 1972 and a similar VGIIa isolate was identified from a *Eucalyptus* tree in California in 1990 (2, 17). Although the travel history of the Washington patient is unknown, it is possible that *C. gattii* VGIIa has actually been present in the PNW for decades before the present emergence but for unknown reasons has only recently emerged or been recognized as a cause of invasive and potentially lethal disease in both humans and animals. Interestingly, whole-genome analysis indicates that while the 1972 isolate is almost indistinguishable from the emergent isolates and most closely related to the 1990 environmental isolate from California, the California isolate is less similar to the isolates from the PNW and could be a less virulent predecessor that had been independently diverging (27, 30).

Another interesting aspect of the emergence of *C. gattii* in the PNW is that the clinical manifestations of the disease seem to be different from what was typically seen in North American cases of *C. gattii* infection. The majority of patients in the PNW suffered from a primary pulmonary infection with or without meningoencephalitis (33–36). The major symptoms were cough, dyspnea, and headache rather than the typical neurological symptoms most often associated with the more commonly seen meningoencephalitis, such as blurred vision, neck stiffness, and seizures (33–35). This may be an indication that the different molecular types (now species) actually cause different diseases, it may have something to do with acute versus reactivation disease, or it may be a unique manifestation of the isolates from the PNW, possibly related to the genotypic differences in the PNW isolates that were necessary for them to occupy a new environmental niche (27, 37).

Whether *C. gattii* has always been in the PNW at some very low level and underwent genetic changes that allowed it to emerge or whether it arrived recently and is currently emerging is not known. What is clear is that multiple molecular types of *C. gattii* are currently causing infections in areas where *C. gattii* had not previously been recognized as a significant pathogen. The two clonal strains, VGIIa and VGIIb, have spread slowly southward from VI over the last 10 years along the coastal Douglas fir biogeoclimatic zone and have now been recorded for the first time in northern California, a climatic region more typical of traditional *C. gattii* colonization (24). Whether these strains will be able to expand further within new niches remains to be seen.

COCCIDIOIDOMYCOSIS: EXPANDING ITS GEOGRAPHIC RANGE

Coccidioides species are dimorphic fungi that grow in specific regions within the western hemisphere generally found to have limited rainfall and sandy, alkaline soils (38). The environmental form grows as a hyphal mold that differentiates into arthroconidia (39). When the soil is disrupted, these arthroconidia become aerosolized and when inhaled can cause infection in humans and animals. Once in the lungs, the arthroconidia change into a spherule form containing progeny called endospores, which can propagate when the mature spherule structure ruptures (40, 41). This mycosis that develops in the host is known as coccidioidomycosis (Valley fever). Most people infected with *Coccidioides* are asymptomatic or exhibit only subclinical symptoms (42–45). However, among those who do become ill, the disease can present as a range of syndromes from a self-limited pneumonia (46, 47) to a progressive infection in the lungs (48). In a small number of cases, the disease disseminates to other areas in the body and can become life-threatening (49). Knowledge of the geographic areas where the fungus exists is of great importance for clinical awareness

of Valley fever in those living in or traveling to these areas.

Our early understanding of the epidemiology of this organism and the areas where it is endemic comes from early studies using a "coccidioidin" skin test that evaluates an individual's previous exposure to *Coccidioides*. Much of the work with the coccidioidin skin test was accomplished by the U.S. military. Prior to World War II, the area where *Coccidioides* was endemic was not clearly defined, although many case reports and a few outbreaks had been published. During World War II, the importance of this disease for the U.S. military became prominent when they began year-round aviation training programs in the San Joaquin Valley of California (44). This involved migration of many naive populations into the deserts of the southwestern United States. These arriving military recruits were tested with the coccidioidin skin test (42). It soon became apparent that those with positive skin test reactions did not develop infection (43). It was later confirmed that the cellular immune process usually provided immunity against reinfection (50).

Establishment of the Range of Endemicity in the United States

The first description of geographic distribution of coccidioidomycosis in the United States was accomplished through a large evaluation of the prevalence of coccidioidin sensitivity. During the mid- 1940s to early 1950s, coccidioidin skin tests were performed on approximately 110,000 persons from three populations: Navy recruits, college students, and student nurses. In order to establish geographic range, the study included only those participants who were lifetime single-county residents, white men and women between 17 and 21 years old (51). The authors then plotted the proportion of those remaining 48,676 participants by positive skin test reactions and county of residence. The study identified Arizona, California, Nevada,

New Mexico, Utah, and Texas as states where coccidioidomycosis was endemic, with the highest rates of skin test positivity (50 to 70%) in California's southern San Joaquin Valley, Arizona's Sonoran Desert, and Texas's Rio Grande Valley. This created the basis for the map of the area of endemicity that has been used for decades (51); however, recent evidence now demonstrates that *Coccidioides* exists beyond these previously described geographic areas (Fig. 1).

Outbreaks at archeological excavations have identified specific locations outside of the traditional area of endemicity where groups have had close contact with soil and dust exposure in the process of identifying artifacts. One such outbreak, where 11 cases of coccidioidomycosis occurred among a group of 23 students, occurred in 1968 in Capay Valley of Yolo County, CA, at an ancient Native American burial ground approx-

imately 40 miles northwest of Sacramento and at least 50 miles beyond the originally recognized area of endemicity (52). Two years later another outbreak occurred, this time in the foothills of the Sierra range, near Chico, Butte County, CA, approximately 70 miles north of the recognized area of endemicity. Among the 103 archeology students, at least 61 developed compatible clinical illnesses, of which 27 were confirmed by serological test or skin test conversion. Additionally, culture was able to confirm the presence of the *Coccidioides* in the soil (53).

In 2001, 10 of the 18 workers and archeologists at an archeological site in Dinosaur National Monument in northeastern Utah developed clinically compatible symptoms. This was approximately 200 miles north of the historical area of endemicity in Utah. Nine of the 18 cases were confirmed by serology (54). These outbreaks clearly sup-

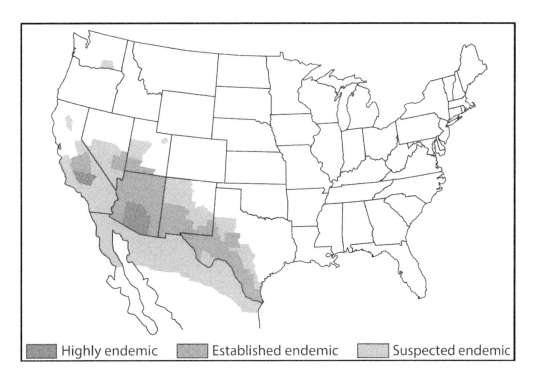

FIGURE 1 Areas where coccidioidomycosis is known and suspected to be endemic in the United States and Mexico (58). The map depicts approximate areas where *Coccidioides* in known to live or suspected to live based on studies from the late 1940s and early 1950s and from documented outbreak locations.

port the fact that foci of *Coccidioides* exist beyond the northern border of regions of endemicity in California and Utah, yet it was still unclear how the fungus got there.

The farthest documented presence of *Coccidioides immitis* north of the traditional region of endemicity occurred in the PNW from 2010 to 2011. This investigation began when three unrelated cases of coccidioidomycosis, not believed to have resulted from travel to areas where the disease was endemic, were identified in south-central Washington (55). The first of these cases occurred in June 2010, when a 12 year-old male presented with chest pain and was initially hospitalized for a bacterial pneumonia. His symptoms progressed, and upon readmission, *Coccidioides* was cultured from pleural fluid. The boy's only travel outside of Washington and a neighboring county in Oregon was a 2-day trip to Santa Maria, CA, in 2008, with no acute illness after the trip. The following month, a 15-year-old male suffered an all-terrain vehicle accident on a dirt track and sustained knee lacerations. His wound became infected, and *Coccidioides* was identified from wound culture. This patient had no recent travel to an area where the organism was endemic. Finally, in May 2011 a 58-year-old male who worked as an excavator in eastern Washington presented with dyspnea and chest pain despite antibiotic treatment. Respiratory cultures were able to confirm coccidioidal pneumonia. His infection progressed to meningitis in March 2012. His only travel to a known area where *Coccidioides* was endemic was a plane change in Arizona some 5 years before his illness (56). After the identification of these cases, retrospective analyses identified coccidioidomycosis cases in two dogs and a horse that had not traveled out of the PNW (56).

COCCIDIOIDES IN THE SOIL

Throughout the course of the investigation into these three cases from Washington, 22 soil samples were collected from likely exposure locations for two cases, even though at the time no reliable methods for detecting *Coccidioides* in environmental samples existed (55). However, in August 2013, a novel PCR developed by the Translational Genomics Research Institute in Flagstaff, AZ, detected *Coccidioides* DNA in six of the samples, and *C. immitis* was isolated by culture from four of those samples at the CDC (55). Whole-genome sequencing revealed that the Washington *C. immitis* isolates were related to strains from California's San Joaquin Valley but represented a distinct phylogenetic clade, making it clear that the fungal strains, although related to those from California, had been in Washington for some time. In addition, whole-genome sequencing showed that the clinical isolate from the 2010 wound infection was genetically indistinguishable from soil isolates from the site of the patient's all-terrain vehicle crash, directly linking the infection with the environmental source (57). These new tools provided clear evidence of the existence of *Coccidioides* well beyond the traditional area where it is endemic, making it critical that we reconsider the geographic range for this fungus.

Whether *Coccidioides* in the PNW represents sporadic environmental distribution of the fungus or, more likely, previous under-recognition of the disease, it is clear that the geographic risk for infection with this organism is much broader than our current understanding. It is critical for health care providers to know the true geographic range for this fungus in order to be able to consider it as a possible diagnosis in patients with symptoms. Early diagnosis and management of cases of coccidioidomycosis in humans and animals are paramount in reducing morbidity and mortality. Public health needs to continue to work on the identification and reporting of cases in order to document the expanding areas where the disease is endemic. The new methods for detection of the fungus in the environment have provided important tools to employ in efforts to redefine the endemicity range of *Coccidioides*. In the future, additional human, animal, and environmental testing is needed to continue to characterize the full extent of the geographic range of *Coccidioides* in order to help guide appropriate educational and awareness efforts for clinicians and the public.

CONCLUSION

Although many fungi are ubiquitous in the environment, certain species that cause serious human disease such as *Cryptococcus gattii* and *Coccidioides immitis* have a limited geographic distribution. When the distribution of these organisms changes, it is incumbent upon public health to investigate and determine the change in geographic distribution, and for clinicians and veterinarians to incorporate the changes into their differential diagnoses. Only through awareness of the disease, understanding its true distribution, and recognition of the burden can we hope to decrease the morbidity and mortality associated with these important fungal diseases.

ACKNOWLEDGMENTS

The findings and conclusions in this report are those of the authors and do not necessarily represent the official position of the Centers for Disease Control and Prevention.

CITATION

Lockhart SR, McCotter OZ, Chiller TM. 2016. Emerging fungal infections in the Pacific Northwest: the unrecognized burden and geographic range of *Cryptococcus gattii* and *Coccidioides immitis*. Microbiol Spectrum 4(3):EI10-0016-2016.

REFERENCES

1. **Kwon-Chung KJ, Varma A.** 2006. Do major species concepts support one, two or more species within *Cryptococcus neoformans*? *FEMS Yeast Res* **6:**574–587.

2. **Ellis D, Pfeiffer T.** 1992. The ecology of *Cryptococcus neoformans. Eur J Epidemiol* **8:**321–325.

3. **Wilson DE, Bennett JE, Bailey JW.** 1968. Serologic grouping of *Cryptococcus neoformans. Proc Soc Exp Biol Med* **127:**820–823.

4. **Bennett JE, Kwon-Chung KJ, Howard DH.** 1977. Epidemiologic differences among serotypes of *Cryptococcus neoformans. Am J Epidemiol* **105:**582–586.

5. **Chaturvedi S, Dyavaiah M, Larsen RA, Chaturvedi V.** 2005. *Cryptococcus gattii* in AIDS patients, southern California. *Emerg Infect Dis* **11:**1686–1692.

6. **Denton JF, Di Salvo AF.** 1968. The prevalence of *Cryptococcus neoformans* in various natural habitats. *Sabouraudia* **6:**213–217.

7. **Fromtling RA, Shadomy S, Shadomy HJ, Dismukes WE.** 1982. Serotype B/C *Cryptococcus neoformans* isolated from patients in nonendemic areas. *J Clin Microbiol* **16:**408–410.

8. **Bottone EJ, Kirschner PA, Salkin IF.** 1986. Isolation of highly encapsulated *Cryptococcus neoformans* serotype B from a patient in New York City. *J Clin Microbiol* **23:**186–188.

9. **Hoang LM, Maguire JA, Doyle P, Fyfe M, Roscoe DL.** 2004. *Cryptococcus neoformans* infections at Vancouver Hospital and Health Sciences Centre (1997–2002): epidemiology, microbiology and histopathology. *J Med Microbiol* **53:**935–940.

10. **Duncan C, Stephen C, Lester S, Bartlett KH.** 2005. Sub-clinical infection and asymptomatic carriage of *Cryptococcus gattii* in dogs and cats during an outbreak of cryptococcosis. *Med Mycol* **43:**511–516.

11. **Duncan C, Schwantje H, Stephen C, Campbell J, Bartlett K.** 2006. *Cryptococcus gattii* in wildlife of Vancouver Island, British Columbia, Canada. *J Wildl Dis* **42:**175–178.

12. **Kidd SE, Bach PJ, Hingston AO, Mak S, Chow Y, MacDougall L, Kronstad JW, Bartlett KH.** 2007. *Cryptococcus gattii* dispersal mechanisms, British Columbia, Canada. *Emerg Infect Dis* **13:**51–57.

13. **Kidd SE, Chow Y, Mak S, Bach PJ, Chen H, Hingston AO, Kronstad JW, Bartlett KH.** 2007. Characterization of environmental sources of the human and animal pathogen *Cryptococcus gattii* in British Columbia, Canada, and the Pacific Northwest of the United States. *Appl Environ Microbiol* **73:**1433–1443.

14. **MacDougall L, Kidd SE, Galanis E, Mak S, Leslie MJ, Cieslak PR, Kronstad JW, Morshed MG, Bartlett KH.** 2007. Spread of *Cryptococcus gattii* in British Columbia,

Canada, and detection in the Pacific Northwest, USA. *Emerg Infect Dis* **13**:42–50.

15. **MacDougall L, Fyfe M.** 2006. Emergence of *Cryptococcus gattii* in a novel environment provides clues to its incubation period. *J Clin Microbiol* **44**:1851–1852.

16. **Bartlett KH, Kidd SE, Kronstad JW.** 2008. The emergence of *Cryptococcus gattii* in British Columbia and the Pacific Northwest. *Curr Infect Dis Rep* **10**:58–65.

17. **Fraser JA, Giles SS, Wenink EC, Geunes-Boyer SG, Wright JR, Diezmann S, Allen A, Stajich JE, Dietrich FS, Perfect JR, Heitman J.** 2005. Same-sex mating and the origin of the Vancouver Island *Cryptococcus gattii* outbreak. *Nature* **437**:1360–1364.

18. **Kidd SE, Hagen F, Tscharke RL, Huynh M, Bartlett KH, Fyfe M, Macdougall L, Boekhout T, Kwon-Chung KJ, Meyer W.** 2004. A rare genotype of *Cryptococcus gattii* caused the cryptococcosis outbreak on Vancouver Island (British Columbia, Canada). *Proc Natl Acad Sci USA* **101**:17258–17263.

19. **Byrnes EJ III, Li W, Ren P, Lewit Y, Voelz K, Fraser JA, Dietrich FS, May RC, Chaturvedi S, Chaturvedi V, Heitman J.** 2011. A diverse population of *Cryptococcus gattii* molecular type VGIII in southern Californian HIV/AIDS patients. *PLoS Pathog* **7**:e1002205.

20. **Hagen F, Khayhan K, Theelen B, Kolecka A, Polacheck I, Sionov E, Falk R, Parnmen S, Lumbsch HT, Boekhout T.** 2015. Recognition of seven species in the *Cryptococcus gattii/Cryptococcus neoformans* species complex. *Fungal Genet Biol* **78**:16–48.

21. **Mak S, Klinkenberg B, Bartlett K, Fyfe M.** 2010. Ecological niche modeling of *Cryptococcus gattii* in British Columbia, Canada. *Environ Health Perspect* **118**:653–658.

22. **Upton A, Fraser JA, Kidd SE, Bretz C, Bartlett KH, Heitman J, Marr KA.** 2007. First contemporary case of human infection with *Cryptococcus gattii* in Puget Sound: evidence for spread of the Vancouver Island outbreak. *J Clin Microbiol* **45**:3086–3088.

23. **Iqbal N, DeBess EE, Wohrle R, Sun B, Nett RJ, Ahlquist AM, Chiller T, Lockhart SR, Cryptococcus gattii Public Health Working Group.** 2010. Correlation of genotype and in vitro susceptibilities of *Cryptococcus gattii* strains from the Pacific Northwest of the United States. *J Clin Microbiol* **48**:539–544.

24. **Lockhart SR, Iqbal N, Harris JR, Grossman NT, DeBess E, Wohrle R, Marsden-Haug N, Vugia DJ.** 2013. *Cryptococcus gattii* in the United States: genotypic diversity of human and veterinary isolates. *PLoS One* **8**:e74737.

25. **Byrnes EJ III, Li W, Lewit Y, Ma H, Voelz K, Ren P, Carter DA, Chaturvedi V, Bildfell RJ, May RC, Heitman J.** 2010. Emergence and pathogenicity of highly virulent *Cryptococcus gattii* genotypes in the northwest United States. *PLoS Pathog* **6**:e1000850.

26. **Byrnes EJ III, Bildfell RJ, Frank SA, Mitchell TG, Marr KA, Heitman J.** 2009. Molecular evidence that the range of the Vancouver Island outbreak of *Cryptococcus gattii* infection has expanded into the Pacific Northwest in the United States. *J Infect Dis* **199**:1081–1086.

27. **Engelthaler DM, Hicks ND, Gillece JD, Roe CC, Schupp JM, Driebe EM, Gilgado F, Carriconde F, Trilles L, Firacative C, Ngamskulrungroj P, Castañeda E, Lazera MS, Melhem MS, Pérez-Bercoff A, Huttley G, Sorrell TC, Voelz K, May RC, Fisher MC, Thompson GR III, Lockhart SR, Keim P, Meyer W.** 2014. *Cryptococcus gattii* in North American Pacific Northwest: whole-population genome analysis provides insights into species evolution and dispersal. *mBio* **5**:e01464-14.

28. **Ngamskulrungroj P, Serena C, Gilgado F, Malik R, Meyer W.** 2011. Global VGIIa isolates are of comparable virulence to the major fatal *Cryptococcus gattii* Vancouver Island outbreak genotype. *Clin Microbiol Infect* **17**:251–258.

29. **Kidd SE, Guo H, Bartlett KH, Xu J, Kronstad JW.** 2005. Comparative gene genealogies indicate that two clonal lineages of *Cryptococcus gattii* in British Columbia resemble strains from other geographical areas. *Eukaryot Cell* **4**:1629–1638.

30. **Billmyre RB, Croll D, Li W, Mieczkowski P, Carter DA, Cuomo CA, Kronstad JW, Heitman J.** 2014. Highly recombinant VGII *Cryptococcus gattii* population develops clonal outbreak clusters through both sexual macroevolution and asexual microevolution. *mBio* **5**:e01494-14.

31. **Hagen F, Ceresini PC, Polacheck I, Ma H, van Nieuwerburgh F, Gabaldón T, Kagan S, Pursall ER, Hoogveld HL, van Iersel LJ, Klau GW, Kelk SM, Stougie L, Bartlett KH, Voelz K, Pryszcz LP, Castañeda E, Lazera M, Meyer W, Deforce D, Meis JF, May RC, Klaassen CH, Boekhout T.** 2013. Ancient dispersal of the human fungal pathogen *Cryptococcus gattii* from the Amazon rainforest. *PLoS One* **8**:e71148.

32. **Kunadharaju R, Choe U, Harris JR, Lockhart SR, Greene JN.** 2013. *Cryptococcus gattii*, Florida, USA, 2011. *Emerg Infect Dis* **19**:519–521.

33. **Galanis E, Hoang L, Kibsey P, Morshed M, Phillips P.** 2009. Clinical presentation, diagnosis and management of *Cryptococcus gattii* cases: lessons learned from British Columbia. *Can J Infect Dis Med Microbiol* **20:**23–28.

34. **Harris JR, Lockhart SR, Debess E, Marsden-Haug N, Goldoft M, Wohrle R, Lee S, Smelser C, Park B, Chiller T.** 2011. *Cryptococcus gattii* in the United States: clinical aspects of infection with an emerging pathogen. *Clin Infect Dis* **53:**1188–1195.

35. **Harris JR, Lockhart SR, Sondermeyer G, Vugia DJ, Crist MB, D'Angelo MT, Sellers B, Franco-Paredes C, Makvandi M, Smelser C, Greene J, Stanek D, Signs K, Nett RJ, Chiller T, Park BJ.** 2013. *Cryptococcus gattii* infections in multiple states outside the US Pacific Northwest. *Emerg Infect Dis* **19:**1620–1626.

36. **Galanis E, Macdougall L, Kidd S, Morshed M, British Columbia Cryptococcus gattii Working Group.** 2010. Epidemiology of *Cryptococcus gattii*, British Columbia, Canada, 1999–2007. *Emerg Infect Dis* **16:**251–257.

37. **Farrer RA, Desjardins CA, Sakthikumar S, Gujja S, Saif S, Zeng Q, Chen Y, Voelz K, Heitman J, May RC, Fisher MC, Cuomo CA.** 2015. Genome evolution and innovation across the four major lineages of *Cryptococcus gattii*. *mBio* **6:**e00868-15.

38. **Fisher FS, Bultman MW, Johnson SM, Pappagianis D, Zaborsky E.** 2007. *Coccidioides* niches and habitat parameters in the southwestern United States: a matter of scale. *Ann NY Acad Sci* **1111:**47–72.

39. **Sun SH, Sekhon SS, Huppert M.** 1979. Electron microscopic studies of saprobic and parasitic forms of *Coccidioides immitis*. *Sabouraudia* **17:**265–273.

40. **Galgani JN.** 1993. Coccidioidomycosis. *West J Med* **159:**153–171.

41. **Einstein HE, Johnson RH.** 1993. Coccidioidomycosis: new aspects of epidemiology and therapy. *Clin Infect Dis* **16:**349–354.

42. **Smith CE, Beard RR, Rosenberger HG, Whiting EG.** 1946. Effect of season and dust control on coccidioidomycosis. *JAMA* **132:**833–838.

43. **Smith CE, Whiting EG, Baker EE, Rosenberger HG, Beard RR, Saito MT.** 1948. The use of coccidioidin. *Am Rev Tuberc* **57:**330–360.

44. **Smith CE, Beard RR.** 1946. Varieties of coccidioidal infection in relation to the epidemiology and control of the diseases. *Am J Public Health Nations Health* **36:**1394–1402.

45. **Smith CE, Beard RR, Saito MT.** 1948. Pathogenesis of coccidioidomycosis with special reference to pulmonary cavitation. *Ann Intern Med* **29:**623–655.

46. **Valdivia L, Nix D, Wright M, Lindberg E, Fagan T, Lieberman D, Stoffer T, Ampel NM, Galgiani JN.** 2006. Coccidioidomycosis as a common cause of community-acquired pneumonia. *Emerg Infect Dis* **12:**958–962.

47. **Kim MM, Blair JE, Carey EJ, Wu Q, Smilack JD.** 2009. Coccidioidal pneumonia, Phoenix, Arizona, USA, 2000–2004. *Emerg Infect Dis* **15:**397–401.

48. **Thompson GR III.** 2011. Pulmonary coccidioidomycosis. *Semin Respir Crit Care Med* **32:**754–763.

49. **Adam RD, Elliott SP, Taljanovic MS.** 2009. The spectrum and presentation of disseminated coccidioidomycosis. *Am J Med* **122:**770–777.

50. **Borchers AT, Gershwin ME.** 2010. The immune response in coccidioidomycosis. *Autoimmun Rev* **10:**94–102.

51. **Edwards PQ, Palmer CE.** 1957. Prevalence of sensitivity to coccidioidin, with special reference to specific and nonspecific reactions to coccidioidin and to histoplasmin. *Dis Chest* **31:**35–60.

52. **Loofbourow JC, Pappagianis D, Cooper TY.** 1969. Endemic coccidioidomycosis in Northern California. An outbreak in the Capay Valley of Yolo County. *Calif Med* **111:**5–9.

53. **Werner SB, Pappagianis D, Heindl I, Mickel A.** 1972. An epidemic of coccidioidomycosis among archeology students in northern California. *N Engl J Med* **286:**507–512.

54. **Petersen LR, Marshall SL, Barton-Dickson C, Hajjeh RA, Lindsley MD, Warnock DW, Panackal AA, Shaffer JB, Haddad MB, Fisher FS, Dennis DT, Morgan J.** 2004. Coccidioidomycosis among workers at an archeological site, northeastern Utah. *Emerg Infect Dis* **10:**637–642.

55. **Marsden-Haug N, Hill H, Litvintseva AP, Engelthaler DM, Driebe EM, Roe CC, Ralston C, Hurst S, Goldoft M, Gade L, Wohrle R, Thompson GR, Brandt ME, Chiller T, Centers for Disease Control and Prevention.** 2014. *Coccidioides immitis* identified in soil outside of its known range—Washington, 2013. *MMWR Morb Mortal Wkly Rep* **63:**450.

56. **Marsden-Haug N, Goldoft M, Ralston C, Limaye AP, Chua J, Hill H, Jecha L, Thompson GR III, Chiller T.** 2013. Coccidioidomycosis acquired in Washington State. *Clin Infect Dis* **56:**847–850.

57. **Litvintseva AP, Marsden-Haug N, Hurst S, Hill H, Gade L, Driebe EM, Ralston C, Roe C, Barker BM, Goldoft M, Keim P, Wohrle R, Thompson GR III, Engelthaler DM, Brandt ME, Chiller T.** 2015. Valley fever: finding

new places for an old disease: *Coccidioides immitis* found in Washington State soil associated with recent human infection. *Clin Infect Dis* **60:**e1–e3.

58. **CDC.** 2016. *Sources of valley fever (coccidioidomycosis).* CDC, Atlanta, GA. http://www.cdc.gov/fungal/diseases/coccidioidomycosis/causes.html. Accessed 6 March 2016.

The Emerging Amphibian Fungal Disease, Chytridiomycosis: A Key Example of the Global Phenomenon of Wildlife Emerging Infectious Diseases

21

JONATHAN E. KOLBY[1,2] and PETER DASZAK[2]

INTRODUCTION: GLOBAL AMPHIBIAN DECLINE

During the latter half of the 20th century, it was noticed that global amphibian populations had entered a state of unusually rapid decline. Hundreds of species have since become categorized as "missing" or "lost," a growing number of which are now believed extinct (1). Amphibians are often regarded as environmental indicator species because of their highly permeable skin and biphasic life cycles, during which most species inhabit aquatic zones as larvae and as adults become semi or wholly terrestrial. This means their overall health is closely tied to that of the landscape. Amphibian declines in recent decades are largely attributed to increases in habitat destruction, pollution, and commercial exploitation, but enigmatic declines and mass mortality events began to be observed in seemingly healthy environments, suggesting that an additional factor with considerable negative impact was also influencing declines (2, 3).

Discovery of *Batrachochytrium dendrobatidis*

In 1998, a mass mortality event occurred in a colony of poison-dart frogs (*Dendrobates* spp.) held in a collection at the National Zoo in Washington, DC.

[1]One Health Research Group, College of Public Health, Medical, and Veterinary Sciences, James Cook University, Townsville, Queensland, Australia; [2]EcoHealth Alliance, New York, NY 10001.

Emerging Infections 10
Edited by W. Michael Scheld, James M. Hughes and Richard J. Whitley
© 2016 American Society for Microbiology, Washington, DC
doi:10.1128/microbiolspec.EI10-0004-2015

During an autopsy, histological examination revealed an unusual fungal infection of the skin. The fungus was soon described as *B. dendrobatidis*, a previously unknown species of parasitic chytrid fungi with a particular appetite for amphibians (4). There are several hundred described species of chytrid fungi, most of which are important decomposers of nonliving organic material in the environment, such as pollen and rotting vegetation. A few exceptions infect living plant or animal cells, with *B. dendrobatidis* becoming the first known species to attack living vertebrate hosts.

Infection with *B. dendrobatidis* and Chytridiomycosis

B. dendrobatidis begins life as an aquatic uniflagellated zoospore released from a mature zoosporangia embedded in the skin of an amphibian (4, 5). *B. dendrobatidis* zoospores are commonly shed into the water, where they can swim short distances and/or are carried by water currents to reach a new host. Upon contact with an amphibian, *B. dendrobatidis* zoospores burrow several layers down into the skin, to the area where keratin is produced. These zoospores remain there, where they grow and mature into new zoosporangia. Through asexual reproduction, multiple new zoospores are produced within the zoosporangia and, when ready, are released from the amphibian's skin via discharge tubules. If the infected amphibian is in a terrestrial location when zoospores are released, they are likely to reinfect that animal and/or be shed onto vegetation or into soil. This growth cycle from zoospore to mature zoosporangium normally takes about five days at optimum temperatures and nutrient conditions.

Infection with *B. dendrobatidis* has various effects upon an amphibian, ranging from asymptomatic presence to the often lethal disease, chytridiomycosis (5). Low host-species specificity threatens potentially thousands of species with disease. As of 2013, 42% of

1,240 amphibian species tested were found to be infected (6). In amphibians susceptible to disease, the presence of *B. dendrobatidis* causes hyperkeratosis and interferes with normal shedding, damaging the animal's ability to osmoregulate and maintain electrolyte balance. In severe infections, this leads to death by cardiac arrest (7). Amphibians also sometimes manifest behavioral symptoms of disease such as lethargy, anorexia, and loss of righting reflex, but these are inconsistent and nonspecific to chytridiomycosis and thus cannot be used alone to confirm infection. The same applies to the presence of amphibian skin lesions sometimes caused by *B. dendrobatidis*. Consequently, diagnosis of chytridiomycosis is challenging and nearly impossible under field conditions. Thus, the presence of seemingly healthy amphibian populations is sometimes misleading. Dead amphibians are infrequently observed in the field despite sometimes high mortality rates (8), because they quickly decompose or become scavenged.

Chytrid Resistance in Nature

While some amphibians readily develop clinical symptoms of chytridiomycosis, others do not express illness. Certain species appear to possess a variable degree of innate resistance to *B. dendrobatidis* infection and/or disease. It is not yet fully understood what provides these species with a greater defense than most others, but it sometimes involves the presence of anti–*B. dendrobatidis* symbiotic bacteria in the skin and/or the amphibian's ability to produce certain skin antimicrobial peptides (9). These species can sometimes resist or clear *B. dendrobatidis* infection or persist with low-intensity infections. Unfortunately, some of these are species known to be invasive outside their native ranges, such as the American bullfrog (*Lithobates catesbeianus*) and African clawed frog (*Xenopus laevis*), and have established feral populations around the world (10). These species serve as asymptomatic *B. dendrobatidis* reservoir hosts that can transmit *B. dendrobatidis* infections to more susceptible species sharing a habitat. The presence of tolerant amphibians in a community of *B. dendrobatidis*–susceptible species can maintain pathogen presence even as vulnerable species decline and become locally extinct.

Detection of *B. dendrobatidis* Infection versus Disease

Distinction between *B. dendrobatidis* presence on a skin swab, *B. dendrobatidis* infection, and the disease chytridiomycosis must be made since these terms are sometimes used interchangeably, but each has a distinct meaning and denotes a different physical presence. The most widely accepted protocol to identify a *B. dendrobatidis*–infected amphibian is the collection of a skin swab sample together with a highly sensitive and specific quantitative PCR diagnostic test (11). This is effective because *B. dendrobatidis* grows within the amphibians' skin and frequently sheds zoospores back out to the skin surface, where swabbing the highly keratinized regions (i.e., pelvic patch and feet) is likely to collect *B. dendrobatidis* particles that are then identifiable by PCR. It is important to remember that PCR-positive skin swab results alone do not show the condition of infection or disease, but rather show the molecular presence of live or dead *B. dendrobatidis*. Since *B. dendrobatidis* particles are shed by infected animals into the environment, it is possible that some skin swabs test positive from contact with *B. dendrobatidis*–contaminated water droplets or soil on an amphibians' skin (12). Still, skin swabs are highly advantageous over traditional histological analysis in that they are noninvasive and sampling can be performed on rare and endangered species, whereas tissue extraction would be potentially harmful to the animals' well-being. Therefore, although PCR-positive results for *B. dendrobatidis* via skin swabs do not truly prove the animal is infected, researchers agree that this is a generally acceptable assumption since the amount of *B. dendrobatidis* detected on swabs can now be quantified and is often quite high compared to detection outside the host in environmental substrates. For absolute confirmation of infection, tissue sampling and histological examination are needed (13). The presence of *B. dendrobatidis* within the amphibian's skin does indicate infection, but unless there are also clinical signs of detriment to the surrounding tissues, it is possible to have *B. dendrobatidis* infection without the disease chytridiomycosis.

Sampling techniques are also now available to detect the presence of *B. dendrobatidis* in the environment, outside the host. Water samples can be collected and filtered to capture environmental DNA, which includes free-floating zoospores and/or *B. dendrobatidis*-infected animal cells shed into the water (14–16). This technique is useful both independently, to screen for areas of *B. dendrobatidis* presence where swabbing surveys are impossible to perform, or complementary to swabbing surveys to develop greater context for interpretation of the survey results. In either case, it should be noted that detection of *B. dendrobatidis* in water filter samples only proves pathogen presence at a location, and not the infection of amphibians at that location.

Effects of *B. dendrobatidis* on Amphibian Populations

The effect of *B. dendrobatidis* on amphibian populations generally varies by species and region, but population decline attributed to this pathogen has now been documented on every continent where amphibians are found (6). Although all 7,000+ species in the class *Amphibia* are potentially vulnerable to infection, *B. dendrobatidis* seems to cause disease most often in members of the order *Anura*, the frogs and toads. Not only is *B. dendrobatidis* capable of impacting a broad range of host species, but it is also believed to be the first wildlife pathogen to have caused widespread species extinctions (17, 18). In recent years, it has been blamed for the extinction of several Australian frogs, including the sharp-snouted day frog (*Taudactylus acutirostris*) (17), the Northern gastric brooding frog (*Rheobatrachus vitellinus*) (19), and the Southern gastric brooding frog (*Rheobatrachus silus*) (19). Although unconfirmed, it is also suspected to have driven extinction of the golden toad (*Incilius periglenes*) in Costa Rica, a formerly common species endemic to the cloud forest of Monteverde that mysteriously vanished in 1989 (20), around the time a wave of *B. dendrobatidis*–associated disease swept through Central America causing a wave of dramatic decline (21, 22). In Africa, it is believed that *B. dendrobatidis* together with habitat degradation catalyzed the precipitous decline of Tanzania's Kihansi spray toad (*Nectophrynoides asperginis*), declared extinct in the wild by 2009 (23). In the United States, chytridiomycosis has driven the loss of California's yellow-legged frogs (*Rana muscosa* and *Rana sierrae*) from 93% of their historical range over the past few decades (24) and the near-extinction of the endangered Wyoming toad (*Bufo baxteri*) (25).

It would be remiss to speak of amphibian extinctions without also mentioning that some species previously declared extinct have later been rediscovered. Some are suspected to have vanished due to *B. dendrobatidis*, while others disappeared for less certain reasons. Instances of the former include the miles robber frog (*Craugastor milesi*) of Honduras (26), the armored mistfrog (*Litoria lorica*) of Australia (27), and the Rancho Grande harlequin frog (*Atelopus cruciger*) of Venezuela (28). These previously common species were suddenly "lost" for approximately 20 years following the arrival of *B. dendrobatidis*. Each was declared extinct, and then rediscovered and now classified as critically endangered. Other species went missing for much longer, and from places where *B. dendrobatidis* was not suspected, such as the Hula painted frog (*Disco-glossus nigriventer*) from Israel (57 years) (29), the Bururi long-fingered frog (*Cardioglossa cyaneospila*) from Burundi (62 years) (30), and the starry shrub frog (*Pseudophilautus stellatus*) from Sri Lanka (160 years) (31). In some instances, the surviving populations are unsurprisingly found in regions or habitats not previously explored, but curiously, most have been close to where the last known sighting was recorded. Although this phenomenon provides hope that other lost species might not yet be extinct, these instances remain the minority. Judging from the population crashes observed in *B. dendrobatidis*'s wake as it has invaded new regions, and particularly Central America (21, 32, 33), it is reasonable to think that a greater number of missing amphibian species are likely extinct or on the verge.

Emerging Infectious Disease or Globally Endemic Pathogen?

The seemingly sudden emergence of *B. dendrobatidis* and its association with global amphibian declines generated uncertainty as to the origin of this pathogen and the reason for disease emergence. A rift within the scientific community developed, and two virtually opposite hypotheses to explain this phenomenon were postulated: (i) the globally endemic pathogen hypothesis and (ii) the emerging infectious disease hypothesis (18). Each conveyed a different reason for disease emergence with a distinct conservation and management undertone. In the former, *B. dendrobatidis* is assumed to have become globally dispersed in historic times, and its presence alone was not a threat to amphibians until recently, when some external influence "changed" *B. dendrobatidis* to become virulent. In this scenario, *B. dendrobatidis* was already everywhere, and something flicked a switch that allowed disease to suddenly emerge from a longstanding commensal relationship with amphibian hosts. The latter hypothesis assumed that the global distribution of *B. dendrobatidis* was heterogeneous and it was still actively spreading, driving a wave of disease as it progressed. Skerratt et al. (18) showed that greater evidence supported the emerging infectious disease hypothesis and advocated the importance of continued surveillance efforts to monitor *B. dendrobatidis*'s spread and for activities that predict and mitigate future biodiversity decline.

Global *B. dendrobatidis* Distribution

Even after 15 years of investigation, the global origin of *B. dendrobatidis* and timeline of emergence remain poorly understood (34). *B. dendrobatidis*'s presence has recently been reported from 52 of 82 countries sampled (6), and it continues to spread (Fig. 1). There remain many countries where sampling for *B. dendrobatidis*'s presence has been limited or not yet performed, and it remains unknown just how many regions have still evaded *B. dendrobatidis* exposure. Demonstrating the presence of *B. dendrobatidis* is relatively straightforward—a few PCR-positive field samples will generally suffice

—but proving the absence of *B. dendrobatidis* requires thousands of negative samples, and yet this still only suggests its absence. At present, only two countries have been systematically surveyed for nearly a decade without *B. dendrobatidis* confirmation: Hong Kong (35) and Madagascar (36).

Multiple *B. dendrobatidis* Strains

The true genetic diversity of *B. dendrobatidis* was not fully appreciated until nearly a decade following its initial discovery as a pathogen affecting amphibians. We now know that there exists a diversity of molecularly distinct *B. dendrobatidis* isolates, some of which seem to be associated with particular regions of the world, possibly due to periodic isolation and mutations (34, 37, 38,). Some isolates have been studied in depth and represent distinct "strains" that consistently vary from others by genotype, morphology, and virulence (34, 38, 39). Laboratory exposure experiments have shown that *B. dendrobatidis* strains from different geographic regions differ in virulence (5, 39–41)

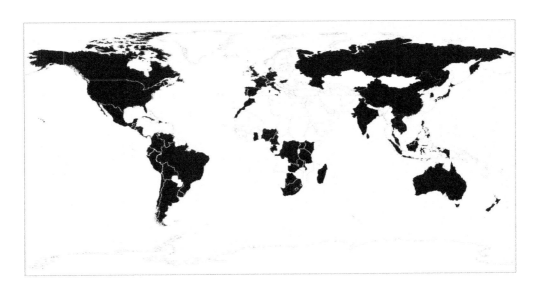

FIGURE 1 Detection of the amphibian chytrid fungus *Batrachochytrium dendrobatidis* as of August 2015, as reported in the literature. Black shading represents one or more confirmed detections of *B. dendrobatidis* illustrated at the country level and should be interpreted conservatively.

and that outcomes of exposure to *B. dendrobatidis* can be difficult to predict, especially without knowing the strain identity and characteristics. For example, exposure to *B. dendrobatidis* collected from Spain and the United Kingdom caused significantly greater mortality in European toad (*Bufo bufo*) tadpoles than did an isolate from Majorca; 37.5% survived Majorcan *B. dendrobatidis* exposure compared to only 7.5% and 2.5% for strains from Spain and the United Kingdom, respectively (39). Time until death following exposure to three Australian *B. dendrobatidis* strains also differed significantly; mean time until 100% mortality in juvenile *Litoria caerulea* varied between strains by nearly 19 days (5).

On a global scale, at least 49 genetically distinct isolates of *B. dendrobatidis* have been described that form five lineages (34). Of these lineages, the hypervirulent *B. dendrobatidis* GPL clade is the most broadly distributed strain identified to date, but diverse local isolates likely remain undetected and untested due to a sampling bias toward areas experiencing rapid amphibian declines (38, 42). The global distribution of each *B. dendrobatidis* strain has not yet been identified due to current limitations in diagnostic abilities. If visualized in greater detail —down to the strain level—the global distribution represented in Fig. 1 would likely be much more complex and dynamic, with dozens of overlapping and competing *B. dendrobatidis* boundaries.

Although *B. dendrobatidis* is a clonal organism, it is believed that sexual recombination may have occurred between two different strains to produce novel hybrid offspring (38, 43). This phenomenon has been proposed twice, first between two unidentified strains to produce the hypervirulent *B. dendrobatidis* GPL clade (38) and again between *B. dendrobatidis* GPL and a regionally endemic strain in Brazil (43). The contemporary human-assisted movement of *B. dendrobatidis*–infected amphibians creates numerous opportunities for native and for-

eign *B. dendrobatidis* isolates to cross historical boundaries, meet, and hybridize. This is of particular concern with respect to animals produced at frog-farming facilities, where groups of amphibians (most often American bullfrogs) are maintained in high densities. These artificially crowded environments provide elevated rates of pathogen transmission, and restocking to replace dead animals might remove a selection pressure that could have otherwise tempered virulence over time.

Global Origin of *B. dendrobatidis*: Initial Hypothesis

To identify the catalyst of this global amphibian disease event, it is important to map the expansion of *B. dendrobatidis*'s distribution over time. *B. dendrobatidis* is an ancient organism, (34), existing for thousands of years without apparent adverse effects. Thus, what sparked the relatively recent emergence of chytridiomycosis? Was it simply the expansion of *B. dendrobatidis*'s range into novel regions where naïve amphibian populations become exposed? Or was this just one factor among many that aligned to catalyze this phenomenon?

An "out of Africa: hypothesis for *B. dendrobatidis*'s origin and global dispersal was developed soon after its discovery, anchored on the detection of *B. dendrobatidis* in a South African specimen of *X. laevis* collected in 1938 (44). In 1935, the discovery of a rudimentary human pregnancy test that involved the use of live *X. laevis* sparked a notable export trade of these frogs to countries around the world, which continued for several decades (44). This species tolerates *B. dendrobatidis* infection without developing chytridiomycosis and is an invasive species outside of Africa, having established feral populations globally after escape or release. These factors, together with their export from Africa shortly preceding global disease emergence framed a compelling argument for Africa as the source of *B. dendrobatidis* and provided a plausible catalyst for this global disease event—the international wildlife trade. The previous paucity of *B. dendrobatidis* distribution records preceding the onset of significant amphibian trade strengthened the appearance that this activity "unlocked" *B. dendrobatidis* from its global origin, but correlation does not imply causation. Recent information now suggests that Africa might not have been the original global source of *B. dendrobatidis*.

Timeline of Emergence

Our ability to map the historic presence of *B. dendrobatidis* and develop a more accurate timeline of emergence is limited by the quality and quantity of amphibian material held in museum collections available for *B. dendrobatidis* sampling. Advances in diagnostic methods have recently allowed *B. dendrobatidis* sampling to be performed on samples collected long ago and now preserved in museum collections, no longer restricting detection to freshly collected samples (45–47). Retrospective surveillance

for the presence of *B. dendrobatidis* has now provided greater insight into its geographic history: it was present in the United States by 1888 (48), in Brazil in 1894 (49), Japan in 1902 (50), North Korea in 1911 (51), and Cameroon in 1933 (52) (Fig. 2). These records collectively show that *B. dendrobatidis*'s presence stretched across at least four continents prior to the 1938 *B. dendrobatidis*–positive detection in *X. laevis* from South Africa. Africa still might be the original source of *B. dendrobatidis*, but the best available data now show that it is equally plausible for the global origin to be North or South America, or even Asia (37, 50). Wherever the true origin lies, viable *B. dendrobatidis* must have successfully traversed oceans multiple times before the 20th century. This is an important amendment to make upon the earlier estimated timeline of *B. dendrobatidis* emergence compared to that of disease emergence. It is now apparent that *B. dendrobatidis* was already globally widespread much earlier than the first observed waves of disease, and this further illustrates that the spread of

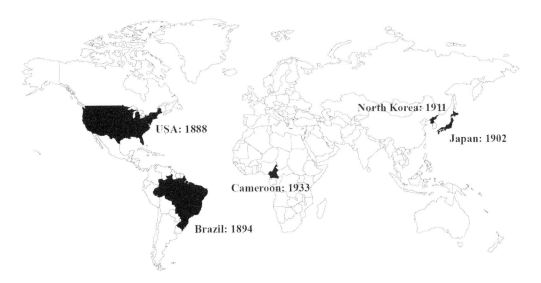

FIGURE 2 Minimum global distribution of amphibian chytrid fungus *Batrachochytrium dendrobatidis* pre-1935. The exportation of *Xenopus laevis* from Africa began in 1935, marking the emergence of the modern international amphibian trade. Black shading represents *B. dendrobatidis* detection in archived museum specimens. Shaded countries and year of *B. dendrobatidis* presence include United States (1888), Brazil (1894), Japan (1902), North Korea (1911), and Cameroon (1933).

B. dendrobatidis is not always associated with the spread of chytridiomycosis.

MODES OF *B. DENDROBATIDIS* DISPERSAL

While the global origin of *B. dendrobatidis* and timeline of emergence remain obscure, significant research effort has been devoted to understanding mechanisms of contemporary dispersal to identify potential *B. dendrobatidis* mitigation opportunities. The spread of *B. dendrobatidis* involves multiple simultaneous pathways, each varying in likelihood, quantity of pathogen transported, and expected consequence. These mechanisms can be generalized into three main categories: (i) anthropogenic-assisted spread, (ii) natural spread by wildlife, and (iii) natural spread by environmental forces.

Anthropogenic-Assisted Spread: International Amphibian Trade

Contemporary global spread of *B. dendrobatidis* is closely associated with international trade in millions of live amphibians annually, facilitating dispersal between countries and across oceans (43, 53–55). Notable global amphibian commerce first emerged around 1935, sparked by the development of a rudimentary human pregnancy test requiring the use of African clawed frogs (*X. laevis*). International trade in live amphibians escalated over the following decades, with animals becoming popularly traded as exotic pets, biomedical research subjects, and food sources (54, 55). Since highly traded species involve those identified as *B. dendrobatidis* reservoir hosts, it is not surprising that surveys of American bullfrogs (*L. catesbeianus*) imported to the United States have demonstrated *B. dendrobatidis* prevalence of 41 to 62% at markets sampled (43) and 70% in *X. laevis* upon importation for the pet trade (55).

Following importation, *B. dendrobatidis* may spill over into the wild and expose native amphibians, by either the accidental or intentional release of amphibians, and especially in instances where these animals survive and become established. This has been documented on numerous occasions with respect to American bullfrogs and African clawed frogs, both of which are considered invasive species and have developed feral populations both in the United States and globally (10). When invasive species invade new regions, they also bring their pathogens along for the ride and provide them with a greater chance to infect local wildlife than would a less adaptable and persistent host.

Additionally, the shipping materials used to transport or house *B. dendrobatidis*–positive amphibians are liable also to transmit infection to new animals if reused or spread *B. dendrobatidis* into the environment if disposed of untreated (56). These *B. dendrobatidis*–contaminated materials commonly include water or soil, cardboard or plastic boxes, and dead animals. If not treated properly to kill *B. dendrobatidis* prior to disposal, wastewater discarded into storm sewers can introduce pathogens directly into local waterways (57), and solid waste can provide new acute sources of transmission in terrestrial locations.

In recent decades the global trade in live amphibians has grown exponentially, and nearly 5 million live amphibians are now imported into the United States annually, all in the absence of required disease screening or quarantine measures. To remedy this situation, and in recognition of the emerging global disease concern, chytridiomycosis was listed as a notifiable disease by the World Organization for Animal Health (OIE) in 2009 (58). OIE notifiable listing requires its 174 member countries to conduct surveillance for *B. dendrobatidis* within in their borders, report confirmed cases, and implement measures to control its spread. Unfortunately, at the time of writing (August 2015), few if any countries have formally integrated these recommendations into legislation and are following this procedure.

Anthropogenic-Assisted Spread: International Trade (Nonamphibian)

The spread of *B. dendrobatidis* through international trade is not limited to the trade in amphibians. Contrary to conventional perception, *B. dendrobatidis* may be vectored by trade activities in the absence of amphibian hosts. In recent years, alternative nonamphibian *B. dendrobatidis* hosts have been identified, including crayfish (*Procambarus* spp. and *Orconectes virilis*) (59, 60) and the nematode worm *Caenorhabditis elegans* (61). Both crayfish and nematodes became infected following laboratory exposure to *B. dendrobatidis* and also suffered associated disease and mortality. Crayfish are traded live, both for direct consumption and for establishing new aquaculture farms, and the widespread soil-dwelling nematode worm *C. elegans* is likely to be transported within potting substrates spread by the international trade in ornamental plants. This is not meant to suggest that the "silent" dispersal of *B. dendrobatidis* by nonamphibian commerce is of greater concern, but rather demonstrates the complexity involved in tracking the spread of a pathogen now known to be capable of infecting three classes of organisms: *Amphibia*, *Malacostraca*, and *Chromadorea*.

Anthropogenic-Assisted Spread: Fomites

It has been suggested that *B. dendrobatidis* may be spread by people following exposure to affected regions, since the pathogen can survive for some time if protected from complete drying and elevated temperatures (56). Fomites, or nonliving objects that can carry pathogens, may be accidentally spread by human activities. The movement of *B. dendrobatidis*–contaminated footwear by researchers or eco-tourists represents a potentially common opportunity for the translocation of viable propagules between disconnected habitats. This dispersal pathway has not been formally evaluated, but

due to its likelihood, hygiene protocols have been provided to prevent the accidental spread of *B. dendrobatidis* after entering *B. dendrobatidis*–positive locations or performing high-risk activities (56, 62–64). In addition to footwear, *B. dendrobatidis* is also likely spread by other freshwater activity–related fomites, such as recreational boating (nondecontaminated boat hulls) and fishing (bait wastewater).

Nonanthropogenic-Assisted Spread: Dispersal by Wildlife

Within the natural environment and in the absence of human influence, *B. dendrobatidis* spreads through autonomous movement of infected animals. It can be transmitted to other nearby amphibians by direct skin–skin contact (65) during territorial exchanges or when engaged in amplexus—the mating embrace in which a male amphibian grasps a female with his front legs. Additionally, infected animals may carry *B. dendrobatidis* away from water and shed zoospores into the terrestrial environment, leaving a trail of *B. dendrobatidis* on vegetation often shared with other amphibian species (66). This phenomenon may partially explain enigmatic records of this aquatic pathogen in species of terrestrial amphibians that do not enter the water (67–69). It is also possible that the aforementioned crayfish carriers, some of which occasionally disperse over land during periods of heavy rain, may contribute toward the spread of *B. dendrobatidis* between separate water bodies. Aside from these local dispersal opportunities, longer-distance *B. dendrobatidis* spread may involve aerial transport on the feet of waterfowl (70) moving between wetlands.

Nonanthropogenic-Assisted Spread: Dispersal by Environmental Forces

Animals infected with *B. dendrobatidis* frequently shed zoospores into their environment (71, 72). If released into an aquatic habitat, zoospores can swim short distances and/or be carried to new locations by water currents (57). In addition, wind and rain are known to assist the spread of microbes, some of which are pathogenic to animals and plants (73, 74), and may also contribute toward the spread of *B. dendrobatidis*. Recently, *B. dendrobatidis* was detected in rainwater processed by filtration (75), although its viability could not be ascertained from molecular presence alone. Atmospheric and avian dispersal of *B. dendrobatidis* is unpredictable, but occasional viability following aerial transport could help explain *B. dendrobatidis*'s multiple successful transoceanic dispersal events prior to the first commercial cargo flights in the 1930s.

B. DENDROBATIDIS MITIGATION ATTEMPTS AND OPPORTUNITIES

At the time of writing (August 2015), the reason why *B. dendrobatidis* seems to have recently increased in virulence to catalyze this disease event remains unknown. Despite 15 years of investigation, this wildlife pandemic continues to progress largely unabated. There is currently no proven method to eradicate *B. dendrobatidis* from an affected habitat, nor have we been able to control its spread and protect new regions from exposure despite knowledge of an approaching wave of *B. dendrobatidis* and disease. In captivity, there are some options to cure infected amphibians, but there is not yet a single cure-all treatment that can be safely applied to all species. It is becoming increasingly evident that a "silver bullet" solution to stem the tide of *B. dendrobatidis*–driven amphibian declines and extinctions does not exist, despite remarkable efforts. More realistically, the application of multiple case-specific activities may provide the necessary "silver buckshot" solution to prevent amphibian extinctions, although resources are limited with respect to the diversity of species potentially vulnerable to chytridiomycosis.

Government Intervention to Mitigate *B. dendrobatidis* Spread

Although *B. dendrobatidis* spreads through a variety of pathways, it is unquestionable that the international trade in live amphibians is spreading a considerable amount of this pathogen and is contributing toward global amphibian declines and extinctions. In 2009, Defenders of Wildlife submitted a petition to the U.S. Fish and Wildlife Service (USFWS) proposing that all live amphibians be listed as injurious species under the Lacey Act and thus be prohibited from trade into and within the United States, except for specimens proven to be free of *B. dendrobatidis* (76). It is currently impossible to eradicate *B. dendrobatidis* following establishment, so preventing importation of foreign *B. dendrobatidis* strains that may express greater virulence to native amphibians should be considered a high conservation priority. Although expressed as a matter of urgency nearly 6 years ago, the USFWS has yet to announce whether regulations will be proposed to address this concern. Meanwhile, trade continues unabated and continues to introduce *B. dendrobatidis* (55). Similar extended delays between listing petitions and listing actions are not uncommon. Due to cumbersome risk assessment and review processes, most injurious species listings by USFWS have proceeded slowly and failed to prevent establishment of harmful organisms (77–78).

Mitigation of *B. dendrobatidis*'s Impact

Efforts to mitigate the impact of *B. dendrobatidis* can generally be divided into one of two categories: those targeting the reduction of *B. dendrobatidis* on amphibian hosts and those that strive to remove *B. dendrobatidis* from affected habitats. While treatment of infected amphibians is an immediate challenge for highly vulnerable species collected from the wild or already held in captivity, the continued spread of *B. dendrobatidis* in the wild is shrinking the amount of safe amphibian habitat and jeopardizing long-term successful population recovery. Therefore, while efforts to develop captive assurance populations of amphibians facing immediate risks of extinction have been fairly successful, reintroduction attempts have been minimal because contaminated natural habitats continue to be problematic. Effective methods to mitigate *B. dendrobatidis* both on amphibians and in their habitats are needed to protect amphibian biodiversity. An effective *B. dendrobatidis* mitigation program will likely require multiple complementary actions and be case-specific. Fortunately, complete eradication or removal of *B. dendrobatidis* may not be necessary to control disease, because a significant reduction in pathogen abundance might be enough to tip the scale in favor of amphibian survival.

Amphibian: antifungal chemotherapy

An antifungal itraconazole bath has been implemented as a common treatment for infection with *B. dendrobatidis* in amphibians held in captivity. The itraconazole treatment solution (0.01%) applied for 5 minutes once daily for 10 consecutive days can produce a dramatic or complete reduction in *B. dendrobatidis* infection load. Unfortunately, this treatment is toxic to some species and especially to larval life stages (79). Recently, this protocol has been experimentally tested at a much lower dosage concentration (0.0025% versus 0.01%) and for fewer days (6 versus 10) and still found to be effective, but with fewer instances of negative side effects (80). Nikkomycin Z is another antifungal agent also found to be effective against *B. dendrobatidis*, but exposure dosages necessary to mitigate *B. dendrobatidis* might also reduce the survival of amphibians (81). Anti–*B. dendrobatidis* chemotherapeutics are not restricted to antifungals; antibiotics such as chloramphenicol have also been effective in some circumstances (82), although its exposure has been associated with bone marrow suppression and aplastic anemia in cats and human beings, and it requires treatment lasting 2 to 4 weeks, which terres-

trial amphibians might not be able to tolerate (79). Given the various disadvantages associated with all currently described *B. dendrobatidis* treatment methods, itraconazole remains the most widely applied and successful treatment. However, Woodhams et al. (9) expressed concern that its wide use might encourage *B. dendrobatidis* to develop resistance to itraconazole over time.

Amphibian: temperature and desiccation

Since antifungal chemotherapies can produce harmful side effects in certain species and life stages, there has been interest in seeking nonchemotherapeutic treatment to aid survival of infected amphibians. It has long been known that *B. dendrobatidis* is vulnerable to elevated temperatures and desiccation. Extended continuous exposure to temperatures of at least 27°C and above, for varying amounts of time, has cleared *B. dendrobatidis* infection on frogs in captivity (83, 84). While this treatment is relatively cost-effective and easy to provide, its effectiveness varies by species. Many amphibians are adapted to cool environments, and the elevated temperatures necessary to kill *B. dendrobatidis* may likewise harm or kill the infected animals. Recent work also explored manipulation of humidity as another potential mode of controlling *B. dendrobatidis* on infected frogs, since complete drying kills *B. dendrobatidis*. Unfortunately, the experiments found that a drying regime provided to the southern corroboree frog (*Pseudophryne corroboree*) neither increased survival nor reduced infection loads (85). Similar to the species-specific variable effectiveness of heat treatment, it remains plausible that other species tested might likewise respond differently if exposed to reduced levels of humidity. Therefore, heat treatment remains the only proven nonchemotherapeutic treatment for *B. dendrobatidis* infection, but it is limited to heat-tolerant species.

Amphibian: vaccination

Infection with *B. dendrobatidis* suppresses the immune response of most amphibian hosts, except for the minority of experimentally tested species that possess a measurable degree of innate resistance. For the less-fortunate majority of species, methods to abate disease outside of captivity are urgently needed to assist survival of wild animals living in *B. dendrobatidis*–established habitats. Two major attempts to investigate whether amphibians can acquire resistance through vaccination have met with mixed results. One study performed in Australia found that vaccination in the form of prior *B. dendrobatidis* infection, treatment with itraconazole to clear the infection, and then re-exposure had no effect on survival or infection intensities in booroolong frogs (*Litoria booroolongensis*) (86). Meanwhile, a study in the United States exposed Cuban tree frogs to *B. dendrobatidis*, treated them with heat to clear infections, and observed a 20% increase in frog survival over the next five months (87). The latter study provided hope that an effective vaccination-type treatment might someday be developed, but it appears that pre-exposure to *B. dendrobatidis* does not alone trigger enough of an adaptive immune response to protect populations from infection in the wild. Still, like the species-specific variable responses to itraconazole and heat treatment, it is also likely that vaccination might elicit a greater adaptive immune response in some species than others.

Amphibian: probiotics
A diversity of microorganisms inhabit the layer of mucus coating an amphibian's skin, many of which are bacteria. The species composition of these bacterial communities varies between amphibian species and sometimes includes symbiotic bacteria that possess anti–*B. dendrobatidis* properties. When isolated and cultured, these "anti–*B. dendrobatidis*" bacteria can inhibit the growth of *B. dendrobatidis* in the laboratory. The most well-studied bacterial species with such properties is *Janthinobacterium lividum*, which is isolated from the red-backed salamander (*Plethodon cinereus*) (88, 89). The exact mechanism by which *B. dendrobatidis* is inhibited remains unknown but likely involves the production of fungicidal compounds that either interrupt *B. dendrobatidis* reproduction or directly kill *B. dendrobatidis*. Efforts are underway to isolate and culture this and additional bacterial species found to demonstrate similar properties for eventual application as a probiotic treatment. Such treatment would involve a bacterial bath to provide bioaugmentation to amphibian species not normally colonized by anti–*B. dendrobatidis* bacteria or those that carry low levels insufficient to manifest *B. dendrobatidis* resistance. This treatment was tested on the mountain yellow-legged frog (*R. muscosa*), a species that is highly susceptible to chytridiomycosis, and reduced mortality was observed (89). Probiotic treatment does appear to provide susceptible amphibians with some additional defense against disease, but it remains unknown how long these bacteria will continue to remain on the skin of "new" amphibian species. The duration of bacterial persistence will dictate how long amphibians will retain boosted resistance to *B. dendrobatidis*, and this remains to be investigated over the long term in wild frog populations under natural conditions.

Amphibian: selective breeding for disease resistance
In circumstances where amphibian species are threatened with extinction in the wild due to *B. dendrobatidis*, animals are sometimes collected and brought into captivity to establish captive assurance populations. The end goal of these efforts is to breed animals and eventually reintroduce their offspring back into the wild to supplement the remaining dwindling populations. Although several such breeding operations are in progress, few have reintroduced animals due to the challenges posed by the presence of only *B. dendrobatidis*–contaminated habitats within a species' range. The incorporation of selective breeding into these

operations, or assisted evolution, is one possible method that might reduce the risk of disease to animals placed back into an affected habitat. While no attempts to selectively breed amphibians for resistance to *B. dendrobatidis* have been reported in the literature, preliminary evidence from field experiments does suggest this might be possible. In field reintroduction and mark-recapture surveys of the alpine tree frog (*Litoria verreauxii alpina*) in Australia, it was recently observed that susceptibility to chytridiomycosis varied significantly among clutches of offspring, despite being a highly susceptible species (90). Although this represents a potential long-term solution for some species, it remains unknown whether the genetic traits that provide *B. dendrobatidis* resistance can be identified, selected for, and consistently inherited by the offspring.

Habitat-Level Mitigation: Eradication versus Management

Eradication of a newly introduced pathogen is desirable to halt an epidemic and prevent pathogen establishment in a new location. Unfortunately, this has not yet been considered feasible with respect to *B. dendrobatidis*. By the time *B. dendrobatidis* was discovered in 1999, it had already spread to dozens of countries. The global reach of *B. dendrobatidis* soon became apparent, and focus shifted toward identifying ways to abate *B. dendrobatidis* abundance and mitigate the impact of its presence in amphibian habitats rather than eradicate the pathogen entirely.

Habitat: site-level treatment

Although *B. dendrobatidis* eradication has not been approached as a primary management target, it does warrant mention. There are still regions that might not have been exposed to *B. dendrobatidis*, where early intervention to prevent establishment may be possible to protect the area's amphibians. Few concerted efforts to abolish *B. dendro-*

batidis from a location have been seriously considered, and fewer still have been attempted in the natural environment. While antifungal compounds can be introduced to a water body in an effort to kill *B. dendrobatidis* (91), none are specific to *B. dendrobatidis* and thus will cause unintended damage to additional aquatic life, the scope of which is unknown and difficult to predict. Therefore, site-level chemical treatment is not generally embraced as a viable option for *B. dendrobatidis* eradication.

In lieu of chemical application, other more dramatic eradication attempts could include the drainage of entire wetland systems to fight *B. dendrobatidis* with desiccation. Although this may seem extreme, it is often employed to control mosquito vectors of human disease and might likewise be effective to combat *B. dendrobatidis* (9). Pond-level drainage was performed on *B. dendrobatidis*–infected populations of the Majorcan midwife toad (*Alytes muletensis*) inhabiting livestock water cisterns in Europe (92). All tadpoles were removed, held in a laboratory where they were treated with itraconazole to clear *B. dendrobatidis* infections, and the cisterns were completely drained and allowed to dry. When the cisterns naturally filled again with rainwater the following season, the *B. dendrobatidis*–negative tadpoles were reintroduced. Unfortunately, soon after reintroduction, *B. dendrobatidis* reappeared in these animals, demonstrating the importance of our ability to predict and mitigate *B. dendrobatidis* dispersal pathways, which still remain relatively poorly understood.

Another complicating factor in any possible attempt to eradicate *B. dendrobatidis* is a lack of understanding about precisely where it occurs when outside the amphibian host. While we know that *B. dendrobatidis* zoospores are shed into the water, it is uncertain where they are most commonly found: do they remain near the surface of the water column exposed to a potential chemical or physical treatment, or do they settle to the bottom where they may become embedded in mud or layers of dead vegetation, largely shielded from assault? The reality likely straddles both, which would jeopardize the chances for success of any eradication attempt.

Although rapid response and eradication of *B. dendrobatidis* from a newly invaded location has never been attempted, the recent discovery of *B. dendrobatidis* in Madagascar (93–95) might warrant such action. Following nearly a decade of surveillance with only negative detection, *B. dendrobatidis* was detected in amphibians exported to the U.S. pet trade and shortly thereafter in wild amphibian populations within the country. A true eradication effort would require swift and decisive action as quickly as possible following the arrival of *B. dendrobatidis*. Although additional research is needed to identify which strain of *B. dendrobatidis* is present and whether or not it threatens Malagasy amphibians, eradication might still be feasible, if justified, although the window of opportunity is now shrinking.

Habitat: biological control

Although it is a formidable predator with respect to amphibians, *B. dendrobatidis* itself becomes subject to predation and competition for resources with other aquatic organisms when present outside the host. *Daphnia* and other freshwater zooplankton that graze on organisms in the water column may consume *B. dendrobatidis* zoospores and reduce pathogen density (96). In laboratory experiments, predation by *Daphnia* reduced the number of zoospores present in the water sample. In turn, exposure to this water then resulted in a lower rate of *B. dendrobatidis* transmission to tadpoles versus that in which *Daphnia* had not been introduced. Also, the presence and amount of algae in the water containing *B. dendrobatidis* sometimes reduced its abundance, perhaps due to competition for resources if *B. dendrobatidis* was acting as a saprobe by feeding on nonliving organic matter. Therefore, manipulation of the zooplankton community in a contami-

nated habitat might help mitigate the impact of *B. dendrobatidis* on amphibians. Despite these laboratory results, however, it is uncertain whether similar phenomena would occur in the natural environment and whether the abundance of zooplankton could be manipulated on such a grand scale as to yield the desired effect.

Habitat: physical modification

Many factors affect the presence and survival of *B. dendrobatidis* at a particular location, but temperature and moisture are especially important. Scheele at al. (97) described potential methods of *in situ B. dendrobatidis* mitigation by manipulating habitat structure to modify microclimates; for instance, by selectively pruning vegetation to control for the amount of direct sunlight exposure, it might be possible to push temperatures of amphibian basking sites and standing bodies of water slightly beyond conditions optimal for *B. dendrobatidis* growth. Since *B. dendrobatidis* can survive extended exposure to neither elevated temperatures nor drying, this manner of intervention may provide a way to reduce *B. dendrobatidis* densities in natural habitats. By mitigating the presence of *B. dendrobatidis*, this could then help assist an amphibian's own immune response by reducing pathogen burden. This would also help reduce the likelihood of *B. dendrobatidis* survival on the surface of riparian vegetation where infected amphibians shed zoospores as they emerge from the water (66).

A recent field study in Queensland, Australia, found that severe tropical cyclone Yasi reduced *B. dendrobatidis* infection risk at sites that suffered considerable habitat disturbance (98). This cyclone damaged the forest structure at some locations where powerful winds snapped trees and stripped foliage, reducing the canopy cover at certain stream habitats, some of which were part of a long-term *B. dendrobatidis* infection survey. Comparing damaged versus primarily intact survey sites, the amount of canopy cover was inversely related to both temperature and evaporative water loss, suggesting that amphibians at disturbed locations were exposed to conditions less favorable to *B. dendrobatidis* survival than at intact sites, where temperatures remained lower and greater humidity persisted. Accordingly, endangered rainforest frogs (*Litoria rheocola*) sampled at these disturbed sites demonstrated significantly lower risk of *B. dendrobatidis* infection than those at intact sites with greater moisture retention and lower temperatures. These data are encouraging because they suggest that *B. dendrobatidis* management via habitat modification may help reduce pathogen burden at some locations (97, 98).

REMAINING QUESTIONS

Despite past and present efforts, certain aspects of *B. dendrobatidis* ecology and chytridiomycosis remain enigmatic and challenge our ability to effectively mitigate the impact of disease. Although framed within the context of *B. dendrobatidis*, the essence of these questions and uncertainties is equally relevant to any wildlife emerging infectious disease that we have not yet been able to control. These lingering questions include but are not limited to:

- **Persistence of *B. dendrobatidis* outside the host.** *B. dendrobatidis* zoospores are frequently shed from an infected host into the environment, but how long do these zoospores typically survive? Few published studies are available for reference: one found that *B. dendrobatidis* generally became inactive after 48 h in distilled water (99); another detected the presence of infectious zoospores for 7 weeks in autoclaved pond water (100), and a third detected *B. dendrobatidis* survival for three months in sterile, moist river sand without the addition of nutrients (57).
- **Virulence of different *B. dendrobatidis* strains.** What causes certain strains of *B. dendrobatidis* to express greater virulence than others?
- **Variable innate resistance to *B. dendrobatidis* and disease.** Why do some frogs (within a species) tolerate *B. dendrobatidis* infection while others succumb?
- **Long-term global presence but recent emergence of disease.** *B. dendrobatidis* has been spreading globally for over 100 years, so why does chytridiomycosis appear to be a novel phenomenon?
- **History of emergence.** Where did *B. dendrobatidis* originate, and when did it first emerge?
- **Abundance and diversity of nonpathogenic *B. dendrobatidis* strains.** What proportion of *B. dendrobatidis* strains are pathogenic, or does each express virulence when placed in a certain context of exposure (amphibian species exposed, dose of *B. dendrobatidis* inoculum, environmental influences, etc.)?
- **Host spectrum.** Is *B. dendrobatidis* correctly referred to as an amphibian pathogen, or does it affect yet additional classes of organisms?

ADDITIONAL EMERGING INFECTIOUS DISEASES OF WILDLIFE

Although *B. dendrobatidis* is the first emerging infectious disease of wildlife to become pandemic, it will certainly not be the last. The pace of globalization is racing ahead more quickly than our ability to discover and prevent the spread of diseases, and especially those affecting wildlife. Over the past decade, several additional disease events have emerged in the United States that are also now causing dramatic uncontrollable declines in wildlife populations. This includes bat white nose syndrome, spread by the fungus *Pseudogymnoascus destructans*, which infects skin of the muzzle, ears, and wings of hibernating bats. White nose syndrome has caused sudden and widespread mortality, precipitating the death of millions of bats in recent years (101), which has been said to be analogous to chytridiomycosis for amphibians. More recently, the emergence of snake fungal disease has been described, spread by the fungus *Ophidiomyces ophiodiicola*, which infects the skin and causes high rates of mortality and is said to be analogous to bat white nose syndrome in many respects (102). Like *B. dendrobatidis*, it remains uncertain what catalyzed the emergence of these disease events, although the international movement of pathogen-contaminated material is suspected, whether by the trade in live animals or fomites. It is reasonable to assume that additional wildlife pathogens not yet described are already circulating within the international wildlife trade and spillover events may have occurred without our knowledge. The accelerated global spread of *B. dendrobatidis* by the international wildlife trade proceeded unabated for decades before a series of obvious mortality events led to the discovery of *B. dendrobatidis* existed and that our actions had been facilitating a pandemic.

SALAMANDER CHYTRID FUNGUS: THE NEXT AMPHIBIAN "PLAGUE"?

The recent near-extinction of fire salamanders (*Salamandra salamandra*) in The Netherlands led to a surprising and alarming discovery—that a second species of amphibian chytrid fungus exists which specifically attacks salamanders, and it is soon expected to ignite a wave of salamander extinctions in the United States unless immediate intervention occurs (103, 104). This species of "salamander-eating" chytrid fungus (*Batrachochytrium salamandrivorans*) is believed to have originated in Asia, where it appears to have existed for nearly 30 million years until the exportation of infected salamanders by the pet trade recently introduced this pathogen to Europe (104, 105).

Like *B. dendrobatidis*, *B. salamandrivorans* is easily transmitted through skin contact with infected salamanders or by exposure to contaminated materials, such as water, soil, and shipping containers (104). A disease outbreak in The Netherlands resulted in the near extirpation of fire salamanders, which raised the alarm and led to the discovery of this pathogen (103). Initially unaware of the true cause of this mortality phenomenon and then unprepared to quickly mitigate this novel disease event, European scientists already report *B. salamandrivorans* to be spreading uncontrollably in Western Europe, where it has recently been detected in The Netherlands, Belgium, and the United Kingdom (103–105).

Fortunately, recent surveys in the United States have not yet detected the presence of *B. salamandrivorans* (104), but with the importation of nearly 200,000 salamanders from Asia annually (USFWS amphibian import records provided to J. Kolby) and without any required disease screening, an outbreak in the United States similar to that in The Netherlands appears inevitable. Although *B. salamandrivorans*–infected salamanders have not yet been detected in the wild in the United States, it is likely that *B. salamandrivorans*–infected salamanders have been and continue to be imported from Asia. It is now only a matter of time before spillover occurs, precipitating a disease-driven decline in forest biomass and species diversity.

This is the first time advance warning of an impending wildlife disease outbreak in the United States existed prior to discovery of the pathogen within the country. The recent near-extinction of fire salamanders in The Netherlands caused by *B. salamandrivorans* exposure from Asian salamanders in the pet trade has provided a clear call to arms. A rapid proactive response is necessary to prevent similar salamander declines in the United States, the "salamander capital of the world." Research shows that *B. salamandrivorans* is highly lethal to North American salamanders, including the eastern newt (*Notophthalmus viridescens*), striped newt (*Notophthalmus perstriatus*), black-spotted newt (*Notophthalmus meridionalis*), rough skinned newt (*Taricha granulosa*), red-bellied newt (*Taricha rivularis*), and California newt (*Taricha torosa*), and likely additional species not yet tested in the laboratory (106). The USFWS is currently considering regulatory actions to mitigate the spread of *B. salamandrivorans* through the trade in salamanders and is expected to announce their approach in the coming months.

CONCLUSIONS

Scientists first became aware of *B. dendrobatidis* nearly 15 years ago, a fungal pathogen associated with global frog declines, mass mortality events, and extinctions (3, 18). Nearly a decade of exhaustive research to find a silver bullet solution and gain control over this pandemic has been largely unsuccessful (9), leaving the long-term survival of thousands of species in jeopardy. While many questions still surround this disease event, the most straightforward explanation for the apparent recent global emergence of chytridiomycosis is that of pathogen pollution driven by rapid globalization in the absence of wildlife health screening and regulatory intervention. Since the protection of global biodiversity is often valued below that of human and agricultural health, mitigation of wildlife disease is rarely viewed as a national priority unless it is closely linked to short-term economic consequences of inaction. The slow global response to the emergence of *B. dendrobatidis* and the absence of a coordinated international mitigation attempt helped to facilitate the continued spread of this pathogen to dozens of countries and hundreds of amphibian species worldwide.

Legislative barriers continue to provide an impediment to mounting a rapid response to emerging wildlife diseases in the United States, one of the greatest consumers of the international wildlife trade. The majority of laws and regulations administered by the USFWS to regulate the international wildlife trade were developed long before pathogen pollution and the threat of wildlife disease was realized, and thus the legislative toolbox available to intervene in such events is virtually empty. The only potentially applicable existing legislation is the Lacey Act, under which authority a species may be banned from importation and interstate transport if listed as injurious, but this act only allows species of mammals, birds, fish, amphibians, reptiles, mollusks, and crustacea to be considered for listing. This language excludes authority for the listing of microorganisms such as pathogens. Although the animal vector of a pathogen can potentially be listed as injurious as a way to work around this policy gap, this has only ever been approved once, to protect salmonid fish from the importation of fish diseases (18 U. S.C. 42: 50 CFR §16.13).

The relative lack of interest and concern in responding to emerging wildlife diseases is problematic and threatens not only animals, but also human health (107). The majority of recent emerging infectious diseases affecting humans were in fact zoonotic, at an earlier point only affecting wildlife. Some examples include hantavirus in rodents and Marburg and Ebola viruses in nonhuman primates. In a world of rapidly increasing globalization, human and animal health are becoming increasingly connected as wildlife habitats shrink, human–wildlife contact increases, and global commerce carries pathogens past historical boundaries. Therefore, while the investment of greater resources toward mitigation and prevention of wildlife disease events may appear to benefit only wildlife health, it actually contributes toward the longer-term protection of environmental and human health. Despite current and future amphibian declines as a result of chytridiomycosis, there remains much to learn from this disease event. As a case study, *B. dendrobatidis* can offer insight into how to better address the next wildlife disease event that emerges, hopefully more rapidly and with greater international coordination.

CITATION

Kolby JE, Daszak P. 2016. The emerging amphibian fungal disease, chytridiomycosis: a key example of the global phenomenon of wildlife emerging infectious diseases. Microbiol Spectrum 4(3):EI10-0004-2015.

REFERENCES

1. **Stuart SN, Chanson JS, Cox NA, Young BE, Rodrigues AS, Fischman DL, Waller RW.** 2004. Status and trends of amphibian declines and extinctions worldwide. *Science* **306**:1783–1786.

2. **Laurance WF, McDonald KR, Speare R.** 1996. Epidemic disease and the catastrophic decline of Australian rainforest frogs. *Conserv Biol* **10**:406–413.

3. **Berger L, Speare R, Daszak P, Green DE, Cunningham AA, Goggin CL, Slocombe R, Ragan MA, Hyatt AD, McDonald KR, Hines HB, Lips KR, Marantelli G, Parkes H.** 1998. Chytridiomycosis causes amphibian mortality associated with population declines in the rain forests of Australia and Central America. *Proc Natl Acad Sci USA* **95**:9031–9036.

4. **Longcore JE, Pessier AP, Nichols DK.** 1999. *Batrachochytrium dendrobatidis* gen et *sp nov*, a chytrid pathogenic to amphibians. *Mycologia* **91**:219–227.

5. **Berger L, Marantelli G, Skerratt LF, Speare R.** 2005. Virulence of the amphibian chytrid fungus *Batrachochytium dendrobatidis* varies with the strain. *Dis Aquat Organ* **68**:47–50.

6. **Olson DH, Aanensen DM, Ronnenberg KL, Powell CI, Walker SF, Bielby J, Garner TWJ, Weaver G, Fisher MC, Bd Mapping Group.** 2013. Mapping the global emergence of *Batrachochytrium dendrobatidis*, the amphibian chytrid fungus. *PLoS One* **8**:e56802. doi:10.1371/journal.pone.0056802.

7. **Voyles J, Young S, Berger L, Campbell C, Voyles WF, Dinudom A, Cook D, Webb R, Alford RA, Skerratt LF, Speare R.** 2009. Pathogenesis of chytridiomycosis, a cause of catastrophic amphibian declines. *Science* **326**:582–585.

8. **Scheele BC, Hunter DA, Skerratt LF, Brannelly LA, Driscoll DA.** 2015. Low impact of chytridiomycosis on frog recruitment enables persistence in refuges despite high adult mortality. *Biol Conserv* **182**:36–43.

9. **Woodhams DC, Bosch J, Briggs CJ, Cashins S, Davis LR, Lauer A, Muths E, Puschendorf R, Schmidt BR, Sheafor B, Voyles J.** 2011. Mitigating amphibian disease: strategies to maintain wild populations and control chytridiomycosis. *Front Zool* **8**:8.

10. **Kraus F.** 2009. Alien reptiles and amphibians: a scientific compendium and analysis. Springer Science and Business Media B.V., Dordrecht, The Netherlands.

11. **Hyatt AD, Boyle DG, Olsen V, Boyle DB, Berger L, Obendorf D, Dalton A, Kriger K, Heros M, Hines H, Phillott R, Campbell R, Marantelli G, Gleason F, Coiling A.** 2007. Diagnostic assays and sampling protocols for the detection of *Batrachochytrium dendrobatidis*. *Dis Aquat Organ* **73**:175–192.

12. **Kriger KM, Ashton KJ, Hines HB, Hero JM.** 2007. On the biological relevance of a single *Batrachochytrium dendrobatidis* zoospore: a reply to Smith. *Dis Aquat Organ* **73**:257–260.

13. **Skerratt LF, Mende D, McDonald KR, Garland S, Livingstone J, Berger L, Speare R.** Validation of diagnostic tests in wildlife: the case of chytridiomycosis in wild amphibians. *J Herpetol* **45**:444–450.

14. **Kirshtein JD, Anderson CW, Wood JS, Longcore JE, Voytek MA.** 2007. Quantitative PCR detection of *Batrachochytrium dendrobatidis* DNA from sediments and water. *Dis Aquat Organ* **77**:11–15.

15. **Walker SF, Salas MB, Jenkins D, Garner TW, Cunningham AA, Hyatt AD, Bosch J, Fisher MC.** 2007. Environmental detection of *Batrachochytrium dendrobatidis* in a temperate climate. *Dis Aquat Organ* **77**:105–112.

16. **Chestnut T, Anderson C, Popa R, Blaustein AR, Voytek M, Olson DH, Kirshtein J.** 2014. Heterogeneous occupancy and density estimates of the pathogenic fungus *Batrachochytrium dendrobatidis* in waters of North America. *PLoS One* **9**:e106790. doi:10.1371/journal.pone.0106790.

17. **Schloegel LM, Hero JM, Berger L, Speare R, McDonald K, Daszak P.** 2006. The decline of the sharp-snouted day frog (*Taudactylus acutirostris*): the first documented case of extinction by infection in a free-ranging wildlife species? *J Herpetol* **3**:35–40.

18. **Skerratt L, Berger L, Speare R, Cashins S, McDonald KR, Phillot AD, Hines HB, Kenyon N.** 2007. Spread of chytridiomycosis has caused the rapid global decline and extinction of frogs. *J Herpetol* **4**:125–134.

19. **Retallick RW, McCallum H, Speare R.** 2004. Endemic infection of the amphibian chytrid fungus in a frog community post-decline. *PLoS Biol* **2**:e351. doi:10.1371/journal.pbio.0020351.

20. **Richards-Hrdlicka KL.** 2013. Preserved specimens of the extinct golden toad of Monteverde (*Cranopsis periglenes*) tested negative for the amphibian chytrid fungus (*Batrachochytrium dendrobatidis*). *J Herpetol* **47**:456–458.

21. **La Marca E, Lips KR, Lotters S, Puschendorf R, Ibanez R, Rueda-Almonacid JV, Schulte R, Marty C, Castro F, Manzanilla-Puppo J, Garcia-Perez JE, Bolanos F, Chaves G, Pounds JA, Toral E, Young BE.** 2005. Catastrophic population declines and extinctions in neotropical harlequin frogs (*Bufonidae: atelopus*). *Biotropica* **37**:190–201.

22. **Lips KR, Diffendorfer J, Mendelson JR III, Sears MW.** 2008. Riding the wave: reconciling the roles of disease and climate change in amphibian declines. *PLoS Biol* **6**:e72. doi:10.1371/journal.pbio.0060072.

23. **IUCN SSC Amphibian Specialist Group.** 2015. *Nectophrynoides asperginis*. The IUCN Red List of Threatened Species. Version 2015.2. www.iucnredlist.org.

24. **Vredenburg VT, Knapp RA, Tunstall TS, Briggs CJ.** 2010. Dynamics of an emerging disease drive large-scale amphibian population extinctions. *Proc Natl Acad Sci USA* **107**:9689–9694.

25. **Odum RA, Corn PS.** 2005. *Bufo baxteri*, Porter, 1968, Wyoming toad, p 390–392. *In* Lannoo MJ (ed), *Amphibian Declines: The Conservation Status of United States Species*. University of California Press, Berkeley, CA.

26. **Kolby JE, McCranie JR.** 2009. Discovery of a surviving population of the montane streamside frog *Craugastor milesi* (Schmidt). *Herpetol Rev* **40**:282–283.

27. **Daskin JH, Alford RA, Puschendorf R.** 2011. Short-term exposure towarm microhabitats could explain amphibian persistence with *Batrachochytrium dendrobatidis*. *PLoS One* **6**:e26215. doi:10.1371/journal.pone.0026215.

28. **Manzanilla J, La Marca E, Heyer R, Fernández-Badillo E.** 2004. *Atelopus cruciger*. The IUCN Red List of Threatened Species. Version 20152. www.iucnredlist.org.

29. **Biton R, Geffen E, Vences M, Cohen O, Bailon S, Rabinovich R, Malka Y, Oron T, Boistel R, Brumfeld V, Gafny S.** 2013. The rediscovered Hula painted frog is a living fossil. *Nat Commun* **4**:1959.

30. **Owens B.** 2012. Long-fingered African frog rediscovered after 62 years. Available at: http://blogs.nature.com/news/2012/03/long-fingered-african-frog-rediscovered-after-62-years.html.

31. **Wickramasinghe LJM, Vidanapathirana DR, Airyarathne S, Rajeev G, Chanaka A, Pastorini J, Chathuranga G, Wickramasinghe N.** 2013. Lost and found: one of the world's most elusive amphibians, *Pseudophilautus stellatus* (Kelaart 1853) rediscovered. *Zootaxa* **3620**:112–128.

32. **Lips KR, Brem F, Brenes R, Reeve JD, Alford RA, Voyles J, Carey C, Livo L, Pessier AP, Collins JP.** 2006. Emerging infectious disease and the loss of biodiversity in a neotropical amphibian community. *Proc Natl Acad Sci USA* **103**:3165–3170.

33. **Catenazzi A, Lehr E, Rodriguez LO, Vredenburg VT.** 2011. *Batrachochytrium dendrobatidis* and the collapse of anuran species richness and abundance in the Upper Manu National Park, southeastern Peru. *Conserv Biol* **25**:382–391.

34. **Rosenblum EB, James TY, Zamudio KR, Poorten TJ, Ilut D, Rodriguez D, Eastman JM, Richards-Hrdlicka K, Joneson S, Jenkinson TS, Longcore JE, Parra Olea G, Toledo LF, Arellano ML, Medina EM, Restrepo S, Flechas SV, Berger L, Briggs CJ, Stajich JE.** 2013. Complex history of the amphibian-killing chytrid fungus revealed with genome resequencing data. *Proc Natl Acad Sci USA* **110**:9385–9390.

35. **Rowley JJ, Alford RA.** 2007. Behaviour of Australian rainforest stream frogs may affect the transmission of chytridiomycosis. *Dis Aquat Organ* **77**:1–9.

36. **Weldon C, Crottini A, Bollen A, Rabemananjara FCE, Copsey J, Garcia G, Andreone F.** 2013. Pre-emptive national monitoring plan for detecting the amphibian chytrid fungus in Madagascar. *EcoHealth* **10**:234–240.

37. **James TY, Litvintseva AP, Vilgalys R, Morgan JAT, Taylor JW, Fisher MC, Berger L, Weldon C, du Preez L, Longcore JE.** 2009. Rapid global expansion of the fungal disease chytridiomycosis into declining and healthy amphibian populations. *PLoS Pathog* **5**:e1000458. doi:10.1371/journal.ppat.1000458.

38. **Farrer RA, Weinert LA, Bielby J, Garner TW, Balloux F, Clare F, Bosch J, Cunningham AA, Weldon C, du Preez LH, Anderson L, Pond SL, Shahar-Golan R, Henk DA, Fisher MC.** 2011. Multiple emergences of genetically diverse amphibian-infecting chytrids include a globalized hypervirulent recombinant lineage. *Proc Natl Acad Sci USA* **108**:18732–18736.

39. **Fisher MC, Bosch J, Yin Z, Stead DA, Walker J, Selway L, Brown AJ, Walker LA, Gow NA, Stajich JE, Garner TW.** 2009. Proteomic and phenotypic profiling of the amphibian pathogen *Batrachochytrium dendrobatidis* shows

that genotype is linked to virulence. *Mol Ecol* **18:**415–429.

40. **Gahl MK, Longcore JE, Houlahan JE.** 2012. Varying responses of northeastern North American amphibians to the chytrid pathogen *Batrachochytrium dendrobatidis*. *Conserv Biol* **26:**135–141.

41. **Gervasi S, Gondhalekar C, Olson DH, Blaustein AR.** 2013. Host identity matters in the amphibian-*Batrachochytrium dendrobatidis* system: fine-scale patterns of variation in responses to a multi-host pathogen. *PLoS One* **8:** e54490. doi:10.1371/journal.pone.0054490.

42. **Rosenblum EB, Voyles J, Poorten TJ, Stajich JE.** 2010. The deadly chytrid fungus: a story of an emerging pathogen. *PLoS Pathog* **6:** e1000550. doi:10.1371/journal.ppat.1000550.

43. **Schloegel LM, Toledo LF, Longcore JE, Greenspan SE, Vieira CA, Lee M, Zhao S, Wangen C, Ferreira CM, Hipolito M, Davies AJ, Cuomo CA, Daszak P, James TY.** 2012. Novel, panzootic and hybrid genotypes of amphibian chytridiomycosis associated with the bullfrog trade. *Mol Ecol* **21:**5162–5177.

44. **Weldon C, du Preez LH, Hyatt AD, Muller R, Spears R.** 2004. Origin of the amphibian chytrid fungus. *Emerg Infect Dis* **10:**2100–2105.

45. **Cheng TL, Rovito SM, Wake DB, Vredenburg VT.** 2011. Coincident mass extirpation of neotropical amphibians with the emergence of the infectious fungal pathogen *Batrachochytrium dendrobatidis*. *Proc Natl Acad Sci USA* **108:** 9502–9507.

46. **Richards-Hrdlicka KL.** 2012. Extracting the amphibian chytrid fungus from formalin-fixed specimens. *Methods Ecol Evol* **3:**842–849.

47. **Adams AJ, LaBonte JP, Ball ML, Richards-Hrdlicka KL, Toothman MH, Briggs CJ.** 2015. DNA extraction method affects the detection of a fungal pathogen in formalin-fixed specimens using qPCR. *PLoS One* **10:**e0135389. doi:10.1371/journal.pone.0135389.

48. **Talley BL, Muletz CR, Vredenburg VT, Fleischer RC, Lips KR.** 2015. A century of *Batrachochytrium dendrobatidis* in Illinois amphibians (1888-1989). *Biol Conserv* **182:**254–261.

49. **Rodriguez D, Becker CG, Pupin NC, Haddad CFB, Zamudio KR.** 2014. Long-term endemism of two highly divergent lineages of the amphibian-killing fungus in the Atlantic Forest of Brazil. *Mol Ecol* **23:**774–787.

50. **Goka K, Yokoyama J, Une Y, Kuroki T, Suzuki K, Nakahara M, Kobayashi A, Inaba S, Mizutani T, Hyatt AD.** 2009. Amphibian chytridiomycosis in Japan: distribution, haplotypes and possible route of entry into Japan. *Mol Ecol* **18:**4757–4774.

51. **Fong JJ, Cheng TL, Bataille A, Pessier AP, Waldman B, Vredenburg VT.** 2015. Early 1900s detection of *Batrachochytrium dendrobatidis* in Korean amphibians. *PLoS One* **10:**e0115656. doi:10.1371/journal.pone.0115656.

52. **Soto-Azat C, Clarke BT, Fisher MC, Walker SF, Cunningham AA.** 2010. Widespread historical presence of *Batrachochytrium dendrobatidis* in African pipid frogs. *Divers Distrib* **16:**126–131.

53. **Fisher MC, Garner TWJ.** 2007. The relationship between the emergence of *Batrachochytrium dendrobatidis*, the international trade in amphibians and introduced amphibian species. *Fungal Biol Rev* **21:**2–9.

54. **Schloegel LM, Picco A, Kilpatrick AM, Hyatt A, Daszak P.** 2009. Magnitude of the US trade in amphibians and presence of *Batrachochytrium dendrobatidis* and ranavirus infection in imported North American bullfrogs (*Rana catesbeiana*). *Biol Conserv* **142:**1420–1426.

55. **Kolby JE, Smith KM, Berger L, Karesh WB, Preston A, Pessier AP, Skerratt LF.** 2014. First evidence of amphibian chytrid fungus (*Batrachochytrium dendrobatidis*) and ranavirus in Hong Kong amphibian trade. *PLoS One* **9:** e90750. doi:10.1371/journal.pone.0090750.

56. **Phillott AD, Speare R, Hines HB, Skerratt LF, Meyer E, McDonald KR, Cashins SD, Mendez D, Berger L.** 2010. Minimising exposure of amphibians to pathogens during field studies. *Dis Aquat Organ* **92:**175–185.

57. **Johnson ML, Speare R.** 2005. Possible modes of dissemination of the amphibian chytrid *Batrachochytrium dendrobatidis* in the environment. *Dis Aquat Organ* **65:**181–186.

58. **Schloegel LM, Daszak P, Cunningham AA, Speare R, Hill B.** 2010. Two amphibian diseases, chytridiomycosis and ranaviral disease, are now globally notifiable to the World Organization for Animal Health (OIE): an assessment. *Dis Aquat Organ* **92:**101–108.

59. **McMahon TA, Brannelly LA, Chatfield MWH, Johnson PTJ, Joseph MB, McKenzie VJ, Richards-Zawacki CL, Venesky MD, Rohr JR.** 2013. Chytrid fungus *Batrachochytrium dendrobatidis* has nonamphibian hosts and releases chemicals that cause pathology in the absence of infection. *Proc Natl Acad Sci USA* **110:**210–215.

60. **Brannelly LA, McMahon TA, Hinton M, Lenger D, Richards-Zawacki CL.** 2015. *Batrachochytrium dendrobatidis* in natural and farmed Louisiana crayfish populations: prevalence and implications. *Dis Aquat Organ* **112:**229–235.

61. **Shapard EJ, Moss AS, San Francisco MJ.** 2012. *Batrachochytrium dendrobatidis* can

infect and cause mortality in the nematode *Caenorhabditis elegans*. *Mycopathologia* **173**: 121–126.

62. **Webb R, Mendez D, Berger L, Speare R.** 2007. Additional disinfectants effective against the amphibian chytrid fungus *Batrachochytrium dendrobatidis*. *Dis Aquat Organ* **74**:13–16.

63. **Cashins SD, Skerratt LF, Alford RA, Campbell RA.** 2008. Sodium hypochlorite denatures the DNA of the amphibian chytrid fungus *Batrachochytrium dendrobatidis*. *Dis Aquat Organ* **80**:63–67.

64. **Mendez D, Webb R, Berger L, Speare R.** 2008. Survival of the amphibian chytrid fungus *Batrachochytrium dendrobatidis* on bare hands and gloves: hygiene implications for amphibian handling. *Dis Aquat Organ* **82**:97–104.

65. **Rowley JJL, Chan SKF, Tang WS, Speare R, Skerratt LF, Alford RA, Cheung KS, Ho CY, Campbell R.** 2007. Survey for the amphibian chytrid *Batrachochytrium dendrobatidis* in Hong Kong in native amphibians and in the international amphibian trade. *Dis Aquat Organ* **78**:87–95.

66. **Kolby JE, Ramirez SD, Berger L, Richards-Hrdlicka KL, Jocque M, Skerratt LF.** 2015a. Terrestrial dispersal and potential environmental transmission of the amphibian chytrid fungus (*Batrachochytrium dendrobatidis*). *PLoS One* **10**: e0125386. doi:10.1371/journal.pone.0125386.

67. **Cummer MR, Green DE, O'Neill EM.** 2005. Aquatic chytrid pathogen detected in a terrestrial plethodontid salamander. *Herpetol Rev* **36**:248–249.

68. **Weinstein SB.** 2009. An aquatic disease on a terrestrial salamander: individual and population level effects of the amphibian chytrid fungus, *Batrachochytrium dendrobatidis*, on *Batrachoseps attenuatus* (*Plethodontidae*). *Copeia* **4**:653–660.

69. **Gower DJ, Doherty-Bone T, Loader SP, Wilkinson M, Kouete MT, Tapley B, Orton F, Daniel OZ, Wynne F, Flach E, Müller H, Menegon M, Stephen I, Browne RK, Fisher MC, Cunningham AA, Garner TW.** 2013. *Batrachochytrium dendrobatidis* infection and lethal chytridiomycosis in caecilian amphibians (*Gymnophiona*). *EcoHealth* **10**:173–183.

70. **Garmyn A, Van Rooij P, Pasmans F, Hellebuyck T, Van Den Broeck W, Haesebrouck F, Martel A.** 2012. Waterfowl: potential environmental reservoirs of the chytrid fungus *Batrachochytrium dendrobatidis*. *PLoS One* **7**:e35038. doi:10.1371/journal.pone.0035038.

71. **Reeder NMM, Pessier AP, Vredenburg VT.** 2012. A reservoir species for the emerging amphibian pathogen *Batrachochytrium dendrobatidis* thrives in a landscape decimated by disease. *PLoS One* **7**:e33567. doi:10.1371/journal.pone.0033567.

72. **Shin J, Bataille A, Kosch TA, Waldman B.** 2014. Swabbing often fails to detect amphibian chytridiomycosis under conditions of low infection load. *PLoS One* **9**:e111091. doi:10.1371/journal.pone.0111091.

73. **Griffin DW.** 2007. Atmospheric movement of microorganisms in clouds of desert dust and implications for human health. *Clin Microbiol Rev* **20**:459–477.

74. **Kellogg CA, Griffin DW.** 2006. Aerobiology and the global transport of desert dust. *Trends Ecol Evol* **21**:638–644.

75. **Kolby JE, Ramirez SD, Berger L, Griffin DW, Jocque M, Skerratt LF.** 2015. Presence of amphibian chytrid fungus (*Batrachochytrium dendrobatidis*) in rainwater suggests aerial dispersal is possible. *Aerobiologia* **31**:411–419.

76. **Defenders of Wildlife (DOW).** 2009. Petition: To List All Live Amphibians in Trade as Injurious Unless Free of *Batrachochytrium dendrobatidis*. 9 September 2009. http://www.defenders.org/publications/petition_to_interior_secretary_salazar.pdf.

77. **Fowler AJ, Lodge DM, Hsia JF.** 2007. Failure of the Lacey Act to protect US ecosystems against animal invasions. *Front Ecol Environ* **5**:353–359.

78. **Simberloff D.** 2005. The politics of assessing risk for biological invasions: the USA as a case study. *Trends Ecol Evol* **20**:216–222.

79. **Pessier AP, Mendelson JR (ed).** 2010. *A Manual for Control of Infectious Diseases in Amphibian Survival Assurance Colonies and Reintroduction Programs*. IUCN/SSC Conservation Breeding Specialist Group, Apple Valley, MN.

80. **Brannelly LA, Richards-Zawacki CL, Pessier AP.** 2012. Clinical trials with itraconazole as a treatment for chytrid fungal infections in amphibians. *Dis Aquat Organ* **101**:95–104.

81. **Holden WM, Fites JS, Reinert LK, Rollins-Smith LA.** 2014. Nikkomycin Z is an effective inhibitor of the chytrid fungus linked to global amphibian declines. *Fungal Biol* **118**:48–60.

82. **Bishop PJ, Speare R, Poulter R, Butler M, Speare BJ, Hyatt A, Olsen V, Haigh A.** 2009. Elimination of the amphibian chytrid fungus *Batrachochytrium dendrobatidis* by Archey's frog *Leiopelma archeyi*. *Dis Aquat Organ* **84**:9–15.

83. **Woodhams DC, Alford RA, Marantelli G.** 2003. Emerging disease of amphibians cured by elevated body temperature. *Dis Aquat Organ* **55**:65–67.

84. Berger L, Speare R, Hines HB, Marantelli G, Hyatt AD, McDonald KR, Skerratt LF, Olsen V, Clarke JM, Gillespie G, Mahony M, Sheppard N, Williams C, Tyler MJ. 2004. Effect of season and temperature on mortality in amphibians due to chytridiomycosis. *Aust Vet J* **82**:434–439.

85. Brannelly L, Berger L, Marantelli G, Skerratt LF. 2015. Low humidity is a failed treatment option for chytridiomycosis in the critically endangered southern corroboree frog. *Wildl Res* **42**:44–49.

86. Cashins SD, Grogan LF, McFadden M, Hunter D, Harlow PS, Berger L, Skerratt LF. 2013. Prior infection does not improve survival against the amphibian disease chytridiomycosis. *PLoS One* **8**:e56747. doi:10.1371/journal.pone.0056747.

87. McMahon TA, Sears BF, Venesky MD, Bessler SM, Brown JM, Deutsch K, Halstead NT, Lentz G, Tenouri N, Young S, Civitello DJ, Ortega N, Fites JS, Reinert LK, Rollins-Smith LA, Raffel TR, Rohr JR. 2014. Amphibians acquire resistance to live and dead fungus overcoming fungal immunosuppression. *Nature* **511**:224–227.

88. Harris RN, James TY, Lauer A, Simon MA, Patel A. 2006. Amphibian pathogen *Batrachochytrium dendrobatidis* is inhibited by the cutaneous bacteria of amphibian species. *J Herpetolol* **3**:53–56.

89. Becker MH, Harris RN. 2010. Cutaneous bacteria of the redback salamander prevent morbidity associated with a lethal disease. *PLoS One* **5**:e10957. doi:10.1371/journal. pone.0010957.

90. Brannelly LA, Hunter DA, Skerratt LF, Scheele BC, Lenger D, McFadden MS, Harlow PS, Berger L. 2015. Chytrid infection and post-release fitness in the reintroduction of an endangered alpine tree frog. *Anim Conserv* [Epub ahead of print.] doi:101111/ acv12230.

91. Geiger CC. 2013. Developing methods to mitigate chytridiomycosis: an emerging disease of amphibians. Dissertation. Institute of Evolutionary Biology and Environmental Studies, University of Zurich, Switzerland.

92. Lubick N. 2010. Ecology: emergency medicine for frogs. *Nature* **465**:680–681.

93. Kolby JE. 2014. Presence of the amphibian chytrid fungus *Batrachochytrium dendrobatidis* in native amphibians exported from Madagascar. *PLoS One* **9**:e89660. doi:10.1371/ journal.pone.0089660.

94. Kolby JE, Smith KM, Ramirez SD, Rabemananjara F, Pessier AP, Brunner JL, Goldberg CS, Berger L, Skerratt LF. 2015. Rapid response to evaluate the presence of amphibian chytrid fungus (*Batrachochytrium dendrobatidis*) and ranavirus in wild amphibian populations in Madagascar. *PLoS One* **10**: e0125330. doi:10.1371/journal.pone.0125330.

95. Bletz MC, Rosa GM, Andreone F, Courtois EA, Schmeller DS, Rabibisoa NHC, Rabemananjara FCE, Raharivololoniaina L, Vences M, Weldon C, Edmonds D, Raxworthy CJ, Harris RN, Fisher MC, Crottini A. 2015. Widespread presence of the pathogenic fungus *Batrachochytrium dendrobatidis* in wild amphibian communities in Madagascar. *Sci Rep* **5**:8633.

96. Searle CL, Mendelson JR III, Green LE, Duffy MA. 2013. Daphnia predation on the amphibian chytrid fungus and its impacts on disease risk in tadpoles. *Ecol Evol* **3**:4129–4138.

97. Scheele BC, Hunter DA, Grogan LF, Berger L, Kolby JE, McFadden MS, Marantelli G, Skerratt LF, Driscoll DA. 2014. Interventions for reducing extinction risk in chytridiomycosis-threatened amphibians. *Conserv Biol* **28**:1195– 1205.

98. Roznik EA, Sapsford SJ, Pike DA, Schwarzkopf L, Alford RA. 2015. Natural disturbance reduces disease risk in endangered rainforest frog populations. *Sci Rep* **5**:13472.

99. Berger L. 2001. Diseases in Australian frogs. Dissertation. James Cook University, Townsville, Australia.

100. Johnson ML, Speare R. 2003. Survival of *Batrachochytrium dendrobatidis* in water: quarantine and disease control implications. *Emerg Infect Dis* **9**:922–925.

101. Blehert DS. 2012. Fungal disease and the developing story of bat white-nose syndrome. *PLoS Pathog* **8**:e1002779. doi:10.1371/journal. ppat.1002779.

102. Allender MC, Raudabaugh DB, Gleason FH, Miller AN. 2015. The natural history, ecology, and epidemiology of *Ophidiomyces ophiodiicola* and its potential impact on free-ranging snake populations. *Fungal Ecol* **17**:187–196.

103. Spitzen-van der Sluijs A, Spikmans F, Bosman W, de Zeeuw M, van der Meij T, Goverse E, Kik M, Pasmans F, Martel A. 2013. Rapid enigmatic decline drives the fire salamander (*Salamandra salamndra*) to the edge of extinction in The Netherlands. *Amphib-Reptil* **34**:233– 239.

104. Martel A, Blooi M, Adriaensen C, Van Rooij P, Beukema W, Fisher MC, Farrer RA, Schmidt BR, Tobler U, Goka K, Lips KR, Muletz C, Zamudio KR, Bosch J, Lötters S, Wombwell E, Garner TWJ, Cunningham AA, Spitzen-van der Sluijs A, Salvidio S, Ducatelle R,

Nishikawa K, Nguyen TTT, Kolby JE, Van Bocxlaer I, Bossuyt F, Pasmans F.** 2014. Wildlife disease. Recent introduction of a chytrid fungus endangers Western Palearctic salamanders. *Science* **346:**630–631.

105. **Cunningham AA, Beckmann K, Perkins M, Fitzpatrick L, Cromie R, Redbond J, O'Brien MF, Ghosh P, Shelton J, Fisher MC.** 2015. Emerging disease in UK amphibians. *Vet Rec* **176:**468.

106. **Martel A, Spitzen-van der Sluijs A, Blooi M, Bert W, Ducatelle R, Fisher MC, Woeltjes A, Bosman W, Chiers K, Bossuyt F, Pasmans F.** 2013. *Batrachochytrium salamandrivorans* sp. nov. causes lethal chytridiomycosis in amphibians. *Proc Natl Acad Sci USA* **110:**15325–15329.

107. **Daszak P, Cunningham AA, Hyatt AD.** 2000. Emerging infectious diseases of wildlife: threats to biodiversity and human health. *Science* **287:**443–449.

Artemisinin-Resistant *Plasmodium falciparum* Malaria

22

RICK M. FAIRHURST[1] and ARJEN M. DONDORP[2,3]

ARTEMISININS AND ARTEMISININ COMBINATION THERAPIES

According to the World Health Organization (WHO), 3.2 billion people remain at risk of malaria, and an estimated 214 million new cases of malaria and 438,000 deaths occurred in 2015 (1). Reducing this disease burden continues to rely heavily on the availability and proper use of effective antimalarial drugs. Artemisinin and its derivatives (artesunate, artemether, and dihydroartemisinin [DHA]), referred to collectively as artemisinins, are sesquiterpene lactones with potent activity against nearly all blood stages of *Plasmodium falciparum* parasites. These include asexual stages (rings, trophozoites, and schizonts), which cause the clinical manifestations of malaria, and sexual stages (immature gametocytes), which give rise to the mature gametocytes that transmit infection through *Anopheles* mosquitoes to other humans. These blood stages, but not others (merozoites, which invade red blood cells [RBCs], and mature gametocytes), are susceptible to artemisinins because they actively digest hemoglobin as they develop within RBCs. It is believed that the heme-associated iron released from this process cleaves the endoperoxide moiety of

[1]Laboratory of Malaria and Vector Research, National Institute of Allergy and Infectious Diseases, National Institutes of Health, Rockville, MD 20852; [2]Mahidol-Oxford Tropical Medicine Research Unit, Faculty of Tropical Medicine, Mahidol University, Bangkok 10400, Thailand; [3]Centre for Tropical Medicine, Nuffield Department of Medicine, University of Oxford, Oxford OX3 7BN, United Kingdom.

Emerging Infections 10
Edited by W. Michael Scheld, James M. Hughes and Richard J. Whitley
© 2016 American Society for Microbiology, Washington, DC
doi:10.1128/microbiolspec.EI10-0013-2016

artemisinins, thereby forming the reactive oxygen species that target nucleophilic groups in parasite proteins and lipids. In an unbiased chemical proteomics analysis (2), Wang et al. found that artemisinin covalently binds 124 parasite proteins, many of which are involved in biological processes that are essential for parasite survival, and they suggested that this constellation of chemical reactions kills parasites.

In patients with *P. falciparum* malaria, this killing process can be studied only in the peripheral blood, where rings develop and circulate within RBCs for about 16 to 24 h before they disappear from blood films by developing into trophozoites and sequestering in microvessels. When rings are exposed to artemisinins, they condense into pyknotic forms resembling Howell-Jolly body inclusions that are efficiently cleared from the bloodstream by "pitting" (3, 4). This process squeezes pyknotic parasites out of their host RBCs as they pass through tight endothelial slits in the spleen and returns the resealed "once-infected" RBCs to the peripheral blood. When sequestered forms (trophozoites, schizonts, and immature gametocytes) are exposed to artemisinins, they are killed *in situ* within microvessels. Since artemisinins achieve 10,000-fold reductions in parasite density in the first 48 h after treatment and potently and rapidly kill rings before they sequester and cause symptoms, parenteral artesunate is highly efficacious in reducing the morbidity and mortality of malaria in Southeast Asia (SEA) (5) and sub-Saharan Africa (SSA) (6).

Artemisinin combination therapies (ACTs) are now the recommended first-line treatments for uncomplicated *P. falciparum* malaria worldwide. ACTs are coformulations of a fast-acting, highly potent artemisinin and a slow-acting, less potent partner drug (e. g., mefloquine, piperaquine, or lumefantrine) that are given orally over 3 days. The principle behind ACTs is that the artemisinin component kills the vast majority of parasites over several days by one mechanism, and the partner drug eliminates residual parasites over several weeks by a different mechanism. The artemisinin and partner drug are believed to protect each other from the development of resistance. For example, by rapidly killing large numbers of parasites, artemisinin reduces the chance that the within-host parasite population will spontaneously develop a mutation that confers partner drug resistance. Should parasites spontaneously develop resistance to artemisinin, on the other hand, the partner drug would be expected to eliminate them. In areas where both artemisinin and the partner drug are highly efficacious, ACTs have helped to achieve substantial reductions in malaria morbidity, mortality, and transmission, even in SSA.

PARASITE CLEARANCE HALF-LIFE

In patients treated with artemisinins or ACTs, artemisinin-sensitive parasites rapidly undergo pyknosis and pitting and thus show fast parasite clearance rates. In patients with an initial parasite density of $\geq$10,000 per ×l of whole blood, these rates are estimated by measuring parasite density frequently until parasites are undetectable, log-transforming these densities and plotting them against time, identifying the linear portion of the resultant parasite clearance curve (7) using a Parasite Clearance Estimator tool (8, 9), and then calculating the parasite clearance half-life from the slope of this line. In Ratanakiri, Cambodia, where parasites are sensitive to artemisinins and ACTs and where levels of transmission and acquired immunity are relatively low, the geometric mean (interquartile range [IQR]) parasite clearance half-life in 120 individuals was recently determined to be 2.81 (2.31 to 3.48) h (10). Since parasite clearance half-lives are log-normally distributed, sporadic identification of higher values (e.g., 6 h) does not necessarily signify artemisinin resistance but represents the tail-end of the half-life distribution.

In Kenieroba, Mali, where parasites are also sensitive to artemisinins and ACT partner drugs but where levels of transmission and age-dependent immunity are relatively high (11), the geometric mean (IQR) parasite clearance half-life in 261 children was recently determined to be 1.93 (1.56 to 2.35) h (12). In these children, the parasite clearance half-life decreased significantly with increasing age (i.e., there was a 4.1-min reduction in half-life for every 1-year increase in age), suggesting that age-dependent immunity was involved in clearing ring-infected RBCs within hours of artesunate exposure (12). In the same study population (13), older children cleared their parasites mostly by a nonpitting mechanism, suggesting that they possessed an immune response that could rapidly clear ring-infected RBCs, while younger children cleared their parasites mostly by pitting, suggesting that they lacked such an immune response. The contribution of pitting-independent mechanisms to parasite clearance has not yet been adequately investigated in SEA, where age is generally not a good surrogate for acquired immunity.

ARTEMISININ RESISTANCE

Clinical Phenotype

Artemisinin resistance was first reported as a 100-fold reduction in parasite clearance rate in Pailin, western Cambodia, in 2009 (14) (Fig. 1). Since then, artemisinin resistance has been defined as a parasite clearance half-life of ≥5 h following treatment with artesunate monotherapy or an ACT (15). Although the tail end of the log-linear distribution of parasite half-lives for artemisinin-sensitive parasites exceeds this 5-h cutoff, it has proven to be a useful measure for monitoring artemisinin resistance in the SEA context (10). In SEA, it has also been defined as an increase in parasite clearance half-life, based on a bimodal distribution of geometric mean (IQR) half-life values: 3.0 (2.4 to 3.9) h for

artemisinin-sensitive parasites and 6.5 (5.7 to 7.4) h for artemisinin-resistant parasites (16). Slow parasite clearance represents a "partial" resistance that is expressed only in early-ring-stage parasites (17–19). This clinical phenotype has now been documented elsewhere in Cambodia (10, 20) and in Thailand (10, 21), Vietnam (10, 22, 23), Myanmar (10, 24), Laos (25), and China (26). It is important to emphasize that this phenotype does not signify "complete" resistance, as a 3-day course of artemisinin has never been considered a curative regimen; whether a 7-day course of artemisinin is still curative in SEA has not yet been investigated. Patients with slow parasite clearance almost always clear their infections following an ACT, unless their parasites are also resistant to its partner drug (e.g., piperaquine in Cambodia and mefloquine in Thailand) (27, 28).

In SEA, parasite clearance half-life is not significantly modified by age (21); hemoglobin E, a polymorphism carried by up to 50% of individuals in Cambodia (20); initial parasite density (20, 21); or a somewhat lower drug exposure (i.e., parasite clearance was similar is patients receiving either 4 or 2 mg/kg [of body weight] of artesunate) (10). While immunity likely plays a role in parasite clearance in SEA, this has not yet been adequately studied, mostly because age is a poor surrogate of acquired immunity and no *in vitro* correlate of parasite-clearing immunity has been established for this region. Since parasite clearance is influenced by acquired immunity in areas of SSA where malaria is endemic, new data are needed to define age-stratified, site-specific half-life values for suspected artemisinin resistance in the future. In any area where endemic malaria is being eliminated through mass drug treatments and bed net use, future reductions in immunity may cause parasite clearance half-lives to lengthen over time but would not necessarily signify emerging artemisinin resistance.

Since assessment of the parasite clearance half-life requires frequent blood sampling,

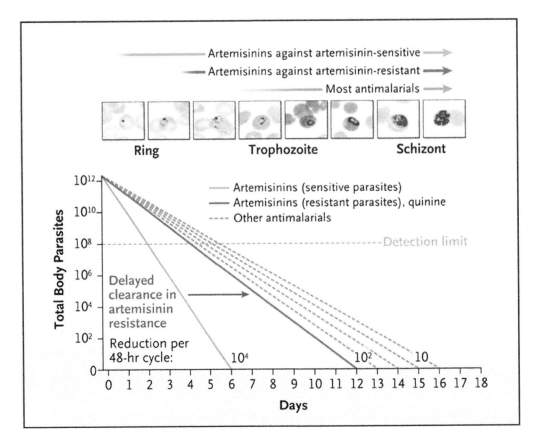

FIGURE 1 Dynamics of parasite clearance by artemisinins and other antimalarial drugs. In sensitive *Plasmodium falciparum* infections, fast-acting and rapidly cleared artemisinins reduce the parasite load by a factor of 10,000 per 48-h asexual-stage parasite cycle. In partially resistant *P. falciparum* infections, artemisinins reduce the parasite load by only by a factor of 100 per cycle, a parasite clearance rate similar to that of slower-acting drugs, such as quinine. Another unique and beneficial feature of artemisinins is their broad stage specificity, but this seems to be compromised in resistant parasites in SEA. Parasites that are at the early ring stage during the brief exposure to rapidly eliminated artemisinins have reduced susceptibility, resulting in delayed parasite clearance following treatment with an artesunate monotherapy or ACT. Reproduced from reference 76 with permission.

the proportion of patients with detectable parasitemia by microscopy at about 72 h ("day 3 positivity") after starting an ACT is often used as a measure of slow parasite clearance in field settings. Although this measure depends strongly on the initial parasitemia and the sensitivity of the detection method at 72 h, and is less accurate, day 3 positivity of >10% has proven to be useful for the initial detection of artemisinin resistance at the population level in SEA (16). In SSA, where parasite clearance is considerably faster because of acquired immunity, the day

3 positivity threshold value will need to be recalibrated.

Laboratory Phenotype

Until recently, it had been difficult to study artemisinin resistance in the laboratory. This is because parasite clearance half-lives correlate poorly with artesunate or DHA 50% inhibitory concentrations (IC_{50}s) (typically between 0 and 8 nM) in "standard" drug susceptibility assays, in which predominantly ring-stage parasites are exposed to low nanomolar concentrations of drug and their DNA content (a surrogate for growth) is measured 48 to 72 h later. Given this finding, and the need to define more precisely the ring stage at which the artemisinin resistance phenotype is expressed, the 0- to 3-h ring-stage survival assay (RSA^{0-3h}) was developed and validated (18). In this *in vitro* assay, parasite clinical isolates are adapted to culture for several weeks, synchronized at the early ring stage (0 to 3 h after invasion of RBCs), exposed to a pharmacologically relevant dose of DHA (700 nM for 6 h), and then cultured for 66 h. The percentage of parasites surviving DHA exposure is then calculated as the ratio of parasites surviving exposure to DHA versus those surviving exposure to dimethyl sulfoxide, the DHA solvent.

The RSA^{0-3h} discriminates two groups of parasites, one with <1% survival and another with ≥1% survival, which are generally defined to be artemisinin sensitive and artemisinin resistant, respectively (18, 29–31). Importantly, this assay is unable to discriminate these two groups of parasites at the middle and late ring stages (9 to 12 h and 18 to 21 h after invasion of RBCs, respectively) (18), indicating that artemisinin resistance is an early-ring-stage phenotype. This finding may account for occasional discrepancies between parasite clearance half-life in patients and percent survival in the RSA^{0-3h} (18). For example, parasite isolates that are artemisinin resistant in the RSA^{0-3h} may have cleared rapidly in patients because they were circulating as middle to late ring stages during the time that parasite clearance was being measured. When the RSA was performed *ex vivo* on unsynchronized ring-stage parasites taken directly from Cambodian patients, percent survival values also fell into two groups (<1% and ≥1%) and correlated strongly with parasite clearance half-lives in the same patients (18).

Genetic Determinants

Two genome-wide association studies of parasite clearance half-life implicated two regions of parasite chromosome 13 in artemisinin resistance (32, 33). The specific genetic determinant remained elusive, however, until Ariey et al. (29) exposed a Tanzanian parasite line to increasing doses of artemisinin *in vitro* over several years and successfully induced artemisinin resistance, as defined by increased percent survival in the RSA^{0-3h} (<1% to 12%). By comparing the whole-genome sequences of drug-pressured and unpressured parasite lines, they identified a single nucleotide polymorphism in the *PF3D7_1343700* gene on chromosome 13, encoding a M476I substitution in the propeller domain of a kelch protein ("K13"). When compared with the known mammalian ortholog Keap1, K13 comprises a *Plasmodium*-specific domain, a BTB-POZ domain, and a six-blade propeller domain (Fig. 2). Ariey et al. validated K13 propeller polymorphism as a molecular marker of artemisinin resistance by showing that 18 different K13-propeller mutations were present in parasites from this country (with each parasite clone carrying only one mutation), that the predominant C580Y mutation had rapidly increased in prevalence where artemisinin resistance had become common in western Cambodia, and that the C580Y, Y493H, and R539T mutations were associated with long parasite clearance half-life and elevated percent survival in the RSA^{0-3h}. While these data established that K13-propeller polymorphism is a genetic marker of artemisinin resistance in Cambodia, additional studies were needed to demonstrate causality.

Since some kelch proteins sense and respond to oxidative stress, and artemisinins are pro-oxidant drugs, it was hypothesized that K13-propeller mutations mediate artemisinin resistance. To test this possibility, Straimer et al. (31) used zing finger nuclease technology to edit the *K13* gene in contemporary Cambodian parasite isolates. When three different K13-propeller mutations (C580Y, R539T, and I543T) were edited to wild-type sequences, the artemisinin resistance phenotype (i.e., elevated percent

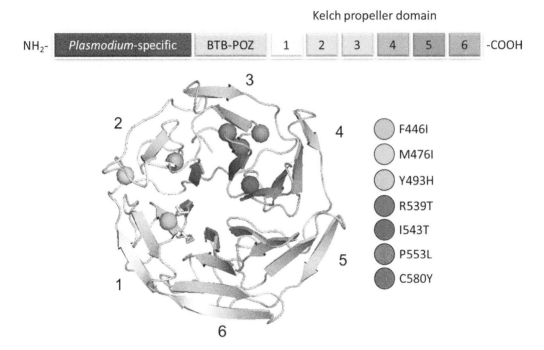

FIGURE 2 *Plasmodium falciparum* **kelch13 (K13) protein. The parasite K13 protein consists of *Plasmodium*-specific sequences, a BTB-POZ domain, and six kelch domains that are predicted to form a six-blade propeller. In the structural model, the original M476I mutation discovered by Ariey et al. (29) and six other mutations associated with artemisinin resistance in SEA are shown. Reproduced from reference 88 with permission.**

survival in the RSA^{0-3h}) was completely lost. When wild-type sequence in the much older SEA parasite line Dd2 was edited to five different K13 propeller mutations, increasing percent survival values (Y493H < C580Y < M476I < R539T < I543T) were observed. Interestingly, the introduction of C580Y conferred higher levels of resistance to contemporary parasite isolates from Cambodia than to older parasite lines from SEA. Together, these data suggest that different K13-propeller mutations confer different levels of artemisinin resistance and that these levels are influenced by parasite genetic background. C580Y also conferred artemisinin resistance to the African parasite line NF54 (34).

Population genetics studies of artemisinin resistance (35, 36) have made several unusual and novel discoveries. First, 11 parasite "founder" populations were identified in Cambodia and Vietnam. These clonal subpopulations are extremely genetically differentiated from each other and from the core populations of each country, suggesting that they recently passed through a bottleneck and subsequently expanded. Second, seven of the founders were artemisinin-resistant in patients (35, 36), and three of these were confirmed as artemisinin resistant in the RSA^{0-3h} (30), suggesting that they were naturally selected by artemisinin pressure. Third, each of the seven artemisinin-resistant founders carried a single K13-propeller mutation, with C580Y emerging independently on three different Cambodian founders, and also shared a common genetic background consisting of four single nucleotide polymorphisms in genes encoding apicoplast ribosomal protein s10 (*arps10*; V127M), ferredoxin (*fd*; D193Y), multidrug resistance 2 transporter (*mdr2*; T484I), and chloroquine resistance transporter (*crt*; N326S) (36). The roles of these mutations in the evolution of these founders are unknown, but they likely increase fitness by compensating for putative deleterious effects of K13-propeller mutations, augmenting the level of artemisinin resistance, mediating resistance to previously or currently used antimalarial drugs (i.e., chloroquine, sulfadoxine, pyrimethamine, mefloquine, and piperaquine), increasing the transmission of parasites to *Anopheles* mosquitoes, or some combination of these effects.

Molecular Mechanisms

Several K13-propeller mutations confer artemisinin resistance to various parasite clinical isolates and laboratory lines (31, 34),

but their molecular mechanisms have not yet been defined. Since some mammalian kelch proteins detect cellular stressors, like oxidants, it was readily hypothesized that K13-propeller mutations mediate resistance to artemisinins (29). One hypothetical model (Fig. 3) speculates that in artemisinin-sensitive parasites, wild-type K13 constitutively binds a putative transcription factor in the parasite cytosol and delivers it to ubiquitin ligase, which polyubiquitinates the transcription factor and thus targets it for proteosomal degradation. In the presence of oxidative stress, a conformational change in wild-type K13 liberates the transcription factor, enabling it to avoid degradation, accumulate in the nucleus, and upregulate genes involved in antioxidant and other protective responses. In this model, the pro-oxidant activity of artemisinins is simply too potent and rapid

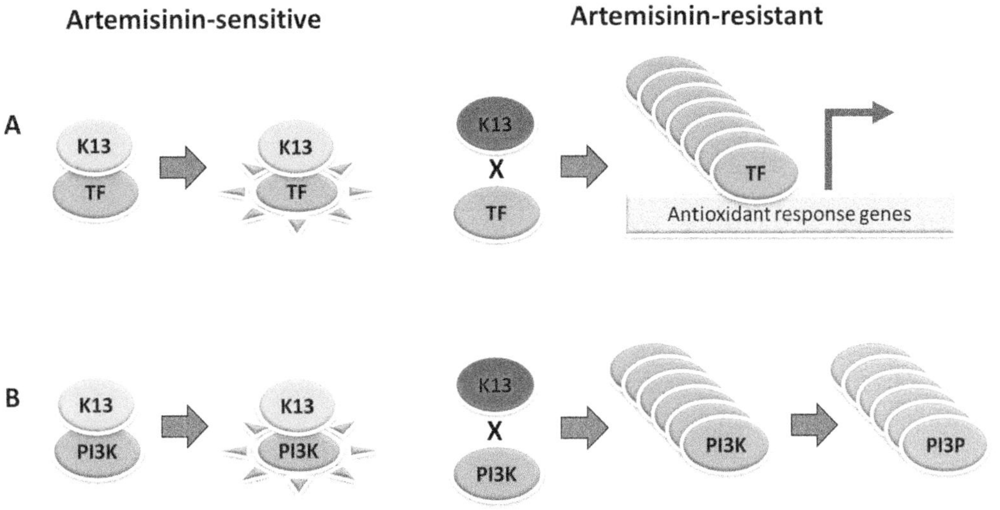

FIGURE 3 Recently proposed mechanisms of artemisinin sensitivity and resistance in *Plasmodium falciparum*. (A) In artemisinin-sensitive parasites, wild-type K13 (green) binds a putative transcription factor and targets it for degradation. In artemisinin-resistant parasites, mutant K13 (red) fails to bind this transcription factor, which translocates to the nucleus and upregulates genes involved in the antioxidant response. In this "pre-prepared" state, parasites are better able to handle the oxidative stress that is exerted by activated artemisinins, for example, by repairing and replenishing oxidant-damaged proteins. (B) In artemisinin-sensitive parasites, wild-type K13 (green) binds PI3K and targets it for degradation. In artemisinin-resistant parasites, mutant K13 (red) fails to bind PI3K, leading to increased PI3K activity and PI3P levels. In this "prepared" state, high PI3P levels are presumably able to promote the survival of parasites exposed to artemisinins, for example, by mediating membrane fusion events involved in parasite growth. Reproduced from reference 88 with permission.

for wild-type parasites to combat and survive. In artemisinin-resistant parasites, on the other hand, K13-propeller mutations constitutively prevent the binding of K13 to the transcription factor, leading to a baseline gene expression pattern that prepares parasites to withstand the sudden oxidative damage caused by artemisinins.

In a large population transcriptomics study of *P. falciparum* clinical isolates in SEA (37), Mok et al. have provided some evidence to support this model. Using a panel of stage-specific reference transcriptomes, they identified a cluster of 549 parasites that were collected from patients at the early ring stage of parasite development, that is, when the artemisinin resistance phenotype is expressed. In correlating the transcriptional profiles of these isolates *ex vivo* with the clearance half-lives of these parasites in patients, they were able to link artemisinin resistance to an upregulated "unfolded protein response" pathway involving two major chaperone complexes: *Plasmodium* reactive oxidative stress complex and TCP-1 ring complex. The transcriptional profiles of artemisinin-resistant isolates also showed evidence of delayed progression through the intraerythrocytic lifecycle upon *ex vivo* cultivation. Both transcriptional phenotypes are closely associated with K13-propeller polymorphism and may enable parasites to survive artemisinin by repairing and replenishing their oxidatively damaged proteins before advancing through the cell cycle. More research is needed to integrate these findings with those of additional studies, which report that artemisinin-resistant parasites show enhanced responses to cellular stress (19) and altered patterns of intraerythrocytic development (38).

Additional progress in exploring artemisinin resistance mechanisms was recently reported by Mbengue et al. (39), who propose that artemisinin targets *P. falciparum* phosphatidylinositol-3-kinase (PI3K) and that PI3K is the binding partner of K13. Their model of artemisinin mode of action (Fig. 3) proposes that the interaction between wild-type K13 and PI3K targets the latter for proteosomal degradation. Since these parasites have low basal levels of PI3-phosphate (PI3P), the product of PI3K activity, they are highly sensitive to artemisinin-induced inhibition of PI3K. Without a functional PI3K, parasites cannot generate the high PI3P levels they need for growth (PI3P is involved in membrane biogenesis and fusion events and increases in amount as parasites develop from rings to schizonts). Their model of artemisinin resistance speculates that because mutant K13 fails to bind PI3K, PI3K accumulates and produces high basal levels of PI3P. With subsequent exposure to artemisinin, high basal levels of PI3P enable the continuous PI3P-dependent growth of artemisinin-resistant parasites while they recover from the effects of PI3K inhibition. Further studies are needed to integrate this model with that of the aforementioned transcriptomics study (37) and to reconcile disparate artemisinin modes of action: nonspecific oxidation of >100 parasite proteins (2) and specific inhibition of a single parasite enzyme (39).

Molecular Epidemiology

Several studies have confirmed that some K13-propeller mutations are also markers of slow parasite clearance outside Cambodia, in Thailand, Vietnam, Myanmar, and China (10, 26, 40, 41). Retrospective data from Cambodia, Thailand, and Myanmar indicate that these mutations arose as early as 2001. Molecular surveillance studies have greatly expanded the map of K13-propeller polymorphism to include additional areas of Cambodia (42–44), Thailand (45, 46), Myanmar (47–49), China (48, 50), Laos (51), Bangladesh (52), and India (53). While some of these mutations have already been associated with slow parasite clearance in patients at other sites, most have not and require validation. Currently, C580Y predominates along the Cambodia-Thailand (29, 41–44, 54) and Thailand-Myanmar (29, 41, 47) borders, and F446I predominates along the China-Myanmar and the Myanmar-India borders (26, 47, 49, 50). It is not known how C580Y has essentially approached fixation in western Cambodia given that it confers lower percent survival in the RSA$^{0\text{-}3h}$ than R539T and I543T (29–31).

Multiple studies in SSA have detected dozens of K13-propeller mutations, many of which have not yet been observed in SEA, at very low frequency in 18 countries: Cameroon, Central African Republic, Chad, Comoros Archipelago, Democratic Republic of the Congo, Ethiopia, Gabon, Gambia, Ghana, Kenya, Madagascar, Malawi, Mali, Rwanda, Senegal, Togo, Uganda, and Zambia (55–66). The most frequent mutation in SSA is A578S; however, haplotype analysis does not show evidence of selection of this mutation in the African *P. falciparum* population, and this mutation is present naturally in *Plasmodium vivax* and *Plasmodium knowlesi* (67). A recent global survey of *P. falciparum* genome sequences found that in SSA, K13-propeller mutations have originated locally and that K13 shows a normal pattern of sequence variation relative to other genes in African parasites (67). In SEA, on the other hand, K13-propeller sequences contain a great excess of nonsynonymous mutations, many of which cause radical amino acid changes. Together, these findings suggest that while K13-propeller mutations are not being strongly selected at this time, there is a considerable amount of baseline variation that could enable resistance to rapidly emerge in the future. Table 1 lists all 124 K13-propeller mutations discovered to date, according to their geographic location (SEA, SSA, or both) and association with artemisinin resistance.

One recent study reported the independent emergence of C580Y in Guyana, South America, but did not investigate its potential association with long parasite clearance half-life or increased percent survival in the RSA$^{0\text{-}3h}$ (68).

Mosquito Transmission

Until recently, information on the transmission potential of artemisinin-resistant *P. falciparum* to native or nonnative *Anopheles* species was largely absent. Given that some parasite isolates do not infect some *Anopheles* species, it had been hypothesized that some *Anopheles* species may prevent the spread of artemisinin-resistant parasites. An alternative possibility is that artemisinin-resistant parasites are spreading so fast in SEA because they infect most or all native *Anopheles* species. In support of the latter hypothesis, St. Laurent et al. have provided evidence that parasite clones from three artemisinin-resistant founder populations in western Cambodia (each carrying a different K13-propeller mutation) are able to infect both *Anopheles dirus* and *Anopheles minimus*, two divergent malaria vectors from SEA, in the laboratory setting (69). Ongoing field studies of wild-caught mosquitoes will determine whether these and about 30 other diverse malaria vectors in SEA transmit artemisinin-resistant parasites. The three founder populations were also able to infect *Anopheles coluzzii*, the major vector of SSA. This finding suggests that *A. coluzzii* will pose no major barrier to the spread of these parasites should they make their way to SSA, where most of the world's malaria mortality, morbidity, and transmission occur.

The finding that these artemisinin-resistant parasite clones infect three highly diverse vector species raises the possibility that they have evolved this ability to enhance their transmission in SEA. Given that genetic polymorphism in the *pfs47* gene can mediate parasite-mosquito compatibility (70) and that *pfs47* is closely linked to *K13* on chromosome 13, it has been hypothesized that *pfs47* polymorphism plays a role in promoting the spread of artemisinin-resistant parasites. In support of this hypothesis, St. Laurent et al. found that although 516 Cambodian isolates carried a total of 22 *pfs47* haplotypes, the three founder populations they tested each

TABLE 1 K13-propeller mutations, according to propeller blade, geographic location, and association with artemisinin resistance[a]

Blade no.	Amino acid									
1	**P441L**	F442	P443S	L444	V445	**F446I**	C447	I448	**G449A**	G449S
	G449D	G450	F451	D452E	G453	V454I	E455	Y456	L457	**N458Y**
	N458I	S459L	M460	E461	L462	L463S	D464H	D464Y	I465T	S466
	Q467	Q468	**C469Y**	C469F	W470	R471	M472	C473	T474I	
2	P475	*M476I*	S477Y	T478P	K479I	K480	**A481V**	Y482	F483S	G484
	S485N	A486	V487I	L488S	N489	N490T	N490H	F491	L492S	*Y493H*
	V494I	F495L		G496F	G497	N498	N499D	Y500	D501G	Y502
	K503	A504T	L505	F506	E507	T508N	E509	V510	Y511M	D512
	R513	L514	R515T	D516Y	V517	W518	Y519	V520I	V520A	S521
	S522C	N523	L524	N525D	I526M					
3	P527H	**R528T**	R529	N530	N531	C532S	G533A	G533S	V534L	V534I
	T535	S536	N537I	**G538V**	*R539T*	I540	Y541	C542Y	*I543T*	G544R
	G545E	Y546	D547	G548S	S549Y	S550	I551	I552C	**P553L**	N554D
	N554H	N554K	V555	E556D	A557S	Y558H	D559	H560	**R561H**	R561C
	M562	K563	A564H	W565	V566I	E567	**V568G**	A569T	P570	L571
	N572	T573S								
4	**P574L**	R575K	R575G	S576L	S577	A578S*	M579	*C580Y*	V581F	A582
	F583	**D584V**	D584N	D584E	N585	K586	I587	Y588	V589I	I590
	G591	G592	T593S	N594	G595S	E596G	R597	L598	N599	S600
	I601	E602	V603	Y604H	E605G	E606	K607	M608L	N609S	K610
	W611	E612D	Q613E	Q613L						
5	**F614L**	P615	Y616	A617T	A617V	L618	L619S	E620	A621F	R622I
	S623C	S624	G625	A626P	A626T	A627	F628	N629Y	Y630F	L631
	N632D	Q633	I634	Y635	V636	V637I	V637A	V637D	G638R	G639V
	G639D	I640	D641	N642	E643	H644	N645	I646	L647	D648
	S649	V650	E651	Q652	Y653	Q654	P655	F656	N657	K658
	R659	W660	Q661	F662	L663	N664	G665			
6	V666A	P667A	P667L	E668	K669	K670	M671	N672	**F673I**	G674
	A675V	A676S	A676D	T677	L678	S679	D680N	S681	Y682	I683
	I684	T685	G686	G687	E688	N689	G690	E691	V692	L693
	N694	S695	C696	H697	F698	F699	S700	P701	D702	T703
	N704	E705	W706	Q707	L708	G709	P710	S711	L712	L713
	V714	P715	R716	F717	G718	**H719N**	S720	V721	L722	I723
	A724	N725	I726							

[a]K13-propeller amino acids (after position 440) predicted by the *P. falciparum* 3D7 reference sequence (version 3) are shown, according to propeller blade number (1 through 6). A total of 124 mutations have been discovered to date. The colors indicate mutations observed only in SEA (blue; $n = 46$), only in SSA (yellow; $n = 62$), and in both regions (green; $n = 16$). Bold type indicates mutations (total of 20) associated with a parasite clearance half-life of ≥5 h in at least one SEA patient with malaria (10, 26, 29, 40–43, 45, 47, 48, 50, 52, 55–58, 60). Italic type indicates mutations (total of five) associated with artemisinin resistance in the *in vitro* RSA^{0-3h} (29–31). The asterisk indicates a mutation associated with a parasite clearance half-life of ≥5 h in three Ugandan children with severe malaria (59). Updated from reference 88.

carried the most common *pfs47* haplotype (representing 33% of all haplotypes) (69). Given that these founders infect the geographically diverse *A. coluzzii* vector from SSA, their shared *pfs47* haplotype may represent a "master key" that enables them to promiscuously infect *Anopheles* species and enhance their spread. To explore this possibility, it will be necessary to test whether these founders can infect vectors in SEA, as well as geographically separated *Anopheles* species in Oceania, SSA, and the Americas. A vaccine strategy that targets this particular *pfs47* haplotype may help reduce the transmission of these artemisinin-resistant parasites in SEA and elsewhere.

Since artemisinins kill rings (which give rise to immature gametocytes) as well as immature gametocytes (which give rise to mature gametocytes), they have helped to reduce malaria transmission (71, 72). A single low dose of primaquine has been shown to reduce parasite transmission to mosquitoes (reviewed in reference 73) and is currently recommended by the WHO to reduce malaria transmission in areas where artemisinin-resistant *P. falciparum* is prevalent (74). This regimen is deemed unlikely to cause serious hemolysis in individuals with any genetic variant of glucose-6-phosphate dehydrogenase deficiency. Given that artemisinin and primaquine both have pro-oxidant activities, it is possible that that single low-dose primaquine may not kill artemisinin-resistant parasites and that new drugs will be needed (75).

REDEFINING ARTEMISININ RESISTANCE: A WORK IN PROGRESS

Some, but not all, K13-propeller genotypes were recently used to refine the definition of artemisinin resistance (51). At the moment, "suspected" artemisinin resistance is defined as a high prevalence of the delayed parasite clearance phenotype or a high prevalence of K13-propeller mutations, and "confirmed" artemisinin resistance is defined as a combination of a delayed parasite clearance phenotype and a K13 resistance-associated mutation in an individual patient. At this time, only 20 of 124 nonsynonymous K13-propeller mutations discovered have been associated with artemisinin resistance: P441L, F446I, G449A, N458Y, C469Y, A481V, Y493H, S522C, G538V, R539T, I543T, P553L, R561H, V568G, P574L, C580Y, D584V, F673I, A675V,

and H719N (Table 1). Of these, only four have been validated *in vivo* and *in vitro*: Y493H, R539T, I543T, and C580Y. These definitions of artemisinin resistance are likely to change slightly as new K13-propeller mutations, and perhaps other genetic variants, are discovered and associated with artemisinin resistance *in vivo* and *in vitro*. This can be achieved by correlating them with delayed parasite clearance in patients, elevated percent survival in the *in vitro* RSA^{0-3h} or *ex vivo* RSA or increased percent survival in the *in vitro* RSA^{0-3h} when introduced into the parasite genome. Any phenotypic definition of artemisinin resistance involving the parasite clearance rate will continue to be confounded by parameters that are difficult to measure or await further investigation, such as the effects of partner drugs, immunity (12, 13), insufficient blood levels of artemisinin or partner drugs, and the presence of associated mutations that have not yet been validated.

CLINICAL IMPACT OF ARTEMISININ RESISTANCE: RAPID FAILURE OF ACTS

The WHO currently recommends monitoring the efficacy of first- and second-line ACTs every 2 years in all countries where *P. falciparum* malaria is endemic. One aim of such studies is to determine the proportion of patients who are parasitemic on day 3, the currently accepted indicator of "suspected" artemisinin resistance in *P. falciparum*. If the day 3 positivity rate is higher than 10%, then a parasite clearance rate study should be conducted to confirm delayed parasite clearance, and *K13* genotyping should be performed to identify the presence of resistance associated or validated mutations. Another aim is to determine the proportion of patients who fail treatment within 28 or 42 days of follow-up (depending on the half-life of the partner drug). If the ACT failure rate exceeds 10%, the national antimalarial treatment policy should be changed. Table 2

TABLE 2 Current status of artemisinin resistance and ACT options for treating uncomplicated *P. falciparum* malaria in the GMS[a]

Country	AL		AM		DP	
	Day 3+	TF	Day 3	TF	Day 3+	TF
Cambodia	>10%	>10%	>10%	<10%	>10%	>10%
Vietnam	ND	ND	ND	ND	>10%	<10%
Laos	>10%	<10%	ND	ND	ND	ND
Thailand	>10%	>10%	>10%	>10%	>10%	<10%
Myanmar	>10%	<10%	>10%	<10%	>10%	<10%

[a]Day 3 positivity (Day 3+) and treatment failure (TF) rates for five GMS countries are shown. TF rates of >10% prompt a change in national antimalarial treatment guidelines. The current first-line ACTs are artemether-mefloquine (AM) (Cambodia), dihydroartemisinin-piperaquine (DP) (Thailand and Laos), artesunate-lumefantrine (AL) (Laos), and either AM, DP, or AL (Myanmar). Adapted from reference 15.

shows the current day 3 positivity and ACT failure rates, and the recommended first-line ACTs, in five SEA countries.

Delayed parasite clearance alone will not necessarily lead to ACT failure. In SEA, a high ACT failure rate has only been observed where resistance to the partner drug is present, regardless of whether artemisinin resistance is present. Over time, however, artemisinin resistance may facilitate the emergence of and select for partner drug resistance (76). This is because the much greater parasite biomass that survives artemisinin exposure is far more likely to develop spontaneous mutations that confer partner drug resistance. To monitor for such an event, we and others have measured the efficacy of DHA-piperaquine in western Cambodia, where the presence of validated resistance mutations is high. Here, DHA-piperaquine is now failing to cure *P. falciparum* malaria in >10% of patients, with 11% to 54% failure rates being reported from 2008 to 2014 from four provinces: Pailin, Pursat, Oddar Meanchey, and Preah Vihear (28, 44, 77). In these studies, a significant risk factor for treatment failure has been the presence of the resistance-associated K13 mutation C580Y. Since high ACT failure rates in SEA have been observed only where partner drug resistance exists, these studies also investigated whether piperaquine resistance had emerged in western Cambodia, as initially suggested by temporal increases in piperaquine IC_{50}s at multiple sites (78; unpublished data) in this region.

In a recent prospective cohort study, Amaratunga et al. identified several characteristics of recrudescent infections following DHA-piperaquine treatment (28). Recrudescent infections were significantly correlated with a resistance-associated K13 mutation, the presence of piperaquine in patient plasma at the time of enrollment, and elevated piperaquine IC_{50} but not with patient age, initial parasite density, or plasma piperaquine concentration at 7 days (a marker of adequate drug exposure). In a prospective *ex vivo* study of piperaquine susceptibility, Duru et al. found that nearly all parasites that recrudesce following DHA-piperaquine treatment show >10% survival in a novel assay in which parasites are exposed to a pharmacologically relevant dose of piperaquine (200 nM for 48 h) and then assessed for survival 24 h later (79). Together, these data indicate that piperaquine resistance has emerged in western Cambodia and that use of DHA-piperaquine in the private sector is no longer an appropriate treatment option. Whether artemisinin resistance has precipitated the emergence of piperaquine resistance, or whether it has helped to further select parasites that were already piperaquine resistant, requires further study. Since piperaquine has a long half-life and was previously used as a monotherapy (like mefloquine), piperaquine resistance may also have emerged independently from artemisinin resistance. Identification of genotypic markers of piperaquine resistance should help to survey its spread in SEA, elucidate its molecular mechanism, and discover new drugs to circumvent it.

ACT FAILURES: POTENTIAL APPROACHES TO TREATMENT AND ELIMINATION

Since ACTs are currently the first-line treatment for uncomplicated *P. falciparum* malaria in all countries where it is endemic, the increasing incidence of ACT failures in SEA is a very real threat to malaria treatment and elimination efforts worldwide (76). In western Cambodia, where first-line DHA-piperaquine treatment fails to cure half of all patients in some areas, alternative treatments are hardly available. The combination of quinine plus doxycycline or tetracycline is still efficacious, but it requires a 7-day course and is poorly tolerated, leading to poor patient adherence. Several new antimalarial compounds are currently under development, including synthetic endoperoxides (80), spiroindolones (81), and imidazolopiperazines (82). Although these are all promising drugs, their further development will require at least another 4 years.

As a stopgap measure, artesunate-mefloquine (the former first-line ACT in all of Cambodia) is now recommended as the first-line treatment for *P. falciparum* malaria in ten of its western provinces where DHA-piperaquine failures are unacceptably high. Several recent findings have supported this recommendation. For example, increases in DHA-piperaquine failures have been accompanied by contemporaneous reductions in mefloquine IC_{50}s and in the prevalence of multiple copies of *pfmdr1*, a genetic marker of mefloquine resistance (83), in the parasite population (44, 54, 78, 84). Moreover, following DHA-piperaquine treatment, recrudescent parasites had lower mefloquine IC_{50}s

than their nonrecrudescent counterparts, and none carried the multicopy *pfmdr1* genotype (28). It is not known whether these findings reflect the recent removal of mefloquine pressure, the addition of piperaquine pressure, or both. Whether artesunate-mefloquine adequately treats patients who have initially failed DHA-piperaquine has not yet been tested in a clinical trial.

To avoid a sharp increase of multidrug-resistant *P. falciparum* malaria in the Greater Mekong Subregion (GMS) and beyond, it will be essential to define alternative treatment strategies using existing antimalarial drugs. There are several possibilities, including extending the present ACT course from 3 days to either 5 or 7 days (depending on the safety and tolerability of the partner drug), sequential administration of two different 3-day ACT regimens (e.g., DHA-piperaquine followed by artesunate-mefloquine), rotating the deployment of DHA-piperaquine and artesunate-mefloquine, deploying multiple first-line therapies simultaneously, and using triple ACTs (TACTs) that combine an artemisinin with two partner drugs. The latter option is currently being trialed by the Tracking Resistance to Artemisinin Collaboration II in areas with high ACT failure rates (Clinicaltrials.gov identifier NCT02453308). In one TACT, DHA-piperaquine is combined with mefloquine since all piperaquine-resistant *P. falciparum* isolates genotyped to date contain a single copy of *pfmdr1* (28, 79), whereas amplification of this gene is the main driver of mefloquine resistance (83). In another TACT, artemether-lumefantrine is combined with amodiaquine since lumefantrine and amodiaquine seem to select alternative mutant alleles of the parasite's *pfcrt* and *pfmdr1* genes (85). Initial efficacy, safety, and tolerability results from Tracking Resistance to Artemisinin Collaboration II look promising; final results are expected in 2017.

Due to the emergence of artemisinin and partner drug resistance in the GMS, the WHO and others now recommend that malaria be eliminated in this region. In 2013, the WHO launched the Emergency Response to Artemisinin Resistance in the GMS (86), which urges partners to coordinate their provision of malaria interventions to all at-risk groups, tighten the coordination and management of field operations, obtain better information for containment of artemisinin resistance, and strengthen regional oversight and support. Despite these emergency efforts, there is concern that *P. falciparum* malaria in the GMS may becoming increasingly resistant to antimalarial drugs, making it effectively untreatable and prone to resurgence. This possibility, and the finding that artemisinin resistance has emerged independently in many areas of the GMS, led the WHO's Malaria Policy Advisory Committee to recommend in 2014 that *P. falciparum* malaria be eliminated in the GMS, prioritizing areas with artemisinin resistance. In response to this, the WHO launched a strategy for malaria elimination in the GMS for 2015 to 2030 (87).

prevailing partner drug in a given area, test whether single low-dose primaquine kills mature artemisinin-resistant gametocytes and blocks their transmission to native mosquito populations, discover measures to interrupt transmission (for example, by developing new gametocytocidal drugs, transmission-blocking vaccines, and mosquito repellents), and identify the best overall strategy to eliminate *P. falciparum* in SEA. In areas where artemisinin resistance is entrenched, additional studies are needed to monitor for the potential worsening of this phenotype, which may manifest as an even slower parasite clearance rate, increased survival of trophozoite and schizont stages, or failure of a 7-day artemisinin regimen to cure patients. In SSA, where several dozen K13-propeller mutations have already been identified in 18 countries, extensive surveillance is needed to detect K13-propeller mutations that are increasing in frequency and investigate incidents of slow-clearing infections.

KNOWLEDGE GAPS AND FUTURE DIRECTIONS

There is still much we do not know about artemisinin-resistant *P. falciparum*. How do K13-propeller mutations alter cell biological processes to cause artemisinin resistance? Do genetic background mutations facilitate the natural selection of artemisinin-resistant parasites? Do artemisinin-resistant parasites have a transmission advantage in the human and mosquito populations of SEA? To prevent the further emergence and spread of artemisinin-resistant parasites in this region, efforts are needed to routinely monitor the prevalence of K13-propeller mutations, ensure that recommended ACTs are effective in areas where the prevalence of K13-propeller mutations is increasing, implement changes in national drug policies in a timely manner, identify ways to treat infections that are resistant to both artemisinin and the

CONCLUSIONS

Throughout SEA, where ACTs are the frontline treatments for *P. falciparum* malaria, artemisinin resistance has repeatedly emerged and spread, and threatens to decrease ACT efficacy and compromise intensified efforts to eliminate multidrug-resistant malaria in this region before it spreads to Africa. Artemisinin resistance is defined as a parasite clearance half-life >5 hours following treatment with artesunate or an ACT in patients, and a parasite survival rate >1% in the RSA^{0-3h} *in vitro*. These phenotypes are caused by SNPs in the parasite's *K13* gene, are associated with an upregulated "unfolded protein response" in the parasite that may antagonize the pro-oxidant activity of artemisinins, and have promoted the selection of PPQ resistance, which has rapidly led to DHA-PPQ failures in western Cambodia. *K13* mutations have been selected on a constellation of several "genetic background" SNPs, which may augment artemisinin resistance, confer partner drug resistance, compensate for putative deleterious effects of *K13* polymorphism, or enhance transmission through native mosquito populations. Given that ACTs are failing fast, new treatment approaches that utilize new combinations of existing antimalarials, such as DHA-PPQ-MQ, or combinations of newer experimental drugs must be urgently tested for efficacy, safety, and tolerability. In the laboratory setting, artemisinin-resistant parasites are able to infect not only native vectors (*Anopheles dirus* and *An. minimus*) of SEA, but also the major non-native vector of Africa (*An. coluzzii*), suggesting that these mosquitoes present no major barrier to the spread of artemisinin-resistant parasites in these two regions. While there is yet no evidence of artemisinin resistance in Africa, it is unlikely that biological barriers will halt its eventual introduction to this continent – where most of the world's malaria transmission, morbidity, and mortality occur.

ACKNOWLEDGMENTS

R. M. Fairhurst is funded by the Intramural Research Program of the NIAID, NIH grant Z01 AI001000-01. A. M. Dondorp is funded by the Wellcome Trust of Great Britain.
    We declare no conflicts of interest.

CITATION

Fairhurst RM, Dondorp AM. 2016. Artemisinin-resistant *Plasmodium falciparum* malaria. Microbiol Spectrum 4(3):EI10-0013-2016.

REFERENCES

1. **World Health Organization.** 2015. *World Malaria Report 2015.* World Health Organization, Geneva, Switzerland. http://apps. who.int/iris/bitstream/10665/200018/1/ 9789241565158_eng.pdf?ua=1. Accessed 20 January 2016.

2. **Wang J, Zhang CJ, Chia WN, Loh CC, Li Z, Lee YM, He Y, Yuan LX, Lim TK, Liu M, Liew CX, Lee YQ, Zhang J, Lu N, Lim CT, Hua ZC, Liu B, Shen HM, Tan KS, Lin Q.** 2015. Haem-activated promiscuous targeting of artemisinin in *Plasmodium falciparum. Nat Commun* **6:**10111.

3. **Chotivanich K, Udomsangpetch R, Dondorp A, Williams T, Angus B, Simpson JA, Pukrittayakamee S, Looareesuwan S, Newbold CI, White NJ.** 2000. The mechanisms of parasite clearance after antimalarial treatment of *Plasmodium falciparum* malaria. *J Infect Dis* **182:**629–633.

4. **Buffet PA, Milon G, Brousse V, Correas JM, Dousset B, Couvelard A, Kianmanesh R, Farges O, Sauvanet A, Paye F, Ungeheuer MN, Ottone C, Khun H, Fiette L, Guigon G, Huerre M, Mercereau-Puijalon O, David PH.** 2006. Ex vivo perfusion of human spleens maintains clearing and processing functions. *Blood* **107:**3745–3752.

5. **South East Asian Quinine Artesunate Malaria (SEAQUAMAT) Trial Group.** 2005. Artesunate versus quinine for treatment of severe falciparum malaria: a randomised trial. *Lancet* **366:**717–725.

6. **Dondorp AM, Fanello CI, Hendriksen IC, Gomes E, Seni A, Chhaganlal KD, Bojang K, Olaosebikan R, Anunobi N, Maitland K, Kivaya E, Agbenyega T, Nguah SB, Evans J, Gesase S, Kahabuka C, Mtove G, Nadjm B, Deen J, Mwanga-Amumpaire J, Nansumba M, Karema C, Umulisa N, Uwimana A, Mokuolu OA, Adedoyin OT, Johnson WB, Tshefu AK, Onyamboko MA, Sakulthaew T, Ngum WP, Silamut K, Stepniewska K, Woodrow CJ, Bethell D, Wills B, Oneko M, Peto TE, von Seidlein L, Day NP, White NJ, AQUAMAT Group.** 2010. Artesunate versus quinine in the treatment of severe falciparum malaria in African children (AQUAMAT): an open-label, randomised trial. *Lancet* **376:**1647–1657.

7. **White NJ.** 2011. The parasite clearance curve. *Malar J* **10:**278.

8. **World Antimalarial Resistance Network.** *Parasite clearance estimator (PCE).* http:// www.wwarn.org/tools-resources/toolkit/analyse/parasite-clearance-estimator-pce. Accessed 20 January 2016.

9. **Flegg JA, Guerin PJ, White NJ, Stepniewska K.** 2011. Standardizing the measurement of parasite clearance in falciparum malaria: the parasite clearance estimator. *Malar J* **10:**339.

10. **Ashley EA, Dhorda M, Fairhurst RM, Amaratunga C, Lim P, Suon S, Sreng S, Anderson JM, Mao S, Sam B, Sopha C, Chuor CM, Nguon C, Sovannaroth S,**

Pukrittayakamee S, Jittamala P, Chotivanich K, Chutasmit K, Suchatsoonthorn C, Runcharoen R, Hien TT, Thuy-Nhien NT, Thanh NV, Phu NH, Htut Y, Han KT, Aye KH, Mokuolu OA, Olaosebikan RR, Folaranmi OO, Mayxay M, Khanthavong M, Hongvanthong B, Newton PN, Onyamboko MA, Fanello CI, Tshefu AK, Mishra N, Valecha N, Phyo AP, Nosten F, Yi P, Tripura R, Borrmann S, Bashraheil M, Peshu J, Faiz MA, Ghose A, Hossain MA, Samad R, Rahman MR, Hasan MM, Islam A, Miotto O, Amato R, MacInnis B, Stalker J, Kwiatkowski DP, Bozdech Z, Jeeyapant A, Cheah PY, Sakulthaew T, Chalk J, Intharabut B, Silamut K, Lee SJ, Vihokhern B, Kunasol C, Imwong M, Tarning J, Taylor WJ, Yeung S, Woodrow CJ, Flegg JA, Das D, Smith J, Venkatesan M, Plowe CV, Stepniewska K, Guerin PJ, Dondorp AM, Day NP, White NJ, Tracking Resistance to Artemisinin Collaboration (TRAC). 2014. Spread of artemisinin resistance in *Plasmodium falciparum* malaria. *N Engl J Med* **371**:411–423.

11. Lopera-Mesa TM, Doumbia S, Konate D, Anderson JM, Doumbouya M, Keita AS, Diakite SA, Traore K, Krause MA, Diouf A, Moretz SE, G ST, Miura K, Gu W, Fay MP, Taylor SM, Long CA, Diakite M, Fairhurst RM. 2015. Impact of red blood cell variants on childhood malaria in Mali: a prospective cohort study. *Lancet Haematol* **2**:e140–e149.

12. Lopera-Mesa TM, Doumbia S, Chiang S, Zeituni AE, Konate DS, Doumbouya M, Keita AS, Stepniewska K, Traore K, Diakite SA, Ndiaye D, Sa JM, Anderson JM, Fay MP, Long CA, Diakite M, Fairhurst RM. 2013. *Plasmodium falciparum* clearance rates in response to artesunate in Malian children with malaria: effect of acquired immunity. *J Infect Dis* **207**:1655–1663.

13. Ndour PA, Lopera-Mesa TM, Diakite SA, Chiang S, Mouri O, Roussel C, Jaureguiberry S, Biligui S, Kendjo E, Claessens A, Ciceron L, Mazier D, Thellier M, Diakite M, Fairhurst RM, Buffet PA. 2015. *Plasmodium falciparum* clearance is rapid and pitting independent in immune Malian children treated with artesunate for malaria. *J Infect Dis* **211**:290–297.

14. Dondorp AM, Nosten F, Yi P, Das D, Phyo AP, Tarning J, Lwin KM, Ariey F, Hanpithakpong W, Lee SJ, Ringwald P, Silamut K, Imwong M, Chotivanich K, Lim P, Herdman T, An SS, Yeung S, Singhasivanon P, Day NP, Lindegardh N, Socheat D, White NJ. 2009. Artemisinin resistance in *Plasmodium falciparum* malaria. *N Engl J Med* **361**:455–467.

15. **World Health Organization.** 2015. *Update on artemisinin and ACT resistance—September 2015.* World Health Organization, Geneva, Switzerland. http://www.who.int/malaria/publications/atoz/update-artemisinin-resistance-sep2015/en/ Accessed 20 January 2016.

16. White LJ, Flegg JA, Phyo AP, Wiladpaingern JH, Bethell D, Plowe C, Anderson T, Nkhoma S, Nair S, Tripura R, Stepniewska K, Pan-Ngum W, Silamut K, Cooper BS, Lubell Y, Ashley EA, Nguon C, Nosten F, White NJ, Dondorp AM. 2015. Defining the in vivo phenotype of artemisinin-resistant falciparum malaria: a modelling approach. *PLoS Med* **12**:e1001823.

17. Witkowski B, Khim N, Chim P, Kim S, Ke S, Kloeung N, Chy S, Duong S, Leang R, Ringwald P, Dondorp AM, Tripura R, Benoit-Vical F, Berry A, Gorgette O, Ariey F, Barale JC, Mercereau-Puijalon O, Menard D. 2013. Reduced artemisinin susceptibility of *Plasmodium falciparum* ring stages in western Cambodia. *Antimicrob Agents Chemother* **57**:914–923.

18. Witkowski B, Amaratunga C, Khim N, Sreng S, Chim P, Kim S, Lim P, Mao S, Sopha C, Sam B, Anderson JM, Duong S, Chuor CM, Taylor WR, Suon S, Mercereau-Puijalon O, Fairhurst RM, Menard D. 2013. Novel phenotypic assays for the detection of artemisinin-resistant *Plasmodium falciparum* malaria in Cambodia: in-vitro and ex-vivo drug-response studies. *Lancet Infect Dis* **13**:1043–1049.

19. Dogovski C, Xie SC, Burgio G, Bridgford J, Mok S, McCaw JM, Chotivanich K, Kenny S, Gnadig N, Straimer J, Bozdech Z, Fidock DA, Simpson JA, Dondorp AM, Foote S, Klonis N, Tilley L. 2015. Targeting the cell stress response of Plasmodium falciparum to overcome artemisinin resistance. *PLoS Biol* **13**:e1002132.

20. Amaratunga C, Sreng S, Suon S, Phelps ES, Stepniewska K, Lim P, Zhou C, Mao S, Anderson JM, Lindegardh N, Jiang H, Song J, Su XZ, White NJ, Dondorp AM, Anderson TJ, Fay MP, Mu J, Duong S, Fairhurst RM. 2012. Artemisinin-resistant *Plasmodium falciparum* in Pursat province, western Cambodia: a parasite clearance rate study. *Lancet Infect Dis* **12**:851–858.

21. Phyo AP, Nkhoma S, Stepniewska K, Ashley EA, Nair S, McGready R, ler Moo C, Al-Saai S, Dondorp AM, Lwin KM, Singhasivanon P, Day NP, White NJ, Anderson TJ, Nosten F. 2012. Emergence of artemisinin-resistant malaria on the western border of Thailand: a longitudinal study. *Lancet* **379**:1960–1966.

22. Thriemer K, Hong NV, Rosanas-Urgell A, Phuc BQ, Ha do M, Pockele E, Guetens P,

Van NV, Duong TT, Amambua-Ngwa A, D'Alessandro U, Erhart A. 2014. Delayed parasite clearance after treatment with dihydroartemisinin-piperaquine in *Plasmodium falciparum* malaria patients in central Vietnam. *Antimicrob Agents Chemother* **58:**7049–7055.

23. Hien TT, Thuy-Nhien NT, Phu NH, Boni MF, Thanh NV, Nha-Ca NT, Thai le H, Thai CQ, Toi PV, Thuan PD, Long le T, Dong le T, Merson L, Dolecek C, Stepniewska K, Ringwald P, White NJ, Farrar J, Wolbers M. 2012. In vivo susceptibility of *Plasmodium falciparum* to artesunate in Binh Phuoc Province, Vietnam. *Malar J* **11:**355.

24. Kyaw MP, Nyunt MH, Chit K, Aye MM, Aye KH, Aye MM, Lindegardh N, Tarning J, Imwong M, Jacob CG, Rasmussen C, Perin J, Ringwald P, Nyunt MM. 2013. Reduced susceptibility of *Plasmodium falciparum* to artesunate in southern Myanmar. *PLoS One* **8:**e57689.

25. World Health Organization. 2014. *Status report on artemisinin resistance—January 2014.* http://www.who.int/malaria/publications/atoz/status_rep_artemisinin_resistance_jan2014.pdf. World Health Organization, Geneva, Switzerland. Accessed 20 January 2016.

26. Huang F, Takala-Harrison S, Jacob CG, Liu H, Sun X, Yang H, Nyunt MM, Adams M, Zhou S, Xia Z, Ringwald P, Bustos MD, Tang L, Plowe CV. 2015. A single mutation in K13 predominates in southern China and is associated with delayed clearance of *Plasmodium falciparum* following artemisinin treatment. *J Infect Dis*. doi:10.1093/infdis/jiv249.

27. Wongsrichanalai C, Meshnick SR. 2008. Declining artesunate-mefloquine efficacy against falciparum malaria on the Cambodia-Thailand border. *Emerg Infect Dis* **14:**716–719.

28. Amaratunga C, Lim P, Suon S, Sreng S, Mao S, Sopha C, Sam B, Dek D, Try V, Amato R, Blessborn D, Song L, Tullo GS, Fay MP, Anderson JM, Tarning J, Fairhurst RM. 2016. Dihydroartemisinin-piperaquine resistance in *Plasmodium falciparum* malaria in Cambodia: a multisite prospective cohort study. *Lancet Infect Dis*. doi:10.1016/S1473-3099(15)00487-9.

29. Ariey F, Witkowski B, Amaratunga C, Beghain J, Langlois AC, Khim N, Kim S, Duru V, Bouchier C, Ma L, Lim P, Leang R, Duong S, Sreng S, Suon S, Chuor CM, Bout DM, Menard S, Rogers WO, Genton B, Fandeur T, Miotto O, Ringwald P, Le Bras J, Berry A, Barale JC, Fairhurst RM, Benoit-Vical F, Mercereau-Puijalon O, Menard D. 2014. A molecular marker of artemisinin-resistant *Plasmodium falciparum* malaria. *Nature* **505:**50–55.

30. Amaratunga C, Witkowski B, Dek D, Try V, Khim N, Miotto O, Menard D, Fairhurst RM. 2014. *Plasmodium falciparum* founder populations in western Cambodia have reduced artemisinin sensitivity in vitro. *Antimicrob Agents Chemother* **58:**4935–4937.

31. Straimer J, Gnadig NF, Witkowski B, Amaratunga C, Duru V, Ramadani AP, Dacheux M, Khim N, Zhang L, Lam S, Gregory PD, Urnov FD, Mercereau-Puijalon O, Benoit-Vical F, Fairhurst RM, Menard D, Fidock DA. 2015. Drug resistance. K13-propeller mutations confer artemisinin resistance in *Plasmodium falciparum* clinical isolates. *Science* **347:**428–431.

32. Takala-Harrison S, Clark TG, Jacob CG, Cummings MP, Miotto O, Dondorp AM, Fukuda MM, Nosten F, Noedl H, Imwong M, Bethell D, Se Y, Lon C, Tyner SD, Saunders DL, Socheat D, Ariey F, Phyo AP, Starzengruber P, Fuehrer HP, Swoboda P, Stepniewska K, Flegg J, Arze C, Cerqueira GC, Silva JC, Ricklefs SM, Porcella SF, Stephens RM, Adams M, Kenefic LJ, Campino S, Auburn S, MacInnis B, Kwiatkowski DP, Su XZ, White NJ, Ringwald P, Plowe CV. 2013. Genetic loci associated with delayed clearance of *Plasmodium falciparum* following artemisinin treatment in Southeast Asia. *Proc Natl Acad Sci U S A* **110:**240–245.

33. Cheeseman IH, Miller BA, Nair S, Nkhoma S, Tan A, Tan JC, Al Saai S, Phyo AP, Moo CL, Lwin KM, McGready R, Ashley E, Imwong M, Stepniewska K, Yi P, Dondorp AM, Mayxay M, Newton PN, White NJ, Nosten F, Ferdig MT, Anderson TJ. 2012. A major genome region underlying artemisinin resistance in malaria. *Science* **336:**79–82.

34. Ghorbal M, Gorman M, Macpherson CR, Martins RM, Scherf A, Lopez-Rubio JJ. 2014. Genome editing in the human malaria parasite *Plasmodium falciparum* using the CRISPR-Cas9 system. *Nat Biotechnol* **32:**819–821.

35. Miotto O, Almagro-Garcia J, Manske M, Macinnis B, Campino S, Rockett KA, Amaratunga C, Lim P, Suon S, Sreng S, Anderson JM, Duong S, Nguon C, Chuor CM, Saunders D, Se Y, Lon C, Fukuda MM, Amenga-Etego L, Hodgson AV, Asoala V, Imwong M, Takala-Harrison S, Nosten F, Su XZ, Ringwald P, Ariey F, Dolecek C, Hien TT, Boni MF, Thai CQ, Amambua-Ngwa A, Conway DJ, Djimde AA, Doumbo OK, Zongo I, Ouedraogo JB, Alcock D, Drury E, Auburn S, Koch O, Sanders M, Hubbart C, Maslen G,

Ruano-Rubio V, Jyothi D, Miles A, O'Brien J, Gamble C, Oyola SO, Rayner JC, Newbold CI, Berriman M, Spencer CC, McVean G, Day NP, White NJ, Bethell D, Dondorp AM, Plowe CV, Fairhurst RM, Kwiatkowski DP. 2013. Multiple populations of artemisinin-resistant *Plasmodium falciparum* in Cambodia. *Nat Genet* **45**:648–655.

36. Miotto O, Amato R, Ashley EA, MacInnis B, Almagro-Garcia J, Amaratunga C, Lim P, Mead D, Oyola SO, Dhorda M, Imwong M, Woodrow C, Manske M, Stalker J, Drury E, Campino S, Amenga-Etego L, Thanh TN, Tran HT, Ringwald P, Bethell D, Nosten F, Phyo AP, Pukrittayakamee S, Chotivanich K, Chuor CM, Nguon C, Suon S, Sreng S, Newton PN, Mayxay M, Khanthavong M, Hongvanthong B, Htut Y, Han KT, Kyaw MP, Faiz MA, Fanello CI, Onyamboko M, Mokuolu OA, Jacob CG, Takala-Harrison S, Plowe CV, Day NP, Dondorp AM, Spencer CC, McVean G, Fairhurst RM, White NJ, Kwiatkowski DP. 2015. Genetic architecture of artemisinin-resistant *Plasmodium falciparum*. *Nat Genet* **47**:226–234.

37. Mok S, Ashley EA, Ferreira PE, Zhu L, Lin Z, Yeo T, Chotivanich K, Imwong M, Pukrittayakamee S, Dhorda M, Nguon C, Lim P, Amaratunga C, Suon S, Hien TT, Htut Y, Faiz MA, Onyamboko MA, Mayxay M, Newton PN, Tripura R, Woodrow CJ, Miotto O, Kwiatkowski DP, Nosten F, Day NP, Preiser PR, White NJ, Dondorp AM, Fairhurst RM, Bozdech Z. 2015. Drug resistance. Population transcriptomics of human malaria parasites reveals the mechanism of artemisinin resistance. *Science* **347**:431–435.

38. Hott A, Casandra D, Sparks KN, Morton LC, Castanares GG, Rutter A, Kyle DE. 2015. Artemisinin-resistant *Plasmodium falciparum* parasites exhibit altered patterns of development in infected erythrocytes. *Antimicrob Agents Chemother* **59**:3156–3167.

39. Mbengue A, Bhattacharjee S, Pandharkar T, Liu H, Estiu G, Stahelin RV, Rizk SS, Njimoh DL, Ryan Y, Chotivanich K, Nguon C, Ghorbal M, Lopez-Rubio JJ, Pfrender M, Emrich S, Mohandas N, Dondorp AM, Wiest O, Haldar K. 2015. A molecular mechanism of artemisinin resistance in *Plasmodium falciparum* malaria. *Nature* **520**:683–687.

40. Nyunt MH, Hlaing T, Oo HW, Tin-Oo LL, Phway HP, Wang B, Zaw NN, Han SS, Tun T, San KK, Kyaw MP, Han ET. 2015. Molecular assessment of artemisinin resistance markers, polymorphisms in the k13 propeller, and a multidrug-resistance gene in the eastern and western border areas of Myanmar. *Clin Infect Dis* **60**:1208–1215.

41. Takala-Harrison S, Jacob CG, Arze C, Cummings MP, Silva JC, Dondorp AM, Fukuda MM, Hien TT, Mayxay M, Noedl H, Nosten F, Kyaw MP, Nhien NT, Imwong M, Bethell D, Se Y, Lon C, Tyner SD, Saunders DL, Ariey F, Mercereau-Puijalon O, Menard D, Newton PN, Khanthavong M, Hongvanthong B, Starzengruber P, Fuehrer HP, Swoboda P, Khan WA, Phyo AP, Nyunt MM, Nyunt MH, Brown TS, Adams M, Pepin CS, Bailey J, Tan JC, Ferdig MT, Clark TG, Miotto O, MacInnis B, Kwiatkowski DP, White NJ, Ringwald P, Plowe CV. 2015. Independent emergence of artemisinin resistance mutations among *Plasmodium falciparum* in Southeast Asia. *J Infect Dis* **211**:670–679.

42. Bosman P, Stassijns J, Nackers F, Canier L, Kim N, Khim S, Alipon SC, Chuor Char M, Chea N, Dysoley L, Van den Bergh R, Etienne W, De Smet M, Menard D, Kindermans JM. 2014. Plasmodium prevalence and artemisinin-resistant falciparum malaria in Preah Vihear Province, Cambodia: a cross-sectional population-based study. *Malar J* **13**:394.

43. Spring MD, Lin JT, Manning JE, Vanachayangkul P, Somethy S, Bun R, Se Y, Chann S, Ittiverakul M, Sia-Ngam P, Kuntawunginn W, Arsanok M, Buathong N, Chaorattanakawee S, Gosi P, Ta-Aksorn W, Chanarat N, Sundrakes S, Kong N, Heng TK, Nou S, Teja-Isavadharm P, Pichyangkul S, Phann ST, Balasubramanian S, Juliano JJ, Meshnick SR, Chour CM, Prom S, Lanteri CA, Lon C, Saunders DL. 2015. Dihydroartemisinin-piperaquine failure associated with a triple mutant including kelch13 C580Y in Cambodia: an observational cohort study. *Lancet Infect Dis* **15**:683–691.

44. Leang R, Taylor WR, Bouth DM, Song L, Tarning J, Char MC, Kim S, Witkowski B, Duru V, Domergue A, Khim N, Ringwald P, Menard D. 2015. Evidence of falciparum malaria multidrug resistance to artemisinin and piperaquine in western Cambodia: dihydroartemisinin-piperaquine open-label multicenter clinical assessment. *Antimicrob Agents Chemother.* doi:10.1128/AAC.00835-15.

45. Talundzic E, Okoth SA, Congpuong K, Plucinski MM, Morton L, Goldman IF, Kachur PS, Wongsrichanalai C, Satimai W, Barnwell JW, Udhayakumar V. 2015. Selection and spread of artemisinin-resistant alleles in Thailand prior to the global artemisinin resistance containment campaign. *PLoS Pathog* **11**:e1004789.

46. **Putaporntip C, Kuamsab N, Kosuwin R, Tantiwattanasub W, Vejakama P, Sueblinvong T, Seethamchai S, Jongwutiwes S, Hughes AL.** 2015. Natural selection of K13 mutants of *Plasmodium falciparum* in response to artemisinin combination therapies in Thailand. *Clin Microbiol Infect.* doi:10.1016/j.cmi.2015.10.027.

47. **Tun KM, Imwong M, Lwin KM, Win AA, Hlaing TM, Hlaing T, Lin K, Kyaw MP, Plewes K, Faiz MA, Dhorda M, Cheah PY, Pukrittayakamee S, Ashley EA, Anderson TJ, Nair S, McDew-White M, Flegg JA, Grist EP, Guerin P, Maude RJ, Smithuis F, Dondorp AM, Day NP, Nosten F, White NJ, Woodrow CJ.** 2015. Spread of artemisinin-resistant *Plasmodium falciparum* in Myanmar: a cross-sectional survey of the K13 molecular marker. *Lancet Infect Dis* **15:**415–421.

48. **Feng J, Zhou D, Lin Y, Xiao H, Yan H, Xia Z.** 2015. Amplification of pfmdr1, pfcrt, pvmdr1, and K13 propeller polymorphisms associated with *Plasmodium falciparum* and *Plasmodium vivax* isolates from the China-Myanmar border. *Antimicrob Agents Chemother* **59:**2554–2559.

49. **Wang Z, Wang Y, Cabrera M, Zhang Y, Gupta B, Wu Y, Kemirembe K, Hu Y, Liang X, Brashear A, Shrestha S, Li X, Miao J, Sun X, Yang Z, Cui L.** 2015. Artemisinin resistance at the China-Myanmar border and association with mutations in the K13 propeller gene. *Antimicrob Agents Chemother* **59:**6952–6959.

50. **Wang Z, Shrestha S, Li X, Miao J, Yuan L, Cabrera M, Grube C, Yang Z, Cui L.** 2015. Prevalence of K13-propeller polymorphisms in *Plasmodium falciparum* from China-Myanmar border in 2007–2012. *Malar J* **14:**168.

51. **World Health Organization.** 2015. *Status report on artemisinin and ACT resistance—September 2015.* World Health Organization, Geneva, Switzerland. http://www.who.int/malaria/publications/atoz/status-rep-artemisinin-resistance-sept2015.pdf. Accessed 20 January 2016.

52. **Mohon AN, Alam MS, Bayih AG, Folefoc A, Shahinas D, Haque R, Pillai DR.** 2014. Mutations in *Plasmodium falciparum* K13 propeller gene from Bangladesh (2009–2013). *Malar J* **13:**431.

53. **Mishra N, Prajapati SK, Kaitholia K, Bharti RS, Srivastava B, Phookan S, Anvikar AR, Dev V, Sonal GS, Dhariwal AC, White NJ, Valecha N.** 2015. Surveillance of artemisinin resistance in *Plasmodium falciparum* in India using the kelch13 molecular marker. *Antimicrob Agents Chemother* **59:**2548–2553.

54. **Imwong M, Jindakhad T, Kunasol C, Sutawong K, Vejakama P, Dondorp AM.** 2015. An outbreak of artemisinin resistant falciparum malaria in Eastern Thailand. *Sci Rep* **5:**17412.

55. **Taylor SM, Parobek CM, DeConti DK, Kayentao K, Coulibaly SO, Greenwood BM, Tagbor H, Williams J, Bojang K, Njie F, Desai M, Kariuki S, Gutman J, Mathanga DP, Martensson A, Ngasala B, Conrad MD, Rosenthal PJ, Tshefu AK, Moormann AM, Vulule JM, Doumbo OK, Ter Kuile FO, Meshnick SR, Bailey JA, Juliano JJ.** 2015. Absence of putative artemisinin resistance mutations among *Plasmodium falciparum* in sub-Saharan Africa: a molecular epidemiologic study. *J Infect Dis* **211:**680–688.

56. **Kamau E, Campino S, Amenga-Etego L, Drury E, Ishengoma D, Johnson K, Mumba D, Kekre M, Yavo W, Mead D, Bouyou-Akotet M, Apinjoh T, Golassa L, Randrianarivelojosia M, Andagalu B, Maiga-Ascofare O, Amambua-Ngwa A, Tindana P, Ghansah A, MacInnis B, Kwiatkowski D, Djimde AA.** 2015. K13-propeller polymorphisms in *Plasmodium falciparum* parasites from sub-Saharan Africa. *J Infect Dis* **211:**1352–1355.

57. **Escobar C, Pateira S, Lobo E, Lobo L, Teodosio R, Dias F, Fernandes N, Arez AP, Varandas L, Nogueira F.** 2015. Polymorphisms in *Plasmodium falciparum* K13-propeller in Angola and Mozambique after the introduction of the ACTs. *PLoS One* **10:**e0119215.

58. **Ouattara A, Kone A, Adams M, Fofana B, Maiga AW, Hampton S, Coulibaly D, Thera MA, Diallo N, Dara A, Sagara I, Gil JP, Bjorkman A, Takala-Harrison S, Doumbo OK, Plowe CV, Djimde AA.** 2015. Polymorphisms in the K13-propeller gene in artemisinin-susceptible *Plasmodium falciparum* parasites from Bougoula-Hameau and Bandiagara, Mali. *Am J Trop Med Hyg* **92:**1202–1206.

59. **Hawkes M, Conroy AL, Opoka RO, Namasopo S, Zhong K, Liles WC, John CC, Kain KC.** 2015. Slow clearance of *Plasmodium falciparum* in severe pediatric malaria, Uganda, 2011–2013. *Emerg Infect Dis* **21:**1237–1239.

60. **Conrad MD, Bigira V, Kapisi J, Muhindo M, Kamya MR, Havlir DV, Dorsey G, Rosenthal PJ.** 2014. Polymorphisms in K13 and falcipain-2 associated with artemisinin resistance are not prevalent in *Plasmodium falciparum* isolated from Ugandan children. *PLoS One* **9:**e105690.

61. **Bayih AG, Getnet G, Alemu A, Getie S, Mohon AN, Pillai DR.** 2016. A unique *Plasmodium falciparum* K13 gene mutation in northwest Ethiopia. *Am J Trop Med Hyg* **94:**132–135.

62. **Maiga-Ascofare O, May J.** 2016. Is the A578S single-nucleotide polymorphism in K13-propeller a marker of emerging resistance to artemisinin among *Plasmodium falciparum* in Africa? *J Infect Dis* **213:**165–166.

63. **Huang B, Deng C, Yang T, Xue L, Wang Q, Huang S, Su XZ, Liu Y, Zheng S, Guan Y, Xu Q, Zhou J, Yuan J, Bacar A, Abdallah KS, Attoumane R, Mliva AM, Zhong Y, Lu F, Song J.** 2015. Polymorphisms of the artemisinin resistant marker (K13) in *Plasmodium falciparum* parasite populations of Grande Comore Island 10 years after artemisinin combination therapy. *Parasit Vectors* **8:**634.

64. **Boussaroque A, Fall B, Madamet M, Camara C, Benoit N, Fall M, Nakoulima A, Dionne P, Fall KB, Diatta B, Dieme Y, Wade B, Pradines B.** 2015. Emergence of mutations in the K13 propeller gene of *Plasmodium falciparum* Isolates from Dakar, Senegal, in 2013-2014. *Antimicrob Agents Chemother* **60:**624–627.

65. **Cooper RA, Conrad MD, Watson QD, Huezo SJ, Ninsiima H, Tumwebaze P, Nsobya SL, Rosenthal PJ.** 2015. Lack of artemisinin resistance in *Plasmodium falciparum* in Uganda based on parasitological and molecular assays. *Antimicrob Agents Chemother* **59:**5061–5064.

66. **Torrentino-Madamet M, Collet L, Lepere JF, Benoit N, Amalvict R, Menard D, Pradines B.** 2015. K13-propeller polymorphisms in *Plasmodium falciparum* isolates from patients in Mayotte in 2013 and 2014. *Antimicrob Agents Chemother* **59:**7878–7881.

67. **MalariaGEN Plasmodium falciparum Community Project.** 2016. Genomic epidemiology of artemisinin resistant malaria. *eLife* **5:** e08714.

68. **Chenet SM, Akinyi Okoth S, Huber CS, Chandrabose J, Lucchi NW, Talundzic E, Krishnalall K, Ceron N, Musset L, Macedo de Oliveira A, Venkatesan M, Rahman R, Barnwell JW, Udhayakumar V.** 2015. Independent emergence of the *Plasmodium falciparum* Kelch propeller domain mutant allele C580Y in Guyana. *J Infect Dis* doi:10.1093/infdis/jiv752.

69. **St Laurent B, Miller B, Burton TA, Amaratunga C, Men S, Sovannaroth S, Fay MP, Miotto O, Gwadz RW, Anderson JM, Fairhurst RM.** 2015. Artemisinin-resistant *Plasmodium falciparum* clinical isolates can infect diverse mosquito vectors of Southeast Asia and Africa. *Nat Commun* **6:**8614.

70. **Molina-Cruz A, Garver LS, Alabaster A, Bangiolo L, Haile A, Winikor J, Ortega C, van Schaijk BC, Sauerwein RW, Taylor-Salmon E, Barillas-Mury C.** 2013. The human malaria parasite Pfs47 gene mediates evasion of the mosquito immune system. *Science* **340:**984–987.

71. **Pukrittayakamee S, Chotivanich K, Chantra A, Clemens R, Looareesuwan S, White NJ.** 2004. Activities of artesunate and primaquine against asexual- and sexual-stage parasites in falciparum malaria. *Antimicrob Agents Chemother* **48:**1329–1334.

72. **Okell LC, Drakeley CJ, Ghani AC, Bousema T, Sutherland CJ.** 2008. Reduction of transmission from malaria patients by artemisinin combination therapies: a pooled analysis of six randomized trials. *Malar J* **7:**125.

73. **White NJ.** 2013. Primaquine to prevent transmission of falciparum malaria. *Lancet Infect Dis* **13:**175–181.

74. **World Health Organization.** 2012. *Updated WHO Policy Recommendation (October 2012): single dose primaquine as a gametocytocide in* Plasmodium falciparum *malaria.* World Health Organization, Geneva, Switzerland. http://www.who.int/malaria/pq_updated_policy_recommendation_en_102012.pdf?ua=1. Accessed 20 January 2016.

75. **Plouffe DM, Wree M, Du AY, Meister S, Li F, Patra K, Lubar A, Okitsu SL, Flannery EL, Kato N, Tanaseichuk O, Comer E, Zhou B, Kuhen K, Zhou Y, Leroy D, Schreiber SL, Scherer CA, Vinetz J, Winzeler EA.** 2015. High-throughput assay and discovery of small molecules that interrupt malaria transmission. *Cell Host Microbe* doi:10.1016/j.chom.2015.12.001.

76. **Dondorp AM, Fairhurst RM, Slutsker L, Macarthur JR, Breman JG, Guerin PJ, Wellems TE, Ringwald P, Newman RD, Plowe CV.** 2011. The threat of artemisinin-resistant malaria. *N Engl J Med* **365:**1073–1075.

77. **Leang R, Barrette A, Bouth DM, Menard D, Abdur R, Duong S, Ringwald P.** 2013. Efficacy of dihydroartemisinin-piperaquine for treatment of uncomplicated *Plasmodium falciparum* and *Plasmodium vivax* in Cambodia, 2008 to 2010. *Antimicrob Agents Chemother* **57:**818–826.

78. **Chaorattanakawee S, Saunders DL, Sea D, Chanarat N, Yingyuen K, Sundrakes S, Saingam P, Buathong N, Sriwichai S, Chann S, Se Y, Yom Y, Heng TK, Kong N, Kuntawunginn W, Tangthongchaiwiriya K, Jacob C, Takala-Harrison S, Plowe C, Lin JT, Chuor CM, Prom S, Tyner SD, Gosi P, Teja-Isavadharm P, Lon C, Lanteri CA.** 2015. Ex vivo drug susceptibility and molecular profiling of clinical *Plasmodium falciparum* isolates from Cambodia in 2008–2013 suggest emerging piperaquine resistance. *Antimicrob Agents Chemother* doi:10.1128/AAC.00366-15.

79. **Duru V, Khim N, Leang R, Kim S, Domergue A, Kloeung N, Ke S, Chy S, Eam R, Khean C, Loch K, Ken M, Lek D, Beghain J, Ariey F, Guerin PJ, Huy R, Mercereau-Puijalon O, Witkowski B, Menard D.** 2015. *Plasmodium falciparum* dihydroartemisinin-piperaquine failures in Cambodia are associated with mutant K13 parasites presenting high survival rates in novel piperaquine in vitro assays: retrospective and prospective investigations. *BMC Med* **13:**305.

80. **Phyo AP, Jittamala P, Nosten FH, Pukrittayakamee S, Imwong M, White NJ, Duparc S, Macintyre F, Baker M, Mohrle JJ.** 2016. Antimalarial activity of artefenomel (OZ439), a novel synthetic antimalarial endoperoxide, in patients with *Plasmodium falciparum* and *Plasmodium vivax* malaria: an open-label phase 2 trial. *Lancet Infect Dis* **16:**61–69.

81. **White NJ, Pukrittayakamee S, Phyo AP, Rueangweerayut R, Nosten F, Jittamala P, Jeeyapant A, Jain JP, Lefevre G, Li R, Magnusson B, Diagana TT, Leong FJ.** 2014. Spiroindolone KAE609 for falciparum and vivax malaria. *N Engl J Med* **371:**403–410.

82. **Leong FJ, Zhao R, Zeng S, Magnusson B, Diagana TT, Pertel P.** 2014. A first-in-human randomized, double-blind, placebo-controlled, single- and multiple-ascending oral dose study of novel Imidazolopiperazine KAF156 to assess its safety, tolerability, and pharmacokinetics in healthy adult volunteers. *Antimicrob Agents Chemother* **58:**6437–6443.

83. **Price RN, Uhlemann AC, Brockman A, McGready R, Ashley E, Phaipun L, Patel R, Laing K, Looareesuwan S, White NJ, Nosten F, Krishna S.** 2004. Mefloquine resistance in *Plasmodium falciparum* and increased pfmdr1 gene copy number. *Lancet* **364:**438–447.

84. **Lim P, Dek D, Try V, Sreng S, Suon S, Fairhurst RM.** 2015. Decreasing pfmdr1 copy number suggests that *Plasmodium falciparum* in western Cambodia is regaining in vitro susceptibility to mefloquine. *Antimicrob Agents Chemother* **59:**2934–2937.

85. **Venkatesan M, Gadalla NB, Stepniewska K, Dahal P, Nsanzabana C, Moriera C, Price RN, Martensson A, Rosenthal PJ, Dorsey G, Sutherland CJ, Guerin P, Davis TM, Menard D, Adam I, Ademowo G, Arze C, Baliraine FN, Berens-Riha N, Bjorkman A, Borrmann S, Checchi F, Desai M, Dhorda M, Djimde AA, El-Sayed BB, Eshetu T, Eyase F, Falade C, Faucher JF, Froberg G, Grivoyannis A, Hamour S, Houze S, Johnson J, Kamugisha E, Kariuki S, Kiechel JR, Kironde F, Kofoed PE, LeBras J, Malmberg M, Mwai L, Ngasala B, Nosten F, Nsobya SL, Nzila A, Oguike M, Otienoburu SD, Ogutu B, Ouédraogo JB, Piola P, Rombo L, Schramm B, Somé AF, Thwing J, Ursing J, Wong RP, Zeynudin A, Zongo I, Plowe CV, Sibley CH, WWARN AL, ASAQ Molecular Marker Study Group.** 2014. Polymorphisms in *Plasmodium falciparum* chloroquine resistance transporter and multidrug resistance 1 genes: parasite risk factors that affect treatment outcomes for *P. falciparum* malaria after artemether-lumefantrine and artesunate-amodiaquine. *Am J Trop Med Hyg* **91:**833–843.

86. **World Health Organization.** 2013. *Emergency Response to Artemisinin Resistance in the Greater Mekong Subregion. Regional Framework for Action 2013–2015.* World Health Organization, Geneva, Switzerland. http://apps.who.int/iris/bitstream/10665/79940/1/9789241505321_eng.pdf. Accessed 8 January 2016.

87. **World Health Organization.** 2015. *Strategy for malaria elimination in the Greater Mekong subregion (2015–2030).* World Health Organization. Geneva, Switzerland. http://www.who.int/malaria/areas/greater_mekong/consultation-elimination-strategy/en/. Accessed 8 January 2016.

88. **Fairhurst RM.** 2015. Understanding artemisinin-resistant malaria: what a difference a year makes. *Curr Opin Infect Dis* **28:**417–425.

Index

16S ribosomal RNA, *Bordetella holmesii*, 246
Acellular vaccines, *Bordetella pertussis*, 322
Acute flaccid myelitis (AFM)
  enterovirus-D68, 110–112, 111, 113
  West Nile virus-associated, 180–181, 184–186, 187, 189
Acute flaccid paralysis, Chikungunya virus (CHIKV), 148
Ad26.ZEBOV vaccine, Ebola virus disease, 62
Advisory Committee on Immunization Practices (ACIP)
  Bordetella pertussis, 322–326
  measles, 132–133, 137
Aedes aegypti mosquitoes
  Chikungunya virus, 143–146, 150
  Zika virus, 165, 167, 170
Aedes albopictus mosquitoes, 144, 150, 170
Aedes apicoargenteus, 167
Aedes furcifer, 167
Aedes luteocephalus, 167
Aedes [Stegomyia] africana, Zika virus, 163, 167
Aedes vittatus, 167
Africa, *see also* West Africa
  Clostridium difficile infection (CDI), 271–272
  nontyphoidal *Salmonella* (NTS) infection, 341–342, 350–351
  Zika virus, 163–164, 166–168, 170
AIDS (acquired immunodeficiency syndrome), *see* HIV/AIDS
American Academy of Pediatrics, 324
American Society for Microbiology, 46
Amphibian fungal disease, *see also Batrachochytrium dendrobatidis*; Chytridiomycosis
  Batrachochytrium dendrobatidis and amphibian population, 387–388
  global amphibian decline, 385, 401
  global distribution map, 391
Amphotericin B, fungal infections, 368
Anaplasma capra, 301–302
Anaplasmataceae family, 301, 302, 304
Anaplasmosis, 295, 301–302
Animal models
  Chikungunya virus (CHIKV), 147, 150, 153, 155
  Middle East respiratory syndrome (MERS), 87–88

Animal reservoir
  Bordetella holmesii, 248
  Middle East respiratory syndrome (MERS), 84–85
Anopheles mosquitoes, artemisinin-resistant parasites, 409, 415, 417–419
Antibacterial agents, *Clostridium difficile* infection (CDI), 276–278
Antibiotics
  Bordetella holmesii, 246–248
  Bordetella pertussis, 319–320
  Cronobacter infection, 258–259
Antibodies
  Chikungunya virus (CHIKV), 153–154
  Clostridium difficile infection (CDI), 278
  Ebola virus disease (EVD), 56–58
  medical countermeasures, 56–58
Antifungal chemotherapy, amphibian, 395
Antimalarials, *see also* Artemisinin-resistant *Plasmodium falciparum* malaria
  parasite clearance, 410–411, 412
Antimicrobial resistance
  Neisseria gonorrhoeae, 215–220
  nontyphoidal *Salmonella* (NTS), 341–343, 345, 348–350
  World Health Organization, 208, 221
Antimicrobials
  Bordetella pertussis, 319–320
  Global Gonococcal Antimicrobial Surveillance Programme (Global GASP), 221–222
  Gonococcal Isolate Surveillance Project (GISP) testing panel, 223–224
  gonorrhea treatment, 226–228
Antitoxin, *Clostridium difficile* infection (CDI), 278–279
Antivirals
  Chikungunya virus (CHIKV), 152–155
  enterovirus, 113–114
  host-targeted, for CHIKV, 154–155
  influenza viruses, 126, 128, 129
  Middle East respiratory syndrome coronavirus (MERS-CoV), 93
  Virus-targeted, for CHIKV, 153
Arabian Peninsula, Middle East respiratory syndrome (MERS), 75, 77, 82–83, 86, 90, 94

Arboviruses, *see also* West Nile virus (WNV)
arthropod-borne viruses, 175, 176
Argasidae (soft ticks), 295
Artemisinin-resistant *Plasmodium falciparum* malaria
artemisinin and artemisinin combination therapies (ACT), 409–410
artemisinin resistance, 411–419
clinical impact of artemisinin resistance, 419–421
clinical phenotype, 411–412
failures with ACTs, 421–422
future research, 422
genetic determinants, 413–415
K13-propeller mutations, 418
laboratory phenotype, 412–413
molecular epidemiology, 416–417
molecular mechanisms, 415–416
mosquito transmission, 417–419
parasite clearance by artemisinins and antimalarials, 412
parasite clearance half-life, 410–411
P. falciparum kelch13 protein, 414
redefining artemisinin resistance, 419
treatment options, 420
Asia, *Clostridium difficile* infection (CDI), 268–271
Assessment-Feedback-Incentives-eXchange of information (AFIX) system, 133
Australia
Clostridium difficile infection (CDI), 270–271
treatments for uncomplicated *Neisseria gonorrhoeae* infections, 221
Automated microbial identification devices, *Bordetella holmesii*, 246
AVI Biopharma (Sarepta) molecules, Ebola virus disease, 58–59
Azoles, fungal infections, 370

Bacteremia, *Bordetella holmesii*, 243–244, 247
Bacteriotherapy, *Clostridium difficile* infection (CDI), 279–281
Batrachochytrium dendrobatidis
amphibian populations, 387–388
anthropogenic-assisted spread, 392, 393
detection of, infection *vs.* disease, 387
detection of amphibian chytrid fungus, 389
discovery of, 385–386
emergence of, and global amphibian decline, 388–389
global distribution, 389
global origin of, 390–391
infection with, 386
modes of dispersal, 392–394
multiple strains of, 389–390
nonanthropogenic-assisted spread, 393–394
questions and uncertainties, 399
timeline of emergence, 391–392
Batrachochytrium dendrobatidis dispersal

anthropogenic-assisted spread, 392–393
environmental forces, 393–394
fomites, 393
international amphibian trade, 392
international nonamphibian trade, 393
nonanthropogenic-assisted spread, 393–394
wildlife, 393
Batrachochytrium dendrobatidis mitigation
amphibian antifungal chemotherapy, 395
amphibian probiotics, 396
amphibian selective breeding for resistance, 396–397
amphibian temperature and desiccation, 395
amphibian vaccination, 395–396
attempts and opportunities, 394–399
government intervention, 394
habitat biological control, 398
habitat-level, 397–399
habitat physical modification, 398–399
habitat site-level treatment, 397–398
mitigation of *B. dendrobatidis*'s impact, 394–397
Batrachochytrium salamandrivorans, 400–401
Bat white nose syndrome, 399–400
Bavarian Nordic, 62
BCX4430 (Biocryst), Ebola virus disease, 59
Biomedical Advanced Research and Development Authority (BARDA), 57, 59, 61
Bordetella bronchiseptica, 245
biochemical characteristics, 240, 241
infections, 317
Bordetella genus, 239
biochemical characteristics, 240, 241
infections, 314–317
organism, 312–314
Bordetella holmesii, 239–240
16S ribosomal RNA sequencing, 246
antibiotic prophylaxis, 248
automated microbial identification devices, 246
bacteremia, 243–244, 247
biochemical characteristics, 240, 241
clinical features, 243–244
colonies on sheep blood agar plate, 241
culture, 245
diagnosis, 244–246
epidemiology, 248–249
genome, 240–241
genome map, 242
gram stain of, 240
incidence, 248–249
infections, 317
invasive infections, 244, 247
loop-mediated isothermal amplification assay, 245–246
management, 248
microbiology, 240–243
morphological characteristics, 240
pathogenic factors, 242–243

pertussis-like respiratory infections, 243
polymerase chain reaction (PCR), 245
prevalence, 248–249
prevention, 247–248
reservoir, 248
respiratory infections, 247
spectrometry, 246
systematic misidentification as *B. pertussis*, 239, 248, 249
transmission, 248
treatment, 246–247
vaccination, 247–248
Bordetella parapertussis
biochemical characteristics, 240, 241
infections, 316–317
Bordetella pertussis
antibiotics, 319–320
antimicrobial treatment, 320
biochemical characteristics, 240, 241
clinical syndrome, 314–316
diagnosis, 318–319
differential diagnosis, 318
epidemiology, 317–318
genome map, 242
immunization, 321–324
immunization schedule, recommendations and contraindications, 322–324
infections, 314–316
pathogenesis, 313–314
pathogenic factors, 242–243
pertussis, 311–312
polymerase chain reaction (PCR), 245
post-exposure prophylaxis, 320
prevention, 321–324
respiratory infection, 243, 247
resurgence of pertussis, 324–326
supportive care, 320–321
systematic misidentification of *B. holmesii* as, 239, 248, 249
treatment, 319–321
vaccines, 321–324
virulence factors, 313–314
Borrelioses, 295, 302–304
Brincidofovir, Ebola virus disease, 20, 21
Bundibugyo ebolavirus, 41

California, measles, 136–139
Cambodia, artemisinin-resistant *Plasmodium falciparum* malaria, 411, 413–414, 416–417, 420
Canada
treatments for uncomplicated *Neisseria gonorrhoeae* infections, 221
West Nile virus (WNV), 177
Candidatus Neoehrlichia mikurensis (*C. N. mikurensis*), 299, 301, 302
Carbapenemases

clinical context of, 202–203
detection challenges, 205–206
epidemiologies of major, 203, 205
global epidemiology of KPC, OXA–48 and NDM, 204
impact of genetic context on mobility, 206–208
KPC (*Klebsiella pneumoniae* carbapenemase), 202, 203, 208
NDM (New Delhi metallo-β-lactamase), 202, 203, 205, 208
OXA-48-like (oxacillinase-48-like), 202, 203, 205, 207–208
schematic of mechanisms of mobility, 207
Caribbean, Chikungunya virus (CHIKV), 144–145
Case fatality rate (CFR), Ebola virus disease, 3–4, 10, 13, 15, 19
Case management, Ebola virus disease, 26
CDC (Centers for Disease Control and Prevention), 6, 17, 24
Bordetella holmesii, 239
Ebola virus disease, 6, 17, 24, 47
enterovirus-D68, 106–107
fungal infections, 359–360
Gonococcal Isolate Surveillance Project (GISP), 222–225
gonorrhea as public health concern, 214–215
Sexually Transmitted Diseases (STD) Treatment Guidelines, 222–223
West Nile virus (WNV), 178, 179
CDI, *see Clostridium difficile* infection (CDI)
Cephalosporin resistance, *Neisseria gonorrhoeae*, 216, 219–220
ChAd3-EBOZ vaccine, Ebola virus disease, 61–62
Chikungunya virus (CHIKV)
Aedes aegypti mosquitoes, 143–146, 150
antibody therapies, 153–154
antivirals against, 152–155
CHIKV disease, 146–148
emergence, 143–146
host-targeted antivirals, 154–155
joint and muscle disease, 146–148
mortality associated with infection, 148
neurologic involvement, 148
reemergence, 143–146, 155
therapeutics, 148–155
therapies for chronic CHIKV disease, 155
treating acute CHIKV disease, 152–153
vaccines, 148, 149–152
virus-targeted antivirals, 153
Children
nontyphoidal *Salmonella* (NTS) infection, 343–344
pediatric West Nile virus infection, 186–187
Children's Mercy Hospital, enterovirus-D68, 106, 114–115

Chytridiomycosis, *see also Batrachochytrium dendrobatidis*
    Batrachochytrium dendrobatidis infection, 386
    detection of *B. dendrobatidis* infection *vs.* disease, 387
    global emergence of, 390–391, 401–402
    resistance in nature, 386–387
    salamander fungus, 400–401
    susceptibility to, 397
    World Organization for Animal Health (OIE), 392
    yellow-legged frog (*Rana muscosa*), 388, 396
Clinical and Laboratory and Standards Institute (CLSI)
    carbapenemase detection, 205
    Gonococcal Isolate Surveillance Project (GISP) antimicrobial testing, 223–224
Clostridium difficile infection (CDI)
    Africa, 271–272
    antibacterial agents, 276–278
    antitoxin, 278–279
    Asia, 268–271
    Australia, 270–271
    bacteriotherapy, 279–281
    clinical presentation, 272–274
    colectomy, 282
    diagnosis, 274–276
    diverting loop ileostomy with lavage, 282
    East Asia, 268–269
    epidemiology, 266–272
    Europe, 267
    fecal microbiota transplant, 279–280
    fidaxomicin, 277–278
    immunoglobulin (IG), 279
    Latin America, 267–268
    management, 276–283
    metronidazole, 276–277
    monoclonal antibodies, 278
    mortality, 274
    nontoxigenic *C. difficile* (NTCD), 281
    North America, 267
    pathophysiology, 265–266
    probiotics, 280–281
    recurrent disease, 274
    risk factors, 272–273
    severity of disease, 273–274
    South Asia, 270
    Southeast Asia, 269–270
    surgical interventions, 281–282
    tolevamer, 278–279
    vaccine, 282–283
    vancomycin, 277
Coccidioides immitis, geographic distribution, 380, 381
Coccidioides posadasii, 375
Coccidioidomycosis
    geographic range, 378–380
    map of United States and Mexico, 379

    range of endemicity in U.S., 378–380
    in soil, 380–381
Colectomy, *Clostridium difficile* infection (CDI), 282
Community preparedness, emerging infectious diseases, 46–48
Convalescent blood and plasma, Ebola virus disease, 20, 57–58
Coronavirus
    antivirals, 93
    human coronavirus-Erasmus Medical Center (HCoV-EMC), 73, 76
    MERS (Middle East respiratory syndrome), 76, 78–80
    MERS-CoV case definition, 89, 90, 91
    severe acute respiratory syndrome (SARS), 75
Countermeasures, *see* Medical countermeasures (MCMs)
Cronobacter genus, 255–256
    antibiotic susceptibility, 258–259
    classification, 256
    clinical associations, 257–258
    environmental sources, 256–257
    epidemiology, 256–257
    pathogenesis, 258
    virulence, 258
Crucell subsidiary (Johnson & Johnson), 62
Cryptococcus gattii, 375, 381
    emergence in North America, 376–378
Culex pipiens, West Nile virus (WNV), 176
Culex quinquefasciatus, West Nile virus (WNV), 176
Culex tarsalis, West Nile virus (WNV), 176
Culture, *Bordetella holmesii*, 245

Disney amusement parks, measles, 132, 137, 139
Diverting loop ileostomy with lavage, *Clostridium difficile* infection (CDI), 282
Drug Quality and Security Act (2013), 371
DTaP vaccine (diphtheria-tetanus toxoids-acellular pertussis), *Bordetella pertussis*, 311–313, 322–324
DTP vaccine (diphtheria-tetanus-pertussis), *Bordetella pertussis*, 311–312, 322, 324

East Asia, *Clostridium difficile* infection (CDI), 268–269
Ebola virus disease (EVD)
    case fatality rate (CFR), 3–4, 10, 13, 15, 19
    case management, 26
    clinical management, 13–14
    clinical presentation, 12–13
    Ebola treatment units (ETUs), 6, 8, 10–11, 13, 17–18, 21–22, 24, 26
    experimental therapeutics, 18–22, 41–42
    experimental vaccines, 22–23, 42–43
    factors contributing to 2013–2015 outbreak, 47
    field surveillance, 26
    funding for global preparedness and response, 11

future challenges, 26–27
health-care worker infections, 16–18
infection prevention and control, 5, 16–18
information technology, 26
international community response, 5–6
laboratory-confirmed outbreaks (1976–2016), 3–4
labor problem, 6–8
map of 2013–2016 outbreak, 2
medical countermeasure development, 54–62
new diagnostic methods, 23–26
patient bed capacity and requirements, 8
patient care, 40–41
personal protective equipment (PPE), 5, 16–18, 44–46
population density, 8–9
registered clinical trials, 20
resource-poor countries, 5
response to control measures, 8–11
sequelae, virus persistence and recrudescence, 14–16
travel frequency, 8–9
virus persistence after onset, 16
West Africa 2013 outbreak, 1–2, 5–12
Ehrlichia muris-like (EML), 299, 301
Ehrlichioses, 295, 301
Elderly patients, *Cronobacter* spp., 255–259
Enterobacteriaceae, see also Carbapenemases
carbapenem-resistant, 201–202
clinical context of carbapenemase enzymes, 202–203
Cronobacter as member, 255
epidemiologies of carbapenemases, 203, 205
mechanisms of mobility of carbapenemase genes in, 206–208
Enteroviruses, 105
biological characteristics, 105–106
pathogenesis, 105–106
Environmental Protection Agency (EPA), 46, 170
Epidemiology
Bordetella holmesii, 248–249
Bordetella pertussis, 317–318
changing, in United States, 136–138
Clostridium difficile infection (CDI), 266–272
Coccidioides species, 378
Cronobacter spp., 256–257
Ebola virus disease (EVD), 7, 15, 25–27
enterovirus-D68 (EV-D68), 106–108, 109
fungal infections, 360–362
KPC (*Klebsiella pneumoniae* carbapenemase), 203, 204
Middle East respiratory syndrome coronavirus (MERS-CoV), 75, 82–85, 90, 93–94
NDM (New Delhi metallo-β-lactamase), 204, 205
nontyphoidal *Salmonella* (NTS) disease, 342
OXA-48-like (oxacillinase), 203, 204, 207–208
Plasmodium falciparum mutations, 416–417
West Nile virus (WNV), 177, 179

WNV infection in humans, 180–181
Zika virus, 164, 165–166, 170
Escherichia coli, 202, 206–208
Europe
Clostridium difficile infection (CDI), 267
treatments for uncomplicated *Neisseria gonorrhoeae* infections, 221
West Nile virus (WNV), 176–177, 179–180
EVD, *see* Ebola virus disease (EVD)
EV-D68 (enterovirus-D68), 106
acute flaccid myelitis, 110–112, 113, 114
clinical features, 108, 110–112
diagnostics, 112–113
epidemiology, 106–108, 109
lessons learned from 2014 outbreak, 114–115
potential neurologic disease, 110–112
respiratory disease, 108, 110, 113
treatment and prevention, 113–114
Exophiala dermatitidis, 361
Experimental therapeutics, Ebola virus disease (EVD), 18–22, 41–42
Experimental vaccines, Ebola virus disease, 22–23
Exserohilum rostratum, see also Fungal infections
azoles for treatment, 370
cerebrospinal fluid (CSF), 366, 367
growth in culture, 366
histopathology, 366
infection, 359–360, 371
mycology, 362
voriconazole, 368

Favipiravir (Toyama Chemical), Ebola virus disease, 20, 21, 59
Fecal microbiota transplant, *Clostridium difficile* infection (CDI), 279–280
Fidaxomicin, *Clostridium difficile* infection (CDI), 277–278
Fire salamanders, 400–401
Flavivirus, see Zika virus
Fluoroquinolone resistance, *Neisseria gonorrhoeae*, 216, 218
Food and Drug Administration (FDA)
carbapenemase detection, 205
fungal infections, 360, 371
Fungal infections
amphotericin B, 368
azoles, 370
cerebrospinal fluid (CSF) (1,3) beta-D-glucan, 367
clinical aspects, 363–366
Coccidioides immitis, 378–381
contaminated methylprednisolone, 359
Cryptococcus gattii, 376–378
culture, 366
diagnosis, 366–367
epidemiology, 360–362
histopathology, 366–367
long-term outcomes, 365–366

Fungal infections (*continued*)
  meningitis, 363–364
  mycological aspects, 362
  peripheral osteoarticular infections, 365
  polymerase chain reaction (PCR), 366
  recurrence risk, 370–371
  spinal and paraspinal infections, 364–365
  treatment, 367–370
  voriconazole, 368–370
Fungal meningitis, 359–362, 363–364, 371

Gabon, Ebola virus disease outbreaks, 3–4
GlaxoSmithKline (GSK), 62
Global Gonococcal Antimicrobial Surveillance
  Programme (Global GASP), 221–222
Gonococcal Isolate Surveillance Project (GISP),
  222–225
Gonorrhea, *see also Neisseria gonorrhoeae*
  antimicrobials for treating, 226
  current treatment for, 225–226
  future treatments for, 226–228
  international responses to difficult-to-treat or
    untreatable, 220–222
  Neisseria gonorrhoeae and, 213–215
  public health concern, 214–215, 228
GS-5734 (Gilead), Ebola virus disease, 60
Guinea
  bush taxis in, 10
  Ebola virus disease, 1, 4, 5–10, 15, 19–23, 25
  population density and size, 9

H1N1 influenza virus, 5, 46, 124–125, 128
H2N2 influenza virus, 124, 125
H3N2 influenza virus, 125, 125, 127
Habitat treatment, *Batrachochytrium dendrobatidis*
  eradication, 397–399
Haemophilus influenzae, 342
Haemophilus influenzae type b, 133
Hemagglutinin (HA), influenza A virus, 122, 126–127
HIV/AIDS
  Clostridium difficile infection (CDI), 272, 280
  Cryptococcus gattii, 376
  Ebola virus, 2, 11, 15
  gonorrhea, 214, 221, 224
  nontyphoidal *Salmonella*, 342–346, 349–351
  respiratory infections, 317
Hospital preparedness, emerging infectious
  diseases, 46–48
Human coronavirus-Erasmus Medical Center
  (HCoV-EMC), 73, 76
Human immunodeficiency virus, *see* HIV/AIDS

Immune response, Middle East respiratory
  syndrome coronavirus (MERS-CoV), 92
Immunization, *see also* Vaccination; Vaccines
  Advisory Committee on Immunization Practices
    (ACIP), 132–133, 137, 322–326

Bordetella pertussis, 321–324
B. pertussis schedule, recommendations and
  contraindications, 322–324
measles program, 139–140
measles surveys, 133
National Immunization Survey, 133, 136
Immunoglobulin (IG), *Clostridium difficile* infection
  (CDI), 279
Infection control
  Ebola virus disease (EVD), 5, 16–18
  Middle East respiratory syndrome (MERS),
    85–86
Infectious diseases
  Ebola virus disease, 39–40, 48–49
  experimental therapeutics, 41–42
  hospital and community preparedness for
    emerging, 46–48
  infection control, 43–46
  patient care, 40–41
  schematic of Serious Communicable Diseases
    Unit (SCDU), 45
  vaccines, 42–43
Infectious Diseases Society of America (IDSA),
  Clostridium difficile infection (CDI),
  273–275
Influenza A virus
  adaptation, 125
  biology, 122–123
  ecology, 123–124
  gene functions, 122
  impact of adaptation on pathogenicity,
    126–128
  life cycle in cells, 123
  neuraminidase (NA), 127
  non-structured protein 1 (NS–1), 128
  pandemics, 124–125
  pandemic timeline, 125
  PB1-F2 protein of, 127–128
  rapid evolution, 125–126
Influenza viruses
  biology and ecology of, 121–124
  pandemic threat, 121, 128–129
International Committee on the Taxonomy of
  Viruses, 76, 106
International community, response to Ebola virus
  disease, 5–6
Invasive infections
  Bordetella holmesii, 244, 247
  nontyphoidal *Salmonella* (NTS) in adults, 344
  NTS infection in children, 343–344
  West Nile neuroinvasive disease, 179, 182–186
Itraconazole, amphibian treatment, 395, 396, 397
Ixodidae (hard ticks), 295, 297, 300–303

Japanese encephalitis, 175, 189–190
Joint disease, Chikungunya virus (CHIKV),
  146–148

Kawasaki's disease, 138
Klebsiella pneumoniae, 201, 203, 206–208
Kunjin virus, 175, 179–180

Lacey Act, 394, 401
Laos, artemisinin-resistant *Plasmodium falciparum*
    malaria, 411, 416, 420
Latin America, *Clostridium difficile* infection (CDI),
    267–268
Liberia, Ebola virus disease, 1, 4–7, 8–11, 13–14, 23, 25
Loop-mediated isothermal amplification assay,
    Bordetella holmesii, 245–246

MabWorks, 57
Macrolides
    Bordetella holmesii, 246–248
    Neisseria gonorrhoeae, 216, 218–219
Malaria, *see also* Artemisinin-resistant *Plasmodium*
    falciparum malaria
    artemisinin resistance, 411–419
    artemisinins and combination therapies, 409–410
    DHA-piperaquine treatment, 420–421
    nontyphoidal *Salmonella* (NTS) infection,
        343–344, 350
    parasite clearance half-life, 410–411
Marburg virus, 53–54, 59, 62, 167
Matrix-assisted laser desorption ionization-time-of-
    flight mass spectrometry (MALDI-TOF
    MS), *Bordetella holmesii*, 246
Measles
    characteristics of recent outbreaks, 136
    comparing key variables, 137
    epidemiological context, 138–139
    immunization program, 139–140
    immunization surveys, 133
    policy changes, 139
    public opinion, 139
    road to elimination, 132–133
    safety of vaccines, 135–136
    transmission, 131–132
    United States (1962–2014), 132
    United States after elimination of, 133–135
Measles-mumps-rubella (MMR) vaccine, 131–133,
    135–137, 139
Medical countermeasures (MCMs)
    Ad26.ZEBOV (Crucell/Johnson & Johnson), 62
    antibodies, 56–58
    AVI–7537, AVI–7539 and AVI–6002 (Sarepta),
        58–59
    BCX4430 (Biocryst), 59
    ChAd3-EBOZ, 61–62
    convalescent blood and plasma, 57–58
    development during 2014–2015 epidemic, 54–62
    emerging infectious diseases, 62–63
    favipiravir (Toyama Chemical), 59
    GS-5734 (Gilead), 60
    MIL-77, 57

MVA-BN Filo (Bavarian Nordic), 62
    safety and efficacy of, 64–65
    supportive care, 55
    therapeutics, 56–60
    TKM-Ebola and TKM-Ebola-Guinea, 60
    vaccines, 60–62
    VSV-ZEBOV, 60–61
    ZMapp, 56–57
Meningitis
    fungal infections, 359–362, 363–364, 371
    neonatal, and *Cronobacter* spp., 255, 257–259
    West Nile meningitis (WNM), 181, 182–183, 188
Merck, 61, 62
MERS, *see* Middle East respiratory syndrome
    (MERS)
Methylprednisolone, *see also* Fungal infections
    compounded drugs, 360, 370
    contaminated, 359–360, 362, 365
    fungal infections associated with contaminated,
        361
Metronidazole, *Clostridium difficile* infection (CDI),
    276–277
Mexico, coccidioidomycosis, 379
Middle East respiratory syndrome (MERS), 46
    animal models, 87–88
    animal reservoir, 84–85
    antivirals, 93
    case definition for MERS-CoV, 89, 90, 91
    cases of MERS coronavirus (MERS-CoV), 76
    characteristics of, 74
    chronology of key events, 75
    clinical features, 75–76
    clinical findings, 88–89
    clinical management, 93
    comparison to severe acute respiratory syndrome
        (SARS), 74
    first patients, 73, 75
    global map of countries with, 77
    immune response, 92
    infection control recommendations for
        healthcare facilities, 85–86
    MERS-CoV, 78–80
    outbreak of, 76–78
    preventing travel-associated transmission, 86–87
    risk factors, 80–82
    transmission, 82–84
    vaccines, 93–94
    virologic diagnosis, 89–92
MIL-77 (MabWorks), Ebola virus disease, 57
Monoclonal antibodies, *Clostridium difficile*
    infection (CDI), 278
Mortality, *Clostridium difficile* infection (CDI), 274
Muscle disease, Chikungunya virus (CHIKV),
    146–148
MVA-BN Filo vaccine, Ebola virus disease, 62
Myanmar, artemisinin-resistant *Plasmodium*
    falciparum malaria, 411, 416–417, 420

National Ebola Training and Education Center, 48
National Immunization Survey, 133, 136
National Notifiable Disease Surveillance System, 312
Necrotizing enterocolitis (NEC), *Cronobacter* spp., 255, 257, 259
Neisseria gonorrhoeae, see also Gonorrhea
  antimicrobial resistance in, 215–220
  cephalosporin resistance, 216, 219–220
  fluoroquinolone resistance, 216, 218
  Gonococcal Isolate Surveillance Project (GISP), 222–225
  gonorrhea and, 213–215
  key components of WHO global action plan, 221
  macrolide resistance, 216, 218–219
  mechanisms of antimicrobial resistance, 215
  penicillin resistance, 216, 216–217
  prevalence of resistance in, 225
  spectinomycin resistance, 216, 217–218
  sulfonamide resistance, 215–216
  tetracycline resistance, 216, 217
  treatments for uncomplicated, 221
Neonatal diseases, *Cronobacter* spp., 255–258
Neonatal meningitis, *Cronobacter* spp., 255, 257–259
Neurologic disease, enterovirus-D68 (EV-D68), 110–112, 113
NewLink Genetics, 61
Nontoxigenic *Clostridium difficile* (NTCD), 281
Nontyphoidal *Salmonella* (NTS), 341–343
  antimicrobial resistance, 341–343, 345, 348–350
  clinical features, 343–344
  diagnosis, 342
  interventions, 350–351
  invasive NTS infection in adults, 344
  invasive NTS infection in children, 343–344
  microbiology, 344–346
  risk factors, 343–344
  sources, 346–348
  transmission, 346–348
  vaccines, 350–351
North America
  Clostridium difficile infection (CDI), 267
  Cryptococcus gattii, 376–378

Ophidiomyces ophiodiicola, 400

Pan American Health Organization (PAHO), 135, 165
Pandemics
  influenza A virus, 124–126
  influenza virus threat, 121, 128–129
  rapid evolution, 125–126
  timeline for influenza A strains, 125
Paraspinal infections, fungal, 364–365
Patient care, Ebola virus disease, 40–41
PCR, *see* Polymerase chain reaction (PCR)
Penicillin resistance, *Neisseria gonorrhoeae*, 216–217

Peripheral osteoarticular infections, 365
Pertussis, 311–312, *see also Bordetella pertussis*
  reported cases, 312
  resurgence, 324–326
Plasmodium falciparum, see also Artemisinin-resistant *Plasmodium falciparum* malaria
  mechanisms of artemisinin sensitivity and resistance, 415–416
  treatment failures, 421–422
Polymerase chain reaction (PCR)
  Bordetella holmesii, 245
  Clostridium difficile infection (CDI), 269–271, 274–276
  Ebola virus disease, 24–26
  fungus detection, 366
Pregnancy, Zika virus, 167–168, 170
Pregnancy Risk Assessment Monitoring System, 325
Probiotics
  amphibian, 396
  Clostridium difficile infection (CDI), 280–281
Profectus BioSciences, 62
Program for Monitoring Emerging Diseases (ProMED), 73, 75
Prophylaxis
  Bordetella pertussis, 320
  Bordetella holmesii, 248
  Zika virus, 170
Pseudogymnoascus destructans, 399–400
Pseudomembranous colitis (PMC)
  clinical presentation, 272–273
  Clostridium difficile infection (CDI), 265–266
  fecal microbiota transplant (FMT), 279
  pathology of, 266
  South Korea, 269
  vancomycin, 277
Public Health Agency of Canada, 56, 61, 107

Registered clinical trials, Ebola virus disease, 20
Repellents, West Nile virus (WNV), 190
Republic of Korea, Middle East respiratory syndrome (MERS), 75, 77, 80–81, 83, 94
Respiratory disease, enterovirus-D68, 108, 110, 113
Respiratory infections, *Bordetella holmesii*, 243, 247
Reverse transcription PCR (RT–PCR)
  Middle East respiratory syndrome coronavirus (MERS-CoV), 75, 89–90, 92
  Zika virus, 169
Rickettsiaceae family, 299, 304, *see also* Tick-borne bacterial pathogens
  Candidatus Rickettsia tarasevichiae, 299, 300
  emerging tick-borne rickettsioses, 299–301
  Rickettsia sp. Atlantic rainforest or Bahia strain, 296, 300–301
  Tick-borne spotted fever group, 296–299

Salamandra salamandra, 400–401
Salmonella, 341–343, *see also* Nontyphoidal
    Salmonella (NTS)
  Enteritidis serotype, 342, 344–347, 349, 351
  infection, 341–343
  microbiology, 344–346
  serotypes, 344–346
  sources, 346–348
  transmission, 346–348
  Typhimurium serotype, 344–347, 349, 351
SARS (severe acute respiratory syndrome), 46
Saudi Arabia, Middle East respiratory syndrome
    (MERS), 73, 75, 76, 77
Selective breeding, amphibians, 396–397
Serious Communicable Diseases Unit (SCDU),
    44–46
Severe acute respiratory syndrome (SARS), 74, 75
Sexual transmission
  Marburg virus disease, 167
  Zika virus, 166, 167, 167–170
Sierra Leone, Ebola virus disease, 1, 4–10, 21, 24
Snake fungal disease, 400
Society for Healthcare Epidemiology of America,
    273, 275
Soil, coccidioides in, 380–381
South Asia, *Clostridium difficile* infection (CDI), 270
Southeast Asia, *Clostridium difficile* infection (CDI),
    269–270
Spectinomycin resistance, *Neisseria gonorrhoeae*,
    216, 217–218
Spinal infections, fungal, 364–365
Staphylococcus aureus, 201, 206
Stevens-Johnson syndrome, 138
Sudan, Ebola virus disease outbreaks, 3–4, 53–54
Sulfonamide resistance, *Neisseria gonorrhoeae*,
    215–216
Surgical interventions, *Clostridium difficile*
    infection (CDI), 281–282
Swine flu, 5

Tanzania, Chikungunya virus (CHIKV), 143–144
Tdap vaccine (reduced-dose acellular pertussis),
    Bordetella pertussis, 312, 313, 322–326
Tekmira Pharmaceuticals, Ebola virus disease, 60
Tetracycline resistance, *Neisseria gonorrhoeae*, 216,
    217
Thailand
  artemisinin-resistant *Plasmodium falciparum*
    malaria, 411, 416–417, 420
  Chikungunya virus (CHIKV), 144
Therapeutics, *see also* Medical countermeasures
    (MCMs)
  Chikungunya virus (CHIKV), 148–155
  Ebola virus disease (EVD), 18–22, 41–42, 56–60
  Zika virus, 170
Tick-borne bacterial pathogens
  anaplasmosis, 295, 301, 301–302, 303

Borrelia miyamotoi, 303
borrelioses, 302–304
ehrlichioses, 301
EML (*Ehrlichia muris*-like), 299, 301
neoehrlichiosis, 301, 302
new *Borrelia* spp., 303–304
Rickettsiae agents of human disease, 296–299
Rickettsia sp. Atlantic rainforest or Bahia strain,
    296, 300–301
rickettsioses, 299–301
Ticks, 295, 299
TKM-100802, Ebola virus disease, 42, 60
TKM 130803, Ebola virus disease, 20, 21
TKM-Ebola, Ebola virus disease, 60
Tolevamer, *Clostridium difficile* infection (CDI),
    278–279
Toyama Chemical, favipiravir, 59
Transmission
  Artemisinin-resistance *Plasmodium falciparum*,
    417–419
  Batrachochytrium dendrobatidis, 390, 392, 398
  Bordetella holmesii, 248
  Marburg virus disease, 167
  measles, 131–132
  Middle East respiratory syndrome (MERS),
    82–84
  Neisseria gonorrhoeae, 213–214, 220
  nonmosquito routes for West Nile virus,
    176–177
  nontyphoidal *Salmonella*, 346–348
  Zika virus, 165–170
Travelers
  Chikungunya virus (CHIKV), 144–145, 152
  Coccidioides immitis, 380
  Ebola virus disease, 8–9
  Middle East respiratory syndrome (MERS),
    86–87
  Zika virus, 165, 170

Uganda
  Ebola virus disease outbreaks, 1, 3–4
  Zika virus, 163, 164
United States
  acute flaccid myelitis (AFM), 111–112
  antimicrobials for treating gonorrhea, 225–226
  changing epidemiology in, 136–138
  characteristics of recent measles outbreaks, 136
  Cryptococcus gattii, 376–378
  decade following measles elimination, 133–135
  enterovirus-D68 (EV-D68) outbreak, 106–108,
    109, 114–115
  measles (1962–2014), 132
  reported cases, 134
  treatments for uncomplicated *Neisseria*
    gonorrhoeae infections, 221
  West Nile virus (WNV), 177–179
  Zika virus, 165

U.S. Environmental Protection Agency (EPA), 46, 170
U.S. Fish and Wildlife Service (USFWS), 394, 400–401

Vaccination, *see also* Immunization
    amphibian, 395–396
    public opinion and policy changes, 139
Vaccine Preventable Disease Public Health
        Laboratory Reference Centers (VPD RCs), 138
Vaccines, *see also* Immunization
    Bordetella holmesii, 247–248
    Bordetella pertussis, 321–324
    Chikungunya virus (CHIKV), 148, 149–152
    Clostridium difficile infection (CDI), 282–283
    Ebola virus disease, 22–23, 42–43, 60–62
    Haemophilus influenzae, 342
    influenza A virus, 126, 129
    malaria, 344, 350
    Middle East respiratory syndrome coronavirus
        (MERS-CoV), 93–94
    Middle East respiratory syndrome (MERS), 93–94
    nontyphoidal *Salmonella* (NTS), 350–351
    quest for gonococcal, 221, 228
    safety and efficacy, 64
    safety of, 135–136
    Streptococcus pneumoniae, 342
    West Nile virus, 190
Vaccines for Children (VFC), measles, 132, 133, 139
Vancomycin, *Clostridium difficile* infection (CDI), 277
Vesicular stomatitis virus (VSV), Ebola virus, 43
Vietnam, artemisinin-resistant *Plasmodium
        falciparum* malaria, 411, 414, 416–417, 420
Voriconazole, fungal infections, 368–370
VSV-ZEBOV vaccine, 60–61

West Africa, *see also* Africa; Ebola virus disease
        (EVD)
    Ebola virus disease (EVD) outbreak, 5–12
    map, 2
West Nile encephalitis (WNE), 181, 182–184,
        187–189
West Nile meningitis (WNM), 181, 182–183, 188
West Nile virus neuroinvasive disease (WNND),
        178, 180–181, 186
West Nile virus (WNV)
    clinical manifestations of human infection,
        181–186
    diagnosis, 187–188
    ecology, 176–180
    epidemiology of human illness, 180–181
    genome, 175
    genomic sequencing, 175–176
    geographic distribution, 177–180

incidence reported to CDC, 178
lineage 1 virus, 176, 179
lineage 2 virus, 176, 179
long-term outcomes, 187
magnetic resonance imaging of cervical spinal
        cord, 185
magnetic resonance imaging of patient's brain
        with WNE, 183
management, 188–189
neuroinvasive disease, 179, 182–186
nonmosquito transmission routes, 176–177
pathogenesis of human infection, 180
pediatric infection, 186–187
prevention, 189–190
reported cases in United States, 178
risk factors for severe disease and death, 180–181
vaccines, 190
virology, 175–176
weakness and paralysis, 184–186
WMV-associated acute flaccid myelitis, 180–181,
        184–186, 187, 189
Whole-cell vaccines, *Bordetella pertussis*, 321
Wildlife emerging infectious diseases, *see
        also*Batrachochytrium dendrobatidis*;
        Chytridiomycosis
    amphibians and *Batrachochytrium dendrobatidis*,
        385–392
    fungus *Pseudogymnoascus destructans*, 399–400
World Health Organization (WHO)
    agenda for change, 48
    antimicrobial resistance, 208
    Ebola virus disease, 5, 7
    Global Gonococcal Antimicrobial Surveillance
        Programme (Global GASP), 221–222
    global health preparedness and response, 11
    global plan for antimicrobial resistance in
        Neisseria gonorrhoeae, 221
    gonorrhea as public health concern, 214–215, 228
    malaria recommendations, 409, 419, 421–422
    measles, 135
    Middle East respiratory syndrome (MERS),
        76–77
World Organization for Animal Health (OIE), 392

Zaire, Ebola virus disease outbreaks, 3–4, 53–54
Zaire ebolavirus, 41
Zaki, Ali Mohamed, 73, 75
Zika virus
    clinical manifestations, 167–168
    complications of disease, 168–169
    diagnosis, 169
    differential diagnosis, 169–170
    disease, 163–164
    epidemiology, 164, 165–166, 170
    etiology, 164
    flavivirus, 163, 170–171
    intrauterine transmission, 166

occurrence of infection, 164–165
pathogenesis, 169
prophylaxis, 170
sexual transmission, 166, 167–170

therapy, 170
transmission, 165–167
vertical transmission, 167
ZMapp, Ebola virus disease, 19, 20, 21, 42, 56–57